Contents

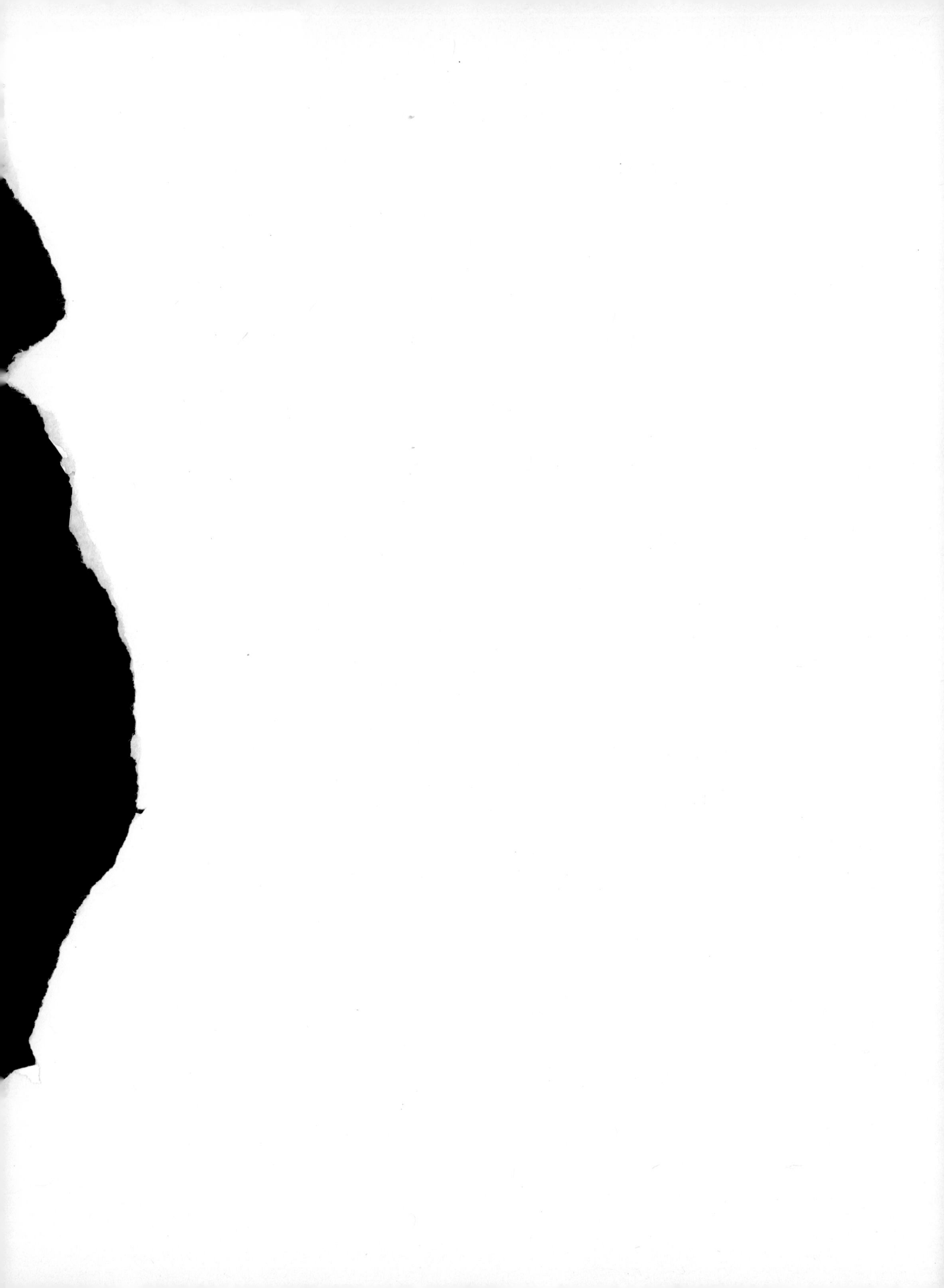

Vascular Medicine and Endovascular Interventions

Edited by

Thom W. Rooke, MD
Consultant, Division of Cardiovascular Diseases and Head, Section of Vascular Medicine, Mayo Clinic; John and Posy Krehbiel Professor of Medicine, Mayo Medical School, College of Medicine; Rochester, Minnesota

Associate Editors

Timothy M. Sullivan, MD
Vascular and Endovascular Surgery, North Central Heart Institute, Sioux Falls, South Dakota

Michael R. Jaff, DO
Director, Vascular Medicine, Massachusetts General Hospital; Assistant Professor of Medicine, Harvard Medical School; Boston, Massachusetts

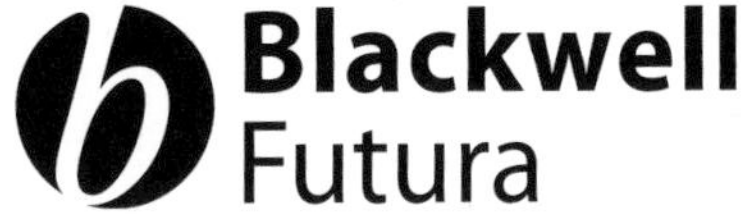

ISBN 9781405158275

Library of Congress Cataloging-in-Publication Data

Vascular medicine and endovascular interventions / edited by Thom W. Rooke, associate editors, Timothy M. Sullivan, Michael R. Jaff.
p. ; cm.
Includes bibliographical references and index.
ISBN-13: 978-1-4051-5827-5
ISBN-10: 1-4051-5827-1
1. Blood-vessels--Diseases--Examinations, questions, etc. 2. Blood-vessels--Diseases--Treatment--Examinations, questions, etc. 3. Blood-vessels--Endoscopic surgery--Examinations, questions, etc. I. Rooke, Thom W. II. Sullivan, Timothy M. (Timothy Michael), 1959- III. Jaff, Michael R. IV. Society for Vascular Medicine and Biology.
[DNLM: 1. Vascular Diseases--therapy--Examination Questions.
WG 18.2 V3305 2007]

RC691.V42 2007
616.1'30076--dc22 2007008008

Dedication

The editors wish to dedicate this book to Jay Coffman, Norman Hertzer, Jack Spittell, Jesse Young, and the other members of the "Greatest Generation" of vascular physicians and surgeons. Without your guidance, patience, and mentorship, our participation in this field would have been impossible.

Thom W. Rooke, MD
Timothy M. Sullivan, MD
Michael R. Jaff, DO

Vascular Medicine and Endovascular Interventions

List of Contributors

J. Michael Bacharach, MD, MPH
Department of Cardiology, North Central Heart Institute; Department of Vascular Medicine and Cardiology, Avera Heart Hospital of South Dakota; Clinical Associate Professor, University of South Dakota School of Medicine; Sioux Falls, South Dakota

John R. Bartholomew, MD
Section Head, Vascular Medicine, Department of Cardiovascular Medicine, Cleveland Clinic Foundation, Cleveland, Ohio

Mark C. Bates, MD
Director, Circulatory Dynamics Lab, Professor, Department of Surgery, Robert C. Byrd Health Sciences Center of West Virginia University–Charleston Division; Charleston Area Medical Center; Charleston, West Virginia

Joshua A. Beckman, MD
Director, Cardiovascular Fellowship Program, Cardiovascular Division, Brigham and Women's Hospital; Assistant Professor of Medicine, Harvard Medical School; Boston, Massachusetts

Haraldur Bjarnason, MD
Chair, Division of Vascular/Interventional Radiology, Mayo Clinic; Associate Professor of Radiology, Mayo Medical School, College of Medicine; Rochester, Minnesota

Daniel G. Clair, MD
Chair, Department of Vascular Surgery, Cleveland Clinic Foundation, Cleveland, Ohio

Anthony J. Comerota, MD
Director, Jobst Vascular Center, Toledo, Ohio; Adjunct Professor of Surgery, University of Michigan, Ann Arbor, Michigan

Mark A. Creager, MD
Director, Vascular Center, Professor of Medicine, Harvard Medical School; Simon C. Fireman Scholar in Cardiovascular Medicine, Brigham and Women's Hospital; Boston, Massachusetts

Mark D. P. Davis, MD
Chair, Division of Clinical Dermatology, Mayo Clinic; Professor of Dermatology, Mayo Medical School, College of Medicine; Rochester, Minnesota

John A. Heit, MD
Consultant, Divisions of Cardiovascular Diseases, Hematology, and Laboratory Genetics, Mayo Clinic; Professor of Medicine, Mayo Medical School, College of Medicine; Rochester, Minnesota

William R. Hiatt, MD
Department of Medicine, University of Colorado School of Medicine; Section of Vascular Medicine, Divisions of Geriatrics and Cardiology, and the Colorado Prevention Center; Denver, Colorado

Michael R. Jaff, DO
Director, Vascular Medicine, Massachusetts General Hospital; Assistant Professor of Medicine, Harvard Medical School; Boston, Massachusetts

Scott Kinlay, MBBS, PhD
Director, Cardiac Catheterization Laboratory and Vascular Medicine, Veterans Affairs Medical Center; Director of Intravascular Imaging, Brigham and Women's Hospital; Boston, Massachusetts

Alan B. Lumsden, MD
Department of Cardiovascular Surgery, Methodist DeBakey Heart Center, The Methodist Hospital; Professor of Surgery, Baylor College of Medicine; Houston, Texas

Jon S. Matsumura, MD
Division of Vascular Surgery, Associate Professor of Surgery, Northwestern University, Feinberg School of Medicine, Chicago, Illinois

Robert D. McBane, MD
Consultant, Division of Cardiovascular Diseases and Director, Thrombophilia Center, Mayo Clinic; Associate Professor of Medicine, Mayo Medical School, College of Medicine; Rochester, Minnesota

Mary M. McDermott, MD
Division of General Internal Medicine, Associate Professor of Medicine, Northwestern University, Feinberg School of Medicine, Chicago, Illinois

Ian R. McPhail, MD
Consultant, Division of Cardiovascular Diseases, Mayo Clinic; Instructor in Medicine, Mayo Medical School, College of Medicine; Rochester, Minnesota

Imran Mohiuddin, MD
Department of Cardiovascular Surgery, Methodist DeBakey Heart Center, The Methodist Hospital, Houston, Texas

Emile R. Mohler, III, MD
Consultant, Cardiovascular Medicine, Associate Professor of Medicine, University of Pennsylvania School of Medicine, Philadelphia, Pennsylvania

Gregory L. Moneta, MD
Chief, Division of Vascular Surgery, Professor of Surgery, Oregon Health and Science University, Portland, Oregon

Jeffrey W. Olin, DO
Director of Vascular Medicine, Professor of Medicine, Zena and Michael A. Wiener Cardiovascular Institute, Mount Sinai School of Medicine, New York, New York

Eric K. Peden, MD
Department of Cardiovascular Surgery, Methodist DeBakey Heart Center, The Methodist Hospital, Houston, Texas

Suman Rathbun, MD
Department of Medicine, Cardiovascular Section, Associate Professor of Medicine, University of Oklahoma, Oklahoma City, Oklahoma

Michael Reardon, MD
Department of Cardiovascular Surgery, Methodist DeBakey Heart Center, The Methodist Hospital, Houston, Texas

Robert M. Schainfeld, DO
Chief, Section of Vascular Medicine, Assistant Professor of Medicine, Tufts University School of Medicine, Boston, Massachusetts

Roger F. J. Shepherd, MBBCh
Consultant, Division of Cardiovascular Diseases, Mayo Clinic; Assistant Professor of Medicine, Mayo Medical School, College of Medicine; Rochester, Minnesota

David P. Slovut, MD, PhD
Departments of Vascular Medicine and Cardiology, St. Mary's/ Duluth Clinic Heart Center, Duluth, Minnesota

Timothy M. Sullivan, MD
Vascular and Endovascular Surgery, North Central Heart Institute, Sioux Falls, South Dakota

Paul W. Wennberg, MD
Consultant, Division of Cardiovascular Diseases, Mayo Clinic; Assistant Professor of Medicine, Mayo Medical School, College of Medicine; Rochester, Minnesota

Christopher J. White, MD
Chairman, Department of Cardiology, Ochsner Clinic Foundation, New Orleans, Louisiana

Brenda K. Zierler, PhD, RN
Associate Professor, Department of Biobehavioral Nursing and Health Systems School of Nursing, Adjunct Associate Professor, Health Sciences, University of Washington Medical Center, Seattle, Washington

R. Eugene Zierler, MD
Department of Surgery, Director, Vascular Diagnostic Laboratory, Professor of Surgery, University of Washington Medical Center, Seattle, Washington

Acknowledgments

The editors wish to acknowledge the spectacular contributions of Alyssa C. Biorn, PhD (editor), Roberta Schwartz (project manager), Barb Golenzer (editorial assistant), Ann Lemke (proofreader), and Kelley Shook (secretary).

1 Vascular Biology

Scott Kinlay, MBBS, PhD, FACC, FRACP

"Vascular Biology" applies to processes affecting arteries, veins, and other blood vessels. This chapter will focus on the physiology and pathophysiology of arteries. Vein function and dysfunction will be discussed in later chapters.

Anatomy and Function of Blood Vessels in Health

Arteries are grouped, in descending size, into large elastic arteries, smaller muscular arteries, and arterioles. Arterioles regulate blood flow into the capillaries, which are endothelial tubes designed to facilitate the exchange of nutrients and byproducts of metabolism. Veins function as low-pressure reservoirs and return blood to the heart.

Arteries have three layers: the intima, media, and adventitia (Fig. 1.1). The intima consists of the vascular endothelium, which is a single layer of cells and a thin layer of connective tissue, and is separated from the media by the internal elastic lamina made of elastin and fibrous tissue. The media consists of fibrous tissue, vascular smooth muscle, and elastin; the media is separated from the adventitia by the external elastic lamina. The adventitia consists of collagen and fibrous tissue that forms loose connective tissue.

Three Layers of Arteries

- Intima (single layer of endothelial cells)
- Media (vascular smooth muscle and connective tissue)
- Adventitia (loose connective tissue)

The connective tissue of large arteries contains more elastin, whereas smaller arteries have more collagen. The elastic properties of healthy large arteries, such as the ascending aorta, help to cushion the stroke volume, decrease the work of ejection by the left ventricle, and maintain pressure during diastole. The smaller arterioles and resistance arteries are able to regulate peripheral resistance by changing vascular smooth muscle tone to alter the lumen size.

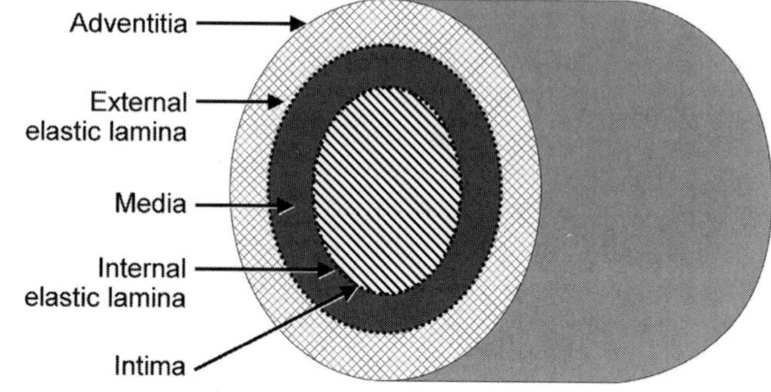

Fig. 1.1 Diagram showing the three layers of an artery.

- Elastic arteries (e.g., the aorta) cushion the stroke volume and reduce ventricular work
- Smaller, more muscular arteries regulate peripheral resistance and blood flow

Endothelial Function

The healthy endothelium is an autocrine and paracrine organ that produces substances that decrease vascular smooth muscle tone and inhibit inflammation and thrombosis. These substances include nitric oxide, prostacyclin, other endothelium-dependent vasodilators, and plasminogen activators. In disease states or after injury by factors such as abnormal strain, temperature, or risk factors for atherosclerosis, the endothelium produces substances that increase vascular tone, promote inflammation, and enhance thrombosis. These substances

include cytokines, growth factors, endothelins, and plasminogen inhibitors.

- Endothelium is an autocrine/paracrine organ
- The endothelium produces substances that affect vascular tone, inflammation, and thrombosis

Endothelium-Derived Vasodilators

The principal vasodilators produced by the endothelium include nitric oxide, prostacyclin, and endothelium-derived hyperpolarizing factor (EDHF). Of these, nitric oxide has a central role in mediating many functions of the endothelium aside from vasodilation.

Nitric Oxide

Nitric oxide is generated in the endothelium from the amino acid L-arginine by nitric oxide synthase (NOS). Nitric oxide production is accelerated by several physiologic stimuli, including shear stress at the endothelial surface (from blood flow) and in response to thrombin, serotonin, and acetylcholine (Fig. 1.2). These stimuli activate NOS by several mechanisms, including phosphorylation of the enzyme, increased intracellular calcium concentrations, and binding of calmodulin. NOS associates closely with invaginations in the endothelial luminal surface called caveolae (Fig. 1.3). A specific caveolar protein, caveolin-1, inactivates NOS by competing for binding with the calcium-calmodulin complex, which activates the enzyme.

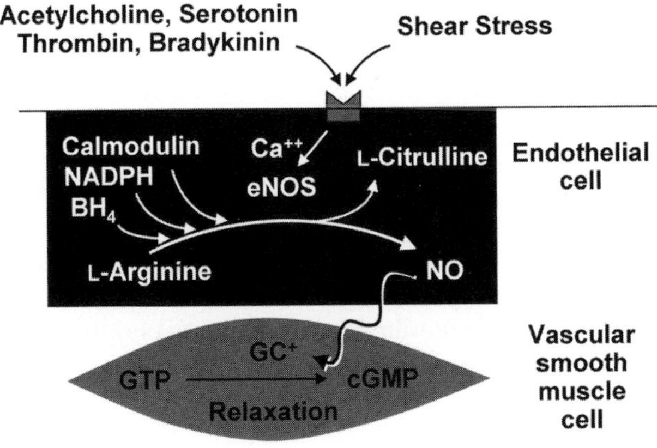

Fig. 1.2 The healthy endothelium responds to several different stimuli that increase nitric oxide (NO) production by increasing the activity of endothelial nitric oxide synthase (eNOS). eNOS function requires several cofactors, including tetrahydrobiopterin (BH_4), NADPH (nicotinamide adenine dinucleotide phosphate), and calmodulin. NO diffuses across the artery wall to activate guanylate cyclase (GC) in vascular smooth muscle; GC converts guanosine triphosphate (GTP) to cyclic guanosine monophosphate (cGMP), which relaxes smooth muscle and causes vasodilation. (From Kinlay S, Selwyn AP, Ganz P. Endothelium as a target of the risk factors in cardiovascular disease. In: Panza JO, Cannon RO III, editors. Endothelium, nitric oxide, and atherosclerosis: from basic mechanisms to clinical implications. Armonk [NY]: Futura Publishing Company, Inc.; 1999. p. 227-41. Used with permission.)

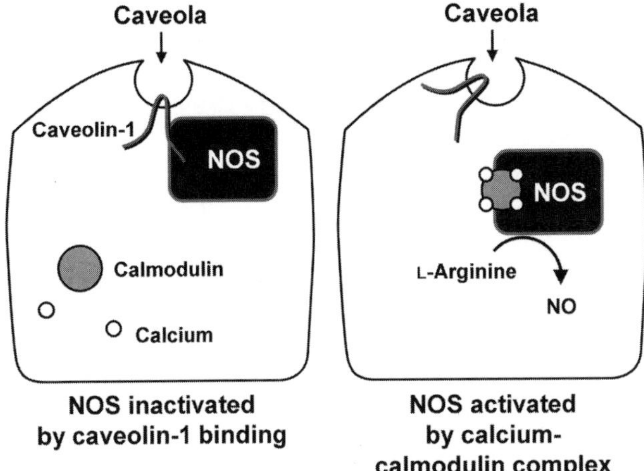

Fig. 1.3 Nitric oxide synthase (NOS) is associated with luminal clefts on the surface of endothelial cells called caveolae. Caveolin-1 is a caveolar protein that inactivates NOS. The calcium-calmodulin complex competes with caveolin-1 for binding to NOS and activates NOS to produce nitric oxide (NO). (From Kinlay S, Libby P, Ganz P. Endothelial function and coronary artery disease. Curr Opin Lipidol. 2001;12:383-9. Used with permission.)

Nitric oxide diffuses through the artery wall and enters vascular smooth muscle cells in the media, where it increases the activity of guanylate cyclase and the concentration of cyclic guanosine monophosphate (cGMP) (Fig. 1.2). The increased level of cGMP relaxes vascular smooth muscle and leads to vasodilation. Because shear stress is related to blood velocity, increased blood velocity also increases nitric oxide production and causes vasodilation, which in turn decreases blood velocity toward its original value. In contrast, decreased blood velocity decreases the stimulus for nitric oxide production, promotes vasoconstriction, and thereby increases blood velocity back toward its original value. In this way, the endothelium regulates vasomotor tone so as to keep blood velocity and shear stress at the endothelial surface within a narrow range. This regulation prevents sluggish blood flow that might promote thrombus formation and high shear that could injure the arterial intima.

- Shear stress, thrombin, serotonin, and acetylcholine are some factors that stimulate NOS
- NOS resides in endothelial clefts called caveolae
- Nitric oxide diffuses through the artery wall to activate guanylate cyclase and increase cGMP, which relaxes smooth muscle and dilates arteries

Prostacyclin

Prostacyclin is another endothelial product that induces

arterial dilation. It is produced from arachidonic acid by cyclooxygenase in response to shear stress or certain factors that also increase nitric oxide production. Prostacyclin activates adenylate cyclase to increase production of cyclic adenosine monophosphate (cAMP). In most vascular beds prostacyclin has only a small role in regulating vasomotor tone, but it is more important in inhibiting platelet aggregation.

- Prostacyclin activates adenylate cyclase to increase cAMP concentration

Other Endothelium-Derived Relaxing Factors

The existence of other endothelium-derived relaxing factors is supported by a residual vasodilation response to various stimuli after blocking nitric oxide and prostacyclin generation. One of these factors, EDHF, appears to be more important in the small arteries than the large conduit arteries; however, the structure of EDHF has yet to be identified. The lack of consistent inhibitors of EDHF that can be safely used in humans has thwarted its clinical study.

- EDHF appears to be a more important vasodilator of small arteries than of conduit arteries

Endothelium-Derived Vasoconstrictors

Although several locally produced substances can cause vasoconstriction, most are platelet-derived products, including serotonin and thrombin. However, the endothelium also produces substances that constrict vascular smooth muscle, of which the most important is endothelin.

Endothelin is one of the most potent vasoconstrictors known. It was first discovered as a product secreted by endothelial cells. Endothelin is a peptide that is generated by successive cleavage of a large polypeptide ("big endothelin") within the endothelium. Three isotypes of endothelin have been described (endothelins 1, 2, and 3); however, endothelin-1 is the most abundant in vascular tissue. Endothelin-1 is also produced by activated macrophages and vascular smooth muscle cells, particularly in atherosclerosis.

Endothelin acts on the endothelin A receptors on vascular smooth muscle to stimulate vasoconstriction and vascular smooth muscle cell proliferation. Endothelin B receptors on the abluminal surface of endothelial cells mediate increased production of nitric oxide, but only in healthy cells. Nevertheless, the net action of endothelin-1 is vasoconstriction in most vascular beds.

Stimuli for endothelin production include thrombin, angiotensin II, and epinephrine. The production of endothelin is inhibited by nitric oxide and, conversely, endothelin inhibits the production of nitric oxide. Endothelin and nitric oxide participate in a "yin-yang" relationship to regulate vasomotor tone, with the net effect depending on the health of the endothelium.

- Endothelin-1 is one of the most potent vasoconstrictors known
- Endothelin-1 is produced by endothelial cells, activated macrophages, and vascular smooth muscle cells
- Endothelin-1 activates endothelin A receptors on vascular smooth muscle to stimulate vasoconstriction

Endothelium as a Regulator of Arterial Inflammation

Nitric oxide also is important for regulating inflammation associated with arterial injury. Nitric oxide inhibits the expression of monocyte chemoattractant protein (MCP)-1 and macrophage colony-stimulating factor (M-CSF). By inhibiting the transcription factor NF-κB, nitric oxide prevents the activation of several proatherogenic processes, including the expression of cellular adhesion molecules (Fig. 1.4). These processes are tightly controlled by the balance of antioxidants and pro-oxidant molecules in the cell. All stages of atherosclerosis exhibit activation of the endothelium, which releases the checks on the proatherogenic processes to increase the recruitment of inflammatory cells into the endothelium.

- Nitric oxide reduces inflammation by inhibition of MCP-1 and activation of NF-κB

Endothelium as a Regulator of Arterial Thrombosis

The final common pathway of many atherosclerotic processes is thrombus and occlusion of the arterial lumen. The healthy endothelium produces several antithrombotic substances, including heparans and the fibrinolytic tissue plasminogen activator. In atherosclerotic arteries, the balance of tissue plasminogen activators to inhibitors, such as plasminogen activator inhibitor (PAI), is reversed. Other factors that promote thrombus formation include decreased nitric oxide concentration in platelets, which promotes platelet activation.

Atherosclerotic Risk Factors and Abnormal Vascular Biology

Endothelial injury is a hallmark of early atherogenesis. Although physical injury such as balloon angioplasty or hypertension can disrupt the endothelium, many of the conventional atherosclerotic risk factors initiate athero-

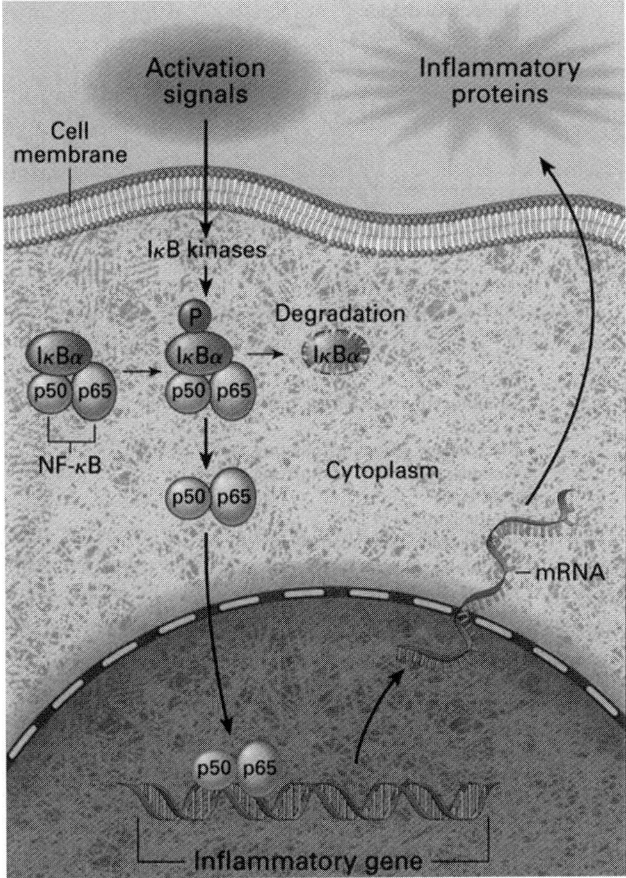

Fig. 1.4 The transcription factor NF-κB is kept inactive (by IκB) in the cytoplasm of healthy cells. Numerous activation signals, such as a decrease in nitric oxide bioavailability or increased oxidant stress, lead to activation of NF-κB, which then migrates to the nucleus and increases the transcription of many proinflammatory molecules. (From Barnes PJ, Karin M. Nuclear factor-κB: a pivotal transcription factor in chronic inflammatory diseases. N Engl J Med. 1997;336:1066-71. Used with permission.)

sclerosis by disturbing the normal homeostatic functions of the endothelium and vascular wall. Pathologic studies have tended to divide the stages of atherosclerosis into lesion initiation, fatty streak, fibroproliferative atheroma, and advanced lesions. However, the cellular events that lead to atherosclerosis occur at different rates and to different extents in different arterial segments of different people.

Lesion Initiation

Endothelial Dysfunction

Endothelial dysfunction is an early feature of atherosclerosis related to all of the conventional cardiovascular risk factors. This is primarily a functional disorder of the endothelium, wherein production and bioavailability of nitric oxide in the artery wall are decreased. Nitric oxide is decreased in regions of low shear stress, such as disturbed blood flow at bifurcations or bends in the artery.

Low-Density Lipoprotein Retention and Oxidative Modification

Low-density lipoprotein (LDL) cholesterol permeates the endothelial cell layer and enters the subendothelial cell matrix. Elevated plasma levels of LDL increase the rate of delivery and retention of LDL in the artery wall. Although very little of the circulating LDL is oxidized, once LDL is in the artery wall, reactive oxygen species deplete antioxidants and oxidize fatty acids on the LDL surface. Elevated glucose levels can also lead to glycosylation of proteins in the artery wall and to advanced glycosylated end products (AGEs). Both modified (oxidized) LDL and AGEs in the artery wall activate the overlying endothelial cells.

- Endothelial dysfunction is an early feature of atherosclerosis
- Endothelial dysfunction results in less nitric oxide in the artery wall
- High plasma LDL concentration increases retention and oxidation of LDL in the artery wall
- Elevated plasma glucose can lead to AGEs in the artery wall
- Oxidized LDL and AGEs activate endothelial cells

High-Density Lipoprotein and Reverse Cholesterol Transport

High-density lipoprotein (HDL) is a significant protective factor for atherosclerosis. HDL contains several antioxidants, including paraoxonase, which may prevent the oxidation of LDL cholesterol.

Reverse cholesterol transport from peripheral tissues to the liver occurs by passive or active transport. HDL can absorb cholesterol passively from the plasma membrane of cells. Active transport occurs by interaction of apolipoprotein A1 on nascent HDL with the ATP-binding cassette transporter A1 (ABCA1) on peripheral tissues, including macrophages. Cholesterol can be removed from mature HDL by HDL-specific scavenger receptors on the liver (SR-B1 receptor). Cholesterol in HDL may be exchanged for triglycerides in intermediate-density lipoprotein (IDL) by cholesterol ester transfer protein (CETP). Transferred cholesterol can be returned to the liver (uptake by the LDL receptor) or delivered to peripheral tissues.

A rare genetic defect in apolipoprotein A1 (ApoA1 Milano) leads to very efficient transfer of cholesterol from the ABCA1 transporter on peripheral tissues and is thought to accelerate reverse cholesterol transport. Recombinant forms of ApoA1 Milano can also enhance this effect and are being developed for therapeutic use. Partial inhibitors

of CETP block cholesterol transfer from HDL to other lipoproteins and may also increase reverse cholesterol transport with obvious therapeutic potential.

- HDL protects against atherosclerosis
- HDL particles have antioxidants and promote reverse cholesterol transport
- HDL returns cholesterol to the liver by direct receptor uptake (SR-B1) and indirectly via transfer to IDL, which is taken up by the LDL receptor on the liver
- CETP inhibitors partially block cholesterol transfer from HDL to IDL and may increase reverse cholesterol transport

Endothelial Cell Activation and Cellular Adhesion Molecules

Endothelial cell activation and the progressive increase in reactive oxidant species in the artery wall (oxidant stress) inhibits the production of nitric oxide by endothelial cells and rapidly converts nitric oxide in the artery wall to inactive metabolites such as peroxynitrate. The decrease in nitric oxide activates transcription factors such as NF-κB, which move into the nucleus to increase the transcription of genes that produce cytokines and cellular adhesion molecules (CAMs) (Fig. 1.4).

CAMs, such as the selectins, intercellular adhesion molecule (ICAM), and vascular cell adhesion molecule (VCAM), are expressed on the luminal surface of endothelial cells. They interact specifically with integrins expressed on the surface of monocytes and T cells (Fig. 1.5). Selectins bind to monocytes to promote a slow rolling of monocytes on the endothelial surface (rolling stage). Selectin binding is followed by firmer interactions between integrins and VCAM or ICAM (adhesion). CAMs, together with chemokines (e.g., MCP-1, oxidized LDL), then promote transmigration of the monocytes through the junctions between endothelial cells into the intima of the artery wall (migration) (Fig. 1.5). This process initiates and promotes inflammatory cell recruitment into the wall.

- Activated endothelial cells exhibit increased activity of the proinflammatory transcription factor NF-κB
- CAMs, including selectins, ICAM, and VCAM, are expressed on the lumen surface of endothelial cells
- The sequence of leukocyte recruitment includes rolling (selectin binding), adhesion (CAM binding), and migration (CAM and cytokine assisted)

Fatty Streak

Like many other cell types, monocytes (which are recruited into the arterial intima and transform into macrophages) have LDL receptors that recognize native LDL and facilitate its uptake in a regulated fashion according to a cell's needs. However, macrophages have scavenger receptors that recognize oxidized LDL; these have a central role in atherosclerosis because they allow the macrophage to take up LDL in an unregulated manner. Retention and oxidation of LDL in the artery wall leads to engorgement of monocytes with oxidatively modified LDL and to formation of foam cells, the hallmarks of the fatty streak (Fig. 1.6). Activated monocytes amplify this process by expressing chemokines (MCP-1) and cytokines (M-CSF).

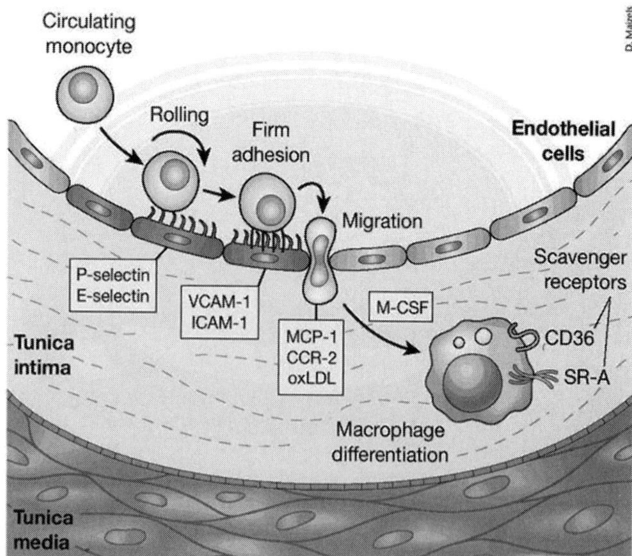

Fig. 1.5 Recruitment of monocytes and lymphocytes into the vessel wall occurs by a coordinated process mediated by selectins (P-selectin, E-selectin) and cellular adhesion molecules (ICAM-1, VCAM-1) on the surface of activated endothelial cells. The three steps are rolling, adhesion, and migration of leukocytes. CCR, chemokine receptor; MCP, monocyte chemoattractant protein; M-CSF, macrophage colony-stimulating factor; oxLDL, oxidized low-density lipoprotein. (From Li AC, Glass CK. The macrophage foam cell as a target for therapeutic intervention. Nat Med. 2002;8:1235-42. Used with permission.)

Foam cells also express angiotensin II receptors and are capable of promoting LDL oxidation. Angiotensin II increases the production of the free radical superoxide by stimulating oxidases on vascular smooth muscle cells. Thus, angiotensin II increases oxidant stress within the artery wall, which promotes atherogenesis.

The macrophage response to oxidized LDL forms part of the rapidly responding innate immunity. Scavenger receptors recognize a diverse range of ligands associated with pathogens and foreign bodies, and other features of the innate defense system, such as C-reactive protein and IgM antibodies to oxidized LDL, are found in atherosclerotic plaques. Although these responses are necessary for eliminating pathogens, the macrophage response has deleterious effects—increased atherosclerotic risk factors.

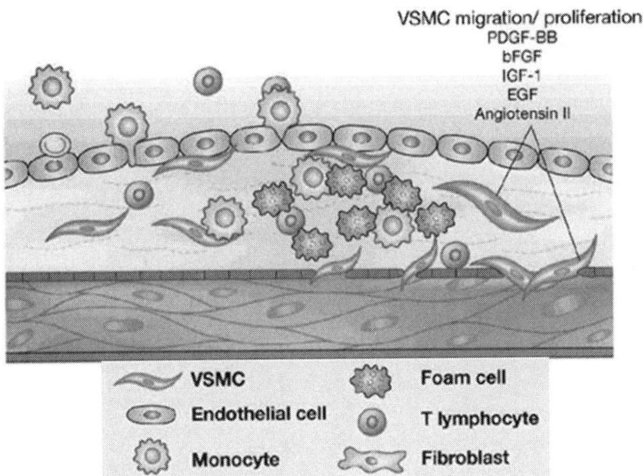

Fig. 1.6 Foam cell formation and the migration of vascular smooth muscle cells (VSMCs) into the intima mark the beginning of the fatty streak. bFGF, basic fibroblast growth factor; EGF, epidermal growth factor; IGF-1, insulin-like growth factor-1; PDGF-BB, platelet-derived growth factor BB. (From Dzau VJ, Braun-Dullaeus RC, Sedding DG. Vascular proliferation and atherosclerosis: new perspectives and therapeutic strategies. Nat Med. 2002;8:1249-56. Used with permission.)

- Monocytes recruited into a plaque mature into macrophages
- Macrophages engorge with modified LDL by scavenger receptor uptake in an unregulated manner and become foam cells
- Chemokines (e.g., MCP-1) and cytokines (e.g., M-CSF) amplify this process
- Angiotensin II increases superoxide production on vascular smooth muscle cells

Fibroproliferative Atheroma

Cytokines, growth factors, and the renin-angiotensin system all stimulate growth of the plaque and the development of more advanced atherosclerotic features.

Cytokines and Signal Amplification

Monocytes recruited early into the plaque produce growth factors and cytokines that stimulate the recruitment of other cell types into the intima, including T cells, B lymphocytes, fibroblasts, and vascular smooth muscle cells. Neutrophils and granulocytes are not features of atherosclerosis.

Smooth muscle cells migrate from the media into the intima and produce extracellular matrix molecules such as collagen I and III, fibronectin, and proteoglycans. These molecules provide biomechanical strength, interact with integrins, and influence plaque stability.

- Monocytes, macrophages, T cells, B cells, fibroblasts, and smooth muscle cells are found in the fibroproliferative atheroma
- Smooth muscle cells produce collagen that provides biomechanical strength to the plaque

T Cell Entry

Lymphocytes interact closely with other cell types to influence plaque development. Both T cells and B cells are recruited into atherosclerotic plaques and form part of the acquired immune response in atherosclerosis. Macrophages activate T cells by presenting antigens (e.g., oxidized LDL) to specific T-cell receptors, with costimulatory signals produced by interactions between CD40 ligand and CD40 on both cells. Interferon-γ, produced by T cells, can regulate the expression of scavenger receptors on macrophages, inhibit the production of matrix by smooth muscle cells, and increase the expression of proteases such as metalloproteases that degrade collagen in the plaque.

- Macrophages activate T cells by presenting antigens (e.g., oxidized LDL) to T-cell receptors
- T cells produce interferon-γ, which inhibits matrix production by smooth muscle cells and increases metalloprotease production by macrophages

Neovascularization

Neovascularization heralds the development of more complex plaques that are associated with clinical events. In normal blood vessels, the vasa vasorum is confined to the adventitia and outer artery wall. During early atherosclerosis development, the vasa vasorum proliferates and forms a disordered network and ultimately extends through the media into the intima (Fig. 1.7). Neovascularization of the intima is associated with focal collections of inflammatory cells and may be a source of intraplaque hemorrhage that could contribute to plaque growth and stenoses.

- More complex plaques have disordered proliferation of the vasa vasorum
- Disruption of these vessels might contribute to intraplaque hemorrhage

Vascular Remodeling and Proteases

Extracellular matrix and collagen in plaque are susceptible to several proteases, including the metalloproteases, which are abundant in plaque, particularly with macrophages. Loss of nitric oxide and the oxidation of nitric oxide to peroxynitrate decrease the activity of the tissue inhibitors of

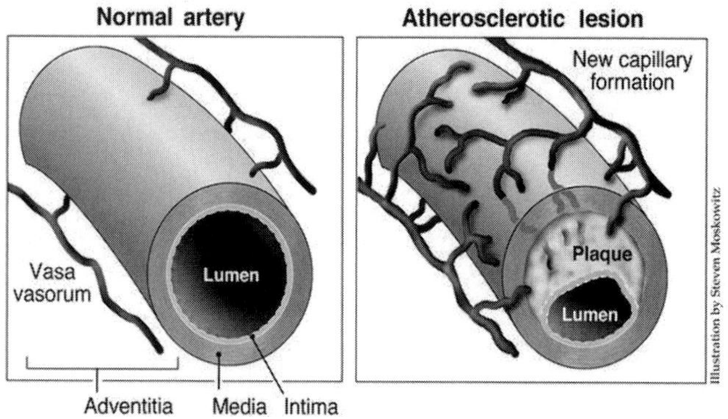

Fig. 1.7 Neovascularization of plaque occurs by disordered growth of penetrating arteries from the vasa vasorum and can potentially lead to intraplaque rupture. (From Moulton KS. Plaque angiogenesis and atherosclerosis. Curr Atheroscler Rep. 2001;3:225-33. Used with permission.)

metalloproteases. The subsequent proteolysis of collagen and fibrous tissue in the plaque promotes plaque instability and the development of complex plaques with thin fibrous caps.

The activation of matrix metalloproteases may prevent the development of flow-limiting lesions in the early stages of atherosclerosis. During atherosclerosis development, the artery remodels to accommodate the growing atherosclerotic plaque and enlarges to preserve the artery lumen (Fig. 1.8). This compensatory enlargement was initially described in cross-sectional pathologic studies and preserves the arterial lumen until plaque exceeds approximately 40% of the total cross-sectional area of the artery. Remodeling also occurs in the opposite direction (negative remodeling) and may contribute to stenoses that limit blood flow. Positive remodeling is associated with greater expression of matrix metalloproteases than negatively remodeled plaques.

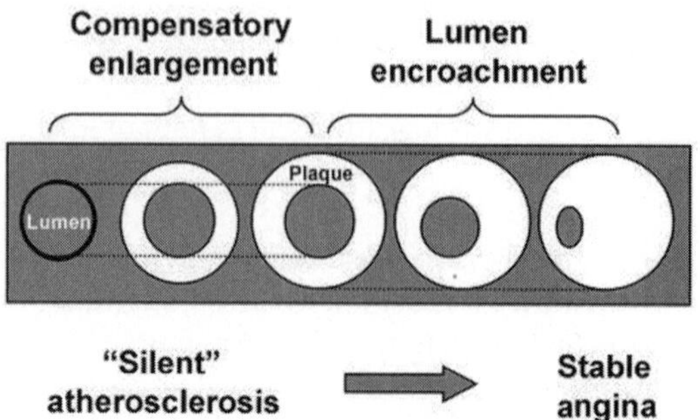

Fig. 1.8 Compensatory enlargement of the artery accommodates atherosclerosis early in its natural history. However, once plaque exceeds approximately 40% of the cross-sectional area of an artery, there is no further enlargement of the vessel, and atherosclerosis encroaches on the lumen. (From Popma JJ, Sawyer M, Selwyn AP, et al. Lipid-lowering therapy after coronary revascularization. Am J Cardiol. 2000;86 Suppl 2:18H-28H. Used with permission.)

Local blood flow and biomechanical forces may regulate vascular remodeling. Laminar flow tends to produce a greater shear stress on the surface of the endothelium than disturbed flow. Regions of low shear stress (on the outer aspects of a bifurcating artery) tend to have greater atheroma and endothelial cell activation than areas of higher shear stress. Areas of higher shear stress are also more likely to exhibit positive remodeling than areas of low shear stress.

- Oxidant stress and T cells stimulate macrophages to produce metalloproteases
- Metalloproteases break down collagen, a process that promotes plaque instability
- During the early stage of plaque growth, the artery is able to prevent lumen encroachment by compensatory enlargement (positive remodeling)
- Positive remodeling is associated with abundant expression of metalloproteases
- Negative remodeling (shrinkage of the lumen) probably contributes to the development of flow-limiting stenoses

Advanced Lesions

Chronic ischemic syndromes during exertion are related to flow-limiting stenoses, whereas acute ischemic syndromes such as the acute coronary syndromes are more often related to thrombosis of disrupted plaques that are minimally narrowed. Several features of advanced plaques cause acute complications related to flow disruption.

Lipid Pool

Unregulated accumulation of cholesterol by macrophages and vascular smooth muscle cells leads to cell apoptosis and release of the cell contents into the extracellular space of the intima. Autopsy studies of acute coronary syndrome have generally identified two types of culprit lesions. The most common form consists of a plaque with a necrotic lipid pool and an overlying thin fibrous cap that has fractured (Fig. 1.9). These plaques typically rupture at the shoulder or edge, where biomechanical forces and inflammatory cell activity are concentrated. A smaller proportion of the lesions result from endothelial cell erosion without frank rupture of the plaque. Loss of endothelial cells can occur by apoptosis induced by inflammatory mediators or by breakdown in the collagens that fix endothelial cells to the underlying matrix.

- Apoptosis of macrophages and vascular smooth muscle cells contributes to the development of the necrotic lipid core of a plaque

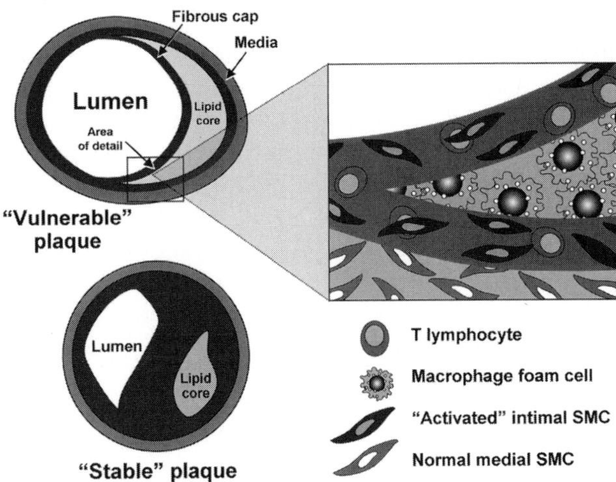

Fig. 1.9 Advanced plaques include the "vulnerable plaque" with inflammatory cell activity and a thin fibrous cap overlying a large lipid pool, which causes only minimal lumen narrowing. Plaques typical of stable exertional angina tend to be rich in fibrous tissue and calcium with a narrow lumen. SMC, smooth muscle cell. (From Libby P. Molecular bases of the acute coronary syndromes. Circulation. 1995;91:2844-50. Used with permission.)

- Most plaques responsible for acute coronary syndromes feature a large lipid core and fracture of an overlying thin fibrous cap
- Endothelial cell erosion contributes to a smaller number of culprit lesions in acute coronary syndromes

Thrombosis

Thrombus occludes the artery lumen in some cases of plaque rupture and is the final common pathway leading to acute ischemic syndromes. Disruption of the endothelial layer exposes the subendothelial tissues and necrotic lipid core, both of which are highly thrombogenic. Tissue factor, a product of foam cells, is also abundant in the lipid core of ruptured plaques and promotes thrombus formation. The endothelium of advanced plaques is dysfunctional and less able to produce nitric oxide, prostacyclins, tissue plasminogen activator, and heparan sulphate. Depletion of these substances activates platelets and thrombotic pathways. Other factors that promote thrombus formation include increased vasomotor tone that may decrease blood flow and elevated circulating plasma PAIs (e.g., PAI-1).

- Disruption of plaque exposes the underlying thrombogenic subendothelial tissues to blood
- Factors that contribute to thrombosis include vasomotor dysfunction, elevated inhibitors of thrombolysis (e.g., PAI-1), and activation of platelets

Calcification

Calcification of the artery wall is a feature of advanced atherosclerosis. Calcification is an active process closely related to remodeling in bone and may be related to intraplaque hemorrhage. Arterial calcification is more often associated with stable plaques than with those with a greater inflammatory component.

- Calcification of arteries is an active process related to remodeling in bone

Asymptomatic Plaque Rupture

Asymptomatic plaque rupture with superficial thrombus is often seen at autopsy. Persons who die suddenly of an acute coronary syndrome due to an identified ruptured plaque often have many more plaques that have ruptured and are clinically silent. Subclinical plaque rupture can contribute to the growth of atherosclerosis and the development of flow-limiting lesions.

Risk Factor Modification

Reversal of several risk factors for atherosclerosis decreases the progression of atherosclerosis and the risk of clinical events. This risk reversal is best studied for LDL reduction by pharmacologic and non-pharmacologic means.

Decreasing LDL cholesterol levels by dietary and pharmacologic methods improves endothelial function and promotes plaque stability. For example, intensive lowering of LDL in humans by apheresis can rapidly improve endothelial vasomotor function within hours. LDL lowering also decreases the density and activity of inflammatory cells in plaque by decreasing recruitment and increasing apoptosis of inflammatory cells. LDL lowering also inhibits various pro-thrombotic pathways, including the tissue factor pathway, within plaque. In most studies of LDL lowering, plaque regression is minimal, indicating that plaque stabilization is the main benefit of lowering of LDL level.

- Risk factor modification, particularly LDL lowering, improves endothelial function, reduces inflammation, and decreases pro-thrombotic factors in plaque
- LDL lowering has little effect on the size of atheroma but has important effects on plaque stabilization

Conclusion

Atherosclerosis is an active process that involves en-

Preface

Vascular medicine has been a relatively unknown specialty, historically limited to major academic medical centers. In these centers, vascular medicine has had a dominant role in the diagnosis and management of all aspects of non-cardiac vascular disease. As the population has aged, the prevalence of all vascular disorders has increased, along with the demand for clinicians dedicated to the clinical evaluation and management of these complex patients.

Before 2006, there were no standards defining the baseline level of knowledge and skill required for clinicians to demonstrate expertise. Recognizing this limitation, several members of the Society for Vascular Medicine and Biology (SVMB) organized a separate entity, the American Board of Vascular Medicine, whose sole charge is to develop and administer certifying examinations in general vascular medicine and endovascular medicine. The first examination was offered in the fall of 2006.

Annual live board review courses presented the knowledge required for potential examinees before the examinations. However, it became readily apparent that the assembly of this information into one document would have tremendous value, not only for potential examinees, but also for physicians from other specialties who were interested in vascular medicine. This textbook has been born out of this need. It is our hope that this compilation of knowledge from experts in the field will result in an expanded pool of skilled clinicians in vascular medicine, which will ultimately lead to better care for our patients.

Michael R. Jaff, DO, Associate Editor

dothelial dysfunction, inflammation, and thrombosis. An understanding of the cellular processes and the effects of therapies has in turn helped our understanding of the clinical complications and prognosis and has helped in the development of new treatment strategies designed to prevent clinical events.

Questions

1. Which of the following statements is most correct?
   a. Endothelial cells migrate into the media during atherosclerosis initiation.
   b. Nitric oxide is produced by endothelial cells.
   c. Endothelin is a potent vasodilator.
   d. Elastic arteries regulate peripheral resistance.
   e. The adventitia contains abundant smooth muscle and connective tissue.

2. Which statement is false?
   a. Prostacyclin inhibits platelet activation.
   b. Nitric oxide inhibits many pro-inflammatory pathways.
   c. The endothelium produces tissue plasminogen activator.
   d. LDL is oxidized in the artery wall.
   e. HDL increases cholesterol deposition in peripheral tissues.

3. Which of the following statements is most true?
   a. An increase in endothelial nitric oxide activates the transcription factor NF-κB.
   b. ICAM is most responsible for monocyte rolling on endothelial cells.
   c. The fatty streak is characterized by foam cells.
   d. The chemokine MCP-1 blocks monocyte migration into the artery wall.
   e. All of the above are true.

4. Features of advanced atherosclerotic plaques include:
   a. Neovascularization of plaque
   b. Lipid pools
   c. T cells
   d. Metalloproteases
   e. All of the above

5. Which of the following statements are true?
   a. Neutrophils are abundant in early atherosclerotic plaques.
   b. T cells stimulate macrophages to produce metalloproteases.
   c. Therapies that lower LDL cholesterol substantially decrease plaque size.
   d. Calcification of arteries generally occurs as a passive process of deposition.
   e. Circulating PAIs such as PAI-1 are increased in patients with atherosclerosis and may promote thrombus formation.

6. Which of the following statements is most true?
   a. Compensatory enlargement of atherosclerotic arteries refers to the enlargement of the vessel lumen over time.
   b. Laminar blood flow imparts a higher shear stress on the endothelium compared with regions of disturbed blood flow.
   c. Negative remodeling of arteries contributes to the shrinkage of atherosclerotic plaques.
   d. Metalloproteases are more often associated with atherosclerotic plaques in regions of negatively remodeled arteries.

Suggested Readings

Aikawa M, Rabkin E, Okada Y, et al. Lipid lowering by diet reduces matrix metalloproteinase activity and increases collagen content of rabbit atheroma: a potential mechanism of lesion stabilization. Circulation. 1998;97:2433-44.

Barnes PJ, Karin M. Nuclear factor-κB: a pivotal transcription factor in chronic inflammatory diseases. N Engl J Med. 1997;336:1066-71.

Beckman JA, Ganz J, Creager MA, et al. Relationship of clinical presentation and calcification of culprit coronary artery stenoses. Arterioscler Thromb Vasc Biol. 2001;21:1618-22.

Brousseau ME, Schaefer EJ, Wolfe ML, et al. Effects of an inhibitor of cholesteryl ester transfer protein on HDL cholesterol. N Engl J Med. 2004;350:1505-15.

Davies MJ. Stability and instability: two faces of coronary atherosclerosis. The Paul Dudley White Lecture 1995. Circulation. 1996;94:2013-20.

Dzau VJ, Braun-Dullaeus RC, Sedding DG. Vascular proliferation and atherosclerosis: new perspectives and therapeutic strategies. Nat Med. 2002;8:1249-56.

Feletou M, Vanhoutte PM. The alternative: EDHF. J Mol Cell Cardiol. 1999;31:15-22.

Glagov S, Weisenberg E, Zarins CK, et al. Compensatory enlargement of human atherosclerotic coronary arteries. N Engl J Med. 1987;316:1371-5.

Kinlay S, Libby P, Ganz P. Endothelial function and coronary artery disease. Curr Opin Lipidol. 2001;12:383-9.

Kinlay S, Selwyn AP, Ganz P. Endothelium as a target of the risk factors in cardiovascular disease. In: Panza JA, Cannon RO III, editors. Endothelium, nitric oxide, and atherosclerosis: from basic mechanisms to clinical implications. Armonk (NY): Futura Publishing Company, Inc.; 1999. p. 227-41.

Kolodgie FD, Gold HK, Burke AP, et al. Intraplaque hemorrhage and progression of coronary atheroma. N Engl J Med. 2003;349:2316-25.

Li AC, Glass CK. The macrophage foam cell as a target for therapeutic intervention. Nat Med. 2002;8:1235-42.
Libby P. Molecular bases of the acute coronary syndromes. Circulation. 1995;91:2844-50.
Libby P. Current concepts of the pathogenesis of the acute coronary syndromes. Circulation. 2001;104:365-72.
Moncada S, Higgs EA, Vane JR. Human arterial and venous tissues generate prostacyclin (prostaglandin x), a potent inhibitor of platelet aggregation. Lancet. 1977;1:18-20.
Moulton KS. Plaque angiogenesis and atherosclerosis. Curr Atheroscler Rep. 2001;3:225-33.
Nichols WW, O'Rourke MF. McDonald's blood flow in arteries: theoretical, experimental and clinical principles. 4th ed. London: Arnold Publishers; 1998. p. 73-97.
Popma JJ, Sawyer M, Selwyn AP, et al. Lipid-lowering therapy after coronary revascularization. Am J Cardiol. 2000;86 Suppl 2:18H-28H.
Yanagisawa M, Kurihara H, Kimura S, et al. A novel potent vasoconstrictor peptide produced by vascular endothelial cells. Nature. 1988;332:411-5.

2 Vasculitis and Connective Tissue Disease*

Emile R. Mohler, III, MD

Vasculitis

The term vasculitis is defined as pathologic inflammation and necrosis of blood vessels. Vasculitis is rare and may occur as a result of an unknown cause (idiopathic) or may be associated with an established disease (secondary). The cause of most vasculitides is thought to be either humoral or cellular immune–related injury. The inflammatory response can lead to narrowing or occlusion of the vascular lumen and ischemia of tissue supplied by a particular vessel. Additionally, aneurysm and possible vessel rupture may occur. Clinical indicators of vasculitis include fever of unknown origin, unexplained arthritis or myositis, suspicious rash (i.e., palpable purpura), mononeuritis multiplex, and glomerulonephritis. Specific classification is often difficult, however, because of overlapping pathologic features and clinical symptoms and because the inciting antigen is unknown in most cases. Generally, vasculitides are classified according to the size of the vessels involved and the histology of the inflammatory cell infiltrate (Table 2.1).

- The cause of most vasculitides is thought to be humoral or a cellular immune–related injury
- Generally, vasculitides are classified according to the vessel size and the histology of the inflammatory cell infiltrate

Table 2.1 Vasculitis Classification

Large vessel	Temporal arteritis
	Takayasu arteritis
Medium vessel	Polyarteritis nodosa
	Kawasaki disease
Small vessel	Churg-Strauss syndrome
	Hypersensitivity vasculitis
	Wegener granulomatosis
	Behçet syndrome

From Mohler ER III. Vasculitis. In: Hiatt WR, Hirsch AT, Regensteiner J, editors. Peripheral arterial disease handbook. Boca Raton (FL): CRC Press; 2001. p. 339-62. Used with permission.

Large Vessel Vasculitis

This group of vasculitides includes temporal (giant cell) arteritis and Takayasu arteritis. Despite distinct clinical patterns, inflammatory giant cells and mononuclear infiltrates characterize both conditions. Figure 2.1 shows a clinical algorithm for diagnosis and treatment of large vessel vasculitis.

Temporal Arteritis

Temporal arteritis typically occurs in patients older than 50 years, is three times more common in women than men, and is most common in whites. Clinical symptoms usually develop slowly and most characteristically manifest as tenderness, erythema, or nodularity over the temporal artery. Other symptoms include fever, headaches, polymyalgia rheumatica, jaw claudication, and visual loss. Branches of the carotid artery are often involved, but any large artery is susceptible. Important but uncommon cardiovascular complications are aneurysm or stenosis of the aorta or its main branches.

Several findings on physical examination are specific for temporal arteritis. Temporal or other cranial arteries may be tender, thickened, visibly swollen, and erythematous. Bruits may be heard on auscultation of the carotid or supra-

*Portions of this chapter have been previously published in Mohler ER III. Vasculitis. In: Hiatt WR, Hirsch AT, Regensteiner J, editors. Peripheral arterial disease handbook. Boca Raton (FL): CRC Press; 2001. p. 339-62. Used with permission.

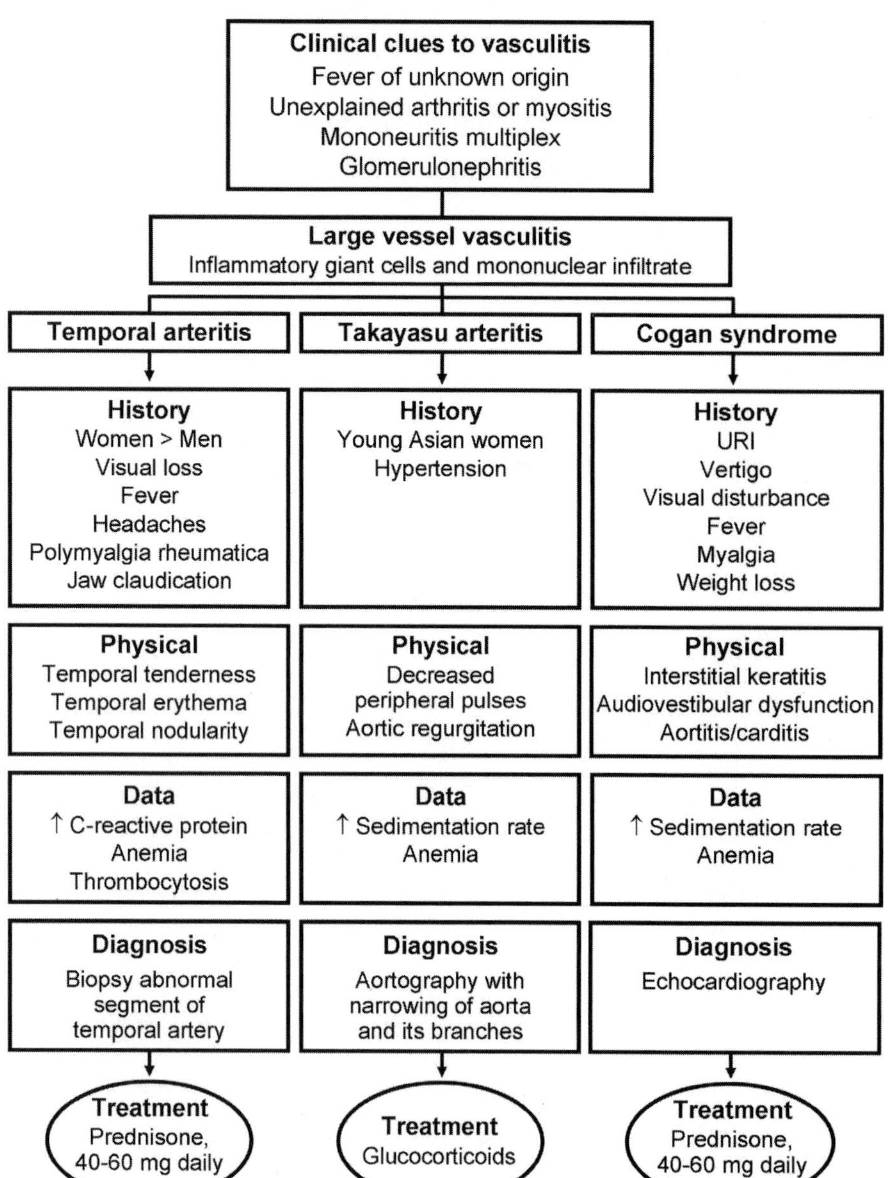

Fig. 2.1 Treatment algorithm for suspected large vessel vasculitis. URI, upper respiratory infection. (From Mohler ER III. Vasculitis. In: Hiatt WR, Hirsch AT, Regensteiner J, editors. Peripheral arterial disease handbook. Boca Raton [FL]: CRC Press; 2001. p. 339-62. Used with permission.)

clavicular areas, over the brachial or axillary arteries, or rarely over the orbits. In patients with polymyalgia rheumatica, active range of motion of the shoulders, neck, and hips is limited because of pain. Approximately 15% to 20% of patients with temporal arteritis have mild to moderate synovitis, especially in the wrists and knees.

Diagnosis of temporal arteritis is made on the basis of several types of studies. Laboratory findings may show elevated erythrocyte sedimentation rate, elevated C-reactive protein, anemia, and thrombocytosis. Recent reports indicate that duplex ultrasonography of the temporal arteries—showing a hypoechoic halo around the occipital artery along with scattered areas of increased peak systolic velocity—may be useful in the diagnosis of temporal arteritis, but not all the reports are favorable. Angiographic examination of the aortic arch and its branches can show abnormalities among those with symptoms or findings of large artery involvement. Computed tomography angiography and magnetic resonance angiography can also detect large artery involvement, but overall vascular changes are not defined as clearly as they are by traditional angiography. Diagnosis is also suspected if biopsy results from a segment of the temporal artery are abnormal.

Treatment of temporal arteritis with corticosteroids (prednisone, 40-60 mg/d) should be initiated immediately after the diagnosis is made; to avoid the possibility of sudden blindness, corticosteroids can be initiated while the diagnosis is pending. Corticosteroids may be withdrawn slowly after clinical and laboratory findings normalize. Levels of the cytokine interleukin-6 are elevated with disease symptoms and decrease with therapy. Temporal arteritis has a tendency to recur, and patients should be monitored closely for disease recurrence after remission.

Takayasu Arteritis

Takayasu arteritis is characterized by thickening and narrowing of the arterial lumen, even to the point of critical stenosis, due to a pathologic inflammatory response (Fig. 2.2). Cardiovascular symptoms include hypertension, decreased peripheral pulses, and aortic regurgitation. This form of vasculitis is most commonly reported in young Asian women and primarily affects large vessels such as the aorta and its main branches. Hypertension may be secondary to coarctation of the aorta or to renal artery stenosis.

The diagnosis of Takayasu arteritis is made by aortography, which typically shows narrowing of affected arteries with a well-developed collateral circulation. The erythrocyte sedimentation rate, as a marker for disease activity, is not universally believed to be reliable. The response to therapy may be monitored by symptomatic improvement, duplex ultrasonography, or magnetic resonance imaging.

Glucocorticoids are considered the first line of therapy for Takayasu arteritis; cytotoxic agents are added for steroid-resistant patients. Invasive vascular procedures such as angioplasty, stent placement, and bypass surgery are reserved for patients in whom disease is refractory to medical management. Indications for invasive intervention include 1) hypertension due to critical renal artery stenosis, 2) clinical features of cerebrovascular ischemia, 3) extremity ischemia limiting normal daily activities, and 4) cardiac ischemia due to coronary artery stenosis.

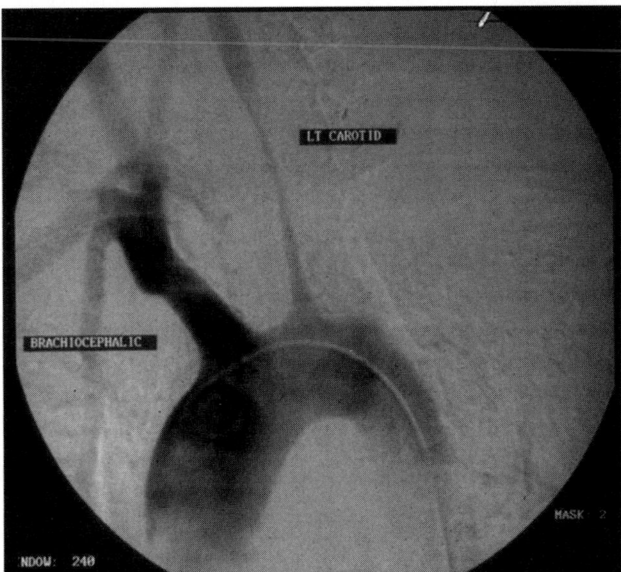

Fig. 2.2 Angiography of the aortic arch and great vessels showing the characteristic narrowing of Takayasu arteritis. (From Mohler ER III. Vasculitis. In: Hiatt WR, Hirsch AT, Regensteiner J, editors. Peripheral arterial disease handbook. Boca Raton [FL]: CRC Press; 2001. p. 339-62. Used with permission.)

Cogan Syndrome

Cogan syndrome is a rare disease of young adults that is predominantly associated with interstitial keratitis and audiovestibular symptoms. However, up to 15% of patients can have vasculitis, usually manifested as aortitis or carditis. Most patients have a preceding upper respiratory tract infection with eye and ear manifestations. This syndrome is named after the ophthalmologist who described the ocular symptoms of interstitial keratitis, which can include decreased visual acuity, photophobia, and impaired lacrimation.

The pathologic findings of aortitis associated with Cogan syndrome typically include a mixed infiltrate of neutrophils and mononuclear cells with disruption of the elastic lamina and vessel wall necrosis. Aortic valve regurgitation may develop (in approximately 10% of patients with Cogan syndrome) due to inflammation involving the valve cusps. In addition to aortic involvement, medium and small arteries can also become inflamed with scar tissue development.

Many findings are possible from the physical examination. Uveitis, optic neuritis, and scleritis can occur in conjunction with the other ocular findings. Audiovestibular dysfunction may occur in close temporal association with interstitial keratitis. Patients may have acute episodes similar to Meniere disease, with symptoms of vertigo, nausea, vomiting, and tinnitus. Somatic symptoms include fever, myalgia, fatigue, or weight loss. The ocular and audiovestibular manifestations are thought to be mediated by organ-specific autoimmunity and are not necessarily a consequence of vasculitis.

Early use of corticosteroids is advocated to ameliorate the ocular and audiovestibular symptoms. Patients may require a hearing aid or cochlear implants because of sensorineural hearing loss. The symptoms of vasculitis are usually controlled with high-dose corticosteroids, but some patients require aortic valve replacement because of severe aortic regurgitation.

Large Vessel Vasculitis

- Temporal arteritis:
  - Typically occurs in patients older than 50 years, in women three times as frequently as in men, and in whites more often than other groups
  - Corticosteroids (prednisone, 40-60 mg/d) should be initiated immediately after the diagnosis is made; if

diagnosis is delayed, empiric use of corticosteroids should be strongly considered

- Takayasu arteritis:
  - Glucocorticoids are considered the first line of therapy, with the addition of cytotoxic agents for steroid-resistant patients
- Cogan syndrome:
  - A rare disease of young adults associated with interstitial keratitis and audiovestibular symptoms
  - 15% of patients can have vasculitis, usually manifested as aortitis or carditis

Medium Vessel Vasculitis

Medium vessel vasculitides include polyarteritis nodosa and Kawasaki disease. Figure 2.3 shows a clinical algorithm for diagnosis and treatment of medium vessel vasculitis.

Polyarteritis Nodosa

Kussmaul and Maier first described polyarteritis nodosa in 1866. It typically presents as a disseminated necrotizing vasculitis involving medium-sized and small muscular arteries. Various clinical features may be observed as a result of frequent multiorgan system involvement; the most common are glomerulonephritis, mesenteric ischemia, polyarthralgia, and overlap syndrome. Other features can include palpable purpura, new-onset hypertension, renal dysfunction, congestive heart failure, and scleritis. Hepa-

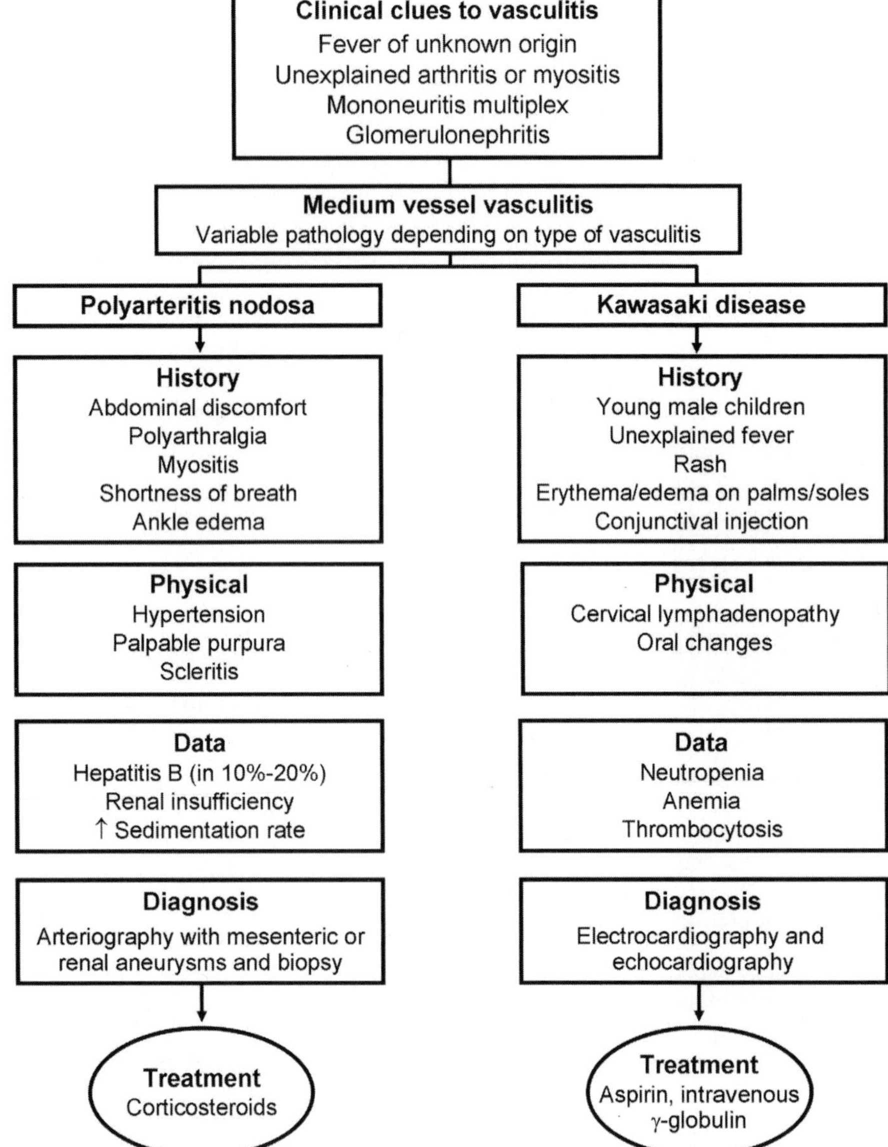

Fig. 2.3 Treatment algorithm for suspected medium vessel vasculitis. (From Mohler ER III. Vasculitis. In: Hiatt WR, Hirsch AT, Regensteiner J, editors. Peripheral arterial disease handbook. Boca Raton [FL]: CRC Press; 2001. p. 339-62. Used with permission.)

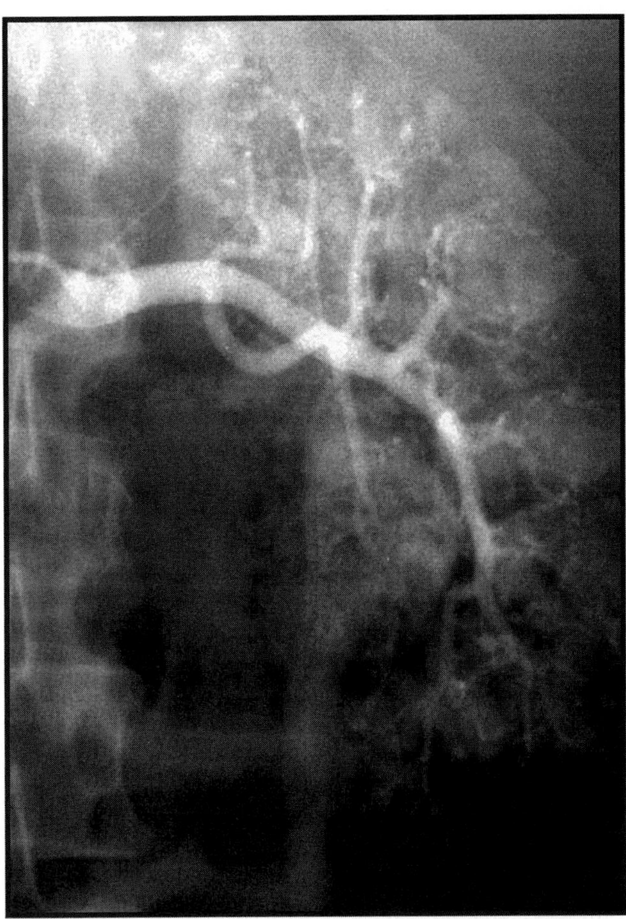

Fig. 2.4 Radiographic contrast angiography of mesenteric arteries with the characteristic aneurysm seen in polyarteritis nodosa. (From Mohler ER III. Vasculitis. In: Hiatt WR, Hirsch AT, Regensteiner J, editors. Peripheral arterial disease handbook. Boca Raton [FL]: CRC Press; 2001. p. 339-62. Used with permission.)

titis B infection is reported in approximately 10% to 20% of patients with polyarteritis nodosa.

The initial arterial injury is thought to begin in the intima, which then progresses to focal transmural inflammatory necrosis. Inflammatory destruction of the media may lead to aneurysm development (Fig. 2.4); aneurysm rupture is a reported source of morbidity and mortality. The diagnosis is usually made by biopsy of involved tissue (which will show the changes noted above) or by arteriographic documentation of mesenteric or renal artery aneurysms. The treatment of polyarteritis nodosa includes corticosteroids and the addition of cyclophosphamide in severe cases.

Kawasaki Disease

Kawasaki disease, also known as mucocutaneous lymph node syndrome, predominantly affects male children and was first described by Tomisaku Kawasaki in 1967. Patients usually have unexplained fever for 5 or more days accompanied by at least four of the five classic physical findings: 1) rash; 2) peripheral extremity changes manifesting as erythema or edema of the palms or soles (acute phase) and periungual desquamation (convalescent phase); 3) bilateral conjunctival injection; 4) oral mucous membrane changes (fissured lips, injected pharynx, strawberry tongue); and 5) cervical lymphadenopathy. Some of the findings of Kawasaki disease can appear similar to those of β-hemolytic streptococcal infection and measles. The disease can involve the large, medium, or small arteries but is most notable for coronary artery involvement. A mononuclear infiltrate with endothelial cell proliferation, elastic laminar disruption, and vessel wall necrosis is characteristic of the arterial disease.

The laboratory findings in Kawasaki disease can include anemia, neutropenia, and elevated platelet count. Electrocardiographic monitoring is important because carditis occurs in up to 50% of patients. Echocardiography is useful in diagnosing coronary artery aneurysms, which can occur within 2 weeks of disease onset. Ruptured coronary aneurysms are rare, but myocardial infarction can result from coronary artery thrombosis. The treatment includes aspirin (80-100 mg/kg per day for 2 weeks) and one high-dose intravenous γ-globulin infusion (2 g/kg) given within the first 10 days of illness. If echocardiography results are normal at 8 weeks, salicylates are discontinued; if echocardiography results are abnormal, salicylates should be continued for at least 1 year.

Medium Vessel Vasculitis

- Polyarteritis nodosa is a disseminated, necrotizing vasculitis involving medium-sized and small muscular arteries
  - Inflammatory destruction of the media may lead to aneurysm development
  - Aneurysm rupture is a reported source of morbidity and mortality
  - Hepatitis B infection is reported in approximately 10%-20% of patients
  - Treatment includes corticosteroids, with cyclophosphamide added in severe cases
- Kawasaki disease can involve the large, medium, or small arteries but is most notable for coronary artery involvement
  - Myocarditis occurs in up to 50% of patients
  - Coronary artery aneurysms can occur within 2 weeks of disease onset
  - Treatment includes aspirin for 2 weeks and a high-dose intravenous γ-globulin infusion within the first 10 days of illness

Small Vessel Vasculitis

Churg-Strauss Syndrome

Churg-Strauss syndrome, also known as allergic granulomatous angiitis, was initially described in 1951; it usually involves the small muscular arteries but also can involve medium-sized arteries. The syndrome usually involves eosinophilia and extravascular granulomas in patients with a history of allergic rhinitis, asthma, or both. However, the disease presentation can be variable and can occur without some of the classic findings. The mean age of onset is 38 years with a male predominance.

Churg-Strauss syndrome typically occurs in three phases. The initial phase is an allergic response manifested by allergic rhinitis, asthma, or both. The second phase involves blood eosinophilia with or without transient pulmonary infiltrates (this may be indistinguishable from Löffler syndrome). The third phase involves systemic necrotizing vasculitis. The asthmatic condition frequently remits during the onset of vasculitis but can occur again later in the disease.

Approximately 75% of patients have pulmonary infiltrates that can appear as patchy peripheral infiltrates, hilar shadows, and even large pulmonary nodules. At least 50% of patients have upper respiratory symptoms including allergic rhinitis and nasal or sinus polyposis. Skin manifestations can include palpable purpura with leukocytoclastic vasculitis. Granulomatous nodules can also develop on the skin. Some patients may have diarrhea secondary to eosinophilia infiltration of the bowel wall with resulting bleeding and nodular masses that can cause gastrointestinal tract obstruction. Bowel ischemia with perforation bleeding or colitis is reported and may be heralded by abdominal pain. The nervous system abnormalities that accompany Churg-Strauss syndrome can mirror those of polyarteritis nodosa and include mononeuritis multiplex, symmetric peripheral neuropathy, ischemic optic neuritis, and cranial nerve palsies. Cardiac involvement can lead to pericarditis or myocardial infarction. Patients sometimes also have urinary tract involvement or focal segmental glomerulonephritis.

The characteristic laboratory findings in Churg-Strauss syndrome include fluctuating levels of eosinophils and increased immunoglobulin (Ig) E levels. In addition, antineutrophil cytoplasmic antibodies (ANCA) and antibodies to myeloperoxidase may be found. A strong correlation between disease activity and eosinophil count is reported.

Diagnosis of Churg-Strauss syndrome relies on the clinical presentation, chest radiography, laboratory studies, and pathologic examination. Several diseases can mimic Churg-Strauss. The differential diagnosis includes Wegener granulomatosis (usually has a more destructive airway component without asthma), Löffler syndrome, sarcoidosis, and allergic bronchopulmonary aspergillosis. Churg-Strauss vasculitis usually responds to corticosteroid administration. Most patients with disease remission have a mean survival of approximately 10 years. The mortality from this condition is usually secondary to pulmonary and cardiac failure. Patients with fulminating vasculitis should be given immunosuppressive drugs if corticosteroids are not successful.

Hypersensitivity Vasculitis

The hypersensitivity vasculitides are vasculitic diseases that previously were reported under various names, including cutaneous necrotizing vasculitis, allergic vasculitis, and leukocytoclastic vasculitis. These diseases characteristically involve inflammation of small vessels (especially venules) with leukocytoclasis (nuclear debris) and cutaneous skin involvement. The clinical syndromes include serum sickness, drug hypersensitivity reactions, Henoch-Schönlein purpura, mixed cryoglobulinemia, and urticarial vasculitis (hypocomplementemic vasculitis).

The onset of hypersensitivity vasculitis is usually abrupt and can occur in both sexes and all age groups. The cutaneous signs of hypersensitivity vasculitis can include palpable purpura (classic finding), petechiae, vesicles, urticaria, papules, pustules, necrotic ulcerations, and nodules. The skin lesions usually appear in groups and are symmetrically distributed on dependent areas. The resolution of lesions can take up to 4 weeks, and hyperpigmentation or scars sometimes occur. Arthralgias or arthritis may develop; the knees are most frequently involved, followed by ankles, wrists, and elbows. Muscular or nervous system involvement can also occur, usually in association with connective tissue diseases or cryoglobulinemia. Gastrointestinal tract involvement suggests Henoch-Schönlein purpura or vasculitis secondary to inflammatory bowel disease. Renal involvement can also occur and should be suspected if hematuria is present.

Laboratory findings may include an elevated erythrocyte sedimentation rate with leukocytosis, eosinophilia, anemia, heme-positive stool, hematuria, proteinuria, cryoglobulinemia, hypocomplementemia, and abnormal liver or renal function tests. IgA-containing immune complexes are characteristically found with Henoch-Schönlein purpura. Patients presenting with symptoms of hypersensitivity vasculitis should be carefully evaluated for underlying systemic illness or exposure to an offending agent.

The pathologic findings in hypersensitivity vasculitis are necrotizing inflammation of vessels less than 1 mm in diameter accompanied by polymorphonuclear cells (less frequently, lymphocytes), which is known as leukocytoclasis (destruction of cells with "nuclear dust"). The diagnosis is confirmed by the presence of a leukocytoclastic pattern involving small vessels at the site of a dermal lesion. The treatment involves removal of the offending agent or treatment of an associated systemic illness. A spontaneous resolution of symptoms is common, although some patients require long-term treatment with corticosteroids for control of disease.

Small Vessel Vasculitis

- Churg-Strauss syndrome:
  - Usually involves the small muscular arteries but can also involve medium-sized arteries
  - Usually includes eosinophilia and extravascular granulomas in patients with a history of allergic rhinitis, asthma, or both
- Hypersensitivity vasculitides:
  - Include serum sickness, drug hypersensitivity reactions, Henoch-Schönlein purpura, mixed cryoglobulinemia, and urticarial vasculitis (hypocomplementemic vasculitis)
  - IgA-containing immune complexes are characteristically found with Henoch-Schönlein purpura

Wegener Granulomatosis

Wegener granulomatosis characteristically involves a necrotizing granulomatous process of the respiratory tract along with glomerulonephritis. It occurs primarily in young and middle-aged persons and has a slight male predominance. Most patients have both upper and lower respiratory tract involvement, although some patients with pulmonary infiltrates may be asymptomatic. In addition to respiratory and renal disease manifestations, cutaneous lesions, ocular disease, peripheral and central nervous system involvement, and cardiovascular inflammation (i.e., carditis) can also develop. The cause of Wegener granulomatosis is unknown.

The pathologic findings can include necrotizing vasculitis of small arteries and veins, necrotizing granulomas, and glomerulonephritis. The vascular lesions usually have fibrinoid necrosis with vessels at different stages of inflammation and healing. The kidney lesions are most commonly focal segmental glomerulonephritis. Wegener granulomatosis is usually distinguished from polyarteritis nodosa by an infiltration of mononuclear cells and frequent involvement of the small veins.

Laboratory findings in Wegener granulomatosis can include an elevated erythrocyte sedimentation rate, leukocytosis, thrombocytosis, and anemia of chronic disease. In most patients (approximately 93%) with diffuse, active disease, the ANCA test is positive but antinuclear antibody tests are negative. The antibodies detected usually are directed against proteinase 3, myeloperoxidase, and occasionally human leukocyte elastase.

The initial evaluation for Wegener granulomatosis should include chest radiography, urinalysis, and blood tests. The differential diagnosis includes other vasculitides, especially systemic lupus erythematosus. Other disorders that should be considered include cholesterol atheroemboli, infective endocarditis, malignancies, fibromuscular dysplasia, and radiation fibrosis. The diagnosis is confirmed with a tissue biopsy of the respiratory tract or kidneys. A biopsy of the lung is the most likely tissue to show classic pathologic findings.

The decision to treat a patient usually is made on the basis of a positive ANCA result in conjunction with biopsy findings. Most patients respond to treatment with cyclophosphamide and corticosteroids. If left untreated, the prognosis of Wegener granulomatosis is poor—90% of patients die within 2 years as a result of respiratory or renal failure. Patients who initially require dialysis because of renal failure may recover enough to discontinue dialysis.

Behçet Syndrome

Behçet syndrome is a rare multisystem inflammatory disorder characterized by recurrent oral aphthous ulcers, genital ulcers, uveitis, and skin lesions. Patients commonly have synovitis and meningoencephalitis. The pathophysiology involves an autoimmune response that can result in vascular injury. The vasa vasorum can be affected by vasculitis in large vessels. Aneurysms and occlusions of large arteries can result in morbid complications. Cerebrovascular accidents, claudication, and renal vascular hypertension secondary to arteritis or thrombosis have been reported with Behçet syndrome. In addition, recurrent thrombophlebitis of superficial and deep veins can occur and can manifest as fever. Neurologic involvement may include cerebral venous thrombosis.

The cause of Behçet syndrome is unknown, but clusters of cases are reported along the ancient Silk Road, which extends from Eastern Asia to the Mediterranean basin. The highest prevalence of this syndrome is in the Eastern Mediterranean region, especially Turkey, and in Japan. An increased prevalence of the HLA-B51 allele matches the disease distribution along the Silk Road and in Japan, but not among white patients who live in Western countries. Microbial infection is implicated in the development of Behçet syndrome because herpes simplex virus DNA and serum antibodies against the virus have been noted in a higher proportion of patients with disease than in controls. Other viruses possibly involved include parvovirus B19 and hepatitis C virus. However, none of these infectious agents have been definitively proven to cause the autoimmune response.

Table 2.2 Criteria for the Diagnosis of Behçet Syndrome*

Finding	Definition
Recurrent oral ulceration	Minor aphthous, major aphthous, or herpetiform ulcers observed by the physician or patient, which have recurred at least three times over a 12-month period
Recurrent genital ulceration	Aphthous ulceration or scarring observed by the physician or patient
Eye lesions	Anterior uveitis, posterior uveitis, or cells in the vitreous on slit-lamp examination; OR retinal vasculitis detection by an ophthalmologist
Skin lesions	Erythema nodosum observed by the physician or patient, pseudofolliculitis, or papulopustular lesions; OR acneiform nodules observed by the physician in a postadolescent patient who is not receiving corticosteroids
Positive pathergy test	Test interpreted as positive by the physician at 24 to 48 hours

*The criteria were proposed by the International Study Group for Behçet's Disease. For the diagnosis to be made, a patient must have recurrent oral ulceration plus at least two of the other findings in the absence of other clinical explanations.
From Sakane T, Takeno M, Suzuki N, et al. Behçet's disease. N Engl J Med. 1999;341:1284-91. Used with permission.

The diagnosis is made on the basis of criteria proposed by the International Study Group for Behçet's Disease (Table 2.2). Valvular and coronary artery disease can occur in some patients. Neutrophil and lymphocyte function are abnormal, which is thought to be responsible for the many immunologic abnormalities that can occur. Useful imaging studies to detect vascular lesions include computed tomography, magnetic resonance imaging, angiography, and ventilation perfusion scintigraphy.

Treatment of Behçet syndrome depends on the clinical manifestations (Table 2.3). Unfortunately, treatment of this form of vasculitis with immunosuppressive agents is not as useful as with other vasculitides. Potential therapies include estradiol, dapsone, colchicine, cyclosporine, and levamisole.

Small Vessel Vasculitis

- Wegener granulomatosis:
  - Involves a necrotizing granulomatous process of the respiratory tract along with glomerulonephritis
  - Most patients (approximately 93%) with diffuse, active disease have a positive ANCA test but a negative antinuclear antibody test
  - Most patients respond to treatment with cyclophosphamide and corticosteroids
- Behçet syndrome:
  - Multisystem inflammatory disorder characterized by recurrent oral aphthous ulcers, genital ulcers, uveitis, and skin lesions

Thromboangiitis Obliterans

Thromboangiitis obliterans (TO), also known as Buerger disease, is a non-atherosclerotic, segmental, inflammatory disease that most commonly affects the small and medium-sized arteries, veins, and nerves of the extremities. This condition is distinguished from other forms of vasculitis by several features. First, pathologic examination shows highly cellular and inflammatory thrombus with relative sparing of the blood vessel wall. Second, the erythrocyte sedimentation rate and serum C-reactive protein level are usually normal. Third, commonly measured autoantibodies (e.g., antinuclear antibody and rheumatoid factor) are normal or negative. Other serologic tests such as circulating immune complexes, complement levels, and cryoglobulins are normal despite an immune reaction in the arterial intima.

Epidemiology

TO is most prevalent in Asia and the Middle East. An incidence of 12.6 per 100,000 persons in the United States was reported in 1986, which is lower than in previous reports. The prevalence of this disease in other parts of the world ranges from 0.5% to 5.6% of patients with peripheral arterial disease in Western Europe, to 45% to 63% of those with peripheral arterial disease in India. The highest prevalence reported (80%) is in Israel among Jews of Ashkenazi ancestry with peripheral arterial disease.

Young men are more commonly affected than women, and the typical age of onset is 40 to 45 years. However, some reports have indicated that the prevalence of TO in women is increasing; women currently comprise 11% to 30% of patients with TO.

The use of tobacco is the sine qua non of disease initiation and progression. TO is more common in countries where tobacco is heavily used, especially among people who use homemade cigarettes with raw tobacco. Most clinicians believe that TO occurs only in smokers, although occasional cases have been reported in users of smokeless tobacco or snuff.

History and Presentation

TO usually begins with ischemia of the distal small arteries and veins, followed by more proximal arterial in-

Table 2.3 Treatment of Behçet Syndrome

Treatment	Dose	Used as first-line therapy	Used as alternative therapy
Topical corticosteroids			
Triamcinolone acetonide ointment	3×/d topically	Oral ulcers	
Betamethasone ointment	3×/d topically	Genital ulcers	
Betamethasone drops	1-2 drops 3×/d topically	Anterior uveitis, retinal vasculitis	
Dexamethasone	1.0-1.5 mg injected below Tenon capsule for an ocular attack	Retinal vasculitis	
Systemic corticosteroids			
Prednisolone	5-20 mg/d orally		Erythema nodosum, anterior uveitis, retinal vasculitis, arthritis
	20-100 mg/d orally	Gastrointestinal lesions, acute meningoencephalitis, chronic progressive central nervous system lesions, arteritis	Retinal vasculitis, venous thrombosis
Methylprednisolone	1,000 mg/d for 3 days IV	Acute meningoencephalitis, chronic progressive central nervous system lesions, arteritis	Gastrointestinal lesions, venous thrombosis
Tropicamide drops	1-2 drops 1-2×/d topically	Anterior uveitis	
Tetracycline	250 mg in water solution 1×/d topically		Oral ulcers
Colchicine	0.5-1.5 mg/d orally	Oral ulcers,* genital ulcers,* pseudofolliculitis,* erythema nodosum, anterior uveitis, retinal vasculitis	Arthritis
Thalidomide	100-300 mg/d orally		Oral ulcers,* genital ulcers,* pseudofolliculitis*
Dapsone	100 mg/d orally		Oral ulcers, genital ulcers, pseudofolliculitis, erythema nodosum
Pentoxifylline	300 mg/d orally		Oral ulcers, genital ulcers, pseudofolliculitis, erythema nodosum
Azathioprine	100 mg/d orally		Retinal vasculitis,* arthritis,* chronic progressive central nervous system lesions, arteritis, venous thrombosis
Chlorambucil	5 mg/d orally		Retinal vasculitis,* acute meningoencephalitis, chronic progressive central nervous system lesions, arteritis, venous thrombosis
Cyclophosphamide	50-100 mg/d orally		Retinal vasculitis, acute meningoencephalitis, chronic progressive central nervous system lesions, arteritis, venous thrombosis
	700-1,000 mg/mo IV		Retinal vasculitis, acute meningoencephalitis, chronic progressive central nervous system lesions, arteritis, venous thrombosis
Methotrexate	7.5-15 mg/wk orally		Retinal vasculitis, arthritis, chronic progressive central nervous system lesions
Cyclosporine†	5 mg/kg of body weight per day orally	Retinal vasculitis*	
Interferon-α	5 million U/d IM or SC		Retinal vasculitis , arthritis
Indomethacin	50-75 mg/d orally	Arthritis	
Sulfasalazine	1-3 g/d orally	Gastrointestinal lesions	Arthritis
Warfarin‡	2-10 mg/d orally	Venous thrombosis	Arteritis
Heparin‡	5,000-20,000 U/d SC	Venous thrombosis	Arteritis
Aspirin§	50-100 mg/d orally	Arteritis, venous thrombosis	Chronic progressive central nervous system lesions
Dipyridamole	300 mg/d orally	Arteritis, venous thrombosis	Chronic progressive central nervous system lesions
Surgery			Gastrointestinal lesions, arteritis, venous thrombosis

IM, intramuscularly; IV, intravenously; SC, subcutaneously.

*The efficacy of this drug for this use has been reported in controlled clinical trials.

†Cyclosporine is contraindicated in patients with acute meningoencephalitis or chronic progressive central nervous system lesions.

‡This drug should be used with caution in patients with pulmonary vascular lesions.

§Low-dose aspirin is used as an antiplatelet agent.

From Sakane T, Takeno M, Suzuki N, et al. Behçet's disease. N Engl J Med. 1999;341:1284-91. Used with permission.

volvement as the disease advances. Patients usually note ischemia of the digits, which may manifest as claudication of the feet, legs, hands, or arms. The disease can progress to include ischemic ulcerations of the fingers or toes with accompanying ischemic pain at rest. In one study of 112 patients, 66% had ischemic ulcerations at the time of presentation. Another study reported that 16% of patients had symptoms in two limbs, 41% had symptoms in three limbs, and 43% had symptoms in all four limbs. Superficial thrombophlebitis can occur and may parallel disease activity. Raynaud syndrome occurs in approximately 40% of patients.

Pathology

Three phases of TO have been described pathologically:
– The acute phase involves development of inflammatory thrombi in arteries and veins, typically of the distal extremities. The thrombus is occlusive, and polymorphonuclear leukocytes, microabscesses, and multinucleated giant cells may be present. However, there is no evidence of fibrinoid necrosis, and the internal elastic lamina is intact.
– The intermediate phase is characterized by progressive organization of the thrombus.
– In the chronic phase, inflammation is no longer present, and only organized thrombus and vascular fibrosis remain. The pathologic appearance in the chronic phase is indistinguishable from all other types of vascular disease.

Although TO most commonly affects the distal extremities, the pathologic findings have been reported in cerebral, coronary, renal, mesenteric, and internal thoracic arteries. Larger vessels such as the aorta, pulmonary arteries, and iliac arteries are also affected in rare instances.

- TO is a non-atherosclerotic, segmental, inflammatory disease that most commonly affects the small- and medium-sized arteries, veins, and nerves of the extremities
- The use of tobacco is the sine qua non of disease initiation and progression
- A positive Allen test in a young smoker with leg ulcerations is suggestive of TO
- No specific laboratory tests can be used to definitively diagnose TO

Diagnosis

TO should be suspected in smokers who present with distal ischemia of the hands, feet, or both. A definitive diagnosis is made if the histopathologic examination identifies an acute phase lesion in a patient with a clinical history of smoking.

Clinical Evaluation

All patients should have a thorough history and detailed vascular examination. A positive Allen test in a young smoker with leg ulcerations is suggestive of TO because it demonstrates small vessel involvement in both the arms and legs. An abnormal Allen test can also occur with other conditions that involve small vessel occlusive disease, such as scleroderma (including CREST syndrome), emboli, hypercoagulable states, repetitive trauma, and other vasculitides. The distal nature of TO and involvement of the legs and arms help distinguish the disorder from atherosclerosis.

Laboratory Tests

No specific laboratory tests can be used to definitively diagnose TO. Patients should have a complete serologic profile including a complete blood count with differential and a chemistry panel including assessment of liver enzymes and renal function. A diagnosis of diabetes mellitus makes the diagnosis of TO unlikely in the absence of a histologic diagnosis of the acute phase lesion.

Evaluation for vasculitis should also be performed and should include tests for antinuclear antibody, rheumatoid factor, complement, screening for scleroderma (anticentromere antibody and Scl-70), and screening for antiphospholipid antibodies and genetic causes of thrombophilia. As mentioned above, these tests are normal or negative in patients with TO. However, anticardiolipin antibodies can be present in some patients with TO.

Imaging Studies

A proximal source of emboli should be ruled out by transthoracic echocardiography. Transesophageal echocardiography is used rarely for screening and only if transthoracic echocardiography suggests a clot.

Arteriography is performed to evaluate for vascular disease in the extremities. Both arms and legs should be examined, even in patients who present with clinical involvement of only one extremity, because of the high prevalence of disease in multiple limbs. Suggestive arteriographic features include 1) involvement of small and medium-sized vessels such as the palmar, plantar, tibial, peroneal, radial, and ulnar arteries; 2) no evidence of atherosclerosis; 3) segmental occlusion distally (diseased arteries interspersed with normal-appearing arteries) and collateralization around areas of occlusion (corkscrew collaterals); and 4) no apparent source of emboli. Although these arteriographic findings are suggestive, they are not pathognomonic because they can be identical to findings for other causes of small vessel occlusive disease such as scleroderma, CREST syndrome, mixed connective tissue disease, and other causes of vasculitis.

Diagnostic Criteria

Several criteria have been proposed for the diagnosis of TO; they are based on a clinical, angiographic, histopathologic, and exclusionary scoring system. One set of criteria includes onset before the age of 45 years in the absence of risk factors for atherosclerotic disease, other than smoking. Most clinicians use the following criteria: age younger than 45 years; current or recent history of tobacco use; distal extremity ischemia (noted objectively on vascular testing); and exclusion of autoimmune and hypercoagulable diseases. Typical arteriographic findings help to exclude proximal atherosclerotic disease and to meet the criteria for TO. A vascular biopsy is usually not necessary unless a patient presents with unusual characteristics such as large artery involvement or is older than 45 years.

Treatment

The most effective treatment of TO is complete discontinuation of cigarette smoking or use of tobacco in any form. The disease is thought to be activated even if patients smoke only one or two cigarettes per day. The correlation between smoking and disease activity is so strong that measurement of urinary nicotine and cotinine (a byproduct of nicotine) should be performed if the disease is still active despite patient claims of tobacco cessation.

Approximately 94% of patients who quit smoking avoid amputation compared with 43% who continue to smoke. Transdermal nicotine patches or nicotine chewing gum may keep the disease active, but bupropion can be used as a smoking cessation aid. Inpatient nicotine dependence treatment is an alternative for recidivist smokers.

Other than discontinuation of tobacco use, there are no definitive treatments for TO. However, several therapies have been investigated. Iloprost (a prostaglandin analog) was investigated in a randomized, double-blind trial of 152 patients treated with either a 6-hour daily intravenous infusion of the drug or low-dose aspirin. The primary outcome measure was total relief of pain at rest and complete healing of all trophic changes. Significant improvement was seen in the iloprost-treated group compared with the aspirin group at 28 days and at 6 months; 18% of patients receiving aspirin required amputation compared with 6% receiving iloprost. A study of oral iloprost did not find it as effective as intravenous administration. The major use of iloprost may be for helping patients with critical limb ischemia during the period when they first stop cigarette smoking.

Thrombolytic therapy has had limited investigation in patients with TO. In one study of 11 patients with longstanding disease who had gangrene or pregangrenous lesions of the toes or feet, treatment with low-dose intraarterial streptokinase resulted in avoidance of or alteration in the level of amputation in 58%. However, further study is required before the precise role of thrombolytic therapy can be defined.

Surgical revascularization usually is not recommended because of the diffuse segmental involvement and distal nature of the disease. Surgical bypass with autologous vein and even omental graft to facilitate limb salvage have been reported. Nevertheless, revascularization is uncommon in the United States because a reasonable vessel for bypass usually is not found and because most patients do well with smoking cessation.

If peripheral vascular surgery is planned, and if preoperative testing suggests the presence of concomitant ischemic heart disease that requires subsequent cardiac catheterization, consideration should be given to performing angiography of the internal thoracic arteries. As noted above, involvement of these arteries occasionally occurs in TO, and planning for coronary bypass surgery is facilitated if their patency is assessed before heart surgery.

Sympathectomy to prevent pain and amputation is a controversial procedure, and results are not definitive. A spinal cord stimulator was used to treat one patient when other measures failed, which resulted in complete healing of finger ulcerations. Administration of intramuscular vascular endothelial growth factor has been reported to improve ulcers in patients with TO, but this treatment remains experimental.

Connective Tissue Diseases

Scleroderma

Scleroderma encompasses a heterogeneous group of conditions linked by the presence of thickened, sclerotic skin lesions. Systemic sclerosis is a subset of scleroderma and includes both diffuse disease and disease limited to the skin. Patients with limited cutaneous scleroderma can have prominent vascular manifestations and may have CREST syndrome (**c**alcinosis, **R**aynaud syndrome, **e**sophageal dysmotility, **s**clerodactyly, and **t**elangiectasia). The manifestations of scleroderma are diverse and can include abnormalities of the vasculature (most notably Raynaud syndrome) and fibrotic or vascular disease involvement of multiple organ systems including the musculoskeletal, renal, pulmonary, cardiac, and gastrointestinal systems. The reported prevalence of scleroderma ranges from 4 to 253 cases per 1 million persons. The incidence in the United States is 14.6 to 50.8 cases per 100,000.

Pathophysiology

Scleroderma is characterized by immune system activation, endothelial dysfunction, and enhanced fibroblast activity. The precise inciting events that lead to development of systemic scleroderma currently are unknown. Data indicate that the effector cell is the activated fibroblast. On a cellular level, several cytokines, including interleukin-2 and transforming growth factor-β, have been implicated in fibroblast activation in patients with scleroderma. These cytokines are released from activated immune cells, fibroblasts, and endothelial cells.

Vascular injury is thought to occur even before fibrosis is clinically obvious, and Raynaud syndrome may be the earliest clinical finding in patients who eventually have development of systemic scleroderma. Most damage occurs at the level of the cutaneous circulation and in the microvasculature of various internal organs. The vascular injury is believed to originate in the endothelial cells. Small arteries and capillaries constrict, with eventual obliteration of the vessel lumen and ensuing ischemia.

Clinical Manifestations

Patients suspected to have scleroderma should be evaluated for multiorgan disease and cutaneous manifestations. The most obvious clinical manifestation of vascular dysfunction among patients with scleroderma is Raynaud syndrome, but vascular injury also results in pulmonary hypertension and scleroderma renal crisis and can have a role in the pathogenesis of cardiac and gastrointestinal diseases. Raynaud syndrome is commonly a reversible vasospasm, but in patients with scleroderma, structural disease of the vessels may develop, with permanently impaired flow. This ischemia may be prolonged and result in digital ulcers or infarcts. In patients with limited scleroderma (including CREST syndrome), Raynaud syndrome may precede other disease manifestations, sometimes by many years. However, in patients with diffuse scleroderma, the onset of Raynaud syndrome often occurs after the appearance of skin or musculoskeletal manifestations.

If organ involvement is present, the disease is typically referred to as "systemic sclerosis" and frequently affects the kidneys, gastrointestinal tract, and lungs. Renal involvement may result in acute renal failure and the abrupt onset of moderate to marked hypertension; some patients, however, remain normotensive. Patients with cardiac involvement can have eventual development of symptomatic pericarditis and myocardial disease primarily consisting of fibrosis without overt coronary artery disease. Arrhythmias are common and thought to be caused by myocardial fibrosis.

Diagnosis

The diagnosis of scleroderma and related disorders is usually made on the basis of characteristic clinical findings. A skin biopsy is not important for confirmation of the diagnosis, although it is sometimes performed to help distinguish scleroderma from other syndromes such as eosinophilic fasciitis or scleromyxedema. Cutaneous features such as calcinosis or telangiectasia are helpful in confirming the diagnosis but are variable and often absent in early stages of disease.

Organ-specific testing may elucidate extracutaneous disease. For example, the diagnosis of scleroderma in a patient with Raynaud syndrome is supported by symptoms of dysphagia or findings of abnormal esophageal motility on barium swallow studies. The demonstration of abnormal capillaries by nailfold microscopy also indicates secondary Raynaud syndrome. The American College of Rheumatology has published diagnostic criteria for systemic scleroderma; the major criterion is proximal sclerodermatous skin changes (proximal to the metacarpophalangeal joints), and the minor criteria are sclerodactyly, digital pitting, scars of fingertips or loss of substance of the distal finger pads, and bibasilar pulmonary fibrosis. The patient should fulfill the major criterion or two of the three minor criteria for a diagnosis of systemic scleroderma.

Serologic testing for autoantibodies can be helpful in the diagnosis and classification of systemic scleroderma. However, none of the serologic tests are sensitive enough to independently exclude disease. The presence of anticentromere and anti–Scl-70 antibodies has been described in patients with systemic sclerosis. Others, such as anti–RNA polymerase or anti–U3-RNP antibodies may also be present. Histologic examination in most patients with scleroderma shows a positive antinuclear staining pattern. The presence of anticentromere antibodies favors the diagnosis of CREST syndrome. Anti–RNA polymerases I and III are found only in patients with systemic sclerosis; ANCAs are not associated with systemic sclerosis. Of note, approximately 10% of patients in whom a diagnosis of systemic sclerosis is eventually made do not have cutaneous disease.

- The diagnosis of scleroderma and related disorders is usually made on the basis of characteristic clinical findings
- The presence of anticentromere and anti–Scl-70 antibodies has been described in patients with systemic sclerosis
- Histologic examination in most patients with scleroderma shows a positive antinuclear staining pattern

The differential diagnosis of scleroderma depends on the most prominent clinical features of the patient. The differential diagnosis of scleroderma-like skin changes with Raynaud syndrome includes other skin diseases due to drugs, toxins, or harmful environmental factors; endocrine disorders, such as diabetes mellitus, hypothyroidism, or amyloidosis; and systemic lupus erythematosus or inflammatory muscle diseases. "Overlap syndrome" is diagnosed if clear-cut scleroderma is present along with sufficient clinical or laboratory features to support a concurrent diagnosis of another connective tissue disease.

Treatment

No available therapy has been proven to reverse the vascular and fibrotic changes in patients with scleroderma. However, several therapies have been investigated for their ability to slow disease progression, improve vascular function, limit mortality, and provide supportive symptomatic care. For patients with Raynaud syndrome, the typical recommended therapies can be used. Endothelin receptor antagonists, such as bosentan, are being studied for the ability to counter vasoconstriction and promote vessel remodeling. Patients with severe, critical digital ischemia may require hospitalization; pain can be relieved with intravenous vasodilatory therapy and systemic anticoagulation. If concomitant infection is present, systemic antibiotics are indicated. Angiographic assessment may be necessary to evaluate for the presence of large vessel disease, and digital sympathectomy can be required to inhibit sympathetic-mediated vasoconstriction.

- No available therapy has been proven to reverse the vascular and fibrotic changes in patients with scleroderma

Drugs such as cyclophosphamide may be beneficial in patients with interstitial lung disease. Methotrexate has been shown to improve skin sores and diffusion capacity. Corticosteroids can be useful in the treatment of myositis and alveolitis, but their use is limited because high doses can precipitate renal crisis. Immunoablation combined with autologous stem cell rescue is currently considered experimental. Angiotensin-converting enzyme inhibitors should be used at the first sign of hypertension, microangiopathic hemolytic anemia, or unexplained renal insufficiency. The early use of angiotensin-converting enzyme inhibitors or angiotensin-receptor blockers is critical in preserving renal function, controlling hypertension, and improving survival during renal crisis.

Systemic Lupus Erythematosus

Systemic lupus erythematosus (SLE) is a chronic inflammatory disease of unknown cause, which can affect the skin, joints, kidneys, lungs, nervous system, serous membranes, and other organs of the body. The clinical course and presentation of SLE are variable and may be characterized by periods of remission and chronic or acute relapses. Women, especially in their 20s and 30s, are affected more frequently than men.

Pathophysiology

The pathophysiology of SLE has not been defined, although many genes that affect immune function, particularly human leukocyte antigen, may augment susceptibility to clinical disease. Most monozygotic twins are discordant for clinical SLE, which strongly suggests that additional factors, probably environmental, trigger the development of autoimmunity in susceptible persons.

Certain medications, such as phenytoin, hydralazine, procainamide, and isoniazid, can produce drug-induced lupus, but this disorder differs from classic SLE in its autoantibody profile (e.g., antihistone antibody–positive) and in sparing the kidneys and central nervous system. Once triggered, the autoimmune reaction in SLE affects many sites through multiple mechanisms, such as deposition of immune complexes, effects of cytokines and other chemical neuromodulators, and direct attack by autoantibodies or active leukocytes. The non-neurologic sites of damage include the renal glomeruli, joints, plural or pericardial serosa, integument, cardiac or vascular endothelium, cardiac valves, and the oral and conjunctival mucosa. Multiple sites may be involved within the nervous system.

- Certain medications can produce drug-induced lupus

In sites of apparent vasculitis, histologic examination shows degenerative changes in small vessels, often with minimal or no inflammatory infiltrates. The chronic effects of immune complex deposition may be one mechanism for SLE vasculopathy; cytokine-mediated effects on vascular endothelium or local brain parenchyma are another. The inflammatory and non-inflammatory SLE vasculopathies can be clinically indistinguishable.

In addition to small vessel vasculopathy, inflammatory changes may occur in large to medium-sized vessels, producing more classic vasculitis. For example, patients may present with clinical stroke syndromes resulting from local thrombosis or artery-to-artery emboli. Other potential causes of stroke in SLE include local thrombosis caused by antiphospholipid antibodies, which can involve small or medium-sized arteries or veins and the venous sinuses. Emboli can occur as a result of Libman-Sacks endocarditis, a sterile endocardial inflammation that produces vegetations on the heart valves, which is seen in greater frequency in the presence of antiphospholipid antibodies. This type of endocarditis also causes a diffuse microembolization pattern that is clinically hard to distinguish from vasculitis or cerebritis.

Clinical Manifestations

A detailed review of the diffuse and varied presentations of SLE is beyond the scope of this chapter. In brief, patients with SLE may present with Raynaud syndrome, which occurred in 16% to 40% of patients in two large series. Approximately 50% of patients have renal involvement that typically develops in the first few years of illness.

Diagnosis

The diagnosis of SLE is made with a combination of clinical features and supportive laboratory studies. A typical presentation is a young woman reporting fatigue, fever, and pleuritic chest pain, who is found to have hypertension, a malar rash, a pleural friction rub, several tender and swollen joints, and mild peripheral edema.

If SLE is suspected, potentially diagnostically useful information can be obtained from tests such as a complete blood count and differential, measurement of serum creatinine and albumin levels, serologic test for syphilis, and urinalysis (24-hour collection for calculation of creatinine clearance and quantitation of proteinuria). Autoantibody testing is also indicated; those that are routinely assayed include antinuclear, antiphospholipid, anti–double-stranded DNA, and anti-Smith antibodies.

- The diagnosis of SLE is made with a combination of clinical features and supportive laboratory studies

Diagnostic imaging may be useful in certain situations but is not routinely obtained unless indicated by specific symptoms, clinical findings, or laboratory abnormalities. For example, plain radiographs of involved joints may be required for joint symptoms. Renal ultrasonography may be used to assess kidney size and cause of renal failure. Computed tomography and magnetic resonance imaging may be obtained to assess neurologic symptoms. Rarely, a biopsy of an involved organ is necessary. Other testing can include electrocardiography for assessment of chest pain, tests to evaluate for pulmonary embolism in patients with pleuritic pain and dyspnea, and diffusion capacity of carbon monoxide to assess suspected pulmonary hemorrhage and estimate the severity of interstitial pneumonitis.

The American College of Rheumatology has published diagnostic criteria for SLE. When tested against other rheumatic diseases, these criteria have a sensitivity and specificity of approximately 96%.

Treatment

The treatment of SLE is organ specific and varies among patients. Several medications are commonly used in the treatment of SLE, including nonsteroidal antiinflammatory drugs, antimalarials, corticosteroids, and immunosuppressant agents such as cyclophosphamide, methotrexate, azathioprine, and mycophenolate.

The major cause of death during the first few years of illness is active disease (renal or cardiovascular) or infection due to immunosuppression. Late deaths are caused by illness (end-stage renal disease) or treatment complications including infection or coronary artery disease. The relationship of SLE to malignancy is unclear; conflicting data have been published. Most studies, but not all, have shown an increased risk of lymphoma, predominantly non-Hodgkin type, whereas the incidence of non-lymphoid malignancies has increased in some series and decreased in others.

Questions

1. What is the most reliable method to determine disease activity in a patient with Takayasu arteritis?
   a. High-sensitivity C-reactive protein test
   b. Erythrocyte sedimentation rate
   c. Interleukin-6 measurement
   d. Physical examination and imaging studies

2. Which of the following may be associated with hepatitis B?
   a. Temporal arteritis
   b. Polyarteritis nodosa
   c. Cogan syndrome
   d. Kawasaki disease

3. Which of the following may resemble Löffler syndrome (pulmonary infiltrates with eosinophilia)?
   a. Takayasu arteritis
   b. Behçet syndrome
   c. Churg-Strauss syndrome
   d. Wegener granulomatosis

4. Which of the following is uniquely positive in systemic sclerosis?
   a. High-sensitivity C-reactive protein
   b. Anti–RNA polymerase I and III
   c. Interleukin-6
   d. ANCA

5. Which statement regarding SLE is false?
   a. Libman-Sacks endocarditis may be present.

b. Drug-induced SLE usually affects the kidneys and central nervous system.
c. Monozygotic twins are usually discordant for SLE.
d. Women are affected more often than men.

Suggested Readings

The European TAO Study Group. Oral iloprost in the treatment of thromboangiitis obliterans (Buerger's disease): a double-blind, randomised, placebo-controlled trial. Eur J Vasc Endovasc Surg. 1998;15:300-7. Erratum in: Eur J Vasc Endovasc Surg. 1998;16:456.

Fiessinger JN, Schafer M. Trial of iloprost versus aspirin treatment for critical limb ischaemia of thromboangiitis obliterans: the TAO Study. Lancet. 1990;335:555-7.

Guillevin L, Lhote F. Treatment of polyarteritis nodosa and microscopic polyangiitis. Arthritis Rheum. 1998;41:2100-5.

Haynes BF, Kaiser-Kupfer MI, Mason P, et al. Cogan syndrome: studies in thirteen patients, long-term follow-up, and a review of the literature. Medicine (Baltimore). 1980;59:426-41.

Hellmann DB. Immunopathogenesis, diagnosis, and treatment of giant cell arteritis, temporal arteritis, polymyalgia rheumatica, and Takayasu's arteritis. Curr Opin Rheumatol. 1993;5:25-32.

Hochberg MC. Updating the American College of Rheumatology revised criteria for the classification of systemic lupus erythematosus. Arthritis Rheum. 1997;40:1725.

Hoffman GS, Kerr GS, Leavitt RY, et al. Wegener granulomatosis: an analysis of 158 patients. Ann Intern Med. 1992;116:488-98.

Hunder GG. Giant cell arteritis in polymyalgia rheumatica. Am J Med. 1997;102:514-6.

Hunder GG, Bloch DA, Michel BA, et al. The American College of Rheumatology 1990 criteria for the classification of giant cell arteritis. Arthritis Rheum. 1990;33:1122-8.

Ishikawa K. Diagnostic approach and proposed criteria for the clinical diagnosis of Takayasu's arteriopathy. J Am Coll Cardiol. 1988;12:964-72.

Lanham JG, Elkon KB, Pusey CD, et al. Systemic vasculitis with asthma and eosinophilia: a clinical approach to the Churg-Strauss syndrome. Medicine (Baltimore). 1984;63:65-81.

Lightfoot RW Jr, Michel BA, Bloch DA, et al. The American College of Rheumatology 1990 criteria for the classification of polyarteritis nodosa. Arthritis Rheum. 1990;33:1088-93.

Newberger JW, Takahashi M, Beiser AS, et al. A single intravenous infusion of gamma globulin as compared with four infusions in the treatment of acute Kawasaki syndrome. N Engl J Med. 1991;324:1633-9.

Olin JW. Thromboangiitis obliterans (Buerger's disease). N Engl J Med. 2000;343:864-9.

Sakane T, Takeno M, Suzuki N, et al. Behçet's disease. N Engl J Med. 1999;341:1284-91.

3 Upper Extremity Arterial Disease: Raynaud Syndrome, Occlusive Arterial Diseases, and Thoracic Outlet Syndrome

Roger F. J. Shepherd, MBBCh

Introduction

Upper extremity arterial disease is a fascinating and often challenging area of vascular medicine. Impaired blood flow to the hands and fingers can be caused by obstruction of the large arteries, smaller digital arteries, or the microvasculature. Resulting digital ischemia can be acute or chronic and can be due to reversible vasospasm, fixed obstructive arterial disease, or both.

Many diverse disorders are associated with upper extremity arterial disease. In addition to atherosclerosis, the vascular clinician must be familiar with various unusual non-atherosclerotic conditions, including connective tissue diseases, vasculitis, thromboangiitis obliterans (TO), hematologic disorders, thoracic outlet syndrome, and occupation-related arterial disease, including the hypothenar hammer syndrome.

Raynaud Syndrome

Definition

Raynaud syndrome is characterized by episodic pallor or cyanosis of one or more fingers occurring in response to cold or emotional stress. Maurice Raynaud first described the digital color changes diagnostic of this syndrome in 1882. A typical vasospastic attack is characterized by the sudden onset of pallor in part or all of one or more digits. Cyanosis follows as static blood in the capillaries becomes desaturated. With relief of vasospasm and return of arterial inflow to the finger, digital rubor results from post-ischemic hyperemia, and the skin color gradually returns to normal. Today, these triphasic color changes are often considered to be the hallmark of Raynaud syndrome.

Many patients have only one or two color changes with episodic pallor or cyanosis of the digits. It is not necessary to have all three (tricolor) changes for a diagnosis of Raynaud syndrome. Vasospastic attacks most commonly involve the fingers but in up to one-third of patients can also affect toes. Less frequently, vasospasm involves the nose, ear, and nipple. Vasospasm can also affect the coronary and cerebral arteries. Patients with Prinzmetal angina are more likely to have Raynaud phenomenon and migraine headaches. In one study of 62 patients with variant angina, 15 had Raynaud phenomenon and 16 had migraine.

- Raynaud syndrome is characterized by episodic pallor or cyanosis of one or more fingers occurring in response to cold or emotional stress

Terminology

Since the days of Maurice Raynaud, all patients with vasospasm, by tradition, have been classified into two groups on the basis of the presence or absence of underlying occlusive arterial disease: Raynaud disease (a primary vasospastic disorder in which no underlying cause is identifiable—idiopathic or pure vasospasm) and Raynaud phenomenon (vasospasm is secondary to some other underlying condition or disease). Unfortunately, in clinical practice, use of these diagnostic terms ("Raynaud disease" or "Raynaud phenomenon") has not been intuitive. They are commonly misunderstood and often mistakenly interchanged. John Porter and others therefore advocated replacing the older terms "disease" and "phenomenon" with "Raynaud syndrome."

"Primary Raynaud syndrome" (idiopathic or pure vasospasm), by Porter's terminology, refers to a primary vasospastic disorder with no identifiable underlying cause; formerly known as "Raynaud disease." "Secondary Raynaud syndrome," by Porter's terminology, refers to vasospasm secondary to some other underlying condition or disease; formerly known as "Raynaud phenomenon." Usually, those with primary Raynaud syndrome (RS) have pure vasospasm and those with secondary RS have underlying occlusive arterial disease predisposing them to vasospastic attacks. This distinction has important clinical utility because it underscores the different pathologic mechanisms, treatment options, and prognoses of these two groups.

For patients with an underlying disease causing RS, both diagnoses should be used (e.g., "TO with secondary RS"). For patients with known occlusive arterial disease causing chronic digital ischemia (as opposed to episodic vasospasm), the diagnosis should not be labeled as "RS" but as the underlying disease, such as atherosclerosis. Many cases of severe, non-episodic, limb-threatening hand ischemia have been misdiagnosed as vasospastic RS. This can cause a delay in the appropriate management of critical non-reversible hand and digital ischemia.

- "Primary Raynaud syndrome" refers to a primary vasospastic disorder with no identifiable underlying cause
- "Secondary Raynaud syndrome" refers to vasospasm secondary to some other underlying condition or disease

Determinants of Blood Flow in the Fingers

Blood flow to the fingers serves two purposes: thermoregulatory and nutritional. Only a very small portion of digital blood flow (less than 10%) is needed to provide nutrients and oxygen to the tissues. Most of the blood flow in the fingers serves an important role in thermoregulation to control body temperature.

Blood vessels that are superficially located in the skin radiate excess heat to the environment, which reduces core body temperature. In response to cold, these arteries constrict to decrease blood flow and conserve body heat. Arteriovenous (AV) anastomoses (connecting the arterial and venous circulation) are present in the fingers and the palms of the hands. These anastomoses shunt blood to venous circulation before it reaches the distal small capillaries. In warm environments the fingers are able to dramatically increase blood flow through these AV fistulas. More than 50 years ago, Greenfield demonstrated that one hand can lose 800 calories of heat per minute, which causes a decrease in esophageal temperature of 0.6°C in 9 minutes.

These AV shunts are under the control of the sympathetic nervous system. In response to cold exposure or body cooling, increased sympathetic tone causes the digital AV shunts to close, and with less blood flow through the fingers, the core body temperature is maintained. Maximum vasoconstriction to cold exposure occurs at skin temperatures of 10°C to 20°C. At lower temperatures, cold-induced vasodilation causes a slight reopening of arteries to allow enough blood flow to the fingers to avoid freezing the fingertips. With continued cold exposure, finger blood flow fluctuates with a regular rhythmic cycle of 30 seconds to 2 minutes. These alternating periods of vasoconstriction and dilation are called "the hunting response."

- Hand blood flow has a substantial effect on body temperature

These changes in blood flow in the fingers due to environmental temperature are effected in part by the central nervous system with input from the cerebral cortex, hypothalamus, and medullary vasomotor centers. The hypothalamus changes body temperature by altering the sympathetic outflow to the digital vessels via the medulla, spinal cord, sympathetic ganglion, and local nerves. The sympathetic nerves innervate vascular smooth muscle in the digital arteries causing digital artery constriction.

During cooling of the finger, abrupt cessation of blood flow can occur due to vasoconstriction. Almost all secondary causes of RS produce some degree of fixed obstruction to blood flow, and cold-induced vasospasm occurs more readily. If a vessel is narrowed because of preexisting large or small vessel disease, a lower "critical closing pressure" results, and a relatively normal vasoconstrictor response to cold or other stimuli can cause temporary vessel closure.

Several systemic diseases may cause decreased digital systolic pressure as a result of "fixed" arterial obstruction or increased blood viscosity. For example, in scleroderma, a combination of intimal hyperplasia, thrombosis, and fibrosis results in arterial narrowing. Abnormal plasma proteins causing hyperviscosity result in reduced blood flow.

Primary Raynaud Syndrome

Incidence

Primary RS is a common disorder. In one large survey conducted in South Carolina, 4.6% of 1,752 randomly selected persons indicated they had experienced symptoms of white or blue color changes of the fingers. The prevalence is higher in cooler climates, especially in European countries including England, Denmark, and France, where incidences as high as 11% in men and 22% in women have been reported.

The age of onset in primary RS ranges from 11 to 45 years. A study of 474 patients with RS reported an average age of 31 years. Older patients can also have primary RS, but onset of symptoms at an older age should arouse suspicion of a secondary underlying cause. Although primary RS is said to predominantly affect young women, occurring more often than in men by a ratio of 4:1, more recent studies have found that men are affected almost as frequently as women with a ratio closer to 1.6:1.

Mechanism of Vasospasm in Primary Raynaud Syndrome

The exact cause of vasospastic attacks in primary RS remains unknown. No structural abnormality of the digital arteries has been demonstrated. Whether primary RS represents an exaggeration of normal thermoregulatory mechanisms or is due to a specific local or systemic abnormality has remained an area of controversy. Raynaud, in 1888, believed that the central nervous system was responsible and that vasospasm resulted from overactivity of the sympathetic nervous system. This seems plausible because the autonomic nervous system maintains arteriolar tone and blood pressure and because emotional stress can bring on vasospastic attacks.

Lewis, in 1929, believed that a local abnormality was present in the digital arteries of patients which caused an increased sensitivity of the blood vessel to cold. In a series of studies, he could produce ischemic attacks in a single finger by local cooling. Nerve blocks or surgical sympathectomy could not prevent these cold-induced attacks. Lewis also found that cooling the proximal finger, but keeping the distal finger warm, caused distal vasospasm. He therefore concluded that the vasospasm was caused by local factors and not entirely sympathetically mediated.

We now recognize that several different factors, acting by local, humoral, and nervous system mechanisms, affect the normal regulation of blood flow to the fingers. Derangement of any of these factors may be responsible for the vasospastic attacks in primary RS. Possible abnormalities in primary RS include alterations in neurotransmitters released from sympathetic nerves; increased activation of β_2-adrenoceptors on the nerve endings; endothelial dysfunction with a shift in the balance from endothelium-derived relaxing to contracting factors; increased platelet serotonin levels or alteration in neurohumoral transmitters released from local nerves; lower systemic blood pressure; or arterial obstruction and changes in blood viscosity.

Secondary Causes of Raynaud Syndrome and Occlusive Arterial Disease

Many disorders are associated with RS (Table 3.1). The two most common secondary causes are connective tissue diseases (CTDs, particularly scleroderma) and atherosclerosis. Less common but important diseases include vasculitis, TO, thromboembolism, and atheroembolism. Diseases unique to the upper extremity include dynamic arterial compression resulting from thoracic outlet syndrome (TOS). Occupational trauma to the hand can cause the hypothenar hammer syndrome or vibration white finger. Prescription drug–induced vasospasm is common. Systemic disorders leading to increased viscosity can cause vasospasm and include myeloma, cryoglobulinemia, and hepatitis antigenemia. Depending on the thoroughness of clinical evaluation and referral bias, more than half of patients referred for evaluation of RS are ultimately found to have an underlying cause.

Table 3.1 Conditions Associated With Secondary Raynaud Syndrome

Disease type	Examples
Connective tissue disease	Scleroderma, CREST syndrome
	Systemic lupus erythematosus
	Rheumatoid arthritis
	Mixed connective tissue disease
	Dermatomyositis
	Small/medium vessel vasculitis
Atherosclerosis and occlusive arterial disease	Atherosclerosis obliterans
	Atheroembolism
	Diabetic distal arterial disease
	Thromboangiitis obliterans (Buerger disease)
Thromboembolism	Cardiac embolism
	Arterial embolism
	Paradoxic embolism
Large vessel vasculitis	Takayasu arteritis
	Extracranial temporal arteritis
Dynamic entrapment	Thoracic outlet syndrome
Occupational arterial trauma	Hypothenar hammer syndrome
	Vibration-induced Raynaud syndrome
Drug-induced vasospasm	β-Blockers
	Vasopressors, epinephrine
	Ergot
	Cocaine
	Amphetamines
	Vinblastine/bleomycin
Infections	Parvovirus
	Sepsis/disseminated intravascular coagulation
	Hepatitis B and C antigenemia
Malignancy	Multiple myeloma
	Leukemia
	Adenocarcinoma
	Astrocytoma
Hematologic	Polycythemia vera
	Thrombocytosis
	Cold agglutinins
	Cryoglobulinemia

Approximately 30% to 60% of patients presenting for evaluation of RS have primary disease. In a large series of 615 patients at the Oregon Health & Science University, more than half had pure vasospastic disease. In those with secondary RS, 27% were found to have a CTD. Scleroderma was the most common CTD, followed by undifferentiated and mixed CTD. Other conditions included atherosclerosis, TO, cancer, and vibration white finger.

- Approximately 30%-60% of patients presenting for evaluation of RS have primary disease

Connective Tissue Diseases

Systemic and Limited Scleroderma

The word "scleroderma" is derived from the words "*skleros*" (meaning "hard") and "*derma*" (meaning "skin"). Scleroderma is characterized by progressive fibrosis of the skin and internal organs. The most characteristic feature of scleroderma is thickening of the skin, especially involving the fingers and hands. In advanced scleroderma, joint contraction leads to a clawlike hand deformity. Ulcers can form at the fingertips and over joints. These ulcers may be refractory to therapy and are slow to heal, which causes considerable ischemic digital pain.

The pathogenesis of arterial disease in scleroderma is not well understood, but it is most likely initiated by proliferation of smooth muscle cells in blood vessel intima, which causes luminal narrowing. Activated platelets release platelet-derived growth factors and thromboxane A_2, which can induce vasoconstriction and stimulate growth of endothelial cells and fibroblasts. Fibrin is deposited within and around vessels, causing vessel obstruction. Small arteries, arterioles, and capillaries are affected by these proliferative structural changes in the vessel wall, which results in tissue ischemia. Digital involvement is disabling, as in limited scleroderma (see below), but death results from cardiac and pulmonary complications in those with systemic scleroderma.

CREST syndrome (or limited scleroderma) takes its name from the 5 main associated symptoms: Calcinosis, RS, Esophageal dysmotility, Sclerodactyly, and Telangiectasis. Calcinosis refers to subcutaneous calcification found in the fingers, forearms, and pressure points. RS occurs in more than 90% of patients with scleroderma and can be the initial presenting symptom in one-third of patients. Esophageal dysmotility leads to dysphagia, regurgitation, and aspiration. Sclerodactyly can present as puffiness of the fingers. Telangiectasis on the fingers and hands is a pathognomonic finding in scleroderma.

Serologic studies may help to confirm the diagnosis of scleroderma and are also useful in screening for occult underlying CTD. Antinuclear antibodies (ANA) are present in 95% of patients with scleroderma but are not specific for scleroderma and can be present in several other CTDs. A positive ANA result raises suspicion for a CTD but on its own does not make the diagnosis. To be clinically significant, a positive ANA should have a titer greater than 1:160 or 1:320. By immunofluorescence, ANA should be >3.0 units (>6.0 units is strongly positive). Autoantibodies specific for scleroderma include those against topoisomerase 1, centromere, Scl-70, RNA polymerase 1, and U3 ribonucleoprotein. The anticentromere antibody is associated with CREST syndrome. As opposed to that in vasculitis, the erythrocyte sedimentation rate is usually normal in systemic scleroderma.

- ANAs are present in 95% of patients with scleroderma but are not specific for scleroderma and can be present in several other CTDs

Mixed and Undifferentiated CTD

Mixed CTD is an overlap syndrome with features of at least two CTDs, usually scleroderma and systemic lupus erythematosus (SLE). Undifferentiated CTD can have a mixture of clinical findings including polyarthritis, RS, and lupus-type features.

- RS is a frequent manifestation of SLE, occurring in up to 80% of patients

Systemic Lupus Erythematosus

SLE is a multisystem disease, most frequently occurring in young females. It can affect many organ systems with features of arthralgias, rash, pericarditis, pleuritis, and glomerulonephritis, usually with a positive ANA. RS occurs in up to 80% of patients with SLE.

Small Vessel Vasculitis

Rheumatoid arthritis and Sjögren syndrome can be associated with a small vessel vasculitis. Other small vessel vasculitides include Wegener granulomatosis, microscopic polyarteritis nodosum, and cutaneous livedo vasculitis. Malignancy can be associated with vasculitis.

Risk of Subsequent CTD Development With Raynaud Syndrome

The onset of RS can precede the clinical onset of a CTD by up to several years. Patients with RS should be told that the risk of future development of a CTD is low but that follow-up evaluation is suggested. Less than 5% of patients (4 of 87 in one study) with primary RS subsequently had CTD development over a 5-year period. Some patients are at higher risk of a CTD developing—especially if they have subtle abnormalities by history, examination, or blood tests, such as a low-positive ANA or abnormal nailfold microscopy. It has been suggested that all patients be followed up for more than 2 years before confirming a diagnosis of primary RS (vs secondary RS).

Atherosclerosis

Atherosclerosis in patients without diabetes mellitus

generally affects the larger, more proximal arteries and is unusual distal to the subclavian level. If proximal atherosclerosis causes digital ischemia, it is more often due to atheroembolism (from an ulcerated plaque in the innominate or subclavian artery) than due to decreased distal perfusion pressure. As in the lower extremities, inflow arterial disease in the upper extremity can cause claudication but is less likely to cause critical ischemia.

RS can be a presenting symptom of TO. TO is a non-atherosclerotic inflammatory disorder involving distal, small, and medium-sized arteries in the fingers and toes, especially affecting male smokers younger than 40 years of age (Fig. 3.1). It can present with features of chronic ischemia with development of painful fingertip necrosis and ulcerations.

- TO is a non-atherosclerotic inflammatory disorder involving distal, small, and medium-sized arteries in the fingers and toes, especially affecting male smokers younger than 40 years

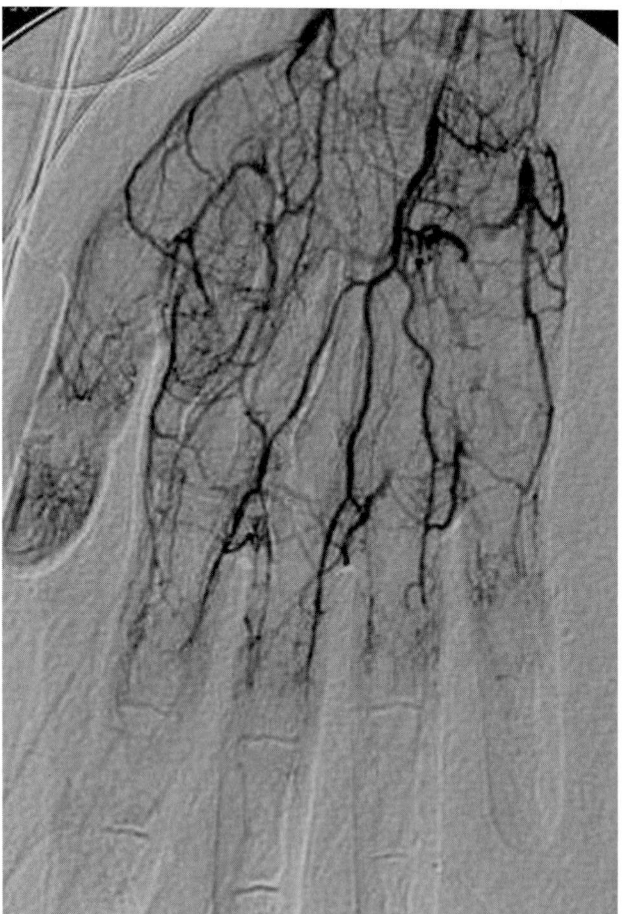

Fig. 3.1 Contrast angiogram in a patient with thromboangiitis obliterans. Thromboangiitis obliterans begins distally, involving small arteries of the toes and fingers in smokers generally younger than 40 years. Angiography may show corkscrew collaterals, but often findings are non-specific, as in this case demonstrating severe occlusive disease of all digital arteries.

Thromboembolism

Most thromboemboli (>70%) traveling to the upper extremities are of cardiac origin. The left atrium is the most common origin of cardiac embolism, usually as a result of atrial fibrillation and stasis of blood in the left atrial appendage. Cardiac embolism can also arise from the left ventricle after a myocardial infarction or less frequently from valvular vegetation occurring in bacterial endocarditis. Most cardiac emboli are relatively large and tend to lodge at bifurcation points in the forearm, in the radial and ulnar arteries. Thromboembolic arterial occlusion should always be considered in a patient with paroxysmal atrial fibrillation or history of cardiac disease.

- Most thromboemboli (>70%) traveling to the upper extremities are of cardiac origin

Hypothenar Hammer Syndrome

The ulnar artery has a superficial course in the palm as it passes laterally to the hook of the hamate bone, which makes it especially vulnerable to localized trauma. Repetitive trauma to the hypothenar eminence of the hand (from using the palm of the hand as a hammer) results in damage to the underlying ulnar artery (Fig. 3.2). Endothelial injury results in intraluminal thrombosis, aneurysm formation, and embolization to one or many fingers. The diagnosis is suggested by a history of repetitive occupational hand trauma in a patient with digital ischemia and a positive Allen test.

The hypothenar hammer syndrome occurs in mechanics, farmers, plumbers, and especially carpenters, who use handheld tools such as wrenches and hammers that exert pressure over the hypothenar eminence of the hand. Palmar and digital occlusive diseases have also been reported in players of professional and recreational sports including golf, tennis, baseball, handball, and volleyball.

Vibration-Induced Raynaud Syndrome

Prolonged use of vibratory tools such as pneumatic hammers or chain saws can cause small-vessel damage to distal vessels. Sympathetic overactivity and endothelial damage are believed to contribute to vibration-induced vasospasm. Chronic vibration may cause structural damage to the artery wall with hypertrophy of the intima and media. The formation of microthrombi can lead to fixed digital ischemia and fingertip necrosis.

Terms that have been used to describe RS caused by chronic vibration include hand-arm vibration syndrome

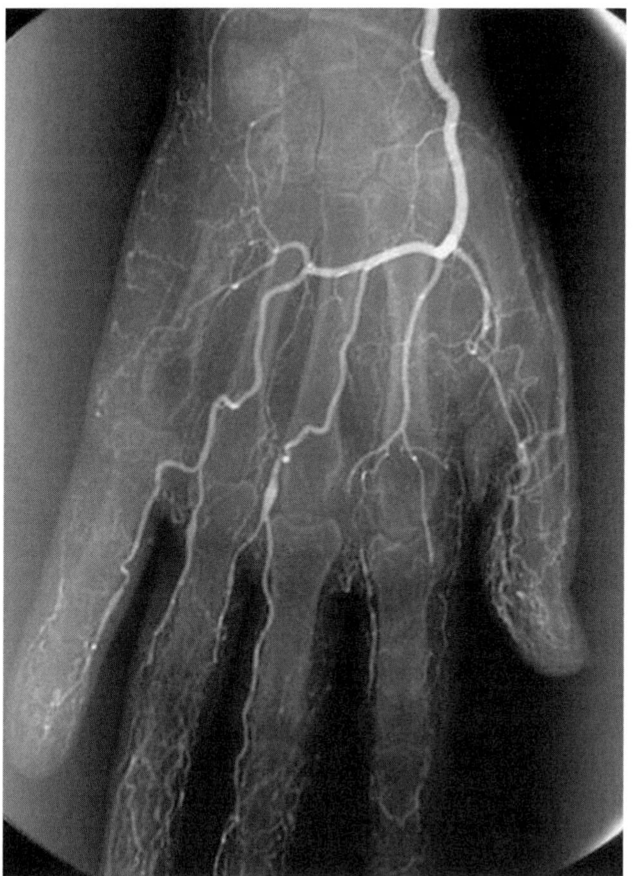

Fig. 3.2 Contrast angiogram demonstrating ulnar artery occlusion with extensive disease of palmar and digital arteries. Diagnostic considerations should include the hypothenar hammer syndrome, thromboangiitis obliterans, connective tissue diseases, and small vessel vasculitis.

and vibration white finger. Vibration-induced RS occurs in many different occupations in which workers use chain saws, grinders, sanders, riveters, jack hammers, and pneumatic hammers. A report from Sweden found the prevalence of vibration white finger in car mechanics to be 25% among those who had worked for 20 years. Whether vibration-induced RS is reversible in earlier stages is unknown. Early symptoms include tingling and numbness from peripheral nerve damage. Preventive measures, which may minimize damage, include wearing gloves, providing a cushioned surface on handles, and avoiding prolonged exposure.

Thoracic Outlet Syndrome

TOS is caused by dynamic compression of neurovascular structures, including the subclavian artery, subclavian vein, and brachial plexus, as they traverse through the thoracic outlet (details regarding TOS discussed below). TOS can be associated with RS, subclavian stenosis, aneurysm formation, thrombosis, and arterial embolization to the hand and fingers. Arterial complications of TOS are often associated with a cervical rib, and severe consequences of arterial disease can occur in healthy patients with no history of atherosclerosis.

Drug-Induced Raynaud Syndrome and Occlusive Diseases

β-Blocking Drugs

β-Blocking drugs are well-established medications for arterial hypertension and cardiac disease. β-Blockers, however, are a common cause of cool fingers and arterial vasospasm due to inhibition of β_2-mediated arterial vasodilation. The incidence of RS among patients with hypertension treated with β-blockers was 40% in a Scandinavian questionnaire-based study. Approximately 5% of patients treated with β-blocking medications for hypertension require withdrawal of the medication or dose reduction because of RS. Vasospasm occurs with selective and non-selective β-blockers. Drugs with combined α- and β-adrenoceptor–blocking activity, such as labetalol, would be expected to cause less symptomatic vasospasm. Despite these concerns, most patients, including many with RS, tolerate β-blockers, and several studies have failed to show any adverse effects of β-blockers on digital blood flow.

- Vasospasm occurs with selective and non-selective β-blockers

Chemotherapy Agents

Vinblastine and bleomycin are used for the treatment of testicular cancer and lymphoma and can induce RS in 2.6% of patients on this therapy. Development of ischemic ulceration has been reported in cases of lung cancer treated with carboplatin and gemcitabine (but other factors may be present). α-Interferon is used in the treatment of leukemia and melanoma. Rare cases of RS with digital ulceration have been reported, occurring within several months to 3 years of therapy.

Other Drugs and Toxins

Ergot preparations, used for migraine, are well known to cause severe upper and lower extremity vasospasm and ischemia with absent pulse. Amphetamine abuse can also cause arterial vasoconstriction. Cocaine abuse has been reported to cause ischemic finger necrosis. The mechanism of vascular damage from cocaine is multifactorial but likely involves initial vasospasm from elevated norepinephrine levels and subsequent arterial thrombosis. Accidental intra-arterial injection of drugs meant for intravenous use can cause severe vasospasm and digital ischemia with gangrene and digital loss.

Infections

Purpura fulminans can cause severe digital ischemia, which often requires amputation. Parvovirus infection has also been associated with severe digital ischemia and secondary RS.

Endocrine Diseases

Hypothyroidism, Graves disease, Addison disease, and Cushing disease are all occasional but rare causes of vasospasm.

Increased Blood Viscosity

Any abnormality that increases blood viscosity results in decreased blood flow. Disorders that affect blood viscosity include cryoglobulinemia, paraproteinemia in myeloma, and polycythemia. Cold-induced precipitation of proteins increases the viscosity of blood. Cryoglobulins occur with malignancies such as lymphomas and some viral infections and can cause skin necrosis and gangrene of fingers, toes, and ears. Hepatitis C, in particular, is associated with secondary cryoglobulinemia. The treatment of cryoglobulinemia is plasmapheresis to remove the cryoglobulin, corticosteroids, and chemotherapy to treat the underlying malignancy.

Malignancy

Digital ischemia is an uncommon but well-recognized paraneoplastic manifestation of malignancy. Possible mechanisms of arterial disease caused by malignancy may include coagulopathy, cryoglobulinemia, or small vessel vasculitis. The most common malignancies associated with RS are: adenocarcinoma of the lung, stomach, colon, pancreas, ovary, testicle, and kidney; hematologic malignancies including myeloma, leukemias, lymphomas, and melanoma; and astrocytoma.

RS associated with malignancy has a sudden onset at an older age, with severe symptoms and asymmetric digital involvement. Many patients (80%) have disease progression to digital infarcts and gangrene. Treatment of the cancer can result in remission of the RS symptoms and digital ischemia.

Physical Examination in Raynaud Syndrome

The diagnosis of RS is often based on the patient's description of a typical vasospastic attack related to cold exposure and involving one or more fingers. A focused physical examination and laboratory testing aid in the determination of primary or secondary disease. Vascular examination for upper extremity arterial disease should start with the heart. Cardiac auscultation may detect an increased P2 pulmonary valve closure sound, which suggests pulmonary hypertension, as can occur in scleroderma. Pulse and heart rhythm examination are important for detection of atrial fibrillation. Valvular heart disease such as mitral stenosis may be apparent on cardiac auscultation.

Palpation of upper extremity pulses should include subclavian, brachial, radial, ulnar, palmar, and digital arteries. Palpation above the clavicle can reveal a cervical rib or an aneurysm of the subclavian artery. A palpable thrill indicates high-grade arterial stenosis. Auscultation over large arteries for a bruit, in particular over the sternoclavicular joint and above the clavicle, can identify arch or proximal arterial disease.

Pulse examination in the hand should include palpation over the hypothenar eminence to identify the ulnar artery and palpation in the palm to identify the superficial palmar arch. A digital artery pulse can be appreciated in both the medial and lateral aspects of each finger. A palpable ulnar pulse at the wrist level only indicates that the ulnar artery is patent at the wrist level. The most common site of occlusion of the ulnar artery is just distal to the wrist, at the hypothenar eminence where the artery crosses over the hook of the hamate bone. The Allen test should be performed in every patient with RS or digital ischemia to detect the presence of ulnar artery occlusion, as occurs in hypothenar hammer syndrome. A positive Allen test identifies ulnar blockage in the hand. A positive reverse Allen test can signify occlusion of the radial artery.

Close inspection of the skin may show telangiectasis of the fingers or hands, or thickening of the skin, which may be suggestive of sclerodactyly, digital ulcerations, pits, mottling, cyanosis, nailfold infarcts, and tight shiny skin. Splinter hemorrhages under the nails are normal findings in manual workers but could also indicate the need to seek a more proximal source of atheroemboli. The main clinical features of primary RS are vasospastic attacks precipitated by exposure to cold or emotional stimuli, symmetrical or bilateral involvement of the extremities, normal vascular examination, symptoms present for a minimum of 2 years, and absence of any other underlying disease.

- A positive Allen test identifies ulnar blockage in the hand

Laboratory Evaluation of Raynaud Syndrome

Non-invasive vascular laboratory testing complements

the history and physical examination. Non-invasive tests can provide objectivity to the clinical evaluation and assist in decision making for medical and surgical treatment. It can also help distinguish between primary and secondary vasospasm by detecting the presence of underlying occlusive disease. Even though attacks of RS are classically brought on by cold exposure, reproducing such attacks in the vascular laboratory is surprisingly difficult, even with digital cooling. The quantitative evaluation of vasospasm has also been difficult, and symptoms do not always correlate with finger skin blood flow measurements. The diagnosis of RS is a clinical diagnosis and should not be made on the basis of a laboratory test. Vascular laboratory studies can help distinguish between primary and secondary disease but should not take the place of a complete history and physical examination.

Segmental Blood Pressure Measurements

Pneumatic cuffs are wrapped around the upper arm, forearm, and wrist, and systolic blood pressure measurements are obtained at each level. Pressures are compared with those at adjacent levels; a pressure differential exceeding 10 to 15 mm Hg may indicate proximal occlusive arterial disease. Wrist-to-brachial artery pressure ratio could be calculated but rarely is; the normal values range widely because of variation in cuff size and arm diameter.

Finger Systolic Blood Pressures

Finger systolic blood pressure measurement is possible using small digital cuffs applied to the proximal finger. Although a decreased systolic pressure may indicate arterial occlusive disease in that finger, the range of normal digital pressure is quite variable and is influenced by temperature. The normal finger brachial index ranges from 0.8 to 1.27. The fingers are especially temperature sensitive, however, and cool fingers can give falsely low indices.

When fingers are very cold, digital indices can be unobtainable because of intense vasoconstriction. Conversely, when the fingers are warm, finger systolic blood pressure may be lower than arm pressure by 10 mm Hg. Non-compressible vessels (similar to the lower extremity) can result in supranormal digital pressures. A difference of more than 15 mm Hg between fingers or an absolute finger systolic blood pressure of less than 70 mm Hg may indicate occlusive disease. Because the digits have dual arteries, early disease with occlusion of one of the digital arteries cannot be detected by finger pressure measurement if the contralateral artery is normal.

The effect of temperature on digital blood pressure can be studied by applying a second cuff on the heated or cooled finger. Nielsen devised a double-inlet plastic cuff for local digital cooling. He found a mild progressive decrease in finger systolic pressure with local cooling in normal young women (up to a 15% decrease in digital systolic pressure at 10°C). During further cooling, 60% of women with primary RS showed digital artery occlusion.

Fingertip Thermography

Skin surface temperature can be used as an indirect index of capillary blood flow in the skin. At temperatures less than 30°C, blood flow is proportional to skin surface temperature. At temperatures higher than 30°C, larger increases in flow may not be appreciated. Patients with vasospasm have increased vascular tone leading to decreased blood flow and decreased surface skin temperature. Measurement of skin temperature can be combined with cold immersion.

Cold Recovery Time

This time-honored test is used to measure the vasoconstrictor and vasodilator response of the fingers to cold exposure. It is based on the principle that patients with RS have greater vasoconstriction in response to cooling of the fingers than do normal subjects. After cold exposure, patients with RS require more time for blood flow to increase, and consequently the fingers take longer to warm back to baseline temperature.

The change in blood flow induced by temperature change can be indirectly assessed by measuring fingertip skin temperatures or by recording laser Doppler flux of the fingertips. Many variations of the cold immersion test exist, with various immersion times and temperatures. A standard protocol is to record baseline digital temperatures at the end of the finger pulp using a temperature probe. The hands are then immersed in 4°C water for 20 seconds. The digital skin temperature is recorded for each finger as the hands and fingers gradually warm up to ambient room temperature. The length of time it takes for the hands to re-warm to baseline is noted by recording finger temperatures or laser Doppler flux at 5-minute intervals until recovery of pre-immersion temperatures. A delay in re-warming suggests a vasospasm tendency. Those with RS typically require more than 10 minutes, and sometimes 30 minutes or longer, for resting finger temperatures to recover, compared with less than 10 minutes for controls. If resting baseline digital temperatures are less than 30°C, the fingers never re-warm in less than 10 minutes after ice water immersion, and no further information is gained from this cold challenge test in these patients. The test cannot distinguish between primary and secondary RS, and some have questioned its ability to diagnose RS at all because of a large overlap with controls.

Laser Doppler Flux

This non-invasive test measures microvascular skin perfusion in the fingers. A laser Doppler probe transmits a low-powered helium-neon light, which is scattered by both static and moving tissue; most of the moving structures are erythrocytes. Laser light hitting moving erythrocytes undergoes a frequency shift according to the Doppler effect. Baseline measurements are highly variable and are affected by emotion, sympathetic tone (which may be increased in an anxious patient), and environmental temperature.

Cold stress testing can be combined with laser Doppler by cooling the fingers with a laser Doppler probe. With cold-induced digital vasoconstriction, decreased skin blood flow and reduced laser Doppler flux occurs. With slow re-warming, laser Doppler flux increases.

Laser Doppler With Thermal Challenge

Laser Doppler can be used to measure relative change in digital skin blood flow with ambient warming of the hand and fingers. Measurement of digital laser Doppler flow at rest and after gentle warming of the hands in a hot-air box provides an excellent indication of primary vasospasm. This test can also assist in distinguishing between obstructive and vasospastic disease. Baseline laser Doppler values are obtained from each digit. The hands are placed in a warming box (at 45°C) for up to 25 minutes or until a finger temperature of 37.0°C is reached. Laser Doppler flows are again determined in each digit.

In general, patients with a history of vasospasm who present with cold fingers have low resting laser Doppler blood flow because of vasoconstricted vessels. After ambient warming, patients with primary RS can have a marked increase in laser Doppler flow in these digits. Failure of Doppler flow to increase after warming of the hands indicates significant arterial occlusive disease. The response of laser Doppler flow to warming correlates well with clinical and angiographic findings.

Scanning laser Doppler has several potential advantages over single-site laser Doppler. Because the Doppler probe does not come in contact with the patient, scanning laser Doppler can be used to assess blood flow at the base of ulcers or other wounds. However, interpretation of results varies considerably, and the applicability of this method appears lower than that of the single-digit Doppler probes.

Imaging Studies

Duplex ultrasonography can image the palmar arch and digital arteries for patency. Doppler ultrasonography also can help to determine completeness of the superficial palmar arch. If no change in Doppler flow occurs over the superficial arch during occlusion of the radial or ulnar artery, the arch is likely to be complete.

Magnetic resonance angiographic imaging of upper extremity arteries is useful for larger arteries, including the aortic arch, arm, and some arteries in the hand. Magnetic resonance angiography can accurately diagnose ulnar artery occlusion in hypothenar hammer syndrome. Contrast angiography, however, remains the gold standard, with better resolution for arterial imaging.

Contrast angiography is the best imaging modality if a detailed examination is necessary to determine the cause of digital ischemia, such as microembolism from an ulcerated plaque, thrombus in an ulnar artery, the corkscrew collaterals of TO, or the tapered arterial narrowing of vasculitis.

Nailfold Capillary Microscopy

Capillaries in the nailfold can be visualized by applying a drop of immersion oil over the cuticle of the finger to make it translucent and imaging with a low-powered microscope (×10-×20) or an ophthalmoscope at 40 diopters. Structural changes in capillary morphology can be seen. Normal capillaries appear as regularly spaced hairpin loops with a venous and arterial limb. The arterial limb has a diameter of 7 to 12 μm. The venous limb has a larger diameter with slower capillary flow. Abnormal capillaries as seen in scleroderma and mixed CTD are enlarged, tortuous, and deformed, with "loop dropout" and avascular areas.

Treatment of Raynaud Syndrome

Management principles may be classified into three groups: non-pharmacologic behavioral therapies, pharmacologic treatment, and interventional-surgical procedures. Potential therapies could specifically target one of the many underlying abnormalities responsible for RS, including the endothelium, autonomic nervous system, or specific neurohumoral and hematologic factors. The approach to therapy for RS should be individualized, depending on the severity of symptoms, frequency of vasospastic attacks, presence of underlying disease, and risk of development of ischemic ulceration, gangrene, or digital loss. For most patients with primary RS, there is no cure. Preventive measures, with education, reassurance, and avoidance of cold exposure, constitute the basis of therapy for most patients.

Behavioral Therapy

In primary RS, many persons have only mild symptoms

that do not require the use of daily vasodilatory medications. RS in these patients is best managed with behavioral modification stressing the concepts of heat conservation and avoiding factors that cause arterial vasoconstriction.

The patient should be educated about the nature and prognosis of primary RS, in particular emphasizing that the underlying arterial circulation is normal and that episodes of pallor and cyanosis are an exaggeration of the normal response of the finger arteries to cold exposure and emotional stress. Patients with primary disease should be reassured that the disorder is benign with little risk of progression, finger ulcers, or digital loss.

Measures to maintain warmth and avoid cold include the use of mittens rather than gloves. The patient should dress appropriately, with long-sleeved garments to avoid exposing extremities to the cold. Chemical hand and feet warmers are inexpensive, disposable, and readily obtained at many sporting goods stores. The concept of "total body warmth" should be emphasized. If the patient feels chilly, the natural response of the body is to constrict flow to the extremities to conserve body heat. Several simple recommendations can be made: 1) avoid or minimize situations likely to cause vasospasm, such as putting the hands in cold water; 2) wear gloves when handling frozen food or taking cold food out of the refrigerator; 3) warm up the car before trips to avoid vasospasm from touching a cold steering wheel; and 4) set the thermostat in the room to a temperature in excess of 70°F.

Patients have more frequent attacks of vasospasm in the winter than in the summer, and some might elect to move to a warmer climate. Medications with potent vasoconstrictor properties include β-blockers and ergotamine preparations used in the treatment of migraine; ergotamines can sometimes cause ergotism with severe and intense vasospasm. Avoidance of these medications, if possible, may decrease the occurrence of vasospasm. Until recently, weight-loss pills contained stimulants including ephedrine, which can cause RS. Abuse of drugs such as cocaine and amphetamines can cause severe arterial constriction that might not be reversible, with permanent arterial damage.

Pharmacologic Therapy

Patients with severe symptoms whose activities of daily living are affected by RS and who have not responded to simple conservative measures might require pharmacologic therapy (Table 3.2). However, it is important to note that medications decrease the intensity and frequency of vasospastic episodes but do not cure the underlying cause of vasospasm. Vasodilator medications are unnecessary for most patients with only mild or moderate symptoms, and behavioral therapy may be more effective for these patients. Only 50% to 75% of people respond to any one medication.

All vasodilators are more effective in patients with primary RS; those with secondary RS have fixed obstructive arterial disease, and vasodilators are less effective or at times ineffective. Potential adverse effects of any medications should be balanced against expected benefit.

Choosing the best medication has been difficult because of the lack of large prospective, randomized, double-blind studies comparing the efficacy of different medications in RS. Most clinical trials rely on patient self-assessment of frequency and severity of RS episodes. Attacks of vasospasm are notoriously difficult to reproduce in the vascular

Table 3.2 Drug Therapy for Raynaud Syndrome

Drug	Dosage	Adverse effects/disadvantages
Calcium-channel blockers		
Nifedipine	30, 60, 90 mg	Hypotension
Amlodipine	2.5-10 mg	Headache
Felodipine	2.5-10 mg	Edema
Isradipine	5, 10 mg	Flushing
Nisoldipine	10, 20, 30, 40 mg	...
α-Blockers		
Tetrazosin	1, 2, 5, 10 mg	Hypotension
Doxazosin	1, 2, 4, 8 mg	Orthostatic syncope
Antiplatelet agents		
Aspirin	81, 325 mg	Bleeding
Clopidogrel	75 mg	...
Endothelin receptor antagonists		Approved only for pulmonary hypertension in scleroderma
Bosentan	62.5, 125 mg	Liver hepatotoxicity, birth defects, expensive
Prostaglandins		IV only, given by continual infusion
Epoprostenol	2 ng·kg^{-1}·min^{-1} IV	Headache, nausea, flushing
Topical nitrates		
Nitroglycerin ointment	Ointment	"Steal phenomenon"

IV, intravenous.

laboratory setting, and laboratory confirmation of clinical response to a medication is often difficult. No currently available drugs are approved by the US Food and Drug Administration for the treatment of RS.

Calcium-Channel Blockers

Calcium-channel blockers inhibit the influx of extracellular calcium ions into smooth muscle cells by blocking specific ion channels in the cell membrane. The smooth muscle contractile process in the artery wall is dependent on extracellular calcium, and a decrease in calcium influx causes vascular smooth muscle relaxation and arterial dilation.

Of the three main classes of calcium-channel blockers, the dihydropyridines (such as nifedipine) are the most potent for relaxing vascular smooth muscle and are consequently better peripheral vasodilators than benzothiazines (such as diltiazem) or phenylalkylamines (such as verapamil). Dihydropyridines, however, are also more likely than other calcium-channel blockers to cause the adverse effects of flushing and peripheral edema, which require withdrawal of the medication. This section will focus only on the dihydropyridines.

Calcium-channel blockers are the most commonly prescribed medications for vasospasm associated with RS. Nifedipine is considered by many to be the drug of first choice if drug treatment of symptoms is required. Multiple studies have documented the effectiveness of dihydropyridine calcium-channel blockers in the treatment of RS. The more than 10 drugs in this class share similar properties. Nifedipine continues to be the gold standard, but most of the newer dihydropyridines, including amlodipine, nicardipine, felodipine, isradipine, and nisoldipine, are likely to be equally efficacious.

Short-acting calcium-channel blockers are no longer recommended because of adverse effects associated with abrupt decreases in blood pressure and an increased risk of hypotensive stroke. Only long-acting or sustained-release preparations of calcium-channel blockers are currently approved for disorders such as arterial hypertension, and the same recommendations apply to the treatment of RS. The most common adverse effects include peripheral edema in up to 25%, headache in up to 20%, facial flushing, and sinus tachycardia. The incidence of adverse effects is dose dependent and increases at larger doses of 60 or 90 mg daily.

Amlodipine is similar to nifedipine but has the theoretical advantage of fewer adverse effects because of its long half-life of more than 24 hours. Studies have shown a decrease in the number of vasospastic episodes with amlodipine compared with placebo.

Nicardipine has been shown to be effective in the treatment of vasospasm and can be administered orally or intravenously. Only a few studies have documented improvement on the basis of a laboratory test. In a randomized, double-blind, crossover, placebo-controlled trial, nicardipine (20 mg twice daily) was better than placebo; the number and severity of RS episodes decreased, and hand disability scores improved. After nicardipine, the time to peak flow after post-ischemic reactive hyperemia was significantly reduced.

Other studies have found no laboratory benefit for oral nicardipine in patients with either primary or secondary RS. Intravenous nicardipine has been shown to raise resting skin temperature in those with primary RS and to improve recovery after cold-induced vasospasm, but these effects are not seen in patients with secondary RS. Felodipine, nisoldipine, and isradipine also have been studied in RS with documented benefit.

Alpha-1 Adrenergic Receptor Blockers

There are two major types of α_1-adrenergic receptor blocking agents (α-blockers). The non-selective α-blockers include phenoxybenzamine and phentolamine, which today are rarely used because of the high incidence of adverse effects including orthostatic hypotension and reflex tachycardia. The selective α-blockers include prazosin and the longer-acting agents terazosin and doxazosin. Prazosin is a short-acting selective α_1 adrenergic antagonist that can decrease the number of attacks in both primary and secondary RS. In double-blind, placebo-controlled, crossover studies, prazosin was reported to be superior to placebo in the treatment of RS. Adverse effects can include postural hypotension (first-dose phenomenon), which usually resolves within several days as tolerance develops. Starting with a lower dose (1 mg) and administering the first dose at bedtime can minimize this effect. The preferred long-acting α-blockers allow once-daily dosing.

Nitrates

Nitrate medications have been used in the treatment of RS as topical, oral, or intravenous preparations. Nitroglycerin is a potent arterial and venous direct-acting vasodilator. A vasodilator medication, such as nitroglycerin ointment 2%, that can be applied to the affected ischemic finger theoretically seems like a reasonable therapeutic option. Although widely used, topical nitroglycerin is rarely effective for distal finger ischemia. Critical digital ischemia almost always denotes severe fixed occlusive disease, which does not respond to vasodilators, and paradoxic worsening of ischemia can occur. Topical nitroglycerin occasionally causes a steal phenomenon by dilating proximal arteries at the expense of distal finger blood flow. Poor dose response characteristics and the occurrence of nitrate-induced headaches generally limit use of oral nitrates. Intravenous nitroglycerin produces systemic vasodilation, as opposed to selectively increasing digital perfusion. Headache, flushing, and hypotension are often limiting adverse effects of parenteral nitroglycerin. In general, nitrates are not considered a first-line therapy for RS.

ACE Inhibitors

Angiotensin-converting enzyme (ACE) inhibitors and angiotensin-2 receptor blockers can be of benefit in both primary and secondary RS. A recent study indicated that losartan 50 mg daily was more effective than nifedipine 40 mg daily in decreasing the frequency of vasospastic episodes in patients with primary RS and those with RS due to systemic sclerosis. ACE inhibitors or angiotensin receptor blockers should also be considered in patients with systemic sclerosis and hypertension to prevent scleroderma renal crisis.

Antiplatelet Therapy

Antiplatelet therapy with aspirin or clopidogrel should be considered for patients with secondary RS caused by atherosclerosis obliterans.

Anticoagulation Therapy

Anticoagulation therapy with intravenous or subcutaneous heparin might prevent extension of thrombosis in patients with acute ischemia. Chronic anticoagulation is generally not of benefit for patients with chronic small vessel occlusive disease because the underlying process is an obliterative and not thrombotic vasculopathy.

Thrombolysis

Thrombolytic agents such as tissue plasminogen activator lyse acute thrombi and acute arterial emboli. This treatment might have a role in some patients with acute small vessel occlusions and has been tried with limited benefit in microvascular disorders.

Novel Drug Therapies

Several new drugs have potential but unproven benefit in RS. Sildenafil, a phosphodiesterase inhibitor, has marked vasodilator properties of benefit for erectile dysfunction but has had limited evaluation in RS. Cilostazol may have antiplatelet properties in addition to vasodilation, but it has not been studied in patients with RS. Fluoxetine is a selective serotonin reuptake inhibitor marketed for the treatment of depression. A decrease in attack frequency and severity was documented in a single study in patients with primary or secondary RS treated with fluoxetine 20 mg daily. Laboratory testing showed improvement in recovery after cold challenge test, with the greatest improvement seen in females with primary RS.

Endothelin-1, a potent neurohormone derived from vascular endothelium, binds to endothelin A and B receptors in the endothelium and smooth muscle, which causes vasoconstriction. Endothelin-1 levels are elevated in patients with pulmonary hypertension. Bosentan is an endothelin-1 receptor antagonist and blocks vasoconstriction caused by endothelin. Bosentan is indicated for the treatment of primary pulmonary hypertension or pulmonary hypertension due to scleroderma. As a potent vasodilator, bosentan has potential benefit in vasospastic disorders. The drug is administered orally (62.5 mg twice daily, then a maintenance dose of 125 mg once daily). Adverse effects include headache, flushing, edema, and elevation of liver transaminases. Bosentan is contraindicated in pregnancy because of teratogenicity, and its use is limited by the expense of the medication ($36,000/year).

Prostaglandins

Some prostaglandins, such as prostacyclin, are potent vasodilators that have been used for patients with critical digital ischemia secondary to fixed occlusive disease. Much of the early experience with this therapy has occurred in Europe with the use of the prostacyclin analog iloprost. Iloprost has been reported to decrease the severity, frequency, and duration of RS episodes and to promote healing of ischemic ulcers. However, effects are not sustained, with no beneficial effects after 1 week.

Epoprostenol is a naturally occurring prostaglandin and metabolite of arachidonic acid with potent vasodilatory and antiplatelet actions. It has been approved for the treatment of primary pulmonary hypertension and pulmonary hypertension associated with scleroderma. Epoprostenol can be beneficial in some patients who have severe RS with digital ischemia, and its use has been associated with an increase in fingertip skin temperature and laser Doppler flow. It is generally administered as a continuous intravenous infusion (0.5-2.0 $ng \cdot kg^{-1} \cdot min^{-1}$) for 1 to 3 days.

Cicaprost is a synthetic oral prostacyclin analog not available in the United States. Studies have failed to show any significant improvement for RS or digital ischemia with oral formulations such as cicaprost.

Food Supplements

Fish oil has the theoretical benefits of decreasing thromboxane A_2 production and increasing prostacyclin synthesis. Its actual benefit for RS, if any, is unknown.

L-Arginine, as a substrate for nitric oxide synthesis, has the theoretical benefit of improving endothelial dysfunction in patients with primary or secondary RS. For example, patients with systemic sclerosis have decreased arterial vasodilation in response to acetylcholine. Unfortunately, most studies of L-arginine (double-blind crossover trials with administration of oral L-arginine, 8 g daily for 28 days), failed to show any improvement in endothelium-dependent vasodilation.

Management of Critical Upper Extremity Ischemia

General measures for management of critical ischemia include the use of a vascular mitten to keep the extremity at body temperature and to protect the finger from trauma. Topical agents are used to prevent infection, and specific wound care products can promote the healing of digital ulcers. Local debridement of dead tissue or removal of the fingernail may be necessary. Amputation of the end of a digit is often a consideration, but primary amputation should be avoided whenever possible because the amputation site can take longer to heal (if it ever does) than the original ulcer.

Sympathectomy

Sympathectomy can be of benefit for some patients with secondary RS and critical ischemia of the digits but is rarely, if ever, indicated for those with primary RS. It may be effective in alleviating pain from atheroembolism and distal tissue infarction, but the benefit is likely to be short lived because of regeneration of nerve fibers. Cervicothoracic sympathectomy can be accomplished by a thoracoscopic procedure instead of thoracotomy, which limits complications such as pneumothorax, phrenic nerve injury, or Horner syndrome. Digital sympathectomy can be performed by orthopedic hand surgeons, and has been successful in the healing of ulcers and improvement of ischemia pain. The main indication for sympathectomy in RS is non-healing digital ulceration refractory to intensive medical therapy. In one study, 26 of 28 patients (93%) had initial resolution or improvement of symptoms, but symptoms recurred in 82% within 16 months after surgery. Despite the rate of recurrence, several patients believed they had some long-term symptomatic improvement.

Devices and Procedures for Treatment of Raynaud Syndrome

Acupuncture

A small randomized trial found acupuncture to be effective in decreasing the frequency and severity of episodes in patients with primary RS. The mechanism of action is believed to be stimulation of sensory nerves causing release of vasodilators such as substance P and calcitonin gene–related peptide.

Transcutaneous Nerve Stimulation

Transcutaneous nerve stimulation may induce vasodilation with varying results in some patients with RS.

Spinal Cord Stimulation

Reduction of pain and promotion of ulcer healing has been reported with use of a spinal cord stimulator in patients with secondary RS. In one small study of 10 patients with RS or reflex sympathetic dystrophy, 90% had substantial relief of chronic pain. Autonomic effects also were seen, as demonstrated by thermographic and plethysmographic changes.

Hyperbaric Oxygen

Hyperbaric oxygen chambers are expensive and limited in availability, but they have been well documented to aid in the healing of ischemic ulceration.

Pneumatic Vascular Pump

Intermittent pneumatic compression is an established therapy for patients with severe limb ischemia who have no other surgical or medical options. Currently, several pneumatic pumps are available from different manufacturers. These are similar to venous pumps used for thromboembolic prophylaxis but with higher compression and more rapid compression cycles. Significant healing of digital ulcers has been documented with the use of pneumatic pumping in patients with scleroderma in whom other conventional therapies have failed.

- Preventive measures, with education, reassurance, and avoidance of cold exposure, constitute the basis of therapy for most patients
- Multiple studies have documented the effectiveness of dihydropyridine calcium-channel blockers in the treatment of RS

Other Vasospastic Disorders Related to Temperature

Erythromelalgia

Erythromelalgia (sometimes known as erythermalgia) is a rare disorder characterized by episodes of burning extremity pain associated with erythema of the skin and markedly increased extremity temperature. It more commonly involves the feet than the hands, is usually bilateral, is brought on by environmental warmth, and pain is always alleviated by local cooling. The term erythromelalgia comes from the words "*erythros*" (red), "*melos*" (extremity), and "*algos*" (pain).

Erythromelalgia is the antithesis of RS: symptoms are caused by warmth and relieved by cold. It can occur secondary to myeloproliferative disorders such as polycythemia vera and essential thrombocytopenia. In many cases, however, the cause is unknown and no underlying disease is found. In a review from Mayo Clinic, fewer than 10% of patients had a history of myeloproliferative disease.

- Erythromelalgia is characterized by episodes of burning extremity pain associated with erythema of the skin and markedly increased extremity temperature

All age groups can be affected, but it commonly affects younger persons (children to young adults). Unlike in reflex sympathetic dystrophy, patients have no history of inciting trauma. Several theories exist as to the pathogenesis of erythromelalgia, including a microcirculatory abnormality with shunting and a local steal, which causes ischemic pain. Recent studies suggest a small-fiber neuropathy. Results of autonomic reflex testing are abnormal, many showing postganglionic sudomotor impairment. An axonal neuropathy has been demonstrated in some who had electromyographic studies.

Erythromelalgia is diagnosed on the basis of clinical history, aided by examination and vascular laboratory documentation of elevated extremity temperature when symptoms are present. During symptoms, laboratory tests can document a mean increase in extremity temperature of 11°C and increased skin blood flow measured by laser Doppler flow.

Treatment is difficult, and several agents have been tried with limited success, including aspirin, nonsteroidal anti-inflammatory agents, β-blockers, α-blockers, tricyclic antidepressants, antihistamines, nitroglycerin, nicotinic acid, and anticonvulsants. Sympathectomy, epidural blocks, biofeedback, hypnosis, and transcutaneous electrical nerve stimulation have been tried without much benefit.

Livedo Reticularis

Livedo reticularis is a lacy, reticular, purplish discoloration of the skin that can be seen in normal persons due to cold-induced vasospasm of small venules in the skin. Benign cold-induced livedo reticularis is intensified by cold exposure and resolves immediately with warming. This pattern can also be seen secondary to atheroembolism (from an ulcerated plaque in locations such as the subclavian or innominate artery), in small vessel vasculitis, and can be induced by β-blockers or chemotherapy agents.

Pernio

Pernio is an inflammatory lesion of the skin that occurs in response to cold. Generally it affects the toes and rarely the fingers, presenting with recurring, erythematous skin lesions, which can turn into superficial ulcers. The ulcers may burn and itch and appear as slightly raised bluish-red blisters that characteristically occur in the winter and resolve during the summer months. This lesion historically has been referred to as "chilblain" because of its similarity to a cold sore, which is a cutaneous inflammatory lesion. Skin biopsy is rarely necessary for diagnosis, but pathologic changes include a localized inflammatory reaction with perivascular lymphocytic infiltration of arterioles and venules of the skin. Acute pernio is self-limiting and most commonly affects young women. The differential diagnosis should include atheromatous embolization, erythema nodosum, SLE, and livedo vasculitis.

- Pernio is an inflammatory lesion of the skin that occurs in response to cold

Thoracic Outlet Syndrome

TOS refers to the symptomatic compression of neurovascular structures as they pass from the upper chest to the arm. The subclavian vein, subclavian artery, and brachial plexus all cross through a limited space as they traverse the thoracic outlet, passing over the first rib and under the clavicle. Extrinsic compression of one or all of these three structures by hypertrophied, anomalous scalene muscles, tendons, bands, or a cervical rib can cause TOS. Although TOS is more common in women, persons with certain occupations or avocations (such as mechanics, wallpaper hangers, cleaners, and athletes involved in upper extremity sports) that require repetitive raising of the arms above the head are predisposed to TOS.

Anatomy of the Thoracic Outlet

The thoracic outlet can be thought of as a triangle with the apex toward the sternum. The clavicle, with underlying subclavius muscle, forms the superior roof and the base is the first thoracic rib. When the arm is in certain positions, the clavicle and first rib can act like a pair of scissors—joined at the manubrium—that opens and closes, compressing structures contained in the thoracic space.

The subclavian vein is the most medial, adjacent to the point where the first rib and clavicular head fuse at the manubrium. The anterior scalene muscle inserts into the first rib just lateral to the vein. The subclavian artery and brachial plexus are lateral to the anterior scalene and pass over the first rib between the anterior scalene and the middle scalene muscle, which is posterior and lateral. The brachial plexus C4-C6 roots are superior and C7-T1 are more inferior.

Several bony, muscular, and tendon insertion anomalies can result in TOS. Ten percent of patients who undergo surgery for TOS have a cervical rib. A cervical rib displaces structures forward—in particular the subclavian artery—predisposing it to injury. (Most persons with an incidentally discovered asymptomatic cervical rib do not need prophylactic rib resection.) Clavicular fracture can cause bony deformity and also intrude into the thoracic outlet space.

Anomalies, based on intraoperative observations (Roos classification), seen in TOS include an incomplete cervical rib, an accessory muscle between the first rib and subclavian artery, a large middle scalene muscle compressing the T1 nerve root, a scalene minimus muscle attached to the first rib behind the scalene tubercle, a band from the middle scalene muscle to costal cartilage, a band traveling under the subclavian vein to its costoclavicular attachment (may cause Paget-Schroetter syndrome), or subclavius muscle hypertrophy that occurs in weight lifters along with hypertrophied scalene muscles. Of patients who had surgery, 10% had a cervical rib, 10% a scalenus minimus muscle, 20% an abnormality of the subclavius tendon insertion, and 43% a defect in scalene musculature.

Types of TOS

There are three forms of TOS, each with different symptoms and a different approach to evaluation and management, depending on the major structure compressed (vein, artery, or nerve).

Neurogenic TOS

Neurogenic TOS is the most common of the three forms, comprising 90% of patients with TOS; much controversy continues about its diagnosis and best management. Patients may initially present to a neurologist for evaluation of positional arm pain and paresthesias, with numbness, tingling, and, infrequently, weakness of the extremity. Pain can involve the posterior shoulder (suprascapular and trapezius muscle area) and pain in the affected arm can be localized or generalized. Weakness is possible from pain, but muscle wasting is unlikely. Compression of the lower brachial plexus (C8, T1) is more common with pain that follows an ulnar distribution in the lateral arm and fingers. Upper trunk (C5, 6, 7) compression occurs less frequently with pain that follows a median nerve distribution.

- Neurogenic TOS is the most common of the three forms, comprising 90% of patients with TOS

The diagnosis of TOS is difficult because it is based on clinical findings that include a history of positional symptoms brought on by overhead activities and confirmatory noninvasive vascular laboratory testing. Electromyography can show decreased nerve conduction velocity, but most often results are normal. Other causes of upper extremity pain, including cervical radiculopathies, ulnar neuropathy, carpal tunnel syndrome, and generalized musculoskeletal pain, such as can occur in fibromyalgia and chronic pain, must be recognized and excluded. The diagnosis is made more difficult because TOS can occur after trauma, and neurogenic TOS is often not recognized for many months after the onset of symptoms.

Physical therapy is the mainstay of therapy for neurogenic TOS. Improvement in posture is of great benefit for older persons with poor muscle tone and conditioning. Shoulder muscle stretching and strengthening exercises, along with nonsteroidal antiinflammatory medications and local heat and cold applications, are of proven benefit for many persons. Surgery is indicated for severe symptoms of incapacitating neurologic dysfunction or pain if it can be clearly demonstrated that symptoms are due to TOS with no other major cause. Decompressive surgery usually involves first rib resection, anterior scalenectomy, or resection of anomalous bands and ligaments. In the past, a supraclavicular approach was taken, but this leaves a scar that is disfiguring in women. Better results are obtained by a transaxillary approach.

Arterial TOS

Arterial complications from TOS are infrequent, but patients may present with vasospasm due to RS or with symptoms resulting from both arterial and nerve compression. Of the many anatomic abnormalities involving the scalene muscles and ligamentous bands, symptomatic arterial compression is most commonly caused by an incomplete or complete cervical rib that displaces the artery forward, stretching it over the rib. Cervical ribs are present in 0.2% to 1% of the population but occur in as many as 80% of those with arterial complications from TOS.

Arterial damage can occur from repetitive subclavian artery compression occurring at the point where it crosses over the first rib or a cervical rib. This arterial damage can predispose patients to aneurysm formation with mural thrombosis and distal embolism to the hand and fingers. Axillary subclavian artery thrombosis due to TOS usually requires surgical intervention with thrombectomy or embolectomy, arterial repair, and excision of the first rib (and cervical rib if present).

Patients with arterial complications of TOS may present with acute upper extremity ischemia due to either proximal arterial obstruction or distal embolization to the hand and fingers. The ischemia is often wrongly attributed to vasospasm due to RS, but persistent pain, pallor, and paresthesias with or without pulses should alert the clinician to the presence of severe ischemia. Prompt evaluation and management are necessary to avoid tissue loss. Treatment can require thrombectomy or thrombolysis of a proximal arterial occlusion or, if distal, embolic arterial obstruction. TOS decompression by first rib resection, arterial repair, or bypass may be required to repair a subclavian aneurysm.

Venous TOS

Paget-Schroetter syndrome refers to axillo-subclavian vein thrombosis resulting from impingement of the subclavian vein as it exits from the chest through the thoracic outlet space. It occurs most commonly in young, otherwise healthy persons and has been called "effort thrombosis" because it occurs in athletes engaged in swimming, basketball, volleyball, or weight lifting. Patients may present with sudden onset of upper extremity swelling, pain, and bluish skin discoloration due to deep vein thrombosis. Most have no prior diagnosis or symptoms of TOS. Anatomic abnormalities can predispose persons to extrinsic subclavian vein compression, but in athletes compression is most often due to hypertrophied anterior scalene and subclavius muscles. The axillary vein, providing venous return from the arm, passes behind the costocoracoid ligament and pectoralis minor tendon insertion, leading to possible vein compression by the pectoralis minor muscle.

- Paget-Schroetter syndrome refers to axillo-subclavian vein thrombosis resulting from impingement of the subclavian vein

Paget-Schroetter syndrome should be suspected in any athlete (in particular weightlifters, swimmers, and baseball or basketball players) presenting with acute upper extremity swelling. TOS should also be suspected in others with unexplained upper extremity deep vein thrombosis not due to a peripherally inserted central catheter or central line. Duplex ultrasonography is the usual initial test to confirm the presence of subclavian deep vein thrombosis. Cervical spine radiography can indicate the presence of a cervical rib, elongated transverse process of T8, or prior clavicular fracture.

Although swelling improves with conservative management (heparin anticoagulation and elastic external compression), many patients have residual disability of the arm with some persistent arm enlargement due to venous hypertension and fatigue aggravated by overhead activities. A more aggressive approach—catheter-directed thrombolysis, with or without mechanical thrombectomy to reopen the vein, followed in 1 to 2 months by transaxillary first rib excision to decompress the thoracic outlet—is most likely to produce long-term benefit with full functional recovery of the extremity and return to normal activities.

Diagnosis of TOS: Role of Provocative Testing

Several maneuvers in the office or in the non-invasive vascular laboratory can assist in making the clinical diagnosis of TOS. A positive thoracic outlet maneuver on its own does not make the diagnosis of TOS because the results can be positive in many normal persons. It helps to objectively correlate symptoms with a demonstration of positional arterial compression at the thoracic outlet level.

The Adson Test (Scalene Maneuver)

This maneuver increases tone in the anterior and middle scalene muscles, leading to interscalene triangle compression. With palpation of the radial pulse, the patient extends the neck, turns the head away from the affected side, and takes a deep breath. Diminution or loss of the radial pulse, or reproduction of symptoms is considered positive. This test is the least sensitive of all the provocative office tests for TOS and is often negative in those with TOS.

The Wright Test (Hyperabduction Test)

This test is usually combined with abduction and external rotation of the arm (passively by the examiner and actively by the patient) with palpation of the radial pulse and auscultation over the subclavian artery. The maneuver is positive if there is loss of radial pulse, an audible subclavian bruit, and replication of symptoms. This is the most sensitive test, but it has low specificity, with up to half of normal asymptomatic persons having a positive test.

The Costoclavicular Maneuver (Military Position)

In this maneuver, the shoulders are drawn back and downward in the military brace position so as to compress the costoclavicular space and structures. A positive test demonstrates loss of radial pulse and reproduction of symptoms.

Exercise Abduction Stress Test

This test uses hyperabduction of the arms (hold-up position); the patient is asked to slowly open and close the hands for a minute or two. A positive test is indicated by symptoms of weakness or numbness and hand pallor after exercise. Symptoms and hand pallor immediately resolve by lowering the arms and moving the shoulders forward. Most believe that this is the most useful office and vascular laboratory test to help substantiate the clinical diagnosis of TOS.

In summary, TOS is an important but controversial syndrome. For those with arterial or venous complications, the diagnosis and management is straightforward, but for most patients with neurogenic TOS, the diagnosis and management can be difficult. Most patients with neurogenic TOS respond to conservative measures with a physical therapy program. Surgical decompression of the thoracic outlet requires excision of the first rib, usually by a transaxillary approach, but this is indicated only for those with arterial or venous complications and less commonly for neurologic pain and dysfunction. Despite successful surgery, not everyone improves after thoracic outlet decompression operations.

Questions

1. A positive Allen test in a mechanic with digital ischemia should suggest which one of the following diagnoses?
a. Raynaud syndrome
b. Thoracic outlet syndrome
c. Hypothenar hammer syndrome
d. CREST syndrome
e. Yellow nail syndrome

2. In which of the following would the erythrocyte sedimentation rate be expected to be normal?
a. Scleroderma
b. Takayasu arteritis
c. Wegener granulomatosis
d. Osteomyelitis
e. Diabetes mellitus with nephrotic syndrome

3. In primary RS, why don't the fingers have ischemic tissue loss or gangrene during prolonged episodes of arterial vasospasm?
a. During vasospastic attacks, digital vessels never actually occlude.
b. During vasospastic attacks, collateral vessels open to provide flow to the distal finger.
c. Arteriovenous anastomoses open during cold exposure to shunt blood back to the venous circulation and increase digital temperature.
d. During cold exposure, vasodilation occurs along with vasoconstriction, allowing a trickle of blood to reach the distal finger to prevent the digits from freezing.

4. Which one of the following is not indicative of primary RS?
a. Vasospastic attacks precipitated by exposure to cold or emotional stimuli
b. Symmetrical or bilateral involvement of the extremities
c. Absence of underlying disease
d. Positive anticentromere antibody

5. A carpenter presents with cold sensitivity of the fingers and a history consistent with RS. Examination reveals a bluish discoloration of the fourth and fifth fingers with splinter hemorrhages. Which of the following tests may help to diagnose the cause of this condition?
a. Allen test
b. Trendelenburg test
c. Exercise abduction stress test
d. Cold water immersion test

6. Which one of the following is true of TOS?
a. The diagnosis of neurogenic TOS should be made in the vascular laboratory by demonstrating positive thoracic outlet maneuvers.
b. An anomalous cervical rib is the most common cause of neurogenic TOS.
c. The Adson test (scalene maneuver) is the most sensitive of all examination maneuvers to document dynamic compression of the subclavian artery at the thoracic outlet level.
d. TOS can be complicated by local aneurysm formation and distal embolization to the fingers.
e. A young patient presenting with "effort thrombosis" of the upper extremity should raise suspicion of possible underlying malignancy.

7. Erythromelalgia is characterized by all of the following except:
a. Increased temperature of the extremity with erythema
b. Severe pain brought on by warmth, relieved by cold
c. Symptoms are worse after exercise and at night
d. May be associated with small fiber neuropathy
e. May occur secondary to myeloproliferative disorders
f. There is often a history of trauma as an inciting event

8. Small blisters on the end of the toes recurring every winter indicate:
a. Pernio
b. Raynaud syndrome
c. Reflex sympathetic dystrophy
d. Acrocyanosis

Suggested Readings

Coffman JD. Raynaud's phenomenon. New York: Oxford University Press; 1989.

Cohen RA. The role of nitric oxide and other endothelium-derived vasoactive substances in vascular disease. Prog Cardiovasc Dis. 1995;38:105-28.

Davis MD, O'Fallon WM, Rogers RS III, et al. Natural history of erythromelalgia: presentation and outcome in 168 patients. Arch Dermatol. 2000;136:330-6.

Edwards JM, Porter JM. Raynaud's syndrome and small vessel arteriopathy. Semin Vasc Surg. 1993;6:56-65.

Greenfield LJ, Rajagopalan S, Olin JW. Upper extremity arterial disease. Cardiol Clin. 2002;20:623-31.

Hummers LK, Wigley FM. Management of Raynaud's phenomenon and digital ischemic lesions in scleroderma. Rheum Dis Clin North Am. 2003;29:293-313.

Joyce JW. Buerger's disease (thromboangiitis obliterans). Rheum Dis Clin North Am. 1990;16:463-70.

Lorelli DR, Shepard AD. Hypothenar hammer syndrome: an uncommon and correctable cause of digital ischemia. J Cardiovasc Surg (Torino). 2002;43:83-5.

Olin JW. Other peripheral arterial diseases. In: Goldman L, Bennett JC, editors. Cecil textbook of medicine. 21st ed. Philadelphia: WB Saunders Company; 2000. p. 362-7.

Olin JW. Thromboangiitis obliterans (Buerger's disease). N Engl J Med. 2000;343:864-9.

Ouriel K. Noninvasive diagnosis of upper extremity vascular disease. Semin Vasc Surg. 1998;11:54-9.

Porter JM, Edwards JM. Occlusive and vasospastic diseases involving distal upper extremity arteries: Raynaud's syndrome. In: Rutherford RB, editor. Vascular Surgery. 4th ed. Philadelphia: WB Saunders Company; 1995. p. 961-76.

Rigberg DA, Freischlag JA. Thoracic outlet syndrome. In: Hallett JW Jr, Mills JL, Earnshaw JJ, et al, editors. Comprehensive vascular and endovascular surgery. Edinburgh: Mosby; 2004. p. 267-84.

Shepherd RF, Shepherd JT. Raynaud's phenomenon. Int Angiol. 1992;11:41-5.

Spittell PC, Spittell JA. Occlusive arterial disease of the hand due to repetitive blunt trauma: a review with illustrative cases. Int J Cardiol. 1993;38:281-92.

Taylor LM Jr. Hypothenar hammer syndrome. J Vasc Surg. 2003;37:697.

Wigley FM. Systemic sclerosis. B. Clinical features. In: Klippel JH, editor. Primer on the rheumatic diseases. 12th ed. Atlanta (GA): Arthritis Foundation; 2001. p. 357-64.

4 Chronic Venous Disease and Lymphatic Disease

Suman Rathbun, MD

Chronic Venous Insufficiency

Natural History

Chronic venous insufficiency (CVI) is one of the most common causes of leg ulcers in the United States and can occur in deep or superficial veins. Pathologic superficial varicose veins occur in about 12% of the population; skin findings that indicate some degree of CVI are found in approximately 20% of adults. CVI results from chronic venous valvular incompetence, chronic deep venous obstruction, or both. Venous insufficiency can be primary, as a result of congenital or acquired connective tissue disorders of the vein wall, or secondary, as a result of direct valve impairment after venous thrombosis. About one-third of patients with CVI have a history of deep vein thrombosis (DVT). Within 5 years after DVT development, up to 80% of patients have signs and symptoms of CVI. CVI and the resulting pathologic features associated with DVT have also been called postphlebitic or post-thrombotic syndrome. CVI can eventually lead to lower extremity edema, hyperpigmentation, cellulitis, dermatitis, and ulceration.

Upper extremity DVT can also occur, especially in the presence of intravenous catheters, which results in obstruction of venous return. However, the incidence of postphlebitic syndrome and CVI of the arm has not been well studied and will not be discussed in this chapter.

- CVI is a common cause of leg ulcers
- CVI is caused by venous valvular incompetence, deep venous obstruction, or both
- CVI after DVT is also known as post-thrombotic or postphlebitic syndrome

Pathophysiology

Deep Venous Insufficiency

The causes of deep venous insufficiency are either chronic deep venous obstruction or chronic venous valvular incompetence.

Obstruction. The most common cause of deep venous outflow obstruction is DVT (Table 4.1). Most veins recanalize after thrombosis, but large veins are more likely than smaller distal veins to remain occluded or partially obstructed. As acute obstruction from DVT above the popliteal vein becomes chronic, distal venous pressure causes increased flow through collateral venous channels that enlarge. Enlargement of vein channels results in venous insufficiency, and perforating veins become incompetent, causing secondary superficial varicose veins. Chronic incompetence of the perforating veins results in stasis changes in the overlying subcutaneous tissue.

Normally, with exercise, arterial flow to the limb increases, which results in an increase in venous return. With venous obstruction, however, exercise increases deep venous pressure, stretches fascial planes, and inhibits effective capillary inflow of nutrients and clearance of metabolic products. A painful syndrome called venous claudication

Table 4.1 Causes of Venous Obstruction

Deep vein thrombosis
May-Thurner syndrome
Malignancy
Pelvic masses including synovial cysts
Bladder distension
Aneurysms of the aortic or lower extremity arteries
Retroperitoneal fibrosis
Tumors of the vein wall
Intraluminal webs or septa
Iatrogenic vein ligation

is the result. Symptoms of pain are relieved with cessation of exercise. Obstruction of isolated segments of small veins below the knee does not produce the same hemodynamic impact as obstruction in more proximal veins.

Non-thrombotic obstruction of the lower extremity veins can also occur but is uncommon. Obstruction can be caused by external compression of the vein or abnormalities in the wall of the vein or within the lumen of the vein. All of these cause an increased resistance to blood flow, which results in the signs and symptoms of chronic vein obstruction with impaired outflow.

In most of the population, the right common iliac artery in the midline, just anterior to the fifth lumbar vertebra, crosses over the left common iliac vein. In general, the overlying pulsating artery does not cause significant obstruction to flow. However, if lumbar lordosis increases or intra-abdominal pressure rises, as occurs during pregnancy, the underlying vein can be compressed, resulting in venous obstruction. This normal anatomic variant may cause a pathologic syndrome of venous obstruction known as May-Thurner syndrome. DVT is a common complication and may explain the higher incidence of left-sided lower leg thrombosis during pregnancy. Another anatomic variant that can lead to venous obstruction is compression of the terminal portion of the external iliac vein by the internal iliac artery.

Malignant disease surrounding the iliac veins can also cause venous obstruction. Cancers of the cervix, ovary, colon, and rectum may spread along the floor of the pelvis and encroach upon the vein. Enlargement of lymph nodes can also externally compress the iliac veins resulting in venous obstruction. Tumors that can spread to the iliac lymph nodes include malignancies of the uterus, cervix, rectum, anal canal, testis, leg, and scrotal skin (malignant melanoma and squamous cell carcinoma).

Other pelvic masses can also obstruct venous outflow. These include masses arising from the hip joint, such as synovial cysts. Bladder distension due to prostatic hypertrophy can compress neighboring iliac veins. In addition, aneurysms of the aortic and iliac arteries have the potential to produce a similar effect.

Retroperitoneal fibrosis is usually found anteriorly, but sometimes spreads across the posterior wall, involving the iliac veins before ultimately reaching the inferior vena cava and aorta. Large tumors of the thigh, including liposarcoma, fibrosarcoma, and aneurysms of the common femoral and femoral arteries can compress the adjacent common femoral and femoral veins. The tendon of the adductor canal may also compress the femoral vein. Iliopectineal bursitis can cause common femoral vein obstruction. Popliteal aneurysms, large popliteal cysts (Baker cyst), popliteal artery entrapment syndrome, or inflamed bursa similarly can impinge on the popliteal vein, which results in venous obstruction.

Vein wall abnormalities include aplasia of the pelvic veins as seen in Klippel-Trénaunay syndrome, a congenital venous disorder that causes CVI. Rare primary tumors of the vein wall such as leiomyosarcoma also cause venous obstruction.

Intraluminal webs or septa of the veins may result in venous obstruction. Webs may occur at the termination of the left common iliac vein where it is compressed by the common iliac artery. These webs can be a result of an inflammatory response to repeated minor trauma rather than a congenital abnormality or residual venous thrombosis. Unintended ligation of the femoral or popliteal vein during surgery for varicose veins is an iatrogenic cause of deep venous obstruction.

- DVT is the most common cause of deep venous obstruction
- Venous claudication develops during exercise when venous outflow is limited by deep venous obstruction
- Obstruction to venous flow caused by the right common iliac artery crossing the left common iliac vein is known as May-Thurner syndrome

Valvular Incompetence. Venous valves are found with greater frequency proceeding distally in the lower extremity. The inferior vena cava has no valves, and valves in the common iliac veins are rare. In more than 90% of the population, venous valves are found distal to the confluence of the femoral and deep femoral veins and more commonly in the proximal popliteal vein. During standing or sitting, venous blood flow is steady and the valve leaflets remain open. After contraction of the calf muscle pump, the intramuscular vein pressure falls to zero, and the valves prevent reflux by maintaining the reduction of venous pressure. Some degree of venous reflux is normal but should not persist for longer than 0.5 second on evaluation by ultrasonography.

The most important cause of CVI is valvular incompetence of the deep veins. Most commonly, this is a result of DVT after the veins become partially or totally recanalized. During the acute and chronic phases of DVT, the fragile valve leaflets become thickened and shortened or they may become embedded in the vein wall, which limits their proper function. The valve is no longer able to allow normal antegrade venous flow or inhibit retrograde flow. Resultant high venous pressures cause distension of veins distally, with elongation, separation, and leakage of the valve leaflets.

Other causes of valvular incompetence include age-related valve changes, congenital absence of valves, trauma to valves, primary valve incompetence (floppy valve cusps), and valve ring dilatation. After the age of 30 years, histologic changes in the venous valves occur, which result in extension and thickening of the elastic membrane.

Congenital absence of deep venous valves is rare and thought to be inherited as an autosomal dominant trait. It is also possible to inherit a decreased number of valves. These patients may present with bilateral leg ulcers in their early teens. Mechanical trauma to the vein wall or infusion of acidic, alkaline, hypotonic, or hypertonic solutions can also damage and impair venous valvular function. In patients with primary floppy valve cusps, the venous valve edge is too long, causing it to evert in an antegrade direction and be incompetent. If normal valve cusps do not meet across the lumen of the vein because of valve ring dilation, the vein becomes incompetent. This more commonly occurs in the superficial veins. Hormonal changes during pregnancy sometimes allow the superficial vein walls to relax and be subject to venous valvular incompetence.

- Valvular incompetence due to DVT is a common cause of CVI
- Absent or reduced number of venous valves can be congenital
- Other causes of valvular incompetence include trauma to the vein wall, infusion of irritant solutions, primary floppy valves, and pregnancy

Regardless of the cause of valvular incompetence, the resulting pathophysiologic features are the same. Valvular incompetence distally, at the level of the popliteal vein or below, is more damaging than reflux in the more proximal deep veins. With valvular incompetence, unidirectional blood flow and emptying of the deep veins does not occur. With calf pump action, blood is shunted partially retrograde; therefore, pressure in the distal veins and deep fascial tissues fails to decrease normally with muscle contraction. As in deep venous obstruction, high pressures cause perforating vein and superficial vein engorgement and valvular dysfunction. This syndrome of deep venous insufficiency with secondary varicose veins, resulting from outward perforator flow during calf pump contraction and inward flow on relaxation with little or no decrease in pressure, is known as "calf pump failure syndrome." Calf pump failure can also occur in the setting of muscle atrophy, neuromuscular disease, or deep fasciotomy that prevents effective muscle contraction.

Chronic valvular incompetence causes inflammation and pericapillary fibrosis, which results in subcutaneous thickening and induration. Erythrocyte lysis causes hemosiderin deposits and characteristic brown pigmentation of the skin. Chronic persistent venous hypertension, interstitial edema, and inflammation eventually cause local hypoxia and malnutrition. Secondary fat necrosis and liposclerosis occur with skin atrophy, eczema, and ulceration. Secondary bacterial invasion can cause cellulitis. Progressive sclerosis of lymph channels can result in secondary lymphedema. At late stages, chronic tissue fibrosis can cause fixation of the ankle joint, leading to muscular atrophy. Rarely, chronic ulceration undergoes malignant transformation to form a Marjolin ulcer.

- Calf pump failure syndrome results from retrograde flow through incompetent perforator veins during calf muscle contraction or ineffective muscle contraction, resulting in secondary varicose veins
- Persistent venous hypertension causes cutaneous changes resulting in liposclerosis and ulceration

Superficial Venous Insufficiency

Superficial varicose veins, one type of superficial venous insufficiency, are enlarged veins within the subcutaneous tissue, usually involving the greater or lesser saphenous veins or their tributaries. Up to 12% of adults have significant varicose veins for which they seek symptomatic relief of discomfort; this incidence is greater if those who seek cosmetic treatment of varicosities are included. The incidence of superficial varicose veins increases with age, especially after the third decade of life, and is twice as common in women as in men. Pregnancy can exacerbate superficial venous insufficiency.

Varicose veins are classified as primary or secondary. Primary varicose veins involve the superficial veins only, whereas in secondary varicose veins, the superficial veins become enlarged secondary to deep vein and perforating vein incompetence. Primary varicose veins are three times more common than secondary varicose veins, and the greater saphenous vein is more commonly involved than the lesser saphenous vein. More than 50% of those with primary varicose veins have a family history of varicosity. The risk may be as high as 90% if both parents have been affected. Persons with occupations requiring prolonged standing are also at higher risk of varicose veins.

Primary varicose veins may be caused by defective anatomy or function of valves in the superficial veins, weakness of vein walls, or the presence of small arteriovenous communications leading to venous enlargement. Secondary varicose veins most commonly arise after DVT that has produced deep valvular incompetence from valve disruption or deep venous obstruction.

Whether primary or secondary, varicose veins are caused by engorgement of normal superficial veins. As enlargement of the vein progresses, the valve leaflets are pulled farther apart, which causes further valve incompetence and increases the hydrostatic pressure of the column of blood in the vein. These high pressures are communicated to the perforator veins, causing reversal of the normal superficial-to-deep venous flow during calf muscle contraction and relaxation. As already described, this inefficient venous emptying eventually causes edema, secondary inflammation, and hyperpigmentation of the skin overlying the varicosities. Complications arising from varicose veins include an increased incidence of DVT and superficial thrombophlebitis.

Venous telangiectasias, another type of superficial venous disorder, are seen as cutaneous clusters of small veins also known as spider veins. Telangiectasias are defined as flat red vessels of 0.1 to 1 mm in diameter. Reticular veins have a bluish hue and are usually 1 to 3 mm in diameter. Patients usually have no pain from these veins and may seek care for their cosmetic appearance. They may be related to hormonal changes in women because they are more common in pregnancy or after menopause, but they can also be a sign of calf pump failure.

- Primary varicose veins involve the superficial veins only
- Secondary varicose veins result from deep venous incompetence and retrograde flow through perforator veins
- Venous telangiectasias do not cause symptoms and may be treated for cosmetic purposes

History

Primary venous valvular insufficiency can be congenital or can be acquired secondary to a connective tissue disorder of the vein wall. Secondary CVI is most commonly a result of DVT and its consequences of obstruction or valvular incompetence. CVI is also caused by repetitive trauma or injury to the veins. Exacerbating conditions include obesity, neuromuscular disorders, arthropathies, pregnancy, cardiac failure, tricuspid regurgitation, occupations requiring prolonged standing, and increasing age. Other comorbid conditions that can complicate CVI include arterial insufficiency, rheumatoid disease, hematologic disorders, diabetes mellitus, and the primary vasculitides.

- Primary venous valvular insufficiency can be congenital or acquired
- CVI may be exacerbated by comorbid conditions such as obesity, neuromuscular disorders, arthropathies, pregnancy, and cardiac failure

Examination

Swelling of the lower extremity that begins at the ankle and progresses to the lower leg and thigh is the most common physical finding of CVI (Fig. 4.1). Other skin changes can also occur, including prominent varicose veins, cyanosis and plethora with dependency, brawny induration, pigmentation, eczema, lipodermatosclerosis, and ulceration. Skin changes are most common just above the medial malleolus, also known as the "gaiter area" (Fig. 4.2). These areas are often tender to palpation. Pain is most common with prolonged standing, with patients reporting tightness and aching of the legs. With exercise, venous claudication pain can develop secondary to ineffective venous return, most commonly in the setting of venous outflow obstruction.

The Trendelenburg and the Perthes tests may be used with high sensitivity to distinguish primary from secondary varicose veins. In the Trendelenburg test, the leg is raised and a tourniquet is applied above the knee to obstruct the superficial veins. When the leg is then lowered as the patient stands, prompt filling of the varicosities suggests reflux through the perforating veins, which indicates an incompetent deep venous system (secondary varicose veins). If the varicose veins take longer than 20 seconds to fill, with prompt filling only after the tourniquet is removed, a diagnosis of primary superficial varicose veins

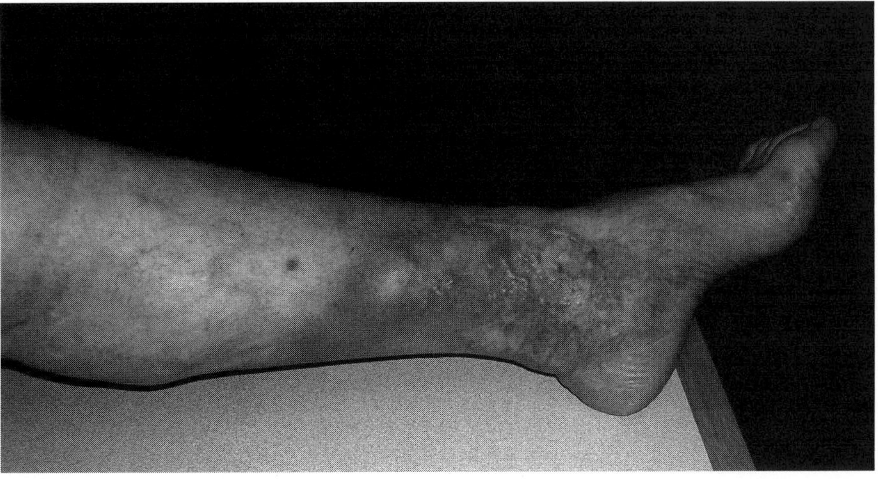

Fig. 4.1 Lipodermatosclerosis and atrophie blanche in a patient with severe left lower extremity venous insufficiency.

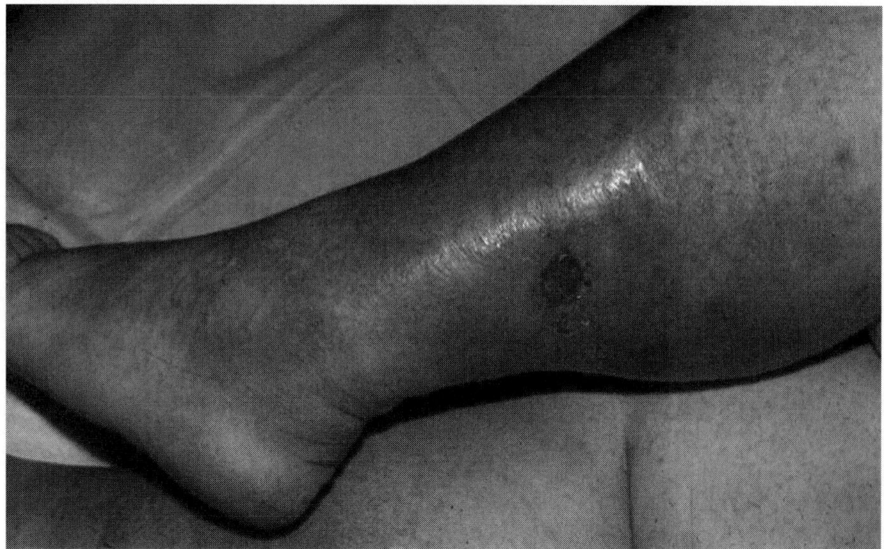

Fig. 4.2 Hyperpigmentation and venous stasis ulcer in a patient with left lower extremity venous insufficiency.

is made. In the Perthes test, a tourniquet is placed at the mid thigh or proximal calf while the leg is elevated. As the patient stands and walks, enlargement of the varicosities below the tourniquet (as blood is forced retrograde through the incompetent perforator veins) is diagnostic of deep venous insufficiency.

- Swelling is the most common physical finding in CVI
- Skin changes are most common in the "gaiter area" above the medial malleolus
- The Trendelenburg and Perthes tests can be used to distinguish deep from superficial varicose veins

The recently updated CEAP (Clinical-Etiology-Anatomy-Pathophysiology) classification is a guide to the systematic, standardized diagnostic evaluation of patients with CVI. Clinical classes are described as follows:

C0– No visible or palpable signs of venous disease
C1– Telangiectasias or reticular veins
C2– Varicose veins; distinguished from reticular veins by a diameter of 3 mm or greater
C3– Edema
C4– Changes in skin and subcutaneous tissue secondary to CVI:
  C4a– Pigmentation or eczema
  C4b– Lipodermatosclerosis or atrophie blanche
C5– Healed venous ulcer
C6– Active venous ulcer

Each clinical class is further characterized by a subscript for the presence of symptoms (S) or the absence of symptoms (A).

E– Etiology (congenital, primary, secondary)
A– Anatomic (superficial, deep)
P– Pathophysiology (reflux, obstruction, both)

The authors of the CEAP classification define the characteristic skin findings:

Atrophie blanche (white atrophy)—Localized, circular, whitish and avascular, atrophic skin areas surrounded by dilated capillaries and sometimes hyperpigmentation. This is a sign of severe CVI and must be distinguished from a healed ulcer.

Corona phlebectatica—Fan-shaped pattern of numerous small intradermal veins on the medial or lateral aspects of the ankle or foot. This is also known as malleolar or ankle flare. It is thought to be an early sign of advanced CVI.

Eczema—Erythematous dermatitis that can progress to blistering, weeping, or scaling eruption of the skin of the leg. It may be a result of uncontrolled CVI or sensitization to local topical therapy.

Edema—Increase in volume of the fluid in the skin and subcutaneous tissue, characteristically indented with pressure.

Lipodermatosclerosis—Localized chronic inflammation and fibrosis of skin and subcutaneous tissues of the lower leg, sometimes associated with scarring or contracture of the Achilles tendon. This is a sign of severe CVI, and patients are susceptible to repeated bouts of cellulitis with staphylococci or streptococci.

Pigmentation—Brownish darkening of the skin, caused by extravasated blood. This usually occurs in the ankle area.

Reticular vein—Dilated bluish subdermal vein, usually 1 to 3 mm in diameter and tortuous. Synonyms include blue veins, subdermal varices, and venulectasias.

Telangiectasia—Confluence of dilated intradermal venules less than 1 mm in diameter. Synonym is spider veins.

Varicose vein—Subcutaneous dilated vein 3 mm in diameter or larger, measured with patient in the upright position. Varicose veins are usually tortuous. Synonyms include varix, varices, and varicosities.

Venous ulcer—Full-thickness defect of the skin, most frequently in the ankle region, that fails to heal spontaneously and is sustained by CVI.

Differential Diagnosis

The differential diagnosis of CVI includes several other conditions that can cause signs and symptoms of CVI.

– Peripheral arterial disease. Arterial insufficiency can cause pain on exercise, pain in the leg at rest, and skin ulceration. Absence of peripheral pulses or measurement of an ankle-brachial index may exclude arterial disease as a complicating factor. Elderly patients commonly have concomitant venous and arterial insufficiency.

– Congestive heart failure. Patients with congestive heart failure, especially with elevated right heart pressure and tricuspid regurgitation, may have edema mimicking the early signs of CVI.

– Myositis and arteritis. Patients can have muscle pain that is exacerbated by exercise and relieved by rest. The muscles can be tender to palpation. Patients usually have an elevated erythrocyte sedimentation rate.

– DVT or superficial thrombophlebitis. New or recurrent DVT can cause a sudden exacerbation in pain, swelling, and calf tenderness that can complicate preexisting CVI. Superficial thrombophlebitis causes inflammation of the vein and surrounding area and palpable cording of the affected vein.

– Arteriovenous fistulae. Arteriovenous fistulae can cause pain, varicose veins, and ulcerations similar to CVI. The diagnosis should be suspected in a young patient with a hot and enlarged limb. Flow murmurs can sometimes be detected over the main limb arteries.

– Lymphedema. Lymphedema may cause ankle swelling that is especially prominent, but usually the skin is healthy with few varicose veins.

– Dermatitis. Primary or secondary dermatitis due to topical preparations can mimic skin findings of CVI. A careful history and examination of other skin area helps to distinguish this entity from CVI. Neomycin, bacitracin, and silver sulfadiazine have been found to cause contact dermatitis. Although avoidance of these compounds is important, minor reactions may be treated with topical corticosteroids.

– Cutaneous vasculitis. White patches and scarring typically occur on the toes or feet without the other signs of CVI.

– Rheumatoid arthritis. Patients may present with acute pain and redness over joints, with immobility.

– Cellulitis. This can be distinguished from acute lipodermatosclerosis by the presence of fever, lymphangitis, and elevated leukocyte count in the blood, or inguinal lymphadenopathy.

– Neurologic disorders. Peripheral neuropathy, musculoskeletal deformity of the ankle, ulcers, and edema can all be caused by neurologic disease.

– Trauma. Mechanical trauma to the skin can produce skin findings and ulcerations similar to CVI. A careful history is crucial in this case.

Diagnostic Testing

Duplex ultrasonography has become the favored technique for evaluation of CVI because of its wide availability and ease of use. It provides information regarding venous anatomy and the direction of venous flow; it has been found to be highly sensitive for evaluation of saphenous reflux, although less sensitive for identification of incompetent perforating veins. Duplex ultrasonography is used initially to identify and characterize the degree of venous flow obstruction from preexisting DVT. For evaluation of venous reflux, the patient is usually examined standing or lying in the reverse Trendelenburg position. In a patient with competent venous valves, manual calf compression produces antegrade venous flow without evidence of flow reversal on relaxation. Reflux is demonstrated by reversal of flow on relaxation after muscle contraction lasting at least 0.5 second, which may be identified by change in direction of flow by Doppler alone or by change in color (typically blue to red) using color flow Doppler. Reflux can usually be elicited by duplex ultrasonography in all vein segments, including the deep veins, superficial veins, and perforator veins in persons with venous insufficiency.

Venography remains the reference standard for evaluation of venous anatomy. Ascending venography is used to show evidence of venous obstruction, recanalization, and collaterals that are a result of DVT. Applying a tourniquet just above or below the knee and noting whether contrast dye fills the superficial veins below the level of the tourniquet can demonstrate valvular reflux through incompetent perforating veins. More commonly, descending venography is used for evaluation of venous reflux. Usually, contrast dye is injected into the common femoral vein above the saphenofemoral junction with the patient in the supine position, allowing visualization of both the deep and superficial veins. Upon tilting the table downward, some contrast dye leaking down the veins of the proximal thigh is normal, but reflux to the level of the knee or distally is abnormal and indicates incompetent valves.

Computed tomography (CT) and magnetic resonance imaging (MRI) have been used to evaluate patients with CVI. CT venography requires less contrast dye compared with ascending venography. Traditional CT often incidentally detects thrombosis in the inferior vena cava or iliac veins. It can be used to show the extent of vascular malformations and involvement of adjacent structures. Because of its advantage in showing tissue detail, MRI is most helpful in distinguishing abnormalities of the veins from abnormalities of the surrounding tissues. Characteristic findings of CVI on MRI include fibrosis, fasciosclerosis, and degenerative changes of the muscle. MR venography can also detect DVT, but its use is limited by expense and availability.

Functional testing with photoplethysmography, air plethysmography, or strain-gauge plethysmography can be used to evaluate efficiency of venous filling and emptying. Venous insufficiency is indicated by lack of a decrease of venous volume in the legs with exercise. Plethysmography detects volume changes in the calf as blood is expelled during exercise and refills at rest. Both venous outflow and reflux can be evaluated; outflow is seen as a rise in the curve, and reflux is determined by the time it takes the curve to return to a steady level, known as the venous refilling time. In normal legs, the venous refilling time should be at least 25 seconds. Refill times less than 25 seconds indicate the presence of deep venous reflux. Application of tourniquets to the superficial veins can help determine the contribution of deep versus superficial venous reflux.

- Duplex ultrasonography is the most common test to evaluate valvular incompetence or deep venous obstruction resulting in CVI
- Ascending or descending venography is used rarely to diagnose venous obstruction or valvular incompetence
- Functional testing using plethysmography is less available but is helpful in determining the extent and nature of venous valvular insufficiency

Treatment

Medical

Edema Reduction. Reduction of edema is the most important element of treatment of CVI to minimize discomfort and tissue changes. Swelling can be reduced by complementary techniques, including leg elevation, external compression therapy with wrapping or stockings, or compression pumping.

When the legs are elevated above the heart, the venous pressure is zero and tissue fluid can be absorbed. While sitting, a patient's feet should be higher than the hips, and while supine, the feet should be elevated higher than the heart. Active calf exercises with the feet elevated also decrease venous pressure by promoting venous drainage toward the heart. Patients should strive for elevation of the legs above heart level for 30 minutes up to four times a day.

Compression therapy with external wraps is used initially to reduce edema before fitting of maintenance compression support hose or is used long term for a patient with an odd-shaped leg. Application of external pressure of 20 mm Hg or more reduces the capillary and venous transmural pressure, lowers capillary permeability and interstitial fluid production, and increases interstitial pressure, thereby reducing edema. In addition, compression therapy can enhance fibrinolysis and venous ulcer healing. Compression therapy has been found to improve the quality of life for patients with CVI. The pressure should be applied maximally at the ankle to just below the knee. Compression stockings of at least 30 mm Hg pressure can be custom fitted and should be worn daily. Compression therapy is contraindicated in patients with known arterial insufficiency and an ankle-brachial index less than 0.7.

Compression pumping or sequential pneumatic compression may be used to reduce edema acutely before applying compression wrapping. There is some evidence that sequential pneumatic compression hastens ulcer healing.

Drug Therapy. Drug therapy for CVI usually involves diuretics and antibiotics. Diuretics can improve swelling in the short term, but the effects are modest and not sustained. Patients with acute lipodermatosclerosis may appear to have cellulitis. However, antibiotics are not useful in treating this condition, and compression therapy is preferred. Horse chestnut seed extract has been given orally to patients with CVI. A recent systematic review of randomized controlled trials indicated decreased pain and leg volume with this extract versus placebo in patients with known CVI. Aspirin in dosages of 300 to 325 mg/d has been found in one trial to accelerate the healing of venous ulcers.

Skin Care. Skin care is important for preventing secondary infection in patients with CVI who have eczematous changes and other cutaneous manifestations. Patients should practice good hygiene and use gentle protective dressings to protect areas most at risk. Exfoliation may be accomplished with 10% to 20% urea cream.

Treatment of Ulcers. Ulcer therapy involves treatment of the limb, surrounding skin, and the ulcer itself and is performed most effectively by a trained wound care specialist. Simple physical measures include elevation of the limb, compression therapy using multilayer bandaging, and weight control. Multilayer bandaging consists of applying an absorbent layer of cotton next to the skin, one or two elastic wraps, and an outer adherent layer to hold the inner bandages in place. An initial regimen for ulcer care involves washing the ulcer and surrounding skin with plain warm water. Debridement of sloughing or scaling skin may be done daily. Wet-to-dry dressings with normal saline on mesh cloth gauze or application of a hydrocolloid may be used to debride the ulcer. Topical antibiotics should be used sparingly because they can cause skin sensitivity. Surrounding eczema may be treated with a dilute corticosteroid cream such as 1% hydrocortisone. An Unna boot, consisting of a paste mixture of zinc oxide, calamine, and gelatin applied to the ulcer with an overlying compression bandage, is commonly used to treat ulcers and usually requires replacement weekly, with most ulcers healing within 4 weeks. Most ulcers smaller than 10 cm^2 can be healed with this regimen.

Larger ulcers can require skin grafting. Split-skin grafting is tedious and expensive because the graft may not "take" initially and can require a prolonged hospital stay. Pinch grafting creates islands of re-epithelialization and promotes ulcer healing by release of growth factors; it can be performed as an outpatient procedure. Artificial skin substitutes have been developed and are used, but data are lacking on their efficacy. As mentioned above, sequential pneumatic compression may hasten ulcer healing.

- Reduction of swelling is the most important treatment in preventing tissue complications of CVI
- Low-dose diuretics have only a modest role in reducing edema
- Small ulcers may be treated effectively by a systematic, medical wound care regimen administered by a trained therapist
- Large ulcers may require attempts at skin grafting with animal or artificial skin grafts

Surgical/Endovascular

Patients with CVI due to venous obstruction represent a minority, but they tend to have the most severe symptoms, including venous claudication, and benefit least from compression therapy. In these patients, venous bypass or stenting may be used. The most widely known femorofemoral crossover venous bypass (Palma operation) uses the contralateral greater saphenous vein with anastomosis to the more patent segment of the common femoral, femoral, or deep femoral vein, thereby relieving venous obstruction. Patency at 5 years has been shown to be greater than 75%. Endovascular techniques with venous angioplasty and stent placement have been used to treat inferior vena cava and iliac vein obstruction. The long-term patency of these techniques is unknown.

Venous valvuloplasty can be performed directly by shortening the redundant floppy valve cusp edges or indirectly by narrowing the dilated valve sinus so the cusps have greater contact. Prosthetic valve transplant has been used to treat CVI but is still experimental.

Vein interruption of incompetent perforating veins decreases venous pressure and is aimed at healing ulcers. The traditional Linton procedure involves subfascial ligation of all the perforating veins from the ankle to the proximal calf. Modified Linton procedures involve a less-extensive incision with selective perforator vein ligation. The SEPS procedure (subfascial endoscopic perforator surgery) has largely replaced the Linton procedure. In SEPS, an endoscope is placed into the posterior compartment of the calf, and perforating veins are interrupted under direct endoscopic visualization. Although SEPS is less invasive than an open procedure, there is still no convincing evidence that it is superior to the best medical therapy for healing of ulcers.

Catheter-based ablation of a varicose greater saphenous vein has been used to treat painful varicose veins and venous ulcers. In radiofrequency endovenous occlusion, radiofrequency energy is delivered through an endovenous electrode to cause controlled heating of the vessel wall, vein shrinkage, or occlusion. Adverse events include a low rate of DVT and subsequent pulmonary embolism, skin burn, clinical phlebitis, and small areas of skin paresthesia that can last 6 to 12 months. Endovenous laser ablation of the greater saphenous vein creates vein occlusion by delivery of laser energy directly into the vein lumen. Heating of the vein wall causes collagen contraction and denudation of the endothelium, which results in vein wall thickening with eventual vein contraction and fibrosis.

Chemical sclerotherapy involves injection of a potent sclerosing agent, most commonly 0.5% to 3% sodium tetradecyl sulphate or 0.5% to 1% polidocanol prepared as foam, into the varicose vein, with angiographic or duplex ultrasonographic visualization. The morbidity of this procedure is low, with reported adverse effects of inflammation and pigmentation. Very rare reports of air embolism causing transient visual disturbances and confusional states with polidocanol microfoam are being investigated in current clinical trials in the United States and Europe. Gradual venous sclerosis and decompression of distal varicosities occurs over 8 to 12 weeks. The success rate is approximately 80%.

- Surgery for CVI involves venous bypass, vein valvuloplasty, or vein interruption aimed at creating improved antegrade venous flow with reduced reflux. Superficial vein surgery may be more effective for preventing ulcer recurrence than for improving ulcer healing
- Vein sclerotherapy, using radiofrequency ablation or laser- or chemical-induced vein sclerosis, is effective in reducing pain from varicose veins and healing venous ulcers

Lymphatic Diseases

Natural History

Lymphedema develops when the production of protein-rich interstitial fluid exceeds its transport proximally through the lymphatic channels. Either an overproduction of lymphatic fluid or a loss of lymphatic fluid transport can thus result in edema. Physiologic quantities of lymphatic fluid are normally returned to the central circulation via lymphatic channels. Disruption in this circulatory equilibrium can occur from changes in intra- or extracellular protein concentrations or altered arteriovenous hemodynamics. For example, elevated venous pressure can cause increased filtration of plasma from the venules into the interstitium. Local inflammation can cause increased capillary permeability with leakage of protein and fluid to the interstitium, causing an increase in lymph production. Both these conditions may result in lymphedema, but lymphedema, by definition, is the result of impaired removal of lymphatic fluid from the interstitium.

Lymphedema is classified as primary or secondary. Primary lymphedema is caused by an inherited defect in lymphatic development and function. About 1 in 10,000 persons younger than 20 years has primary lymphedema. The congenital form of primary lymphedema becomes apparent within the first 2 years of life in approximately 15%. Lymphedema praecox, which is detected from puberty into the early twenties, accounts for about 75% of primary cases. Lymphedema tarda is typically detected after age 35 years and accounts for less than 10% of cases of primary lymphedema. Secondary lymphedema results from acquired destruction of the lymphatic structures. This destruction is most commonly iatrogenic, secondary to node dissection at time of surgery, or occurs after infection. Secondary lymphedema most commonly affects the upper or lower extremities, but visceral lymphatic abnormalities can also occur with or without limb abnormalities.

- Lymphedema is the result of impaired transport of protein-rich lymphatic fluid from the interstitium
- Primary lymphedema is caused by an inherited defect of lymphatic development
- Secondary lymphedema results from acquired destruction of lymphatic structures
- Lymphedema is categorized by its age of onset: congenital, praecox, or tarda

Pathophysiology

Primary (Congenital) Lymphedema

Lymphedema can occur in a familial pattern and when congenital is known as Milroy disease. Although isolated cases of lymphedema are more common, lymphedema can be inherited in an autosomal dominant or recessive pattern. For example, an inherited form of Milroy disease is caused by missense mutations in a gene that encodes the vascular endothelial growth factor (VEGF)-3 receptor expressed in the lymphatic endothelium. Alterations in VEGF-3 receptor expression cause impaired lymphangiogenesis. Meige disease characterizes the autosomal dominantly inherited familial form of lymphedema praecox. It has been associated with mutations in the *FOXC2* gene. Primary lymphedema is associated with other syndromes such as Turner syndrome, Noonan syndrome, yellow nail syndrome, intestinal lymphangiectasia, and arteriovenous malformation.

Pathologically, primary lymphedema may be classified by its lymphographic appearance: hypoplasia (or obstruction) of lymphatics distal to the inguinal nodes; obstruction of pelvic lymphatic vessels with normal distal vessels; distal obstruction of peripheral lymphatics; hyperplasia of lymphatic vessels; or incompetent dilated lymphatic vessels or megalymphatics.

About one-third of all primary cases of lymphedema are caused by agenesis, hypoplasia, or obstruction of distal lymphatic vessels, with normal formation of more proximal channels. Females are more often affected than males, and the swelling is usually bilateral and mild. More than 50% of cases involve obstruction of the proximal lymphatics due to fibrosis. In such cases, the swelling tends to be severe and unilateral. Females are affected at a slightly higher rate. Patients with proximal lymphatic disease are more likely to have progression, which may eventually involve the distal lymphatics as well. Less commonly, bilateral hyperplasia or dilated megalymphatics occurs. This syndrome is more common in males and carries a worse prognosis.

- Milroy disease is the familial form of congenital lymphedema
- Meige disease is the familial form of lymphedema praecox
- Lymphedema may be classified by its lymphographic appearance: aplasia, proximal obstruction, distal obstruction, hyperplasia, and dilated megalymphatics

Secondary (Acquired) Lymphedema

Secondary lymphedema is more common than primary lymphedema and is caused by loss or obstruction of normal lymphatic channels. Secondary lymphedema has many causes (Table 4.2), which may be used to classify the type.

Bacterial Infection. Repeated episodes of cellulitis and lymphangitis can lead to inflammation and fibrosis of the lymphatic channels, eventually causing obstruction.

Table 4.2 Causes of Secondary Lymphedema

Bacterial infection (streptococci)
Parasitic infection (filariasis)
Malignancy
Trauma or tissue damage, including lymph node dissection
Inflammatory diseases (rheumatoid arthritis, dermatitis, psoriasis)
Prolonged immobility
Pregnancy
Factitious

Streptococci that infiltrate through small breaks in the skin are the most common infective organisms.

Parasitic Infection. Worldwide, filariasis is the most common cause of secondary lymphedema (elephantiasis). Filariasis is endemic in Africa, the northern parts of South America, the Caribbean, and India. Causative organisms include *Wuchereria bancrofti*, and *Brugia malayi* or *B timori*. Some *Brugia* species are found in North America and rarely cause lymphatic obstruction. These roundworms are introduced to humans via a mosquito vector, and they induce recurrent lymphangitis with characteristic eosinophilia indicating parasitic infection. They can be identified by blood specimen or complement fixation tests. Treatments include oral diethylcarbamazine or ivermectin.

Malignancy. Cancer that secondarily deposits in the lymph nodes, or primary lymphatic malignancies, such as Hodgkin or non-Hodgkin lymphoma, may cause obstruction of the lymph nodes. Malignancy of the soft tissues of the limbs can infiltrate and occlude lymphatic vessels. In men, lymphatic blockage is most commonly caused by prostate cancer and in women, by lymphoma.

Trauma and Tissue Damage. Lymph node biopsy and excision is one of the most common causes of secondary lymphedema. The incidence of upper extremity lymphedema is high after mastectomy with resection of axillary and chest-wall lymph nodes. Radiation therapy can also cause or exacerbate lymphedema by destroying lymph glands, causing necrosis and fibrosis. Swelling of the limb can occur many years after the surgical procedure, and cancer recurrence must be excluded. Other cancers in which block dissection of the lymph nodes is typical include malignant melanoma, cervical, ovarian, uterine, and vulvar cancers, and cancer of the testis, prostate, penis, and scrotum. Lymphedema can be precipitated by removal of a single enlarged lymph node for diagnostic purposes. Surgical removal of varicose veins in the legs or fat tissue under the arms may also cause lymphedema. Vein harvest for coronary artery bypass grafting or large or circumferential wounds of the leg, including burns, can also lead to lymphedema. Damage to the thoracic duct can cause incompetent lymphatics within the chest and abdomen resulting in chylothorax and chylous ascites.

Inflammatory Disease. Lymphedema occurs as a complication of rheumatoid arthritis, dermatitis, or psoriasis. Granulomatous diseases such as sarcoidosis and tuberculosis may also cause inflammatory changes of the lymph glands.

Other Causes. Edema secondary to prolonged immobility (paralysis) or CVI sometimes produces damage to the lymphatics because of increased capillary and venous pressure. Other causes of secondary lymphedema include factitious lymphedema (edema bleu) induced by application of tourniquets, self-inflicted cellulitis, and chronic subcutaneous inflammation causing lymphatic sclerosis. Lymphedema can also be precipitated by pregnancy or found in pretibial myxedema.

- Secondary lymphedema is more common than primary lymphedema
- Worldwide, parasitic infection with organisms causing filariasis is the most common cause of lymphedema (elephantiasis)

History and Physical Examination

Distribution and Progression

Lymphedema affects the lower extremities more commonly than the upper. Lymphedema of the arm is often accompanied by swelling of the posterior axillary fold. The distribution of swelling in the leg is determined by the site of lymphatic obstruction. If the distal lymphatics are affected, the patient presents with unilateral foot swelling, although both feet may be affected with one side worse. The edema then slowly spreads up the leg. If the obstruction to the lymphatics is more proximal, such as in the ilioinguinal area, swelling of the whole limb occurs, progressing downward, with most of the swelling in the thigh.

Appearance

The swelling that accompanies lymphedema can begin suddenly, but more commonly develops insidiously, worsening over months or years. Pain is rare, but when present should raise suspicion of cellulitis, and other causes of swelling should be evaluated if sudden pain develops in an acutely swollen limb. The skin may pit early in the process. Edema extending into the toes can cause the "square toes" characteristic of lymphedema. Swelling may decrease very slowly with elevation, and diuretics have little effect on reducing the edema. Skin changes include thickening with a peau d'orange appearance in some. The inability to pick up the skin of the base of the toes is called a positive Stemmer sign, which is highly specific but not sensitive for the diagnosis of lymphedema.

Excessive swelling may result in large skin folds separated by deep crevices (Fig. 4.3). Lymphatic fluid may leak

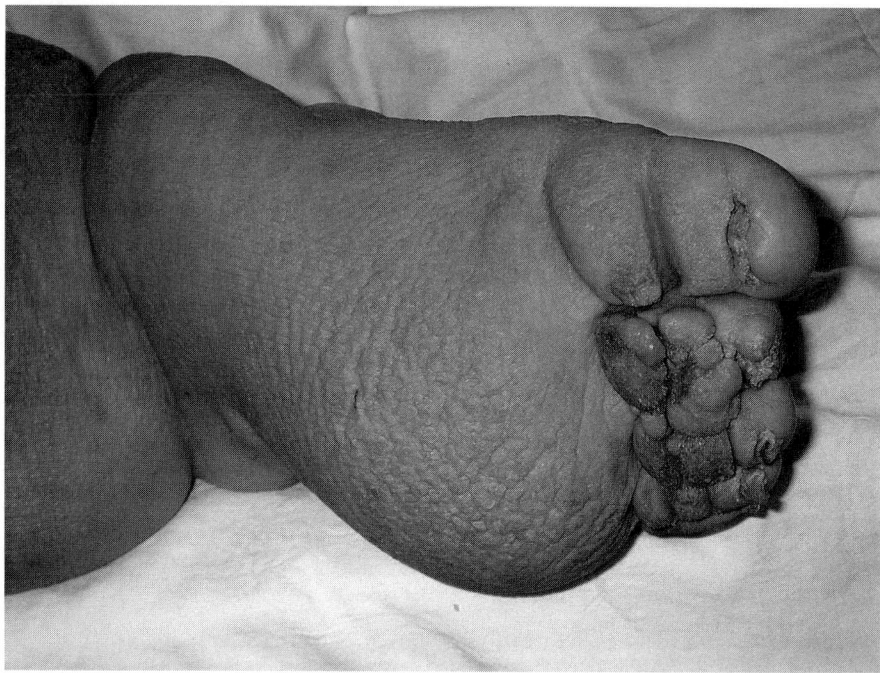

Fig. 4.3 Severe lymphedema of the right lower extremity, which shows the common complications of tinea pedis and onychomycosis.

through the skin via superficial vesicles. Over years, the skin becomes woody and the surrounding skin indurated and fibrotic and may no longer pit. As the proliferation of subcutaneous connective and adipose tissue progresses, the limb becomes grossly enlarged with a cobblestone appearance (elephantiasis).

Complications

With insidious development of lymphedema, pain is most likely minor. The patient may report achiness or heaviness of the limb and skin tightness rather than pain. As swelling becomes severe, function, such as the ability to exercise, can be impaired. Lymphedema sometimes causes psychological morbidity and, if developing in the early teens, may produce reclusiveness and a reluctance to take part in sports. Arm lymphedema can affect vocation, especially if it is in the dominant hand.

Lymphedema can predispose patients to recurrent bacterial infections, most commonly acute streptococcal infection. The patient may present with a history of 12 to 24 hours of generalized malaise followed by the appearance of an erythematous, hot, tender patch in the affected limb. The entire limb may become painful, and red streaks radiating proximally (lymphangitis) may develop. Systemic antibiotics should be taken as early as possible. Cellulitis tends to be recurrent in lymphedema. Fungal infections, especially tinea pedis, can complicate lymphedema (Fig. 4.3). A high percentage of patients with recurrent cellulitis also have tinea pedis. Chylous ascites may reflux into the legs. Although uncommon, long-standing lymphedema can undergo malignant degeneration, resulting in angiosarcomas or lymphangiosarcomas. Other malignancies associated with chronic lymphedema include lymphoma, Kaposi sarcoma, squamous cell cancer, and malignant melanoma.

- The inability to pinch the skin at the base of the toes is a positive Stemmer sign and is highly specific for lymphedema
- Complications of lymphedema include heaviness of the limb, recurrent cellulitis, functional and psychological impairment, cutaneous fungal infections, and, rarely, malignant degeneration

Differential Diagnosis

Lymphedema should be distinguished from other causes of chronic swelling. The differential diagnosis of lymphatic diseases includes several other conditions that can cause similar signs and symptoms.

Venous Disease

Lymphedema must be distinguished from DVT or CVI. Acute DVT presents with sudden pain and swelling and should be excluded by duplex ultrasonography. CVI usually causes pitting edema. Patients have exacerbation of swelling with prolonged sitting or standing, and pruritus may overlie incompetent varicose veins. Skin findings include dusky discoloration from hemosiderin deposition, venous engorgement with dependency, and readily apparent superficial varicosities.

Congestive Heart Failure

Congestive heart failure typically produces dependent pitting edema in both extremities. A history of cardiac disease with physical findings of elevated right heart pressure, including tricuspid regurgitation and jugular venous distension, and confirmatory echocardiographic findings can solidify the diagnosis.

Chronic Limb Dependence

Chronic limb dependence in patients with a sedentary lifestyle or with neurologic disorders can impair calf muscle pump action and venous return, causing edema that is usually confined to below the knee. Patients with cardiorespiratory disorders such as sleep apnea may sleep upright, thereby exacerbating edema by preventing venous drainage by elevation at night.

Myxedema

Myxedema due to thyroid disease can occur when hyaluronic acid–rich proteins are deposited in the dermis, producing edema and decreasing the elasticity of the skin. The process is focal in the pretibial area in thyrotoxicosis and more generalized in hypothyroidism. Other characteristic findings include roughening of the skin of the palms, soles, elbows, and knees, thinning hair, yellow discoloration of the skin, and decreased sweat production.

Lipedema

Lipedema can result from excessive deposition of fat in the subcutaneous tissue, usually occurring in the lower limbs, more commonly in women. The onset is usually at puberty or with pregnancy, suggesting a hormonal etiology. The distribution of fat is characteristic and results in a tourniquet effect around the ankle that spares the feet, with no Stemmer sign, which results in characteristic "skinny" feet. (Lymphedema is distinguished from lipedema by extension of edema into the foot and toes with a positive Stemmer sign.) The deposition of fat is symmetric and the skin remains soft. Weight loss results in loss of fat from non-lipedema areas such as the face, neck, and chest but does not appreciably decrease the size of the lipedema-affected extremity.

Other Conditions

Other conditions can also be distinguished from lymphedema, including reflex sympathetic dystrophy–related swelling, factitious edema, inflammatory skin disease such as eczema or psoriasis, diffuse forms of neurofibromatosis, and congenital gigantism.

Diagnostic Testing

Lymphangiography

Lymphangiography has been used in the past to visualize lymphatic channels. It is performed by injection of dye into the metatarsal web spaces to identify a distal lymphatic vessel. The vessel is subsequently cannulated, and iodinated contrast material is injected. The contrast dye can then be detected radiographically as it ascends through the lymphatic channels. The appearance of the lymphatics by this method can be characterized as follows:

- Aplasia may be indicated; no lymphatics are identified because none are available to cannulate.
- Distal hypoplasia or peripheral obliteration is diagnosed if fewer than five lymphatic channels enter into the inguinal lymph nodes. This is the most common finding in patients with mild distal lymphedema.
- Proximal obstruction is seen if the distal lymphatic channels are normal but the dye does not pass proximally beyond the inguinal lymph nodes because of severe fibrotic obstruction of the proximal lymph nodes. Proximal lymphatic obstruction may progress distally, causing distal lymphatic obliteration.
- An increased number of normally sized lymphatics can be found in males with early-onset lymphedema.
- Megalymphatic channels that are seen as dilated incompetent lymph vessels are usually unilateral and often seen in the pelvis, abdomen, and chest wall, as well as the limbs.
- The thoracic duct may be absent or fragmented, with multiple collateral channels visualized.

Lymphangiography is rarely performed because it requires frequent cut-downs to cannulate the lymphatic channel and causes lymphangitis in some patients.

Lymphoscintigraphy

Lymphoscintigraphy is performed after the indirect injection of a radiocontrast dye into the subcutaneous tissue or skin of the foot or hand. Usually, technetium-labeled colloids are used. Lymphoscintigraphy using a gamma camera provides an assessment of the clearance of large molecules from the interstitium with visualization of the distribution of tracer in the leg and uptake by the lymph nodes. Patterns of lymphatic channels can be similar to those described for lymphangiography. However, in lymphedema from any cause, the proximal progression of tracer is delayed. Accumulation distally produces "dermal backflow" into the dilated channels of the dermis. Lymphoscintigraphy is easy to perform and does not cause lymphangitis.

Imaging

CT or MRI may be used to identify secondary causes of lymphedema such as pelvic tumor or lymphoma. Lymphedema is characteristically seen as a honeycomb pattern on CT. CT can also indicate the extent of volume change and the compartments that are affected.

Ultrasonography

Ultrasonography can visualize the expanded subcutaneous compartments seen in lymphedema. For example, fluid may be found subepidermally in lipodermatosclerosis, deep dermally in heart failure, and uniformly through the dermis in lymphedema. Duplex ultrasonography is most useful for excluding other causes of edema such as DVT.

Other Studies

Chest radiography can indicate signs of chylothorax caused by thoracic duct injury or obstruction, which results in lymphatic dilatation and valvular incompetence. Echocardiography can show other causes of edema, including pulmonary hypertension and heart failure.

- Lymphangiography, although rarely used, shows the characteristic patterns of the lymphatic channels in lymphedema: aplasia, proximal obstruction, distal hypoplasia/obliteration, hyperplasia, or megalymphatics
- Lymphoscintigraphy is the most common test used to diagnose lymphedema. It shows the characteristic patterns of lymphedema as well as dermal backflow
- Other causes of swelling should be excluded by CT, MRI, or ultrasonography of the affected area.

Treatment

Edema Reduction

Limb elevation reduces swelling gradually and is less effective in lymphedema than in other disorders with edema. Elevation enhances the rate of lymphatic drainage only while the lymphatic channels are full; once they have collapsed, the benefit is minimal.

Compression wrapping with multilayer bandaging is designed to generate high pressures during activity—to resist the outward expansion of tissues during muscle contraction—and to maintain low pressures at rest, leading to a decrease in swelling and reversal of skin changes. Short-stretch bandages are preferable to long-stretch bandages.

Multicompartmental sequential compression devices or pumps have been used to improve short- and long-term outcomes in patients with lymphedema. The pump produces synchronized centripetal extrinsic compression of the lymphatics, causing propulsion of lymphatic fluid proximally. Non-synchronized pumps result in bidirectional flow of lymphatic fluid that can exacerbate distal lymphedema. Pumping may be used short term to decrease edema before application of wrapping or compression garments.

Diuretics have very little effect in decreasing the swelling associated with lymphedema. Diuretic use may concentrate protein in the interstitial space, thereby hardening the tissue.

Gene therapy to active VEGF-3 has led to development of functioning lymphatic channels in mouse models. This therapy is currently being investigated.

- Edema reduction, using limb elevation, compression wrapping, and pumping, is the most important component of lymphedema treatment
- Diuretics are of little use in the treatment of lymphedema

Maintenance Therapy

Compression support garments are used to maintain reduction in edema rather than to decrease it markedly. For good compliance, the patient should be carefully fitted for the compression garment after limb edema is maximally reduced. Management of lymphedema usually requires compression sleeves of at least 20 mm Hg for arms and at least 30 mm Hg for legs. Caution is required in patients with known arterial insufficiency. Other garments using foam-filled cylinders that may be applied at night are available.

Manual lymph drainage is a form of lymphatic massage performed and taught by trained therapists to direct lymph away from congested lymphatic areas. Manual lymph drainage focuses on the subcutaneous tissue rather than the muscle in quadrants where the lymphatic plexus is located.

Compression pumping, if used long term, can improve the cutaneous and functional outcomes of patients with lymphedema. Typically, it is used for 30 to 60 minutes once or twice daily on the affected limb.

- Maintenance reduction of lymphedema is accomplished through daily use of compression support garments, manual lymph drainage, and compression pumping

Preventive Measures

Limb protection can be accomplished by application of compression wraps or preventive elastic compression garments and prevents introduction of infection through the skin of the vulnerable limb. Tight jewelry, venipuncture, and injections should be avoided in the affected limb. An electric rather than manual razor should be used to remove unwanted hair.

Exercise is sometimes helpful in decreasing lymphedema. Isotonic exercises such as walking can decrease swelling. Swimming is particularly helpful because the hydrostatic pressure of the surrounding water mimics decompressive therapy. In patients with chylous obstruction, a no-fat diet with supplemental medium-chain triglycerides and vitamins can decrease the amount of chyle produced.

Skin care is important in preventing cellulitis. The skin should be washed daily with a mild antiseptic soap. An emollient can be applied twice daily to prevent fissuring and cracking of the skin. Nails should be trimmed regularly and well-fitting shoes worn. Fungal infections of the skin should be treated with topical antifungal agents.

Antibiotics for bacterial infection are given at first suspicion of cellulitis. Oral penicillin or erythromycin is the agent of first choice. If there is no improvement in 48 hours, the patient should be admitted for intravenous antibiotics. In patients with recurrent cellulitis, prophylactic maintenance antibiotics may be required. Penicillin 500 mg daily is one accepted regimen. Alternatively, benzathine penicillin, 1.2 million units given intramuscularly monthly, has been shown to significantly decrease the number of recurrent bacterial infections. Aggressive treatment of superficial fungal infection with topical or systemic antifungal agents is warranted to prevent chronic inflammation and susceptibility to recurrent cellulitis.

Tumor surveillance for malignant deterioration should occur at routine visits. The patient should report any changes of the skin that could indicate malignant transformation of the blood or lymphatic vessels.

- Attention to skin care using physical protection, emollients, and antibiotics for prevention and treatment of cellulitis and fungal infection decreases the complications of lymphedema
- Aerobic isotonic exercise may improve edema
- Patients should report any skin changes that could indicate malignant transformation

Surgical Procedures

Surgery should be reserved as a last resort for patients with limbs so large and deformed that they cause functional impairment. Surgical procedures include lymphaticovenous anastomosis to allow lymphatic fluid below the obstruction to flow directly into the venous system; excisional procedures involving resection of a portion of the skin and subcutaneous tissue to decrease limb diameter; and liposuction for patients in whom excessive adipose formation in the subdermis is a major contributor to the excess volume of the lymphedematous extremity.

Questions

1. Calf pump failure syndrome refers to:
  a. Injury to the calf muscle resulting in pain with ambulation
  b. Swelling in the calf muscle secondary to congestive heart failure
  c. Secondary varicose veins resulting from retrograde venous flow through incompetent perforator veins
  d. Congenital absence of the calf muscle pump

2. Which of the following statements about May-Thurner syndrome is correct?
  a. It is caused by the left iliac artery.
  b. It may predispose to right lower extremity venous thrombosis.
  c. It may arise during pregnancy.
  d. Everybody has May-Thurner syndrome.

3. A 42-year-old woman presents to your office reporting painful varicose veins. She works as a ward nurse on the night shift and has 3 healthy children; she has no other significant medical history. She reports no trauma to her legs. Physical examination shows mild hyperpigmentation of the ankles with minimal edema (left leg worse than right) and a prominent varicose vein in the distribution of the greater saphenous vein that compresses easily with palpation and is not tender. Spider veins are noticeable on the medial thigh. The best course of action is:
  a. Schedule the patient for chemical sclerotherapy to remove the painful vein
  b. Perform venography to exclude DVT
  c. Perform the Trendelenburg test at the bedside
  d. Prescribe bed rest and analgesics until the vein pain resolves

4. Which one of the following statements is true?
  a. For treatment of CVI, diuretics are the therapy of choice.
  b. Reduction of edema is the most important component of treatment for venous insufficiency.
  c. Small, shallow, venous ulcers should be treated with skin grafting before they have an opportunity to enlarge.

d. The SEPS procedure involves open subfascial ligation of incompetent superficial varicose veins.

5. Worldwide, the most common cause of lymphedema is:
a. Cat-scratch disease
b. Preexisting CVI
c. Filariasis
d. Milroy disease

6. A 17-year-old girl is referred to you for leg swelling. Her mother reports that the girl has been overweight since beginning puberty at 10 years of age, but during the last year, her daughter has noticed that her left leg is swollen, especially at the ankle. She has no pain with rest or ambulation but is reluctant to wear shorts in the summer. Physical examination indicates a well-developed obese adolescent with pitting edema of the left ankle and foot. The dorsum of the foot is swollen but warm to the touch, with no erythema or tenderness on palpation. Noticeable superficial fungal infection is present between the toes. Handheld Doppler examination indicates normal arterial results, phasic flow in the popliteal vein, and no evidence of deep venous reflux. Which one of the following statements is true?
a. If the patient feels discomfort when you pinch her toes, she most likely has lymphedema.
b. Because the patient is obese, excess adipose tissue causing enlargement of one extremity is normal, and no further evaluation is warranted.
c. The swelling will likely resolve on its own as the patient reaches adulthood.
d. The patient is susceptible to recurrent bacterial infections of the skin.

Suggested Readings

Andreozzi GM, Cordova R, Scomparin MA, et al, Quality of Life Working Group on Vascular Medicine of SIAPAV. Effects of elastic stocking on quality of life of patients with chronic venous insufficiency: an Italian pilot study on Triveneto Region. Int Angiol. 2005;24:325-9.

Barwell JR, Davies CE, Deacon J, et al. Comparison of surgery and compression with compression alone in chronic venous ulceration (ESCHAR study): randomised controlled trial. Lancet. 2004;363:1854-9.

Bradbury AW, Ruckley CV. Chronic venous insufficiency. In: Creager MA, editor. Atlas of vascular disease. 2nd ed. Philadelphia: Current Medicine, Inc; 2003. p. 229-40.

Browse N, Burnand KG, Mortimer PS. Diseases of the lymphatics. London: Arnold; 2003. p. 102-78.

Browse NL, Burnand KG, Irvine AT, et al. Diseases of the veins. 2nd ed. London: Arnold; 1999. p. 385-427; 443-503; 571-603.

Cooke JP, Rooke TW. Lymphedema. In: Loscalzo J, Creager MA, Dzau VJ, editors. Vascular medicine: a textbook of vascular biology and diseases. 2nd ed. Boston: Little, Brown and Company; 1996. p. 1133-46.

Cornu-Thenard A, Boivin P, Baud JM, et al. Importance of the familial factor in varicose disease: clinical study of 134 families. J Dermatol Surg Oncol. 1994;20:318-26.

Donaldson MC. Chronic venous disorders. In: Loscalzo J, Creager MA, Dzau VJ, editors. Vascular medicine: a textbook of vascular biology and diseases. 2nd ed. Boston: Little, Brown and Company; 1996. p. 1081-102.

Eklof B, Rutherford RB, Bergan JJ, et al, American Venous Forum International Ad Hoc Committee for Revision of the CEAP Classification. Revision of the CEAP classification for chronic venous disorders: consensus statement. J Vasc Surg. 2004;40:1248-52.

Guex JJ, Allaert FA, Gillet JL, et al. Immediate and midterm complications of sclerotherapy: report of a prospective multicenter registry of 12,173 sclerotherapy sessions. Dermatol Surg. 2005;31:123-8.

Karkkainen MJ, Saaristo A, Jussila L, et al. A model for gene therapy of human hereditary lymphedema. Proc Natl Acad Sci U S A. 2001 Oct 23;98:12677-82. Epub 2001 Oct 9.

Khaira HS, Parnell A. Colour flow duplex in the assessment of varicose veins. Clin Radiol. 1995;50:583-4.

Layton AM, Ibbotson SH, Davies JA, et al. Randomised trial of oral aspirin for chronic venous leg ulcers. Lancet. 1994;344:164-5.

List-Hellwig E, Meents H. Magnetic resonance imaging and computed tomography in advanced chronic venous insufficiency. Curr Probl Dermatol. 1999;27:109-13.

Pittler MH, Ernst E. Horse chestnut seed extract for chronic venous insufficiency. Cochrane Database Syst Rev. 2002;1: CD003230. Update in: Cochrane Database Syst Rev. 2004;2: CD003230.

Rockson S. Lymphatic disease. In: Creager MA, editor. Atlas of vascular disease. 2nd ed. Philadelphia: Current Medicine, Inc; 2003. p. 241-53.

Venous disease primer. American College of Phlebology [homepage on the Internet]. California: ACP Headquarters [cited 2006 Sept 1]. Available from: http://www.phlebology.org/.

5 Thrombophilia*

John A. Heit, MD

Introduction

Symptomatic thrombosis is caused by dysregulation of the normal hemostatic response to vessel wall "injury" that occurs with exposure to a clinical risk factor (e.g., surgery, trauma, or hospitalization for acute medical illness). Vessel wall injury may be anatomic (e.g., venous endothelial microtears within vein valve cusps due to stasis or rupture of a lipid-rich atherosclerotic plaque) or "non-anatomic" (e.g., cytokine-mediated endothelial expression of adhesion molecules or downregulation of thrombomodulin expression, related to the "acute inflammatory response"). However, the vast majority of persons exposed to a clinical risk factor do not have development of symptomatic thrombosis. We now recognize that clinical thrombosis is a multifactorial and complex disease that becomes manifest when a person with an underlying predisposition to thrombosis ("thrombophilia[s]") is exposed to additional risk factors. Emerging evidence suggests that individual variation in the regulation of the procoagulant, anticoagulant, fibrinolytic, and acute inflammation or innate immunity pathways most likely accounts for the development of clinical thrombosis in exposed persons.

Thrombophilia is defined as a predisposition to thrombosis. Thrombophilia is not a disease per se, but may be associated with a disease (e.g., cancer), with drug exposure (e.g., oral contraceptives), or with a specific condition (e.g., pregnancy or post partum—"acquired thrombophilia" [Table 5.1]); thrombophilia may also be inherited (Table 5.2). This concept is important because disease susceptibility does not imply an absolute requirement for primary or secondary prevention or for treatment. In most persons with a thrombophilia, thrombosis does not develop. Thus, thrombophilia(s) must be considered in the context of other risk factors for incident thrombosis or predictors of recur-

*Portions of this manuscript have been previously published in Heit JA. Venous thromboembolism: disease burden, outcomes and risk factors. J Thromb Haemost. 2005;3:1611-7. Used with permission. Supported in part by research grants HL66216, HL83141, HL83797, and RR19457 from the National Institutes of Health and research grant TS1255 from the Centers for Disease Control and Prevention, United States Public Health Service; and by Mayo Foundation.

Table 5.1 Acquired or Secondary Thrombophilia

Definite causes of thrombophilia
Active malignant neoplasm
Chemotherapy (L-asparaginase, thalidomide, antiangiogenesis therapy)
Myeloproliferative disorders
Heparin-induced thrombocytopenia and thrombosis
Nephrotic syndrome
Intravascular coagulation and fibrinolysis/disseminated intravascular coagulation
Thrombotic thrombocytopenic purpura
Sickle cell disease
Oral contraceptives
Estrogen therapy
Pregnancy/postpartum state
Tamoxifen and raloxifene therapy (selective estrogen receptor modulator)
Antiphospholipid antibodies (lupus anticoagulant, anticardiolipin antibody, anti–β2-glycoprotein-1 antibody)
Paroxysmal nocturnal hemoglobinuria
Wegener granulomatosis
Probable causes of thrombophilia
Inflammatory bowel disease
Thromboangiitis obliterans (Buerger disease)
Behçet syndrome
Varicose veins
Systemic lupus erythematosus
Venous vascular anomalies (Klippel-Trénaunay syndrome)
Progesterone therapy
Infertility treatments
Hyperhomocysteinemia
Human immunodeficiency virus infection
Dehydration

Table 5.2 Hereditary (Familial or Primary) Thrombophilia

Definite causes of thrombophilia
Antithrombin III deficiency
Protein C deficiency
Protein S deficiency
Activated protein C resistance
Factor V Leiden mutation
Prothrombin G20210A mutation
Homocystinuria
Probable causes of thrombophilia
Increased plasma factors I (fibrinogen), II (prothrombin), VIII, IX, and XI
Hyperhomocysteinemia
Dysfibrinogenemia
Hypoplasminogenemia and dysplasminogenemia
Hypofibrinolysis
Reduced protein Z and Z-dependent protease inhibitor
Reduced tissue factor pathway inhibitor
Possible causes of thrombophilia
Tissue plasminogen activator deficiency
Increased plasminogen activator inhibitor levels
Methylene tetrahydrofolate reductase polymorphisms
Factor XIII polymorphisms
Increased thrombin-activatable fibrinolysis inhibitor

rent thrombosis, when estimating the need for primary or secondary prophylaxis, respectively. With rare exceptions, the therapy for acute thrombosis is no different for persons with and without a recognized thrombophilia.

- Thrombophilia is a predisposition or susceptibility to thrombosis
- Thrombophilia is not a disease, but may be associated with a disease, drug exposure, or a condition, or may be inherited
- When estimating the need for primary or secondary prophylaxis, thrombophilia(s) must be considered in the context of other risk factors for incident thrombosis or predictors of recurrent thrombosis, respectively
- With rare exceptions, therapy for acute thrombosis is the same for those with and without a recognized thrombophilia

Thrombophilia may present clinically as one or more of several thrombotic manifestations or "phenotypes" (Table 5.3). The predominant clinical manifestation of thrombophilia is venous thromboembolism (VTE). Although it is biologically plausible to hypothesize that patients with atherosclerotic arterial occlusive disease and an underlying thrombophilia who have an atherosclerotic plaque rupture are more likely to have a symptomatic thrombosis, most clinical studies have failed to show a consistent association between thrombophilia and myocardial infarction or stroke.

Table 5.3 Clinical Manifestations of Thrombophilia

Definite manifestations
Purpura fulminans (neonatalis or adult)
Superficial or deep vein thrombosis, pulmonary embolism
Thrombosis of "unusual" venous circulations (cerebral, hepatic, mesenteric, and renal veins; possibly arm, portal, and ovarian veins; not retinal vein or artery)
Warfarin-induced skin necrosis
Possible manifestations
Arterial thrombosis (stroke, acute myocardial infarction)
(Recurrent) fetal loss
Intrauterine growth restriction
Stillbirth
Severe gestational hypertension (preeclampsia)
Abruptio placentae

Unfortunately, no single laboratory assay or simple set of assays can identify all thrombophilias. Consequently, a battery of complex and potentially expensive assays is usually required. Many of the analytes measured in the laboratory are affected by other conditions (e.g., warfarin decreases protein C and S levels), such that the correct interpretation of the results can be complicated and always requires clinical correlation. Detailed descriptions of the known thrombophilias are included in this chapter, as well as information on special coagulation laboratory interpretation.

- The predominant clinical manifestation of thrombophilia is VTE

Indications for Thrombophilia Testing: Why Should I Test for Thrombophilia?

There are no absolute indications for clinical diagnostic thrombophilia testing. Potential relative indications could include the following:
– Selected screening of populations that are potentially "enriched" for thrombophilia (e.g., asymptomatic or symptomatic family members of patients with a known familial thrombophilia, especially first-degree relatives);
– Selected screening of populations at increased risk for thrombosis (e.g., before pregnancy, use of oral contraception or estrogen therapy, before high-risk surgery, or during chemotherapy with angiogenesis inhibitors);
– Testing of symptomatic patients with an incident thrombotic event (e.g., incident VTE, stillbirth or another com-

plication of pregnancy, incident arterial thrombosis in a young person without other arterial disease);
– Testing of symptomatic patients with recurrent thrombosis, "idiopathic" thrombosis, thrombosis at a young age (e.g., ≤40 years for venous thrombosis, ≤50 years for arterial thrombosis) or thrombosis in unusual vascular territory (e.g., cerebral vein, portal vein, hepatic vein, mesenteric vein, or artery).

With the exception of general population screening, which is not recommended, all of these potential indications are controversial and must be considered in the context of the clinical presentation.

Counseling and Screening Asymptomatic Family Members

Thrombophilia testing, especially genetic testing, of asymptomatic family members should be done with caution. Family members (and patients) should receive genetic counseling before genetic testing, and such testing should only be performed after obtaining consent. Counseling should include the reasons for testing, such as the potential for avoiding clinical thrombosis by risk factor modification or prophylaxis (both for the family member as well as his or her children), and the reasons for not testing, such as stigmatization and mental anguish, the potential effect on obtaining personal health insurance or employment, and the possibility of non-paternity.

Thrombophilia testing should only be done if the results are likely to change medical management. The risk of idiopathic ("unprovoked") thrombosis associated with a thrombophilia, although increased, is still insufficient to warrant chronic primary prophylaxis (e.g., warfarin anticoagulation therapy), even for thrombophilias with high penetrance (e.g., antithrombin deficiency or homozygous factor V Leiden carriers) with the possible exception of paroxysmal nocturnal hemoglobinuria. Thus, primary "prophylaxis" typically involves either avoidance or modification of risk exposure or specific prophylactic measures if such exposures are unavoidable.

When counseling a family member (or patient) regarding the risk of thrombosis associated with a thrombophilia, it is most useful to provide the "absolute" risk or incidence of thrombosis among persons with that particular thrombophilia. For example, the relative risk of VTE among women who are factor V Leiden carriers and using oral contraceptives is increased about 30-fold; however, the incidence is only about 300 per 100,000 woman-years, or about 0.3% per woman-year. Thus, the absolute risk provides information on both the baseline risk of VTE (about 10-46 per 100,000 woman-years for women of reproductive age) as well as the relative risk (about 30 for female factor V Leiden carriers using oral contraceptives).

Estimation of the absolute risk of thrombosis should especially account for the effect of age on the baseline incidence of VTE. For example, among women of perimenopausal age (50-54 years), the incidence of VTE is 123 per 100,000 woman-years, which increases exponentially with increasing age (Fig. 5.1). Among female factor V Leiden carriers of perimenopausal age, the relative risk of VTE associated with hormone therapy may be increased 7- to 15-fold. However, whereas the relative risk for VTE is less with the use of hormone therapy than with use of oral contraceptives, the absolute risk is substantially higher (≈900-1,800 per 100,000 woman-years, ≈1%-2% per woman-year) because of the increased incidence with age. Given recent studies questioning the benefit of postmenopausal hormone therapy, most women likely would choose to avoid such therapy if they were known to be factor V Leiden car-

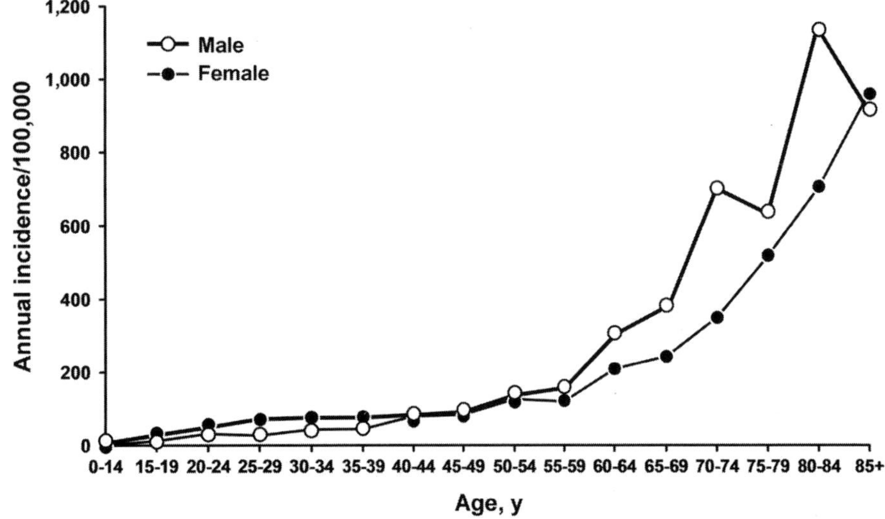

Fig. 5.1 Annual incidence of venous thromboembolism by age and sex. (From Silverstein MD, Heit JA, Mohr DN, et al. Trends in the incidence of deep vein thrombosis and pulmonary embolism: a 25-year population-based study. Arch Intern Med. 1998;158:585-93. Used with permission.)

riers. Thus, it may be relatively cost-effective to perform thrombophilia screening of an asymptomatic perimenopausal or postmenopausal woman with a known family history of thrombophilia who is considering hormone therapy.

Primary Prevention of Incident VTE

Primary prevention of VTE, either by risk factor modification or by appropriate prophylaxis for patients at risk, is essential to improve survival and prevent complications. However, despite improved prophylaxis regimens and more widespread use of prophylaxis, the overall incidence of VTE has been relatively constant at about 1 per 1,000 since 1979.

To avoid or modify risk or appropriately target prophylaxis, patients at risk for VTE must first be identified. In the absence of a central venous catheter or active cancer, the incidence of VTE among children and adolescents is very low (<1 per 100,000 for age ≤15 years). The incidence increases exponentially after age 50 years, eventually reaching about 1,000 per 100,000 for persons aged 85 years or older. The incidence of VTE increases significantly with age for both idiopathic and secondary VTE, which suggests that the risk associated with advancing age may be due to the biology of aging rather than simply to an increased exposure to VTE risk factors with advancing age. The incidence is slightly higher for women during childbearing years and for men after age 50 years. The incidence of VTE also varies by race. Compared with white Americans, black Americans have a 30% higher incidence and Asian and Native Americans have up to a 70% lower incidence; Hispanics have an incidence intermediate between whites and Asian Americans.

Additional independent risk factors for VTE are shown in Table 5.4. Compared with persons in the community, hospitalized patients have a greater than 150-fold increased incidence of acute VTE. The population-attributable risk provides an estimate of the burden of disease in the community that is attributable to a particular risk factor. For example, the risk factors of hospitalization and nursing home residence together account for almost 60% of all incident VTE events occurring in the community. Thus, hospital confinement provides an important opportunity to substantially decrease VTE incidence. Of note, hospitalization for medical illness and surgery account for almost equal proportions of VTE (22% and 24%, respectively), which emphasizes the need to provide prophylaxis to both of these risk groups.

- Primary "prophylaxis" involves either avoidance or modification of risk exposure or specific prophylactic measures if such exposures are unavoidable

Table 5.4 Independent Risk Factors for Deep Vein Thrombosis or Pulmonary Embolism

Baseline characteristic	Odds ratio	95% Confidence interval
Hospitalization		
For acute medical illness	7.98	4.49-14.18
For major surgery	21.72	9.44-49.93
Trauma	12.69	4.06-39.66
Malignancy		
Without chemotherapy	4.05	1.93-8.52
With chemotherapy	6.53	2.11-20.23
Prior central venous catheter or transvenous pacemaker	5.55	1.57-19.58
Prior superficial vein thrombosis	4.32	1.76-10.61
Neurologic disease with extremity paresis	3.04	1.25-7.38
Serious liver disease	0.10	0.01-0.71

From Heit JA, Silverstein MD, Mohr DN, et al. Risk factors for deep vein thrombosis and pulmonary embolism: a population-based case-control study. Arch Intern Med. 2000;160:809-15. Used with permission.

- Compared with persons in the community, hospitalized patients have a greater than 150-fold increased incidence of acute VTE
- Hospitalization for medical illness and surgery account for almost equal proportions of VTE (22% and 24%, respectively), which emphasizes the need to provide prophylaxis to both of these risk groups

The risk among surgical patients can be further stratified on the basis of patient age, type of surgery, and presence of active cancer. The incidence of postoperative VTE is increased for surgical patients aged 65 years and older. High-risk surgical procedures include neurosurgery, major orthopedic surgery of the leg, renal transplantation, cardiovascular surgery, and thoracic, abdominal, or pelvic surgery for malignancy. After controlling for age, type of surgery, and cancer, additional independent risk factors for incident VTE after major surgery include increasing body mass index, intensive care unit confinement for more than 6 days, immobility, infection, and varicose veins. The risk from surgery may be less with neuraxial (spinal or epidural) anesthesia than with general anesthesia.

Independent risk factors for incident VTE among patients hospitalized for acute medical illness include increasing age and body mass index, active cancer, neurologic disease with extremity paresis, immobility, fracture, and prior superficial vein thrombosis. Active cancer accounts for almost 20% of incident VTE events occurring in the community. VTE risk among patients with active cancer can be further stratified by tumor site, presence of distant metastases, and active chemotherapy. Although all of these patients are at risk, the risk appears to be higher for pancreatic cancer, lymphoma, malignant brain tumors, cancer of the liver, leukemia, and colorectal and other digestive cancers, and for patients with distant metastases. Those receiving immunosuppressive or cytotoxic chemotherapy, such as L-asparaginase, thalidomide, angiogenesis inhibitors, tamoxifen, and erythropoietin, are at even higher risk for VTE.

Patients with a central venous catheter or transvenous pacemaker now account for about 9% of those with incident VTE in the community. However, warfarin and low-molecular-weight heparin (LMWH) prophylaxis are not effective in preventing catheter-induced venous thrombosis and are not recommended. Prior superficial vein thrombosis is an independent risk factor for subsequent deep vein thrombosis (DVT) or pulmonary embolism (PE) remote from the episode of superficial thrombophlebitis. The risk of DVT imparted by varicose veins is uncertain and appears to be higher among persons younger than 40 years. Long-haul air travel (>6 hours) is associated with a slightly increased risk for VTE, which is preventable with elastic stockings. Studies regarding the protective effect of coenzyme A reductase inhibitor (statin) therapy against VTE have provided conflicting results. In addition, the risk associated with atherosclerosis, or other risk factors for atherosclerosis such as diabetes mellitus, remains uncertain. Body mass index, current or past tobacco smoking, chronic obstructive pulmonary disease, and renal failure are not independent risk factors for VTE. The risk associated with congestive heart failure, independent of hospitalization, is low.

Among women, additional risk factors for VTE include oral contraceptive use and hormone therapy, pregnancy, and the postpartum period. The greatest risk may occur during early use of oral contraceptives and hormone therapy. This risk may be lower for second-generation oral contraceptives or progesterone alone compared with first- or third-generation oral contraceptives. For women with disabling perimenopausal symptoms that cannot be controlled with non-estrogen therapy, esterified oral estrogen or transdermal estrogen therapy may confer less risk than oral conjugated equine estrogen therapy. Although VTE can occur anytime during pregnancy, the highest incidence is during the first 2 postpartum weeks, especially for older mothers. Independent risk factors for pregnancy-associated VTE include tobacco smoking and prior superficial vein thrombosis. Women receiving therapy with the selective estrogen receptor modulators tamoxifen and raloxifene also are at increased risk for VTE.

Recent family-based studies indicate that VTE is highly heritable and follows a complex mode of inheritance involving environmental interaction. Inherited decreases in natural plasma anticoagulants (antithrombin III, protein C, or protein S) have long been recognized as uncommon but potent risk factors for VTE. More recent findings of other decreased natural anticoagulants or anticoagulant cofactors, impaired downregulation of the procoagulant system (e.g., activated protein C resistance, factor V Leiden), increased plasma concentrations of procoagulant factors (e.g., factors I [fibrinogen], II [prothrombin], VIII, IX, and XI), increased basal procoagulant activity, impaired fibrinolysis, and increased basal innate immunity activity and reactivity have added to the list of inherited or acquired disorders predisposing persons to thrombosis. These plasma hemostasis-related factors or markers of coagulation activation correlate with increased thrombotic risk and are highly heritable. Inherited thrombophilias interact with such clinical risk factors as oral contraceptives, pregnancy, hormone therapy, surgery, and cancer to compound the risk of incident VTE. Similarly, genetic interaction increases the risk of incident VTE. Thus, it may be reasonable to consider thrombophilia testing of asymptomatic family members with a known history of familial thrombophilia.

Secondary Prevention of Recurrent VTE

VTE recurs frequently; about 30% of patients have recurrence within ten years (Table 5.5). A recent modeling study suggested that more than 900,000 incident or recurrent VTE events occurred in the United States in 2002. The hazard of recurrence varies with the time since the incident event and is highest within the first 6 to 12 months. Additional independent predictors of recurrence include male sex, increasing patient age and body mass index, neurologic disease with extremity paresis, and active malignancy (Table 5.6). Other predictors of recurrence include: "idiopathic" VTE; a persistent lupus anticoagulant or high-titer antiphospholipid antibody; antithrombin, protein C, or protein S deficiency; compound heterozygous carriers for

Table 5.5 Cumulative Incidence and Hazard of Venous Thromboembolism Recurrence

	Venous thromboembolism recurrence	
Time to recurrence	**Cumulative recurrence, %**	**Hazard of recurrence, per 1,000 person-days (SD)**
0 days	0.0	0
7 days	1.6	170 (30)
30 days	5.2	130 (20)
90 days	8.3	30 (5)
180 days	10.1	20 (4)
1 year	12.9	20 (2)
2 years	16.6	10 (1)
5 years	22.8	6 (1)
10 years	30.4	5 (1)

Modified from Heit JA, Mohr DN, Silverstein MD, et al. Predictors of recurrence after deep vein thrombosis and pulmonary embolism: a population-based cohort study. Arch Intern Med. 2000;160:761-8. Used with permission.

Table 5.6 Independent Predictors of Venous Thromboembolism Recurrence

Characteristic	Hazard ratio	95% Confidence interval
Age*	1.17	1.11-1.24
Body mass index†	1.24	1.04-1.47
Neurologic disease with extremity paresis	1.87	1.28-2.73
Active malignancy		
With chemotherapy	4.24	2.58-6.95
Without chemotherapy	2.21	1.60-3.06

*Per decade increase in age.
†Per 10 kg/m² increase in body mass index.
From Heit JA, Mohr DN, Silverstein MD, et al. Predictors of recurrence after deep vein thrombosis and pulmonary embolism: a population-based cohort study. Arch Intern Med. 2000;160:761-8. Used with permission.

more than one familial thrombophilia (e.g., heterozygous for the factor V Leiden and prothrombin G20210A mutations) or homozygous carriers; decreased tissue-factor pathway inhibitor levels; persistent residual DVT; and possibly increased procoagulant factor VIII and factor IX levels.

- VTE recurs frequently; about 30% of patients have recurrence within 10 years

Data regarding the risk of recurrent VTE among isolated heterozygous carriers of either the factor V Leiden or the prothrombin G20210A mutation are conflicting. In a recent meta-analysis that pooled results from ten studies involving 3,104 patients with incident VTE, the factor V Leiden mutation was present in 21.4% of patients and was associated with an increased risk of recurrent VTE. Similarly, pooled results from nine studies involving 2,903 patients showed that the prothrombin G20210A mutation was present in 9.7% and was associated with an increased risk of recurrence. The estimated population-attributable risk of recurrence was 9.0% and 6.7% for the factor V Leiden and the prothrombin G20210A mutations, respectively.

An increased D-dimer level measured at least 1 month after discontinuing warfarin therapy may be a predictor of DVT recurrence independent of residual venous obstruction. Secondary prophylaxis with anticoagulation therapy should be considered for patients with these characteristics. Although the incident event type (DVT alone vs PE) is not a predictor of recurrence, any recurrence is significantly more likely to be the same as the incident event type. Because the 7-day case fatality rate is significantly higher for recurrent PE (34%) than for recurrent DVT alone (4%), secondary prophylaxis should be considered for incident PE, especially for patients with chronically reduced cardiopulmonary functional reserve.

Diagnostic Thrombophilia Testing: Who Should Be Tested?

Current Recommendations

Currently recommended indications for thrombophilia testing include idiopathic or recurrent VTE; a first episode of VTE at a "young" age (≤40 years); a family history of VTE (in particular, a first-degree relative with thrombosis at a young age); venous thrombosis in an unusual vascular territory (e.g., cerebral, hepatic, mesenteric, or renal vein thrombosis); and neonatal purpura fulminans or warfarin-induced skin necrosis. If two or more of these thrombosis characteristics are present, the prevalence of antithrombin, protein C, or protein S deficiency, and the factor V Leiden and prothrombin G20210A mutations are increased. Consequently, a "complete" laboratory investigation (described below) is recommended for patients who meet these criteria, whereas more selective testing (e.g., for activated protein C resistance and factor V Leiden and prothrombin G20210A mutations) is recommended for other patients.

The prevalence of hereditary thrombophilia is substantial among patients with a first VTE (Table 5.7). Because knowledge of a hereditary thrombophilia may be important for estimating the risk of VTE recurrence, testing for a hereditary thrombophilia should be considered for patients with a first thrombosis, not limited to patients with recurrent VTE. Moreover, although patients with idiopathic or recurrent VTE may have a higher prevalence of a recognized thrombophilia, these patients should be considered for secondary prophylaxis regardless of the results of thrombophilia testing. In addition, the prevalence of hereditary thrombophilia, such as activated protein C resistance, is substantial among patients with a first episode of VTE at an older age (Table 5.8). Therefore, testing for a hereditary thrombophilia should not be limited to patients with a first episode of VTE before age 40 to 50 years. Although persons with deficiency of antithrombin III, protein C, or protein S are more likely to have thrombosis at a younger age, genetic interaction (e.g., factor V Leiden or prothrombin G20210A mutation combined with either antithrombin, protein C, or protein S deficiency) compounds the risk of thrombosis such that testing among older patients should not be limited to activated protein C resistance (factor V Leiden) or the prothrombin G20210A mutation.

- Currently recommended indications for thrombophilia testing include idiopathic or recurrent VTE; a first episode of VTE at a "young" age (≤40 years); a family history of VTE (in particular, a first-degree relative with thrombosis at a young age); venous thrombosis in an unusual vascular territory (e.g., cerebral, hepatic, me-

Table 5.7 Familial or Acquired Thrombophilia: Estimated Prevalence, and Incidence and Relative Risk of Incident or Recurrent VTE by Type of Thrombophilia

	Prevalence, %*			Incident VTE		Recurrent VTE	
Thrombophilia	**Normal**	**Incident VTE**	**Recurrent VTE**	**Incidence† (95% CI)**	**Relative risk (95% CI)**	**Incidence† (95% CI)**	**Relative risk (95% CI)**
Antithrombin III deficiency	0.02-0.04	1-2	2-5	500 (320-730)	17.5 (9.1-33.8)	10,500 (3,800-23,000)	2.5
Protein C deficiency	0.02-0.05	2-5	5-10	310 (530-930)	11.3 (5.7-22.3)	5,100 (2,500-9,400)	2.5
Protein S deficiency	0.01-1	1-3	5-10	710 (530-930)	32.4 (16.7-62.9)	6,500 (2,800-11,800)	2.5
Factor V Leiden‡	3-7	12-20	30-50	150 (80-260)	4.3§ (1.9-9.7)	3,500 (1,900-6,100)	1.3 (1.0-3.3)
Prothrombin G20210A‡	1-3	3-8	15-20	350	1.9 (0.9-4.1)	...	1.4 (0.9-2.0)
Combined thrombophilias	...	...	...	840 (560-1,220)	32.4 (16.7-62.9)	5,000 (2,000-10,300)	...
Hyperhomocysteinemia	...	...	...	...	...	...	2.5
Antiphospholipid Ab	...	...	...	...	...	...	2.5
Factor VIII (>200 IU/dL)	...	...	...	...	...	...	1.8 (1.0-3.3)

Ab, antibody; CI, confidence interval; VTE, venous thromboembolism.
*In whites.
†Per 100,000 person-years.
‡Heterozygous carriers.
§Homozygous carriers, relative risk=80.

Table 5.8 Age-Specific Annual Incidence and Relative Risk of First Lifetime VTE Among Factor V Leiden Carriers

		VTE	
Study	**Age, y**	**Incidence* (95% CI)**	**Relative risk† (95% CI)**
Ridker et al 1997	40-49	0	...
	50-59	197 (72-428)	2.7
	60-69	258 (95-561)	2.7
	≥70	783 (358-1,486)	4.2
Middeldorp et al 1998	15-30	250 (120-490)	≈15
	31-45	470 (230-860)	4.3
	46-60	820 (350-1,610)	2.4
	>60	1,100 (240-3,330)	2.8
Simioni et al 1999	<15	0	...
	16-30	182 (59-424)	3.6
	31-45	264 (86-616)	3.7
	46-60	380 (104-973)	1.4
	>60	730 (150-2,128)	≈700
Heit et al 2005	15-29	0 (0-112)	0 (0-1.22)
	30-44	61 (7-219)	1.96 (0.24-7.04)
	45-59	244 (98-502)	1.73 (0.70-3.56)
	≥60	764 (428-1,260)	3.61 (2.02-5.95)

CI, confidence interval; VTE, venous thromboembolism.
*VTE incidence per 100,000 person-years.
†Compared with factor V Leiden non-carriers.

senteric, or renal vein thrombosis); and neonatal purpura fulminans or warfarin-induced skin necrosis
- The prevalence of hereditary thrombophilia is substantial among patients with a first VTE

Recent evidence suggests that a family history of VTE does not increase the likelihood of a recognized familial thrombophilia. The cumulative lifetime incidence (penetrance) of thrombosis among carriers of the most common familial thrombophilia (factor V Leiden) is only about 10%. Therefore, most patients with an inherited thrombophilia do not have a family history of thrombosis. Consequently, thrombophilia testing should not be limited to symptomatic patients with a family history of VTE.

The most common presentations of familial thrombophilia are DVT of the leg veins and PE. Except for catheter-induced thrombosis, all VTE is most likely associated with an underlying thrombophilia. Therefore, limiting testing of patients with thrombosis in unusual vascular territories will miss most patients with an identifiable familial (or acquired) thrombophilia.

Several additional issues should be considered regarding testing for a possible thrombophilia. For example, the prevalence of hereditary thrombophilia among patients with VTE differs substantially by ethnic ancestry, but variable testing based on ethnic ancestry has not been directly addressed. The factor V Leiden and prothrombin 20210 mutation carrier frequencies among asymptomatic African, Asian, and Native Americans, as well as African Americans with VTE, are extremely low, such that test selection for hereditary thrombophilia most likely should be tailored to patient ethnic ancestry. The risk of VTE during pregnancy or the postpartum period, and the risk of recurrent fetal loss, is increased among patients with acquired or hereditary thrombophilia. Women with VTE during pregnancy or post partum or recurrent fetal loss should be tested. Recent evidence suggests that patients with acute VTE in the presence of active malignancy are also more likely to have an underlying thrombophilia (e.g., factor V Leiden). Nevertheless, thrombophilia testing for patients with thrombosis associated with active cancer or another risk exposure (e.g., surgery, hospitalization for acute medical illness, trauma, neurologic disease with extremity paresis, or upper extremity thrombosis in the presence of a central venous catheter or transvenous pacemaker) is controversial.

Suggested Revised Recommendations

All patients with VTE—regardless of age, sex, race, location of venous thrombosis, initial or recurrent event, or family history of VTE—should be tested for an acquired or hereditary thrombophilia. Women with recurrent fetal loss or complications of pregnancy and patients with unexplained arterial thrombosis also should be tested. These recommendations are controversial and not universally accepted.

- Most patients with an inherited thrombophilia do not have a family history of thrombosis
- Women with VTE during pregnancy or post partum or recurrent fetal loss should be tested

Diagnostic Thrombophilia Testing: For What Should I Test?

General Testing

A complete history and physical examination is mandatory in evaluating persons with a recent or remote history of thrombosis, with special attention given to age of onset, location of prior thromboses, and results of objective diagnostic studies documenting thrombotic episodes. An inquiry regarding interval imaging to establish a new baseline image is particularly important when diagnosing recurrent thrombosis in the same vascular territory as a previous thrombosis. For patients with an uncorroborated history of DVT, non-invasive venous vascular laboratory or venous duplex ultrasonographic evidence of venous outflow obstruction (e.g., residual vein thrombosis) or possibly venous valvular incompetence may be helpful in corroborating the clinical history.

Patients should be questioned carefully about diseases, exposures, conditions, or drugs that are associated with thrombosis (Tables 5.1 and 5.4). A family history of thrombosis may provide insight for a potential familial thrombophilia, especially in first-degree relatives. Thrombosis can be the initial manifestation of a malignancy, so a complete review of systems directed at symptoms of occult malignancy is important, including whether indicated screening tests for normal health maintenance (e.g., mammography, colon imaging) are current. Ethnic background should be considered given the extremely low prevalence of the factor V Leiden and prothrombin G20210A mutations in those of African, Asian, or Native American ancestry.

The physical examination should include a careful peripheral pulse examination as well as examination of the extremities for signs of superficial or deep vein thrombosis and vascular anomalies. The skin should be examined for venous stasis syndrome (e.g., leg swelling, stasis pigmentation or dermatitis, or stasis ulcer), varicose veins, and livedo reticularis, skin infarction, or other evidence of microcirculatory occlusive disease. Given the strong association of thrombosis with active cancer, a careful examination for lymphadenopathy, hepatosplenomegaly, and abdominal or rectal mass should be performed, as well as breast and pelvic examinations for women, and testicular and prostate examinations for men.

The laboratory evaluation for patients with thrombosis should be selective and based on the history and physical examination (Table 5.9). Specific tests may include a complete blood count with peripheral smear, serum protein electrophoresis, serum chemistries for electrolytes and liver and renal function, prostate specific antigen, carcinoembryonic antigen, α-fetoprotein, β-human chorionic gonadotropin, cancer antigen 125, antinuclear antibodies (double-stranded DNA, rheumatoid factor, extractable nuclear antigen), and urinalysis. Elevations in hematocrit or platelet count may indicate the presence of a myeloproliferative disorder, which can be associated with either venous or arterial thrombosis. Secondary polycythemia can also provide evidence of an underlying occult malignancy. Leukopenia and thrombocytopenia can be found in paroxysmal nocturnal hemoglobinuria, which is characterized by intravascular hemolysis along with thrombotic sequelae. The development of thrombosis and thrombocytopenia concurrent with heparin administration should always prompt consideration of heparin-induced thrombocytopenia. The peripheral smear should be reviewed for evidence of red cell fragmentation that would indicate microangiopathic hemolytic anemia such as occurs with intravascular coagulation and fibrinolysis. In patients with malignancy, chronic intravascular coagulation and fibrinolysis can result in either venous or arterial thrombosis. A leukoerythroblastic picture with nucleated red cells or immature white cells suggests the possibility of marrow infiltration by tumor.

Chest radiography should be performed along with appropriate imaging studies according to standard health maintenance guidelines (e.g., Papanicolaou test, mammography, colon imaging). More detailed imaging, such as angiography or chest, abdominal, or pelvic computed tomography or magnetic resonance imaging should be performed only if other independent reasons exist to suspect an occult malignancy or other arterial disease (in the case of arterial thrombosis). Routine screening for occult cancer in patients presenting with idiopathic VTE has not

Table 5.9 Laboratory Evaluation for Suspected Familial or Acquired Thrombophilia*

General
Blood: CBC, peripheral smear, ESR, chemistries, PSA, β-HCG, CA 125, ANA (dsDNA, rheumatoid factor, ENA)
PA/lateral chest radiography, urinalysis, mammography
Colon imaging, especially if no prior screening (proctosigmoidoscopy, colonoscopy)
Chest imaging for smokers (CT, MRI)
Otolaryngology consultation, especially for smokers
UGI/upper endoscopy
Abdominal imaging (CT, MRI, ultrasonography)
Angiography
Special coagulation laboratory testing
Platelets
HITTS testing: plasma anti-PF4/glycosaminoglycan (heparin) antibodies ELISA; platelet ^{14}C-serotonin release assay; heparin-dependent platelet aggregation
Plasma coagulation
Prothrombin time, aPTT (with phospholipid "mixing" procedure if inhibited)
Thrombin time/reptilase time
Dilute Russell viper venom time (with confirm procedures)
Mixing studies (inhibitors)
Specific factor assays (as indicated)
Fibrinolytic system
Fibrinogen
Plasma fibrin D-dimer
Soluble fibrin monomer complex
Natural anticoagulation system
Antithrombin (activity, antigen)
Protein C (activity, antigen)
Protein S (activity, total and free antigen)
APC-resistance ratio (second generation; factor V–deficient plasma mixing study)
Direct genomic DNA mutation testing
Factor V Leiden gene (depending on the result of the APC-resistance ratio)
Prothrombin G20210A
Additional general testing
Anticardiolipin (antiphospholipid) antibodies (IgG and IgM isotypes); anti–β2-glycoprotein-1 antibodies
Plasma homocysteine (basal, postmethionine load)
Additional selective testing
Flow cytometry for PNH
Plasma ADAMTS-13 activity
Plasminogen (activity)

ANA, antinuclear antibody; APC, activated protein C; aPTT, activated partial thromboplastin time; β-HCG, β-human chorionic gonadotropin; CA 125, cancer antigen 125; CBC, complete blood count; CT, computed tomography; dsDNA, double-stranded DNA; ELISA, enzyme-linked immunosorbent assay; ENA, extractable nuclear antigen; ESR, erythrocyte sedimentation rate; HITTS, heparin-induced thrombotic thrombocytopenia syndrome; MRI, magnetic resonance imaging; PA, posteroanterior; PF4, platelet factor 4; PNH, paroxysmal nocturnal hemoglobinuria; PSA, prostate-specific antigen; UGI, upper gastrointestinal tract series.

*Suggested tests that should be performed selectively based on clinical judgment.

been shown to improve cancer-related survival and is not warranted in the absence of clinical features and abnormal basic laboratory findings suggestive of underlying malignancy. Sputum cytology, an otolaryngologic examination, and upper gastrointestinal tract endoscopy should be considered for tobacco smokers or others at risk for esophageal or gastric cancer. In addition to a Papanicolaou test, endometrial sampling should be considered for women at risk of endometrial cancer.

Recommended assays for initial and reflex special coagulation testing for a familial or acquired thrombophilia are provided in Table 5.9. Detailed discussions regarding the interpretation and nuances of specific assays are provided with the description of the biochemistry, molecular biology, and epidemiology of each thrombophilia at the end of this chapter.

- Routine screening for occult cancer in patients presenting with idiopathic VTE has not been shown to improve cancer-related survival and is not warranted in the absence of clinical features and abnormal basic laboratory findings

Arterial Thrombosis

Familial or acquired thrombophilia appears to be an unusual cause of stroke, myocardial infarction, or other organ or skin infarction, except in the presence of antiphospholipid antibodies (e.g., lupus anticoagulant, anticardiolipin antibody, anti–β2-glycoprotein-1 antibodies), heparin-induced thrombocytopenia, myeloproliferative disorders, homocystinuria, and possibly hyperhomocysteinemia. A young patient with organ or skin infarction in the absence of one of the above disorders or risk factors for atherosclerosis (e.g., diabetes mellitus, hypertension, hyperlipidemia, tobacco exposure) or cardioembolism (e.g., cardiac arrhythmia), should be carefully evaluated for occult arterial disease (Table 5.10).

Organ infarction should not be deemed to be caused by a "hypercoagulable disorder" simply because the patient is young or lacks common risk factors for atherosclerosis or arterial thromboembolism. A detailed inquiry into constitutional or specific symptoms of vasculitis (primary or secondary), infection (systemic [e.g., endocarditis] or local [e.g., infected aneurysm with artery-to-artery embolism]), atheroembolism, trauma (accidental, thermal, or occupational), dissection, vasospasm, or vascular anomaly is required. Pulse should also be carefully examined, including an examination for aneurysmal disease. Evidence of microcirculatory occlusive disease of the hand, such as livedo, skin or nailbed infarction, or ulcer, should prompt

Table 5.10 Occult Causes of Arterial Thrombosis

Cardioembolism (atrial fibrillation, left ventricular or atrial septal aneurysm, endocarditis [infectious or non-infectious], ASD or PFO with "paradoxic" embolism, cardiac tumors)
Artery-to-artery embolism (thromboembolism, cholesterol, tumor, infection)
Arterial dissection (large and small vessel)
Fibromuscular dysplasia (cervical and renal arteries)
Cystic adventitial disease
Arterial aneurysmal disease with thrombosis in situ
Trauma
Arterial entrapment (thoracic outlet syndrome, popliteal entrapment, common femoral entrapment at the inguinal ligament)
Vasculitis (primary or secondary)
Thromboangiitis obliterans
Arterial wall infection
Vasospasm
Vascular tumors
Vascular anomalies
Thermal injury (erythromelalgia, chilblain, frostbite)
Occupational trauma (hypothenar hammer syndrome, etc)
Hyperviscosity syndromes
Cold agglutinins
Cryoglobulinemia

ASD, atrial septal defect; PFO, patent foramen ovale.

evaluations for endocarditis (infectious and non-infectious), thoracic outlet syndrome or other causes of repetitive arterial trauma (e.g., hypothenar hammer syndrome), atheroembolism, and thermal injury. Such physical findings in the foot should include a similar search plus an evaluation for abdominal aortic or popliteal artery aneurysmal disease with athero- or thromboembolism.

- Familial or acquired thrombophilia appears to be an unusual cause of stroke, myocardial infarction, or other organ or skin infarction, except in the presence of antiphospholipid antibodies, heparin-induced thrombocytopenia, myeloproliferative disorders, homocystinuria, and possibly hyperhomocysteinemia

Fibromuscular disease typically affects the carotid and renal arteries and may present as stroke or renal infarcts due to carotid and renal artery dissection or embolism, respectively. Because the vascular supply to organs cannot be directly palpated or observed, arteriography is required to evaluate organ infarction. In general, duplex ultrasonography and computed tomography or magnetic resonance imaging angiography do not provide sufficient resolution to exclude these arteriopathies, with the exception of carotid artery disease. Contrast arteriography should be performed by a vascular physician (vascular radiologist, vascular surgeon, or vascular medicine/cardiologist) who is experienced in diagnosing occult vascular disease, including careful and detailed selective arteriography of the involved and upstream vascular territory with selective vasodilator injection and magnified views, if appropriate.

Timing of Diagnostic Thrombophilia Testing: When Should I Test?

Many of the natural anticoagulant and procoagulant plasma proteins are acute-phase reactants. Acute thrombosis can transiently decrease the levels of antithrombin III and occasionally proteins C and S. Consequently, testing should not be performed during the acute phase of thrombosis or during pregnancy. A delay of at least 6 weeks after the acute thrombosis, or after delivery, usually allows sufficient time for acute-phase reactant proteins to return to baseline.

Heparin therapy can lower antithrombin III activity and antigen levels and can impair interpretation of clot-based assays for a lupus anticoagulant. A delay of at least 5 days after heparin is withdrawn before testing is usually feasible. Warfarin therapy decreases the activity and antigen levels of the vitamin K–dependent factors, including proteins C and S. Rarely, warfarin has also been shown to elevate antithrombin III levels into the normal range in those with a hereditary deficiency. Many authorities recommend delaying testing until the effects of warfarin therapy also have resolved. For those in whom temporary discontinuation of anticoagulation is not practical, heparin can be substituted for warfarin. However, the effect of warfarin on protein S levels may not resolve for up to 6 weeks.

The clinical decision regarding secondary prophylaxis may depend on the results of special coagulation testing. Testing for protein C or S deficiency may be done during stable warfarin anticoagulation therapy, with adjustment of the protein C and S levels for the warfarin effect by comparison with the levels of other vitamin K–dependent proteins with similar plasma half-lives (e.g., factors VII and II [prothrombin], respectively). If the levels of protein C or S are within the normal range, the diagnosis of deficiency can be reliably excluded. However, any abnormal result should be confirmed after the patient is off warfarin for a sufficient amount of time to allow the warfarin effect to resolve (if possible), or by testing a first-degree family member. Direct leukocyte genomic DNA testing for the factor V Leiden and prothrombin G20210A mutations is unaffected by anticoagulation therapy; such testing can be performed at any time.

Thrombophilia Diagnostic Testing

- In general, testing should be delayed at least 6-12 weeks after an acute thrombosis

- Testing for antithrombin deficiency and a lupus anticoagulant should be delayed until the patient is off heparin therapy for at least 48-72 hours
- Testing for protein C and protein S deficiency should be delayed until the patient is off warfarin therapy for at least 1 and 4 weeks, respectively
- A diagnosis of a familial thrombophilia should be confirmed by repeated diagnostic testing after ensuring that all acquired causes of deficiency have been excluded or corrected, and by testing symptomatic family members

Diagnostic Thrombophilia Testing: How Should I Manage Patients With Thrombophilia?

Primary Prophylaxis

All patients should receive appropriate antithrombotic prophylaxis when exposed to thrombotic risk factors such as surgery, trauma, or hospitalization for acute medical illness (Table 5.4). Despite the accumulating evidence that an underlying thrombophilia increases the risk of clinical thrombosis among persons exposed to a clinical risk factor, thrombophilia screening for such persons in the absence of a known family history of familial thrombophilia is not recommended at this time. Although the American College of Chest Physicians guidelines place patients with "molecular hypercoagulable disorders" in the "high risk" category for postoperative VTE, current recommendations regarding VTE prophylaxis for surgery or hospitalization for medical illness are based solely on clinical characteristics. In general, prophylaxis regimens are not altered on the basis of a known inherited or acquired thrombophilia. However, given the emerging evidence that a thrombophilia does increase the risk of symptomatic VTE after high-risk surgery, in the absence of contraindications, such patients should be considered for a longer duration of (out-of-hospital) prophylaxis.

At present, general screening of asymptomatic women for a thrombophilia before commencing oral contraceptive therapy or before conception is not recommended. However, it may be appropriate to screen asymptomatic female members of a proband with a known familial thrombophilia. Anticoagulant prophylaxis is recommended for asymptomatic women with antithrombin deficiency during pregnancy and the puerperium.

Acute Therapy

In general, patients with a familial or acquired thrombophilia and a *first* VTE should be managed in standard fashion—with intravenous unfractionated heparin (UFH) at doses sufficient to prolong the activated partial thromboplastin time (aPTT) into the laboratory-specific therapeutic range as referenced to plasma heparin levels (0.2-0.4 U/mL by protamine sulfate titration or 0.3-0.7 IU/mL by anti–factor Xa activity), or with LMWH or fondaparinux. Among patients with impaired renal function (creatinine clearance ≤30 mL/min), peak LMWH levels (obtained 3 hours after subcutaneous injection) should be monitored and the dose adjusted to maintain a heparin level (anti–factor Xa activity) of 0.5-1.0 IU/mL. Fondaparinux is not approved for use among patients with renal insufficiency. Patients with a prolonged baseline aPTT due to a lupus anticoagulant should be treated with LMWH rather than UFH because of difficulty in using the aPTT to monitor and adjust the UFH dose.

Patients with acute DVT may be managed as outpatients. However, a brief hospitalization may be appropriate for edema reduction and fitting of a 30- to 40-mm Hg calf-high graduated compression stocking for patients with severe edema. Compared with patients with DVT alone, patients with PE have significantly worse survival. Such patients may need to be hospitalized at least briefly to ensure that they are hemodynamically stable. Hemodynamically stable patients with PE and normal cardiopulmonary functional reserve may be managed solely as outpatients with LMWH therapy. Subsequent oral anticoagulation therapy should be adjusted to prolong the international normalized ratio (INR) to a target of 2.5, with a therapeutic range of 2.0 to 3.0. Heparin or oral anticoagulation therapy should be overlapped by at least 5 days regardless of the INR and until the INR has been within the therapeutic range for at least 2 consecutive days. Warfarin therapy for patients with lupus anticoagulant should not be monitored with INR point-of-care devices.

Special attention may be required for patients with deficiencies of antithrombin III or protein C. Some patients with antithrombin III deficiency are heparin resistant and may require large doses of UFH to obtain an adequate anticoagulant effect as measured by the aPTT. Antithrombin III concentrate can be used in special circumstances such as recurrent thrombosis despite adequate anticoagulation, unusually severe thrombosis, or difficulty achieving adequate anticoagulation. It is also reasonable to treat antithrombin III–deficient patients with concentrate before major surgeries or in obstetric situations when the risks of bleeding from anticoagulation are unacceptable. Antithrombin III concentrate appears to have a low risk of transmitting bloodborne infections and is supplied as 500 IU/10 mL or 1,000 IU/20 mL. An initial loading dose should be calculated to increase the antithrombin III level to 120%, assuming an expected rise of 1.4% per IU/kg transfused over the baseline antithrombin III level. For example, for a patient with a baseline antithrombin III level of 57%, the calculated dose is (120%–57%)/1.4% =45 IU/kg. The dose should be administered over 10 to 20 minutes, and a 20-minute postinfusion antithrombin level should be measured. In general, plasma antithrombin levels of 80% to 120% can be maintained by administration of 60% of the initial loading dose every 24 hours.

Hereditary protein C deficiency can be associated with warfarin-induced skin necrosis due to a transient hypercoagulable state. The initiation of warfarin at standard doses leads to a decrease in protein C anticoagulant activity to approximately 50% of baseline within 1 day. Consequently, treatment with warfarin should be started only after the patient is fully heparinized, and the dose of the drug should be increased gradually, after starting from a relatively low dose (2 mg). Those with a history of warfarin-induced skin necrosis can be anticoagulated with warfarin after receiving heparin therapy or a source of exogenous protein C either via fresh frozen plasma or an investigational protein C concentrate. This offers a bridge until a stable level of anticoagulation can be achieved.

The total duration of anticoagulation for acute therapy should be individualized based on the circumstances of the thrombotic event. In general, a duration of 6 weeks to 3 months of anticoagulation appears to be adequate for thrombosis related to transient risk factors, whereas patients with persistent risk factors require 3 to 6 months.

- Hereditary protein C deficiency can be associated with warfarin-induced skin necrosis due to a transient hypercoagulable state

Secondary Prophylaxis

It is important to make a distinction between acute therapy and secondary prophylaxis. Acute therapy aims to prevent extension or embolism of an acute thrombosis and must continue for a sufficient duration of time and intensity to ensure that the acute thrombus has either lysed or become organized and the "activated" acute inflammatory/innate immunity system has returned to baseline. As discussed above, the most appropriate duration of acute therapy varies among patients but probably is between 3 and 6 months.

Beyond about 6 months, the aim of continued anticoagulation is not to prevent acute thrombus extension or embolism but to prevent recurrent thrombosis (i.e., secondary prophylaxis). VTE is now viewed as a chronic disease (most likely because all such patients have an underlying, if not recognized, thrombophilia) with episodic recurrence. All randomized clinical trials that have tested different durations of anticoagulation showed that as soon as anticoagulation is stopped, VTE begins to recur. Thus, anticoagulation therapy does not "cure" VTE. Considering the full spectrum of venous thromboembolic disease, the rate of recurrence after withdrawing acute therapy differs depending on the duration of anticoagulation, but this is because the rate of recurrence decreases with increasing time since the incident event, not the duration of acute therapy.

The decision regarding secondary prophylaxis is complex and depends on estimates of the risk of unprovoked VTE recurrence while not receiving secondary prophylaxis, the risk of anticoagulant-related bleeding, and the consequences of both, as well as the patient's preference (Tables 5.6 and 5.7). Secondary prophylaxis after a first episode of VTE is controversial and should be recommended only after careful consideration of the risks and benefits. In general, secondary prophylaxis is not recommended after a first episode, especially if the event was associated with a transient clinical risk factor such as surgery, hospitalization for acute medical illness, trauma, oral contraceptive use, pregnancy, or the puerperium.

Secondary prophylaxis may be recommended for:

- Idiopathic, recurrent, or life-threatening VTE (PE, especially in association with persistently decreased cardiopulmonary functional reserve due to chronic cardiopulmonary disease; phlegmasia with threatened venous gangrene; purpura fulminans);
- Persistent clinical risk factors (active cancer, chronic neurologic disease with extremity paresis, or other persistent secondary causes of thrombophilia [Table 5.1]);
- A persistent lupus anticoagulant and/or high-titer anticardiolipin or anti–β2-glycoprotein-1 antibody;
- Antithrombin, protein C, or protein S deficiency;
- Increased basal factor VIII activity or substantial hyperhomocysteinemia;
- Homozygous carriers or compound heterozygous carriers for more than one familial thrombophilia (factor V Leiden and prothrombin G20210A mutations);
- Possibly a persistently increased plasma fibrin D-dimer or residual venous obstruction.

The risk of recurrence among isolated heterozygous carriers for either the factor V Leiden or prothrombin G20201A mutation is relatively low and most likely insufficient to warrant secondary prophylaxis after a first thrombotic event in the absence of other independent predictors of recurrence. A family history of VTE is not a predictor of an increased risk of recurrence and should not influence the decision regarding secondary prophylaxis. However, the quality of anticoagulation during acute therapy is a predictor of the long-term risk of recurrence. Because of the high risk of recurrent VTE due to warfarin failure among patients with active cancer, the most recent American College of Chest Physicians Consensus Conference on Antithrombotic and Thrombolytic Therapy recommended LMWH as secondary prophylaxis as long as the cancer remains active.

The risks of recurrent VTE must be weighed against the risks of bleeding from anticoagulant (warfarin)-based secondary prophylaxis. The relative risk of major bleeding is increased about 1.5-fold for every 10-year increase in age and about 2-fold for patients with active cancer. Additional risk factors for bleeding include a history of gastrointestinal tract bleeding or stroke, or one or more comorbid conditions, including recent myocardial infarction, anemia (hematocrit <30%), impaired renal function (serum creatinine >1.5 mg/dL), impaired liver function, and thrombocytopenia. Moreover, the ability to perform activities of daily living should be considered because of the increased risk of bleeding associated with falls. The patient's prior anticoagulation experience during acute therapy should also be considered; patients with unexplained wide variation in the INR or noncompliant patients likely should not receive secondary prophylaxis. Finally, the mechanisms by which the anticoagulation effect of warfarin will be monitored and the dose adjusted should be considered; the efficacy and safety of such care when rendered through an "anticoagulation clinic" or when "self-managed" at home are superior to usual medical care. With appropriate patient selection and management, the risk of major bleeding can be reduced to ≤1% per year.

Because the risk of VTE recurrence decreases with time since the incident event, and because the risk of anticoagulant-related bleeding also may vary over time, the need for secondary prophylaxis must be continually reevaluated. It is inappropriate to simply recommend "lifelong" or "indefinite" anticoagulation therapy.

Questions

1. A 48-year-old woman presents with a 3-hour history of progressive headache, nausea, vomiting, aphasia, and confusion. She is an otherwise healthy non-smoker with no hypertension but is using a transdermal estrogen patch for premature menopause. One brother is on chronic anticoagulation therapy for a history of a "blood clot"; two children are well. Magnetic resonance angiography shows left transverse sinus thrombosis with secondary venous infarction of the left temporal lobe. She is treated with intravenous standard heparin, mannitol, and high-dose corticosteroids, but 3 days later, brain herniation develops requiring craniotomy and hematoma evacuation. The heparin is withdrawn. Four days later, the patient reports left calf pain and swelling, and duplex ultrasonography confirms an isolated left calf DVT. Serial duplex ultrasonography performed the next day shows proximal extension to the femoral vein, and an inferior vena cava filter is placed. She is dismissed home 15 days after admission, but returns 3 days later with new dyspnea and pleuritic chest pain, and a ventilation perfusion scan is interpreted as high probability for PE. She is treated with heparin and warfarin therapy.
Which of the following statements is(are) true?
   a. Special coagulation testing is not indicated because the transdermal estrogen patch is the cause of her venous thromboses; moreover, she cannot have a thrombophilia because she had two uncomplicated pregnancies and her first thrombosis occurred after age 40 years.
   b. Special coagulation testing should be requested because the positive family history and thrombosis in an "unusual" venous circulation (e.g., cerebral sinus) indicate an underlying hereditary thrombophilia.
   c. The cerebral sinus thrombosis and recurrent VTE are an absolute indication for lifelong anticoagulation therapy.
   d. All of the above.
   e. None of the above.

2. The patient described above is referred to you for a second opinion regarding a diagnosis of protein S deficiency and management. The following special coagulation studies are available for your review:

Assay	First presentation	Two months later	Reference range
Platelet count, ×10⁹/L	480	296	150-450
PT, s (INR)	11.4 (1.1)	23 (2.3)	10-12
aPTT, s	66	36	24-37
dRVVT, s	24	55	24-35
Thrombin time, s	>150	19	18-25
Reptilase time, s	22	21	17-23
Fibrinogen, mg/dL	701	455	20-440
Factor II activity, %	109	23	72-140
Factor VII activity, %	100	17	65-160
Factor VIII activity, %	299	121	55-145
Plasma fibrin D-dimer, ng/mL	4,000-8,000	<250	<250
Soluble fibrin monomer complex	Negative	...	...
Plasminogen activity, %	137	...	80-123
Antithrombin activity, %	64	90	83-115
Protein C activity, %	112	...	70-130
Protein S			
Total antigen, %	120	97	50-120
Free antigen, %	27	5	50-120
Activity, %	...	9	60-120

dRVVT, diluted Russell viper venom time; PT, prothrombin time.
(Note: The prolonged aPTT and thrombin time and normal reptilase time indicate a heparin effect.)

Which statement is correct?
   a. On the basis of the admission and follow-up special coagulation testing, the patient definitely has congenital protein S deficiency and requires lifelong anticoagulation therapy.

b. A diagnosis of protein S deficiency cannot be made because the first testing was performed while on heparin therapy, and follow-up testing was performed while on warfarin therapy, both of which decrease protein S levels.
c. A diagnosis of protein S deficiency cannot be made because the first testing was performed while the patient was acutely ill and receiving hormone therapy, and follow-up testing was performed while on warfarin therapy, and both circumstances decrease protein S levels.
d. Admission testing indicates decompensated intravascular coagulation and fibrinolysis that has resolved with therapy, which strongly suggests an occult malignancy.
e. The aggressive course of the venous thrombotic disease in this patient is due to "combined" thrombophilias, including thrombocytosis, increased factor VIII activity, and antithrombin and protein S deficiency, which is compounded by hormone therapy.

3. A 17-year-old girl presents to your institution with acute right groin pain and right leg swelling. Three weeks earlier, she underwent an emergent appendectomy elsewhere; the surgery was complicated by intraoperative bleeding and the platelet count was discovered to be 80×10^9/L. Nine years earlier, she had easy bruising and thrombocytopenia diagnosed as idiopathic thrombocytopenic purpura; she reportedly had a "good response" to prednisone therapy. Physical examination reveals right groin tenderness, right leg edema, and livedo reticularis of the legs.
Laboratory investigations:
Complete blood count showed: hemoglobin, 10.3 g/dL; hematocrit, 29.7%; leukocytes, 10.2×10^9/L; and platelet count, 90×10^9/L.
Antinuclear antibody, positive, 1:160, speckled pattern; anti-dsDNA antibody, negative; extractable nuclear antigen, negative; anti–smooth muscle antibody, negative; total complement, normal.
Computed tomography of the abdomen: acute thrombosis of right common femoral, external, and iliac veins and inferior vena cava extending to renal vein level.

Test	Value (reference range)
PT, s	16.2 (10-12)
1:2 mixing normal plasma	14.0
aPTT, s	75 (24-37)
1:2 mixing normal plasma	58
Platelet neutralization procedure	38
Buffer control	65
dRVVT, s	85 (25-34)
1:2 mixing normal plasma	65
dRVVT confirm procedure	36
Thrombin time, s	19 (control, 20)
Fibrinogen, mg/dL	640
Factor II activity, %	114
Factor V activity, %	80
Factor VIII activity, %	≥160
Ristocetin cofactor activity, %	230
von Willebrand factor level, %	260
Antithrombin, protein C, and protein S	Normal
Anticardiolipin antibody (ELISA)	
IgG	Positive, 1:1,024
IgM	Negative

ELISA, enzyme-linked immunosorbent assay.
Interpretation: Lupus anticoagulant and strongly positive IgG isotype anticardiolipin antibody.

The most appropriate acute therapy for her DVT is:
a. LMWH because no aPTT monitoring is required.
b. UFH with monitoring of the aPTT and dose adjustment to maintain the aPTT at 1.5 to 2 times normal.
c. UFH with monitoring of heparin levels and dose adjustment to maintain the factor Xa activity between 0.5 and 1.0 IU/mL.
d. UFH with monitoring of heparin levels and dose adjustment to maintain the anti–factor Xa activity between 0.5 and 1.0 IU/mL.
e. UFH with monitoring of heparin levels and dose adjustment to maintain the factor Xa activity between 0.3 and 0.7 IU/mL.

4. You are asked to see the patient described above for recommendations regarding warfarin anticoagulation therapy. You recommend the following:
a. Indefinite warfarin anticoagulation therapy with monitoring and dose adjustment to maintain the chromogenic factor Xa activity between 20% and 40%.
b. Warfarin anticoagulation therapy for 6 months with monitoring and dose adjustment to maintain the INR at 3.0 to 4.0.
c. Warfarin anticoagulation therapy for 6 months with monitoring and dose adjustment to maintain the INR at 2.0 to 3.0.
d. Warfarin anticoagulation therapy with monitoring and dose adjustment to maintain the chromogenic factor Xa activity between 20% and 40% for 6 months and indefinitely if repeat testing confirms a persistently positive lupus anticoagulant or high-titer anticardiolipin antibody.
e. Indefinite warfarin anticoagulation therapy with monitoring and dose adjustment to maintain the INR at 2.0 to 3.0.

5. A 45-year-old obese, non-diabetic woman presents with right foot pain 2 days after hospital discharge for bariatric surgery performed 8 days earlier. On examination, her foot is cold and pale; dorsalis pedis and posterior tibial pulses are absent. Current medication is only acetaminophen with codeine for pain.
   Laboratory studies:
   Hemoglobin, 14.0 g/dL; platelet count, 15×10^9/L; aPTT, 30 s; PT, 12 s.
   Which of the following actions should you take next?
   a. Begin treatment with aspirin and clopidogrel
   b. Begin treatment with standard heparin
   c. Begin treatment with LMWH
   d. Begin treatment with recombinant hirudin
   e. Transfuse platelets

6. A 58-year-old woman who works as a secretary has, in the past, had two episodes of DVT, one immediately after the birth of her son. Now she is being evaluated for atrial fibrillation that has been refractory to medical treatment. Chronic oral anticoagulation therapy with warfarin (10 mg daily) has been started. Three days after beginning warfarin treatment, a necrotic area with an erythematous border develops on the patient's left flank.
   Which of the following is the most likely cause of these findings?
   a. Lupus anticoagulant
   b. Protein C deficiency
   c. Protein S deficiency
   d. Antithrombin deficiency
   e. Heparin cofactor II deficiency

Suggested Readings

Bauer KA. Management of thrombophilia. J Thromb Haemost. 2003;1:1429-34.

Beyth RJ, Quinn LM, Landefeld CS. Prospective evaluation of an index for predicting the risk of major bleeding in outpatients treated with warfarin. Am J Med. 1998;105:91-9.

Bloemenkamp KW, Rosendaal FR, Helmerhorst FM, et al. Higher risk of venous thrombosis during early use of oral contraceptives in women with inherited clotting defects. Arch Intern Med. 2000;160:49-52.

Blom JW, Doggen CJ, Osanto S, et al. Malignancies, prothrombotic mutations, and the risk of venous thrombosis. JAMA. 2005;293:715-22.

Brenner BR, Nowak-Gottl U, Kosch A, et al. Diagnostic studies for thrombophilia in women on hormonal therapy and during pregnancy, and in children. Arch Pathol Lab Med. 2002;126:1296-303.

Bucur SZ, Levy JH, Despotis GJ, et al. Uses of antithrombin III concentrate in congenital and acquired deficiency states. Transfusion. 1998;38:481-98.

Buller HR, Sohne M, Middeldorp S. Treatment of venous thromboembolism. J Thromb Haemost. 2005;3:1554-60.

Chandler WL, Rodgers GM, Sprouse JT, et al. Elevated hemostatic factor levels as potential risk factors for thrombosis. Arch Pathol Lab Med. 2002;126:1405-14.

Chee YL, Watson HG. Air travel and thrombosis. Br J Haematol. 2005;130:671-80.

Christiansen SC, Cannegieter SC, Koster T, et al. Thrombophilia, clinical factors, and recurrent venous thrombotic events. JAMA. 2005;293:2352-61.

Curb JD, Prentice RL, Bray PF, et al. Venous thrombosis and conjugated equine estrogen in women without a uterus. Arch Intern Med. 2006;166:772-80.

Dizon-Townson D, Miller C, Sibai B, et al, National Institute of Child Health and Human Development Maternal-Fetal Medicine Units Network. The relationship of the factor V Leiden mutation and pregnancy outcomes for mother and fetus. Obstet Gynecol. 2005;106:517-24.

Folsom AR, Aleksic N, Wang L, et al. Protein C, antithrombin, and venous thromboembolism incidence: a prospective population-based study. Arterioscler Thromb Vasc Biol. 2002;22:1018-22.

Folsom AR, Cushman M, Heckbert SR, et al. Prospective study of fibrinolytic markers and venous thromboembolism. J Clin Epidemiol. 2003;56:598-603.

Folsom AR, Cushman M, Tsai MY, et al. A prospective study of venous thromboembolism in relation to factor V Leiden and related factors. Blood. 2002;99:2720-5.

Folsom AR, Cushman M, Tsai MY, et al. Prospective study of the G20210A polymorphism in the prothrombin gene, plasma prothrombin concentration, and incidence of venous thromboembolism. Am J Hematol. 2002;71:285-90.

Forastiero R, Martinuzzo M, Pombo G, et al. A prospective study of antibodies to beta2-glycoprotein I and prothrombin, and risk of thrombosis. J Thromb Haemost. 2005;3:1231-8.

Goodwin AJ, Rosendaal FR, Kottke-Marchant K, et al. A review of the technical, diagnostic, and epidemiologic considerations for protein S assays. Arch Pathol Lab Med. 2002;126:1349-66.

Heit JA, Mohr DN, Silverstein MD, et al. Predictors of recurrence after deep vein thrombosis and pulmonary embolism: a population-based cohort study. Arch Intern Med. 2000;160:761-8.

Heit JA, Silverstein MD, Mohr DN, et al. Predictors of survival after deep vein thrombosis and pulmonary embolism: a population-based, cohort study. Arch Intern Med. 1999;159:445-53.

Heit JA, Silverstein MD, Mohr DN, et al. Risk factors for deep vein thrombosis and pulmonary embolism: a population-based case-control study. Arch Intern Med. 2000;160:809-15.

Heit JA, Sobell JL, Li H, et al. The incidence of venous thromboembolism among Factor V Leiden carriers: a community-based cohort study. J Thromb Haemost. 2005;3:305-11.

Ho WK, Hankey GJ, Quinlan DJ, et al. Risk of recurrent venous thromboembolism in patients with common thrombophilia: a systematic review. Arch Intern Med. 2006;166:729-36.

Key NS, McGlennen RC. Hyperhomocyst(e)inemia and thrombophilia. Arch Pathol Lab Med. 2002;126:1367-75.

Kottke-Marchant K, Comp P. Laboratory issues in diagnosing abnormalities of protein C, thrombomodulin, and endothelial cell protein C receptor. Arch Pathol Lab Med. 2002;126:1337-48.

Kottke-Marchant K, Duncan A. Antithrombin deficiency: issues in laboratory diagnosis. Arch Pathol Lab Med. 2002;126:1326-36.

McGlennen RC, Key NS. Clinical and laboratory management of the prothrombin G20210A mutation. Arch Pathol Lab Med. 2002;126:1319-25.

Middeldorp S, Henkens CM, Koopman MM, et al. The incidence of venous thromboembolism in family members of patients with factor V Leiden mutation and venous thrombosis. Ann Intern Med. 1998;128:15-20.

Press RD, Bauer KA, Kujovich JL, et al. Clinical utility of factor V Leiden (R506Q) testing for the diagnosis and management of thromboembolic disorders. Arch Pathol Lab Med. 2002;126:1304-18.

Ridker PM, Glynn RJ, Miletich JP, et al. Age-specific incidence rates of venous thromboembolism among heterozygous carriers of factor V Leiden mutation. Ann Intern Med. 1997;126:528-31.

Silverstein MD, Heit JA, Mohr DN, et al. Trends in the incidence of deep vein thrombosis and pulmonary embolism: a 25-year population-based study. Arch Intern Med. 1998;158:585-93.

Simioni P, Sanson BJ, Prandoni P, et al. Incidence of venous thromboembolism in families with inherited thrombophilia. Thromb Haemost. 1999;81:198-202.

Smith NL, Heckbert SR, Lemaitre RN, et al. Esterified estrogens and conjugated equine estrogens and the risk of venous thrombosis. JAMA. 2004;292:1581-7.

Van Cott EM, Laposata M, Prins MH. Laboratory evaluation of hypercoagulability with venous or arterial thrombosis. Arch Pathol Lab Med. 2002;126:1281-95.

van Dongen CJ, Vink R, Hutten BA, et al. The incidence of recurrent venous thromboembolism after treatment with vitamin K antagonists in relation to time since first event: a meta-analysis. Arch Intern Med. 2003;163:1285-93.

Vossen CY, Conard J, Fontcuberta J, et al. Familial thrombophilia and lifetime risk of venous thrombosis. J Thromb Haemost. 2004;2:1526-32.

Vossen CY, Preston FE, Conard J, et al. Hereditary thrombophilia and fetal loss: a prospective follow-up study. J Thromb Haemost. 2004;2:592-6.

Vossen CY, Walker ID, Svensson P, et al. Recurrence rate after a first venous thrombosis in patients with familial thrombophilia. Arterioscler Thromb Vasc Biol. 2005 Sept;25:1992-7. Epub 2005 Jun 23.

Wu O, Robertson L, Langhorne P, et al. Oral contraceptives, hormone replacement therapy, thrombophilias and risk of venous thromboembolism: a systematic review: the Thrombosis: Risk and Economic Assessment of Thrombophilia Screening (TREATS) Study. Thromb Haemost. 2005;94:17-25.

Wu O, Robertson L, Twaddle S, et al, The Thrombosis: Risk and Economic Assessment of Thrombophilia Screening (TREATS) Study. Screening for thrombophilia in high-risk situations: a meta-analysis and cost-effectiveness analysis. Br J Haematol. 2005;131:80-90.

6 Venous Thromboembolism

Robert D. McBane, MD

Introduction

Venous thrombosis can involve any vein. However, the most common location is the deep veins of the lower extremities. It is believed that thrombi in these locations arise within the valve cusps of the deep veins of the calf and then propagate cephalad. Virchow, in the late 19th century, postulated that three variables were required for the pathogenesis of deep vein thrombosis (DVT): vascular injury, stasis, and a hypercoagulable state. The most devastating complication of DVT occurs when these thrombi embolize; the vast majority of the emboli are deposited into the pulmonary arteries resulting in pulmonary embolism (PE). In patients with a patent foramen ovale, these emboli infrequently make their way into the arterial circulation and cause stroke or other arterial occlusion, referred to as a paradoxic embolism. This section discusses the clinical presentation, epidemiology, evaluation, and treatment of venous thromboembolism (VTE), a term that includes both DVT and PE.

Three variables required for the pathogenesis of DVT:

- Vascular injury
- Stasis
- Hypercoagulable state

Clinical Presentation

The typical presentation of DVT is the sudden onset of pain, swelling, or painful swelling of one limb. Bilateral DVT is unusual and when present typically signifies an underlying malignancy. The pain is usually described as a cramp, bursting, or "charlie horse" and is confined to the calf, at least initially. The pain can be sufficiently severe as to limit weight bearing or ambulation. Often, pain precedes swelling by several days, but in some patients the swelling is painless. VTE is frequently preceded by major surgery, major trauma, or prolonged immobility, such as a long car ride or plane flight. This is not always the case, however, and a significant minority of patients has no such identifiable acquired risk factors.

Common symptoms of PE include abrupt onset of dyspnea, cough, or syncope. Chest pain is also quite common and may be pleuritic in nature, although not always so. Because most PE arises from the deep veins of the legs, a history of antecedent leg pain or swelling ought to be universal. This is not the case, however, and in many patients no such history can be elicited.

Epidemiology

The incidence of VTE exceeds 1 per 1,000 persons, with approximately 400,000 new cases diagnosed annually in the United States alone. The 30-day mortality of patients with a thrombotic event is 30%, and 20% die suddenly of PE. VTE is therefore the fourth leading cause of death in Western populations and the third leading cause of cardiovascular death behind myocardial infarction and stroke. Of those surviving the thrombotic event, 30% have development of recurrent VTE within 10 years and 20% to 30% will have development of the postphlebitic syndrome over this time period. VTE is typically a disease of the elderly, with the incidence of thrombotic events increasing after age 60 years (Fig. 6.1). The effect of age is important for several reasons: first, more VTE cases should be expected as the population ages; and second, a young person presenting with VTE is relatively uncommon, and in these patients an underlying etiology must be carefully sought.

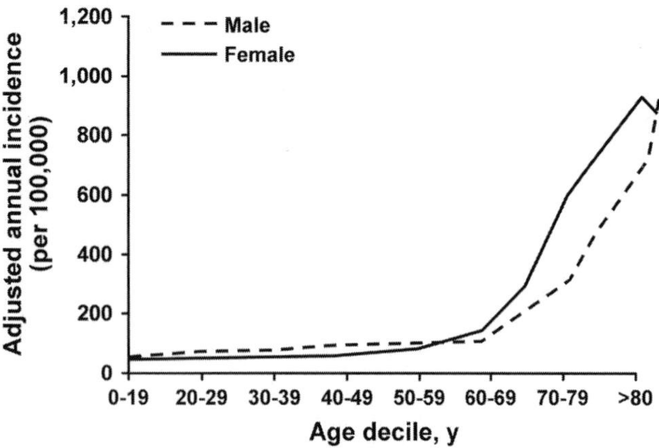

Fig. 6.1 Trends in the incidence of deep vein thrombosis adjusted for age and sex. (Data from Silverstein MD, Heit JA, Mohr DN, et al. Trends in the incidence of deep vein thrombosis and pulmonary embolism: a 25-year population-based study. Arch Intern Med. 1998;158:585-93.)

- VTE is the fourth leading cause of death in Western populations and the third leading cause of cardiovascular death after myocardial infarction and stroke
- Of persons surviving the venous thrombotic event:
  - 30% have recurrent VTE within 10 years
  - 20%-30% have postphlebitic syndrome within 10 years
- The incidence of thrombotic events increases after age 60 years

Acquired Risk Factors

For most patients being evaluated for VTE, the thrombotic event has already occurred. Therefore, the assessment of risk relates not to the prevention of thrombosis but rather to the risk of a recurrent event. This risk assessment helps the clinician stratify patients into high, medium, or low risk and thereby to prescribe the appropriate duration of anticoagulant therapy, balancing the risk of recurrence with the risk of bleeding while receiving the therapy. For an in-depth review of congenital risk factors and laboratory testing for both congenital and acquired thrombophilia, see Chapter 5. Independent acquired risk factors for VTE (in decreasing order of magnitude) include surgery, trauma, hospital or nursing home confinement, malignancy, central venous catheter or pacemaker, superficial venous thrombosis, and neurologic disease with extremity paresis (Table 6.1). Interestingly, liver disease has been found to be protective, possibly because of inadequate production of procoagulant factors, most of which are hepatically synthesized. Many of these risk factors are transient and therefore do not confer a lifelong risk of recurrent VTE. Indeed, for variables such as surgery or major trauma, the risk is clearly increased at the time of the event. However, after convalescence, the risk of recurrent VTE returns to that of the general population.

Table 6.1 Acquired Risk Factors for VTE

Risk	OR	95% CI
Surgery	21.7	9.4-79.0
Trauma	12.7	4.1-39.7
Hospital/NH	8	4.5-14.2
Malignancy	6.5	2.1-20.2
CVP line/PPM	5.6	1.6-19.6
Superficial phlebitis	4.3	1.8-10.6
Paralysis	3	1.3-7.4
Liver disease	0.1	0.0-0.7

CI, confidence interval; CVP, central venous pressure; NH, nursing home; OR, odds ratio; PPM, permanent pacemaker; VTE, venous thromboembolism. Data from Heit JA, Silverstein MD, Mohr DN, et al. Risk factors for deep vein thrombosis and pulmonary embolism: a population-based case-control study. Arch Intern Med. 2000;160:809-15.

Most hospitalized patients have more than one risk factor for venous thrombosis and these risk factors are most likely additive. Although surgery and trauma represent the most important acquired risk factors for VTE, most thrombotic events occur in non-surgical patients. For the non-surgical hospitalized patient, major risk factors include New York Heart Association class III to IV heart failure, chronic obstructive pulmonary disease exacerbation, sepsis, advanced age, prior VTE, cancer, stroke with limb paresis, and bed rest.

Risk Factors in Hospitalized Patients

- Surgery and trauma carry the greatest risk for VTE, but most thrombotic events occur in non-surgical patients
- Major risk factors for non-surgical hospitalized patients include:
  - New York Heart Association class III-IV heart failure
  - Chronic obstructive pulmonary disease exacerbation
  - Sepsis
  - Advanced age
  - History of VTE
  - Cancer
  - Stroke with limb paresis
  - Bed rest

Surgery presents a major risk for VTE, which varies by the type, duration, and indication for surgery, type of anesthesia, associated risk factors, and patient-specific variables including age. The highest risk is associated with orthopedic procedures, especially hip or knee replacement, hip fracture surgery, and trauma surgery including for spinal cord injury. Patient-specific variables include cancer, congenital thrombophilia, history of VTE, obesity, and increasing age (>60 years). In general, spinal or epidural anesthesia carries a lower risk than general anesthesia. Outpatient surgery has a lower associated risk than inpatient surgery. Patients undergoing vascular surgery may have less risk than other surgeries, possibly because of the intraoperative use of heparin therapy. Aortic surgeries carry a higher risk than distal bypass surgeries.

Surgical Risk Factors

- The highest surgical risk is associated with orthopedic procedures:
  - Hip or knee replacement
  - Hip fracture surgery
  - Trauma surgery (especially for spinal cord injury)
- Patient-specific variables include:
  - Cancer
  - Congenital thrombophilia
  - Prior VTE
  - Obesity
  - Increasing age (>60 years)

It is estimated that more than 100 million women worldwide use hormonal contraception. VTE is one of the most disconcerting complications of oral contraception. For women in their teens, twenties, and thirties, the anticipated incidence of VTE ranges from 1 in 100,000 to 1 in 10,000 with increasing age. The risk of VTE for oral contraceptive users is between 3- and 5-fold greater than for non-users (Table 6.2). This risk is exponentially higher in carriers of factor V Leiden or prothrombin G20210A gene mutations. The greatest risk occurs in the first 6 to 12 months of therapy, particularly in first-time users. The risk remains until the third month after discontinuation of therapy. This risk is directly proportional to estrogen dose; several studies have shown that third-generation oral contraceptives have greater VTE risk than second-generation agents. Progesterone-only oral contraceptives are associated with a lower risk than combination preparations.

Data from two large randomized controlled trials enrolling nearly 19,000 women have shown that oral hormone replacement therapy is associated with a 2- to 3-fold increased rate of VTE compared with non-users (Table 6.2). The risk appears to be highest in the first 6 to 12 months of therapy. Limited data suggest that transdermal preparations carry less risk than oral preparations. Inherited thrombophilic states increase the risk of VTE exponentially in hormone replacement therapy users compared with non-users.

Table 6.2 Hormones and VTE

HRT increases VTE risk 2-3 fold
OC increases VTE risk 3-5 fold
VTE risk is greatest in the first 6-12 months of HRT or OC
Risk persists for 3 months after stopping OC
Pregnancy increases VTE risk 3-6 fold
Puerperium is highest pregnancy risk period

HRT, hormone replacement therapy; OC, oral contraception; VTE, venous thromboembolism.

Pregnancy increases the incidence of VTE by 3- to 6-fold, and this incidence is evenly distributed across the three trimesters (Table 6.2). The risk is higher after cesarean than vaginal delivery. The puerperium, which encompasses the 6-week period after delivery, is a higher risk period than pregnancy. This increased risk of VTE might relate to high estrogen levels, venous stasis, pelvic trauma with delivery, and acquired hypercoagulability. This acquired thrombophilia has been attributed to elevated procoagulant variables (fibrinogen, von Willebrand factor, and factor VIII) and to decreased natural anticoagulants such as protein S. Risk factors associated with thrombosis during pregnancy include increasing age, immobility, obesity, and prior VTE. DVT occurs three times more frequently in the left leg than in the right, previously explained by left iliac compression by the right iliac artery.

Inflammatory bowel disease is a generally accepted risk factor for VTE. However, the mechanism underlying this association remains unclear. The reported incidence of VTE in this disease is difficult to ascertain because most studies are limited by referral bias. In one population-based study in Manitoba, the incidence of VTE was 0.5%, which was significantly greater than expected in the general population for both DVT (incidence rate ratio, 3.5; 95% confidence interval [CI], 2.9-4.3) and PE (incidence rate ratio, 3.3; 95% CI, 2.5-4.3). In another study, inflammatory bowel disease resulted in VTE at an earlier age compared with the general population. In this study, however, the overall incidence was comparable.

Thrombosis is a major source of morbidity in patients with nephrotic syndrome. The renal vein is the most common site of venous thrombosis, occurring in approximately 35% of patients with nephrotic syndrome. Thrombosis in other venous segments is seen in 20% of cases. Urinary excretion of antithrombin III, platelet hyperreactivity, and elevated plasma viscosity are pathophysiologic mechanisms of thrombosis in these patients.

The incidence of VTE in patients with an active malignancy could be as high as 11%. Patients with cancer involving the pancreas, gastrointestinal tract, ovary, prostate, and lung are particularly prone to development of VTE; however, all malignancies carry some association. Patients with active malignancy who undergo surgery are at increased risk, with an incidence of thrombosis approaching 40%. Thrombosis may be the first manifestation of malignancy in some persons. Trousseau syndrome, or migratory thrombophlebitis, is a prime example. In a now classic study, the prevalence of malignancy among 153 patients with idiopathic VTE was 3.3% at clinical presentation of the thrombus. During the 2-year follow-up period, a new cancer diagnosis was confirmed in 7.6%, compared with an incidence of 1.9% in patients with secondary thrombosis. If VTE recurred during this time period, the incidence of new malignancy was 17.1%.

Additional Risk Factors

- Nephrotic syndrome:
  - Thrombosis is a major source of morbidity
- Malignancy:
  - The incidence of VTE in patients with an active malignancy may be as high as 11%

Recently, an association between idiopathic VTE and atherosclerosis has been proposed. In a carotid ultrasonography study, the odds ratios for carotid plaques in 153 patients with spontaneous thrombosis were 2.3 (95% CI, 1.4-3.7) versus 146 patients with secondary VTE and 1.8 (95% CI, 1.1-2.9) versus 150 controls. These data have not yet been replicated.

The association between prolonged travel and VTE is controversial. Documented associations have been shown primarily by retrospective studies that assess the history of recent travel in patients with a new VTE. The association appears to be related to duration of travel, with one study showing increased risk only when travel exceeded 10 hours. In another study, only 56 of 135 million travelers flying to Paris had a confirmed PE, for a corresponding rate of 1 per 100 million passengers who traveled less than 6 hours and 1 per 700,000 passengers who traveled more than 6 hours. Most persons with VTE associated with prolonged travel have additional risk factors for thrombosis.

Evaluation

Clinical History and Physical Examination

The history and physical examination historically have not been believed to be helpful in the assessment of VTE. However, as is true in all medicine, a careful history and physical examination are always helpful. Several years ago, the Wells criteria for the clinical diagnosis of DVT were published, followed by similar criteria for PE. These criteria, based on clinical parameters, allow the clinician to quantify at the bedside the pretest likelihood of venous thrombosis. The variables in the criteria, if present, increase the likelihood that the patient has had one or both of these events (Table 6.3). These variables will appear self-evident and need not be memorized. Summed variables from these tables are used to predict the pretest likelihood that the patient has the disease.

Compression Ultrasonography

In many studies, ultrasonography has shown a sensitivity of 85% to 90% and a specificity of 86% to 100% for confirming the diagnosis of proximal DVT involving popliteal, femoral, and iliac veins. Inability to completely compress the venous segment being interrogated confirms the diagnosis of DVT by this method (Fig. 6.2). The detection of

Table 6.3 Clinical Pretest Probability of DVT and PE

DVT		PE	
Points	**Clinical variable**	**Points**	**Clinical variable**
1	Active cancer	3	Clinical symptoms of DVT
1	Paralysis or recent limb casting	3	Alternate explanation less likely than PE
1	Recent immobility >3 days	1.5	Heart rate >100 beats/min
1	Local vein tenderness	1.5	Immobilization or surgery within 4 wk
1	Limb swelling	1.5	Prior VTE
1	Unilateral calf swelling >3 days	1	Hemoptysis
1	Collateral superficial vein	1	Malignancy
−2	Alternative diagnosis likely		
Sum		**Sum**	
>2	High risk	>6	High risk
1-2	Moderate risk	2-6	Moderate risk
<1	Low risk	<2	Low risk

DVT, deep vein thrombosis; PE, pulmonary embolism; VTE, venous thromboembolism.
Left modified from Wells PS, Anderson DR, Bormanis J, et al. Value of assessment of pretest probability of deep-vein thrombosis in clinical management. Lancet. 1997;350:1795-8. Used with permission. Right from Wells PS, Anderson DR, Rodger M, et al. Derivation of a simple clinical model to categorize patients probability of pulmonary embolism: increasing the models utility with the simpliRED D-dimer. Thromb Haemost. 2000;83:416-20. Used with permission.

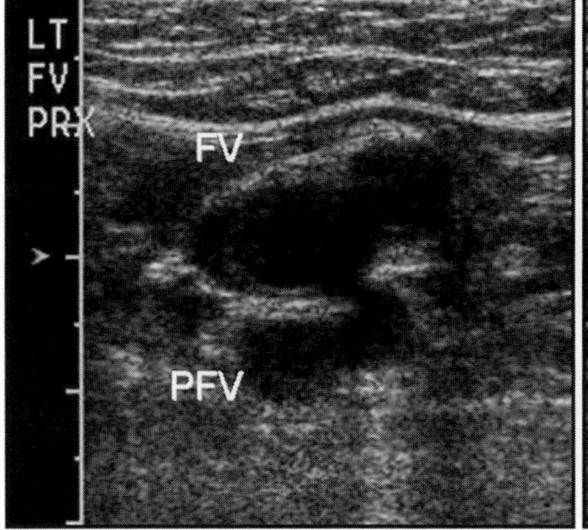

Fig. 6.2 Lower extremity ultrasonography with (*right*) and without (*left*) compression. Arrows represent the non-compressible venous segments with thrombus present. FV, femoral vein; PFV, profunda femoris vein.

calf vein thrombi by this technique is reliable but technically more challenging. Although venography has been considered the gold standard, clinical experience with this test is dwindling as fewer studies are currently being performed.

Computed Tomography

Helical computed tomography (CT) for the diagnosis of embolism has a sensitivity of between 57% and 100% and a specificity of 78% to 100% (Fig. 6.3). These percentages vary by embolism location, ranging from more than 90% for central emboli to much lower for segmental or subsegmental emboli.

Ventilation Perfusion Scanning

Ventilation perfusion scanning is a valuable tool for the diagnosis of PE if the results are definitive. If the results are normal or show a high probability of PE (Fig. 6.4), the clinician can give a definitive diagnosis and preclude further testing. However, many scans yield results interpreted as a "possible," "probable," "indeterminate," or "intermediate" probability of PE, and therefore further imaging is required. In the classic PIOPED study (Prospective Investigation of Pulmonary Embolism Diagnosis), which addressed the utility of ventilation perfusion scanning in the diagnosis of PE, 72% of patients had "intermediate" interpretations and therefore required further testing. When such non-diagnostic imaging results are obtained, the clinician must use CT imaging or pulmonary angiography. The requirement for such additional tests is not ideal because of the time and expense involved.

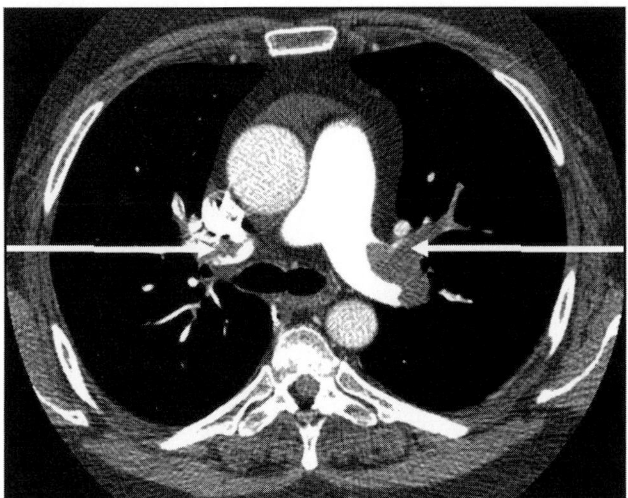

Fig. 6.3 Computed tomography angiography of the chest. Acute pulmonary emboli are noted in both main pulmonary arteries (*arrows*).

Pulmonary Angiography

Pulmonary angiography remains the gold standard for the diagnosis of PE, but it requires expertise in performance and interpretation that is waning in current practice, similar to expertise in venography.

Fibrin D-Dimer Testing

Fibrin D-dimer, the soluble degradation product of fibrin can be measured from a peripheral blood sample using various assays. D-dimer testing has proved to be very sensitive for the detection of ongoing fibrinolysis but is not adequately specific for thrombosis. A negative D-dimer result excludes the presence of thrombosis with a negative predictive value that exceeds 95% and is therefore helpful in excluding the diagnosis of DVT or PE. Unfortunately, many clinical scenarios may give a positive D-dimer result (Table 6.4). A positive D-dimer result carries a poor positive predictive value of no more than 50% and is not helpful clinically.

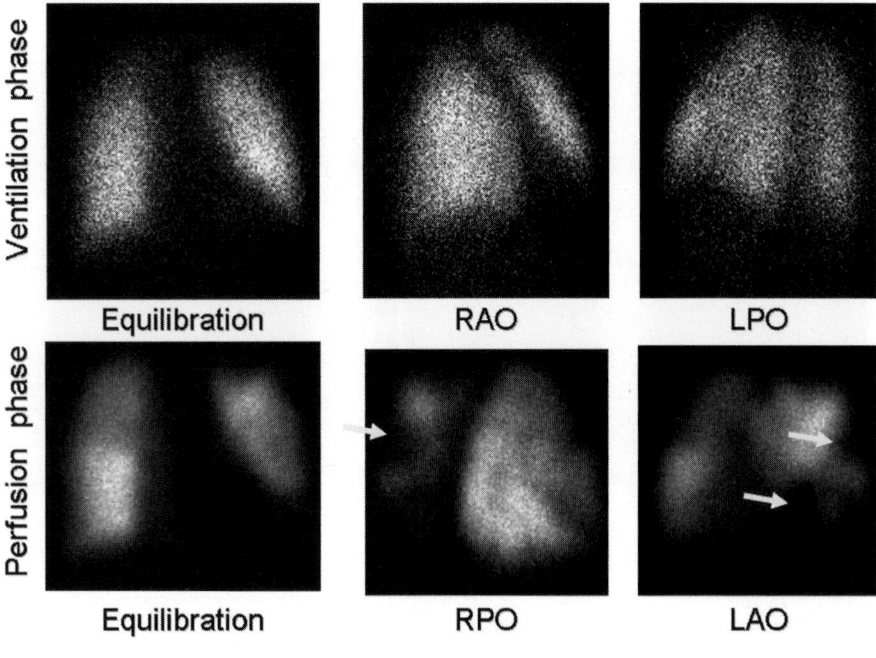

Fig. 6.4 "High probability" ventilation perfusion lung scan. This scan shows evidence of multiple bilateral perfusion mismatches (lower panel, *arrows*) consistent with a high probability of pulmonary embolism. The ventilation phase scan (upper panel) is normally distributed. LAO, left anterior oblique; LPO, left posterior oblique; RAO, right anterior oblique; RPO, right posterior oblique.

Table 6.4 Conditions That Can Give False-Positive D-Dimer Results

Bleeding
Trauma
Surgery
Pregnancy
Abdominal aortic aneurysm
Malignancy

Prevention

In many randomized trials over the past several decades, the use of primary DVT prophylaxis has been proven to reduce the rate of VTE and fatal PE. Furthermore, VTE prophylaxis is widely viewed as cost effective because it decreases adverse patient outcomes. The risk of bleeding if DVT prophylaxis is given is a primary concern, but this risk has not been substantiated by multiple trials of low-dose unfractionated heparin, low-molecular-weight heparin (LMWH), or warfarin. Graduated compression stockings and intermittent pneumatic compression devices have been shown to decrease the incidence of DVT. These mechanical methods, however, have not been shown to reduce the risk of death or PE and in general are less effective than pharmacologic VTE prophylaxis regimens. Aspirin or other antiplatelet prophylaxis has not been satisfactorily shown to adequately prevent VTE and therefore is not recommended for this purpose. Waiting for symptoms of VTE and routine surveillance for asymptomatic DVT are not reliable strategies for preventing clinically relevant incident VTE and are not recommended; a priori prevention is preferable.

In patients undergoing surgical procedures, the decision to provide DVT prophylaxis must be made case by case, factoring in patient-specific risk factors and the general risks of the anticipated procedure. The patient-specific risk factors include age, history of VTE, concurrent malignancy, and congenital thrombophilias. Surgery-specific risk includes the magnitude of the procedure, orthopedic joint replacement or hip fracture surgery, surgery for major trauma or associated spinal cord injury, or malignancy-related surgery. Based on these combined variables, patients are stratified into categories ranging from low to high risk, each with associated prophylaxis recommendations. Alternatively, prophylaxis decisions can be group specific, related to the particular surgery planned. An excellent in-depth review of this topic, including appropriate DVT prophylaxis for many specific surgical procedures, has been published recently.

- The use of primary DVT prophylaxis has been proven to reduce the rate of VTE and fatal PE
- Aspirin or other antiplatelet prophylaxis has not been shown to prevent VTE and is not recommended for this purpose

Treatment

Typical treatment of VTE includes the simultaneous initiation of heparin and warfarin therapy. Optimal therapy includes adequate inhibition of clot propagation, embolization, and death from embolization, while minimizing the risk of hemorrhagic complications. Only US Food and Drug Administration–approved and currently available therapies for clinical use will be highlighted in this section. Although many promising agents await approval, knowledge of these unapproved agents will not be assessed on board examination questions.

Unfractionated Heparin

Heparin is a mainstay of therapy for any thrombotic disorder. Its anticoagulant properties derive from its interaction with antithrombin III (AT) (Fig. 6.5). Heparin induces a conformational change in AT, forming a tertiary structure that enhances the affinity of AT for thrombin by 1,000-fold. Once formed, the thrombin-AT complex is essentially irreversible, which effectively inhibits the action of thrombin.

Heparin is a highly negatively charged proteoglycan extracted from porcine or bovine intestinal mucosa. Unfractionated heparin preparations are heterogeneous, containing heparin chains of variable lengths and molecular weights ranging from 5,000 to 80,000 kDa. A specific pentasaccharide sequence on the heparin molecule is required for heparin binding to AT at the heparin binding site, but only about 25% of the heparin in a preparation contains this pentasaccharide sequence. Non-specific binding to various cells and plasma proteins neutralizes the anticoagulant activity of heparin. Because of these factors and unpredictable distribution volumes and elimination kinetics, therapy with unfractionated heparin must be strictly monitored by serial activated partial thromboplastin time (aPTT) measurement for both safety and efficacy.

The use of unfractionated heparin in the initial treatment of VTE has been shown to decrease morbidity, mortality, and recurrent thrombosis, particularly if therapeutic levels are achieved within the first 24 hours of initiation. This corresponds to prolongation of the baseline aPTT by a factor of 1.5 to 2.5. Several weight-based nomograms have been shown to achieve these levels more rapidly. With use of these nomograms, more than 80% of patients reach the therapeutic range within 24 hours, with a 5% risk of major hemorrhage. At an aPTT greater than 2.5-times baseline, the risk of hemorrhage increases significantly.

When simultaneously using heparin and warfarin, both drugs are continued either until the international normalized ratio (INR) has reached therapeutic levels (2.0-3.0) or for 5 days, whichever is longer. The reason for prolonged heparin therapy is to ensure that procoagulant vitamin K–dependent proteins (factors II, VII, IX, and X) are sufficiently depleted while protecting against thrombosis during this period of hypercoagulability, when vitamin K–dependent anticoagulant (protein C and S) stores are likewise being depleted.

Heparin resistance is relatively common, affecting 25% of persons with VTE. This resistance is defined as a heparin requirement exceeding 35,000 units per day. Several causes of heparin resistance primarily relate to non-specific binding of heparin to plasma proteins and cells. Common culprits include elevated circulating factor VIII and fibrinogen. Other possibilities for heparin resistance include AT deficiency, increased heparin clearance, or medications such as aprotinin or nitroglycerin. Therapeutic options include simply increasing the heparin dose or changing to LMWH or a direct thrombin inhibitor. It is

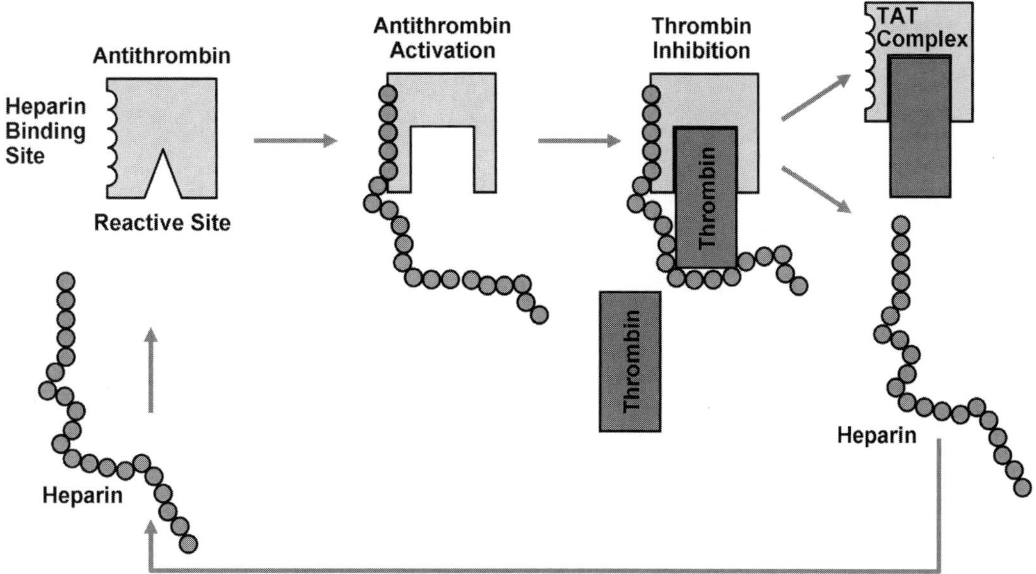

Fig. 6.5 Mechanism of antithrombin activation by heparin. TAT, thrombin–antithrombin III complex.

not appropriate to test for AT deficiency while the patient is receiving heparin, because heparin therapy alone can result in moderate decreases of AT.

Heparin-induced thrombocytopenia (HIT) can complicate heparin therapy in 5% to 7% of patients receiving heparin and typically occurs 5 to 10 days after initiation. Suggested monitoring for this complication includes measuring platelet count every other day. The diagnosis of HIT is suspected if the platelet count decreases by 50% or more, or if thrombocytopenia is present with counts less than $100 \times 10^9/L$. Thrombotic events can occur in up to 50% of cases and the risk can last for 30 days or more after heparin withdrawal. For this reason, an alternative antithrombotic agent must be initiated if the diagnosis of HIT is made and heparin is withdrawn.

Treatment of VTE

- Initiation of heparin and warfarin, both of which are continued until either the INR has reached therapeutic levels (2.0-3.0) or for 5 days, whichever is longer
  - Heparin resistance is relatively common, affecting 25% of those with VTE
  - HIT may complicate heparin therapy in 5%-7% of patients receiving heparin and occurs 5-10 days after initiation
- LMWH given once daily, or in two divided daily doses

Low-Molecular-Weight Heparin

LMWH is produced by depolymerizing unfractionated heparin using chemical or enzymatic methods (Fig. 6.6). This yields a preparation of small heparin fragments of a more uniform molecular weight (4,000-6,000 kDa). LMWH requires AT for activity, but unlike the unfractionated heparin-AT complex, the LMWH-AT complex has a higher specificity for factor Xa than for thrombin. Because LMWH is a smaller molecule, the tertiary structure required for the thrombin-AT interaction cannot be developed and its affinity is therefore increased for factor Xa, which does not require this tertiary intermediate. Because of its uniformity of size and more neutral charge, LMWH has much less non-specific binding, improved bioavailability, and more predictable pharmacology. Dosing is safe and effective when based on patient body weight and does not affect the aPTT.

LMWH given once daily or in two divided daily doses provides effective initial anticoagulant therapy for patients with VTE. Recurrent thrombotic events, major hemorrhage, and mortality rates are equal to or less than those with unfractionated heparin. Weight-based dosing without monitoring makes this drug particularly attractive for the outpatient treatment of DVT. Treatment of PE with LMWH is also very effective; however, initial therapy should begin in the hospital to ensure hemodynamic stability. HIT is a rare complication of LMWH, occurring in less than 1% of patients.

LMWH therapy does not require monitoring under normal circumstances. However, monitoring should be considered for pregnant or morbidly obese patients and for those on prolonged therapy or with renal insufficiency. Under such conditions, it is reasonable to obtain an anti–factor Xa activity level. This should be measured 4 hours after the last LMWH dose; the therapeutic level should be

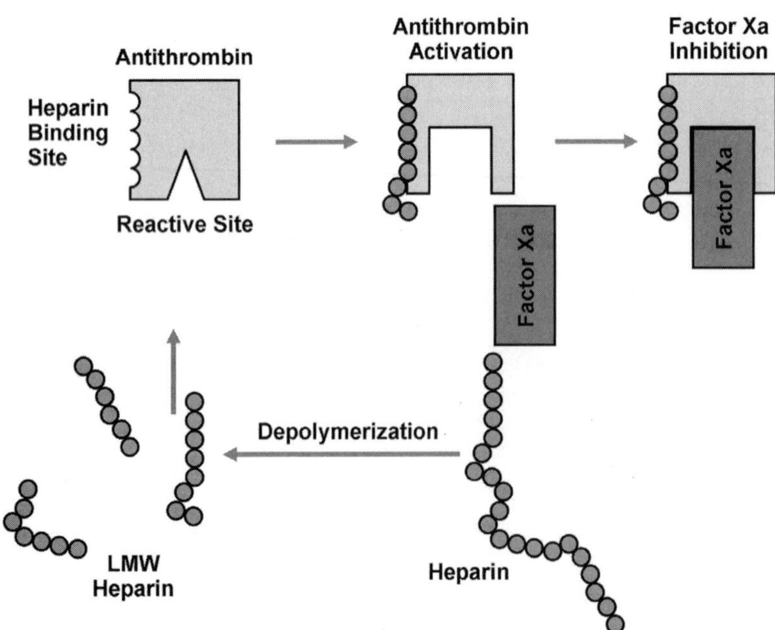

Fig. 6.6 Mechanism of antithrombin activation by low-molecular-weight (LMW) heparin.

0.5 to 1.0 IU/mL if receiving twice-daily dosing or 1.0 to 2.0 IU/mL with once-daily dosing. In most patients, serial monitoring is not necessary.

Fondaparinux

Fondaparinux can be thought of as an ultra-low-molecular-weight heparin. This drug is a synthetic pentasaccharide analog of the sequence necessary for AT activation at the heparin binding site (Fig. 6.7). It is given subcutaneously and has an elimination half-life of 17 to 21 hours. Fondaparinux is eliminated primarily by the kidneys and is most likely contraindicated in patients with severe renal impairment (creatinine clearance <30 mL/min). Because of its very low molecular weight and essentially neutral net charge, this drug does not bind significantly to other plasma proteins and, specifically, does not bind platelet factor 4. Therefore, the risk of HIT developing is negligible. Its net neutral charge also means that fondaparinux is not inhibited by protamine as are unfractionated heparin and LMWH. However, no antidote for bleeding is available for patients receiving this drug.

Fondaparinux, like LMWH, does not require monitoring. Routine coagulation tests such as prothrombin time and aPTT are relatively insensitive measures and unsuitable for monitoring. Like LMWH, the anti–factor Xa activity of fondaparinux can be measured if necessary.

Fondaparinux has been shown to provide superior DVT prophylaxis in the setting of hip fracture surgery. For hip and knee replacement surgeries, fondaparinux was as effective as (in one trial) or more effective than (in two trials) LMWH (enoxaparin) in preventing VTE. Major bleeding occurred in 2% to 3% of patients receiving fondaparinux in these trials compared with 0.2% to 2% for enoxaparin. The MATISSE-DVT trial randomly assigned 2,205 patients to receive either fondaparinux (at one of three doses) or enoxaparin for 5 days while initiating warfarin. At 3 months, the rates of recurrent VTE and major bleeding were similar between the two treatment arms. In the MATISSE-PE trial, patients were randomly assigned to receive either fondaparinux (one of three doses) or unfractionated heparin given intravenously. As in MATISSE-DVT, the rates of recurrent VTE and major bleeding were similar between the two treatment arms at 3 months. Fondaparinux appears to be as effective as LMWH or unfractionated heparin in the initial treatment of VTE.

Warfarin

Warfarin blocks the hepatic carboxylation of vitamin K–dependent coagulation factors (prothrombin and factors VII, IX, and X), thus inhibiting the activation of prothrombin to thrombin. Carboxylation is required for calcium binding and the shape reconfiguration necessary for incorporation of the proteins into activation complexes on the platelet phospholipid bilayer. With either the inhibition of carboxylation or calcium sequestration (e.g., with citrate or ethylenediaminetetraacetic acid), coagulation factor activation is brought to a standstill.

Inhibition of vitamin K reductase activity by warfarin can be overridden by exogenous vitamin K, which is predominantly in the reduced form (Fig. 6.8). Effective anticoagulation requires that these factors be inhibited to 20% to 25% activity. For factor VII, this inhibition can be accomplished within the first day of warfarin initiation. The prothrombin time is very sensitive to factor VII levels and may begin to rise as factor VII is depleted. Factor X and prothrombin, by comparison, have much longer half-lives and may remain relatively normal for several days. Warfarin also blocks the carboxylation of the endogenous anticoagulants protein C and protein S. Protein C has a half-life similar to that of factor VII and is

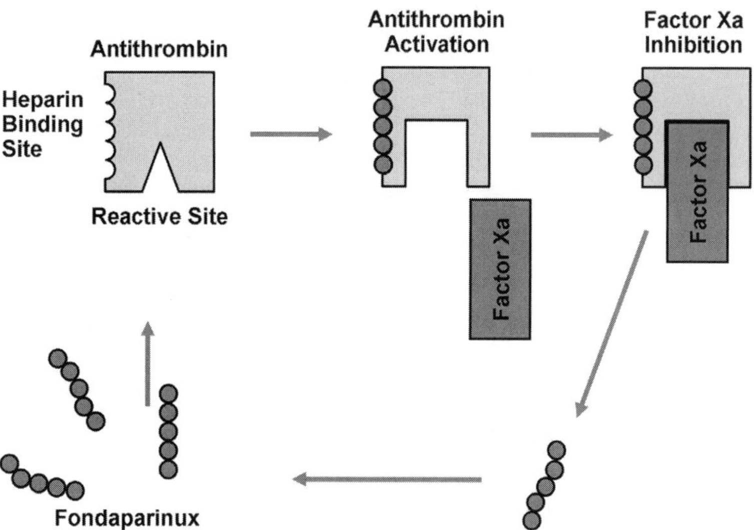

Fig. 6.7 Mechanism of antithrombin activation by fondaparinux.

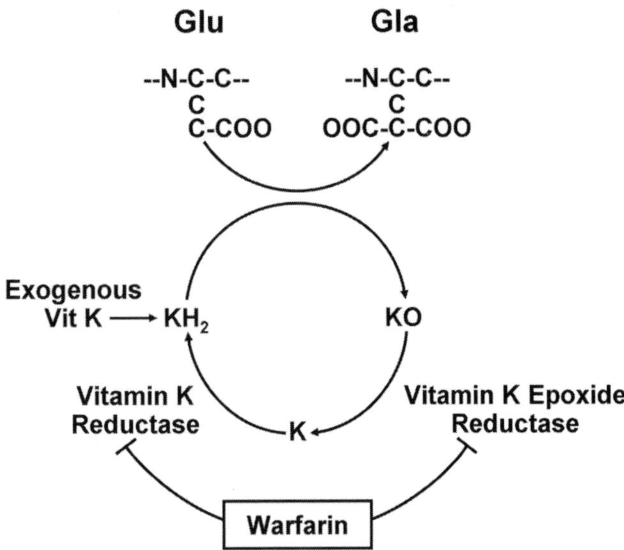

Fig. 6.8 Vitamin K–dependent γ-carboxylation of coagulation proteins. Warfarin inhibits regeneration of the reduced form of vitamin K (KH_2).

depleted quickly (Fig. 6.9). A relative hypercoagulability is therefore observed in the first few days of warfarin initiation, when protein C is depleted but concentrations of factor X and prothrombin are relatively normal. Warfarin therapy is therefore initiated simultaneously with heparin to achieve a goal INR of 2.0 to 3.0. Both warfarin and heparin are continued simultaneously for 5 days or until a therapeutic INR is achieved, whichever is longer.

Determining the duration of therapy for an initial thrombotic event can be difficult. In general, events occurring without provocation (idiopathic thrombosis) should be treated for longer periods (6-12 months), whereas provoked thrombi, such as occur after major surgery, can be treated with a more abbreviated course of therapy (3 months). In patients with idiopathic VTE, the hypothesis that low-intensity warfarin is effective in decreasing recurrent thrombotic events has recently been tested in two major clinical trials, PREVENT (Prevention of Recurrent Venous Thromboembolism) and ELATE (Extended Low-Intensity Anticoagulation for Thrombo-Embolism). These trials compared low-dose warfarin (INR, 1.5-2.0) with placebo (PREVENT) or with conventional warfarin (INR, 2.0-3.0; ELATE), in patients with idiopathic DVT after completing 6 months of conventional therapy. The combined data suggested that continuing warfarin in patients with idiopathic VTE reduces the risk of recurrence by 3- to 10-fold compared with no therapy. Whereas bleeding rates were similar, low-intensity therapy gave no advantage over conventional therapy for patients who elected to continue warfarin beyond 6 months.

- Events occurring without provocation (idiopathic thrombosis) should be treated for longer periods (6-12 months)
- Provoked thrombi, such as those after major surgery, can be treated with a more abbreviated course of therapy (3 months)

The risk of clotting or bleeding while on warfarin depends on several variables, including the adequacy of anticoagulation management. In general, clotting and bleeding rates are highest when management is left to

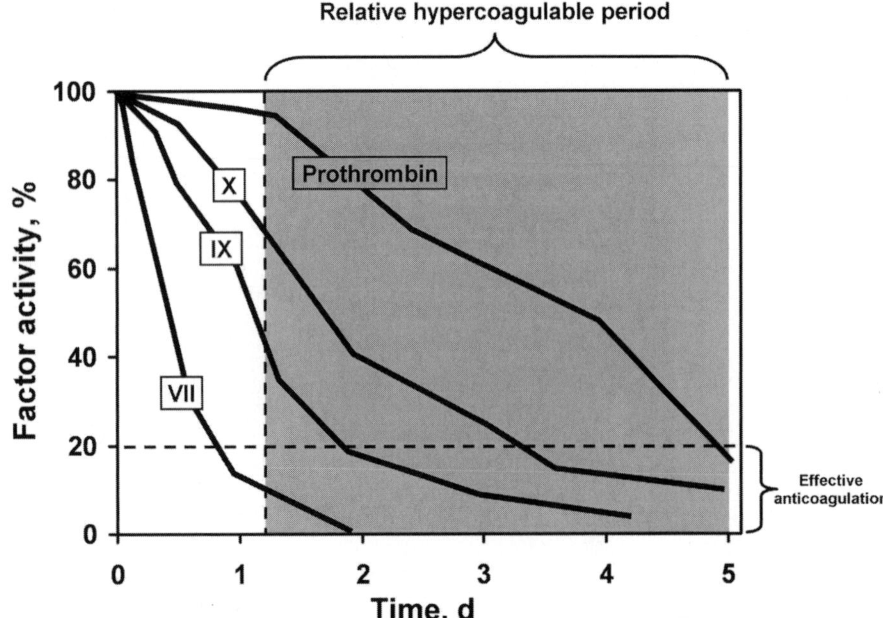

Fig. 6.9 Decrease in vitamin K–dependent coagulation factor (factor VII, IX, X, and prothrombin) activity with initiation of warfarin.

"usual care" by the patient's primary physician (regardless of specialty). In this setting, rates are reported at 5% to 8% annually for either thrombosis or major bleeding. INR management by a specialized anticoagulation clinic was shown to improve these rates to 2% to 5% annually. Decisions to continue anticoagulation with warfarin therefore depend on the bleeding and thrombosis rates expected for the local clinic where the patient receives anticoagulation management.

- "Usual care" rates of either thrombosis or major bleeding are reported at 5%-8% annually
- INR management by a specialized anticoagulation clinic has been shown to improve thrombosis and major bleeding rates to 2%-5% annually

Warfarin skin necrosis is a rare but serious potential complication of initiating anticoagulation therapy, particularly in patients with protein C deficiency. In general, anticoagulation initiation in patients with known protein C deficiency should be accompanied by full therapeutic heparin. This complication typically affects women between the third and tenth day of treatment and usually involves regions of abundant subcutaneous adipose tissue such as breasts, abdomen, buttocks, and thighs. Although not fully established, the pathogenesis of this condition is thought to stem from a disproportionate decrease in protein C levels relative to other procoagulant factors, triggering thrombosis in postcapillary venules, with resultant dermal necrosis. Warfarin skin necrosis is very rare in patients with protein S deficiency but very serious when it occurs.

Inferior Vena Cava Filters

The two indications for inferior vena cava (IVC) filter placement include a contraindication to anticoagulation therapy and anticoagulation failure. After IVC filter placement, the rate of PE is approximately 2% with a fatal complication rate of less than 0.1%. One prospective randomized study found a 2-fold increased risk of recurrent lower extremity venous thrombosis within 2 years of filter placement compared with the control group. Many vascular physicians therefore view filter placement as an indication for lifelong warfarin therapy.

The use of temporary, removable, or "optional" IVC filters (Fig. 6.10, *left*) has greatly increased in recent months and provides an important adjunct for patients who temporarily have a contraindication to anticoagulant therapy. In one study of 192 patients, the rate of PE after placement was 3%. Filter dislodgement, a potential concern for this type of device, occurred in 5% of cases. The rate of filter thrombosis was documented at 16% (Fig. 6.10, *right*). A precise indication for this type of filter has not yet been defined.

Fibrinolytic Therapy

The absolute indication for fibrinolytic therapy for patients with VTE is hemodynamic instability after PE. Whether patients with right ventricular dilatation and dysfunction but preserved hemodynamics should be treated with lytic therapy is controversial. Lytic therapy for lower extremity DVT has been advocated to decrease

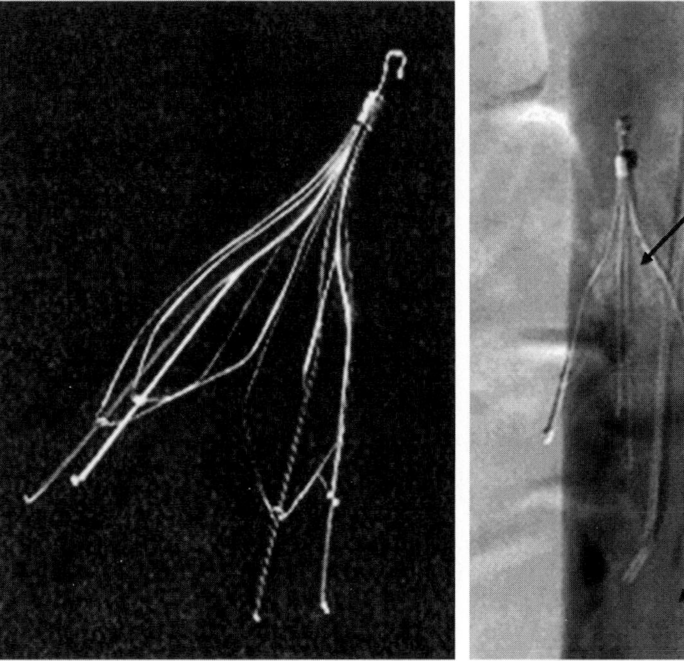

Fig. 6.10 Temporary inferior vena cava (IVC) filter. The right panel depicts an embolism caught in the struts of the filter.

the long-term morbidity of the postphlebitic syndrome. Although many would agree with catheter-directed lytic therapy and angioplasty for iliac vein thrombosis, this approach has not been proven in randomized clinical trials. Systemic fibrinolysis for this indication has largely been abandoned.

Compression Stockings

The postphlebitic syndrome is a chronic sequela of acute DVT and affects approximately 30% of patients within 10 years of the initial thrombotic event. The symptoms of the postphlebitic syndrome include chronic pain and swelling of the affected limb. Approximately 10% of patients have recurrent ulcers. Compression stocking (30-40 mm Hg) use after DVT has been studied prospectively in two randomized trials and shown to reduce the prevalence of the postphlebitic syndrome by 50% if worn for 2 years. No randomized trials have assessed shorter or longer duration of treatment. Furthermore, no trials have assessed venous thrombus location and extent to determine if this recommendation should be applied globally to all patients with lower extremity DVT.

- Indications for IVC filter placement include:
  - Contraindication to anticoagulation
  - Anticoagulation failure
- The absolute indication for fibrinolytic therapy in VTE is hemodynamic instability after PE
- Compression stocking use after DVT has been shown to decrease the prevalence of postphlebitic syndrome by 50% if worn for 2 years

Venous Thrombosis at Unusual Sites

DVT commonly involves the venous vasculature of the lower extremities with or without embolization to pulmonary arteries. In the modern era of central venous catheter use and increasing rates of cardiac device implantation, the incidence of venous thrombosis of the upper extremities is increasing. Venous thrombosis can occur, however, at any location, including cerebral venous sinuses, renal veins, hepatic veins, and other splanchnic veins. Although the diagnosis of venous thrombosis at unusual locations is increasing with the evolution of imaging technology and growing physician awareness, the epidemiology and appropriate treatment remain relatively undefined.

Cerebral Venous Sinus Thrombosis

Cerebral venous sinus thrombosis (CVST) is an uncommon condition with an often striking clinical presentation that affects primarily young to middle-aged women. Although this thrombotic process can involve any combination of venous sinuses or superficial or deep cerebral veins, the superior sagittal and lateral sinuses are most commonly affected and account for 70% of cases (Fig. 6.11).

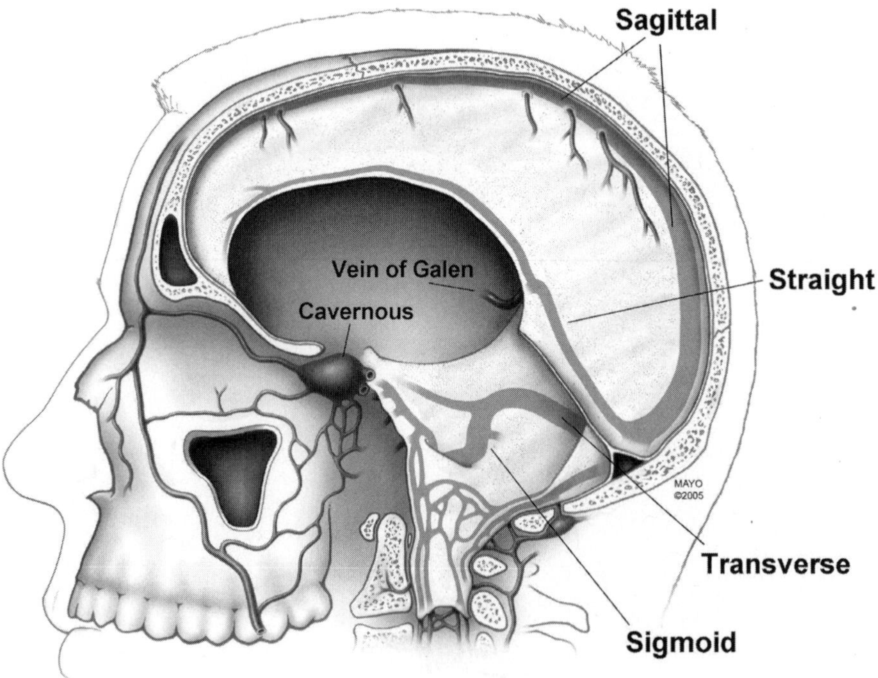

Fig. 6.11 Cerebral venous sinus anatomy. (From Gosk-Bierska I, Wysokinski W, Brown RD Jr, et al. Cerebral venous sinus thrombosis: incidence of venous thrombosis recurrence and survival. Neurology. 2006;67:814-9. Used with permission of Mayo Foundation for Medical Education and Research.)

The epidemiology of CVST depends largely on ascertainment of cases and increases with age. In an autopsy series of 182 deceased patients, the incidence was 9.3% with an average age of 73 years. In comparison, an estimate of peripartum CVST was 11.6/100,000 deliveries in which all patients were younger than 44 years (range, 15-44 years). In a pediatric population, an incidence of 0.67 cases per 100,000 children was found.

The etiology of CVST is diverse, including more than 100 unique causes. Table 6.5 lists the most common causes in decreasing order of frequency. Both acquired and inherited thrombophilias have been implicated, including the antiphospholipid antibody syndrome, factor V Leiden and prothrombin G20210A mutations, protein C and S deficiencies, and AT deficiency. The use of oral contraception is an important contributing variable in affected young women and particularly in those with hereditary thrombophilia. Pregnancy and the puerperium have been recognized as periods vulnerable for this condition. In one study, cesarean delivery, hypertension, coexisting infections, and excessive vomiting were strongly associated with CVST in the postpartum period by multivariate analysis.

The clinical presentation of CVST is broad. Headache, focal neurologic deficits, seizures, or altered consciousness can occur in isolation or in combination and may begin abruptly or evolve over weeks. Focal neurologic deficits, seizures, and impaired consciousness are common and present in 40% of patients. Papilledema is observed in 40% of these patients, yet only 15% of patients are comatose on presentation.

Demonstration of the sinus thrombosis by neuroimaging is crucial for establishing the diagnosis. CT, especially if performed without contrast, can miss the diagnosis of CVST in up to 20% of cases or be misinterpreted as subarachnoid or intraparenchymal hemorrhage. Alterations in blood flow and hemoglobin degradation products in thrombosed veins can produce signal changes on magnetic resonance imaging (MRI) that suggest the diagnosis of CVST, but such findings may be subtle. Thus, the diagnosis of CVST can be missed, particularly in clinically unsuspected cases, unless gadolinium enhancement is used. Although cerebral angiography remains definitive for the diagnosis of CVST, magnetic resonance venography has recently become the imaging technique most widely used to establish the diagnosis.

Therapeutic recommendations for anticoagulant use vary greatly and remain controversial. Although the use of heparin has long been advocated, little evidence supports its use. The optimal dose, duration, and preparation of heparin, whether standard heparin or LMWH, for the treatment of CVST remain to be clarified. Oral anticoagulant therapy has an uncertain role, but it is likely to be reasonable for a limited duration.

Table 6.5 CVST Etiology

Idiopathic
Hormone therapy
Malignancy
Venous malformation
Postoperative
CNS/ENT infections
Dehydration
Pregnancy
Inflammatory bowel disease
Thrombophilia

CNS, central nervous system; CVST, cerebral venous sinus thrombosis; ENT, otolaryngologic.

Renal Vein Thrombosis

The epidemiology of renal vein thrombosis (RVT) in the general population is poorly defined and largely dependent on case ascertainment. Early studies focused primarily on the diagnosis of RVT made at autopsy. Among 29,280 unselected adult autopsies performed at Mayo Clinic from 1929 to 1961, only 17 cases of bilateral RVT were found, for an incidence of approximately 0.6 per 1,000 autopsies. Among these 17 cases, only 2 had nephrotic syndrome, men predominated (2.5:1 vs women), and the average age was 47 years. Several prospective studies have evaluated the incidence of RVT in nephrotic syndrome, and reported incidences range from 1.9% to 42%. Among patients with nephrotic syndrome, membranous glomerulopathy is most often associated with RVT.

Although many studies have focused on the association between RVT and nephrotic syndrome, RVT has many causes (Table 6.6). Primary renal disease is the most common cause, particularly if renal malignancy is added to this group. Both acute and chronic nephropathic conditions can be complicated by venous thrombosis, particularly membranous glomerulonephritis. Renal cell carcinoma has the propensity to invade the venous system and is associated with venous tumor thrombus in 4% to 25% of cases. When present, tumor thrombus heralds a worse prognosis: larger tumors, more advanced grade and stage

Table 6.6 RVT Etiology

Idiopathic
Malignancy
Nephrotic syndrome
Infectious
Postoperative
Dehydration
Inflammatory bowel disease
Hormone therapy
Thrombophilia

RVT, renal vein thrombosis.

of malignancy, and more frequent metastases. Congenital and acquired thrombophilias have been reported, including deficiencies of AT, protein C, and protein S, hyperhomocysteinemia, and the antiphospholipid syndrome; however, these are primarily limited to case reports. Oral contraception, pregnancy, and the puerperium have also been described as causative factors.

The clinical presentation of RVT ranges from a complete lack of symptoms to renal failure. The clinical spectrum of RVT varies depending on the extent and dynamics of venous occlusion, the development of collateral circulation, and underlying disease. Acute complete occlusion, seen more often in neonates and infants with dehydration, causes rapid congestion and hemorrhagic infarction of the affected kidney with subsequent atrophy. If the occlusion occurs gradually, collateral vessels can develop, providing adequate venous drainage and preventing renal damage. Various degrees of upper abdominal pain, flank pain, and hematuria may be the presenting symptoms. Clinical signs and symptoms, however, may be absent, vague, or non-specific.

Duplex ultrasonography is useful in the diagnostic evaluation of RVT with direct visualization of thrombi within the renal vein and IVC, demonstration of renal vein dilatation proximal to the point of occlusion, and increase in renal size during the acute phase of venous congestion. After infarction, renal atrophy results in a small non-functional kidney with abnormal renal structure. Both CT and MRI can provide a definitive diagnosis based on visualization of the clots within the vein and IVC.

The main goals of therapy should be to conserve renal parenchyma and protect renal function. To date, nephrectomy has been abandoned except in an acute life-threatening hemorrhage as a result of capsular rupture, renal cell carcinoma, trauma, and extrinsic compression of the vascular pedicle. A conservative approach, with anticoagulation as the main therapeutic modality, is likely best for most cases in adults. No prospective randomized trials have assessed the effectiveness of anticoagulation therapy in RVT. Renal function can improve markedly in patients with acute RVT who are treated with anticoagulant therapy. Relapses with new episodes of acute RVT have been observed after cessation of anticoagulant therapy. The optimal duration of therapy with anticoagulants is not known for these patients.

Budd-Chiari Syndrome

Budd-Chiari syndrome (BCS) results when hepatic venous drainage is obstructed by various causes, including thrombosis, tumor, primary veno-occlusive disease, or congenital obstruction. Of these, hepatic vein thrombosis is the most common, particularly in Western societies. BCS can be classified according to the location of the venous occlusion: Type 1, the IVC is occluded, with or without obstruction of the hepatic veins; Type 2, occlusion of major hepatic veins; and Type 3, only the small centrilobular venules are involved. Type 3 results primarily from a fibrous obliteration of small intrahepatic venules as a complication of bone marrow transplantation. Depending on the nature and extent of venous obstruction, the clinical course ranges from a slow insidious onset of symptoms to rampant progression of acute hepatic failure.

Precise identification of etiologic factors and their frequency is limited by the rarity of BCS and the lack of large epidemiologic studies. The various implicated causes appear to differ by geographic region. Congenital membranous obstruction of the IVC is the classic cause of BCS in Eastern countries, whereas in Western populations, thrombosis is the predominant cause. The underlying factors associated with hepatic vein thrombosis include inherited or acquired thrombophilic states, myeloproliferative diseases, paroxysmal nocturnal hemoglobinuria, pregnancy, and the use of oral contraception (Table 6.7). Connective tissue diseases and other inflammatory disorders have also been reported as causes, particularly Behçet syndrome.

Hepatic venous obstruction can result from extrinsic compression or endoluminal invasion by malignant tumors. Of these, hepatocellular carcinoma, renal cell carcinoma, and Wilms tumor rank highly. Deficiencies of AT, protein C, and protein S, factor V Leiden and prothrombin G20210A gene mutations, and antiphospholipid antibody syndrome have been reported. However, the contribution of either inherited or acquired thrombophilic states is unclear because of the limited number of epidemiologic studies with complete coagulation testing.

As with venous thrombosis at other atypical locations, the clinical presentation of BCS depends on the extent and rapidity of hepatic venous obstruction. Because hepatic venous outflow is accomplished by three veins, impairment of a single vein can be clinically silent. More extensive venous involvement causes painful hepatic congestion with stretching of the Glisson capsule and hepatomegaly.

Table 6.7 BCS Etiology

Idiopathic
Myeloproliferative disorder
Infectious
Postoperative
Malignancy
Connective tissue disease
Hormone therapy
Pregnancy
Cirrhosis
PNH
Inflammatory bowel disease

BCS, Budd-Chiari syndrome; PNH, paroxysmal nocturnal hemoglobinuria.

Within the confined capsule, sinusoidal congestion with venous hypertension, stasis, and hypoxia may lead to hepatocyte necrosis, hemorrhage, and parenchymal damage. The degree of injury varies from mild hepatic inflammation to fulminant hepatic failure.

Although laboratory testing may be helpful to assess hepatic injury and synthetic function, suspected venous obstruction requires imaging for an accurate diagnosis. Doppler ultrasonography, MRI, and CT all provide the dual advantage of evaluating liver structure and visualizing hepatic vein thrombus with or without IVC thrombosis. Both Doppler ultrasonography and magnetic resonance angiography allow quantitative measurement of flow velocity, flow profile, and directionality.

The primary treatment objectives in BCS are hepatic decompression, functional restoration, and prevention of thrombus propagation and recurrence. Specific treatment depends on the cause and extent of venous obstruction and the reversibility of hepatic injury. Although anticoagulation therapy is often used to prevent venous thrombus propagation and recurrence and to maintain patency of intravascular or surgical shunts, the benefits of chronic anticoagulation therapy remain controversial and have not been proven in randomized controlled trials. Furthermore, the optimal duration and intensity of anticoagulation is unknown. Mechanical or fibrinolytic therapy alone or in combination, to recanalize obstructed hepatic veins, has yielded anecdotal success, but the optimal role in the treatment of BCS remains speculative.

Surgical shunts decompress hepatic venous circulation by diverting hepatic venous outflow through the portal vein into the IVC. This procedure relieves sinusoidal congestion and hemorrhage and decreases hepatocyte necrosis. Potential surgical options include side-to-side portacaval shunt, mesocaval shunt, and an H-graft between the portal vein and IVC. Surgical decompressive therapy has been shown to be superior to chronic anticoagulation and medical management in patients with severe BCS. The long-term success of these surgeries varies, with 5-year survival rates ranging from 57% to 83%. Transjugular intrahepatic portasystemic shunts are another method of mechanically decompressing hepatic venous flow. Using angiographic guidance, a transhepatic parenchymal shunt is created between the intrahepatic portal and hepatic veins and maintained using stents. The procedure to create the transjugular intrahepatic portasystemic shunt, which is physiologically similar to the surgical portacaval shunt, is performed without the risks of general anesthesia or surgery. End-stage liver disease may require orthotopic liver transplantation. In some but not all circumstances, liver transplantation not only corrects hepatic failure and portal hypertension but also removes the underlying cause of hypercoagulability.

Table 6.8 MVT Etiology

Idiopathic
Malignancy
Cirrhosis
Pancreatitis
Myeloproliferative disease
Abdominal surgery
Intra-abdominal sepsis
Hormonal
Inflammatory bowel disease
Connective tissue disease
PNH

MVT, mesenteric vein thrombosis; PNH, paroxysmal nocturnal hemoglobinuria.

Mesenteric Vein Thrombosis

Mesenteric vein thrombosis (MVT) is a rare thrombotic disorder with a broad etiologic spectrum. The first description of MVT as a clinical entity was in 1935. Since then, imaging studies have clarified some of the pathophysiology and clinical presentation of this disorder. The mean age at presentation is 50 years, but MVT can occur in any patient from the neonate to the nonagenarian. Causes cited include malignancy, underlying liver disease, pancreatitis, and recent surgery (Table 6.8). Congenital and acquired thrombophilic states (e.g., protein C or S deficiency, factor V Leiden mutation), pregnancy, and the puerperium are also regarded as risk factors, but in most cases the cause remains unknown.

The clinical presentation of MVT varies considerably, depending on the acuity and extent of venous thrombotic occlusion. Often, the diagnosis is made only after variceal bleeding or ascites—resulting from portal hypertension—brings the patient to clinical attention. More serious presentations of acute extensive thrombosis can lead to bowel infarction and an acute abdomen. The presentation, however, may be more insidious, with jaundice, asterixis, or weight loss, particularly if associated with an underlying abdominal malignancy.

The diagnosis can be difficult and requires a high degree of clinical suspicion. Imaging of the mesenteric venous system with duplex ultrasonography, CT, or MRI identifies the thrombosed mesenteric venous segments.

Treatment decisions depend on the extent and severity of venous compromise at clinical presentation. Surgery with bowel resection is required in the most profound cases of bowel infarction. Anticoagulant therapy with heparin and warfarin is warranted after hemostasis is ensured.

Retinal Vein Thrombosis

Retinal vein thrombosis (RtVT) is unique among the venous thrombotic disorders of unusual locations in that

Table 6.9 RtVT Etiology

Hypertension
Diabetes mellitus
CAD
Connective tissue disease
Leukemia/lymphoma
Glaucoma
Alcohol abuse
Oral contraceptives
Inflammatory bowel disease
Thrombophilia
Idiopathic

CAD, coronary artery disease; RtVT, retinal vein thrombosis.

both the underlying etiologic spectrum and treatment are distinct from other thrombotic disorders. The major risk factors include variables typical for atherosclerosis rather than venous thrombosis (Table 6.9). Retinal arterial hypertension and atherosclerosis cause retinal vein compression and stasis as a potential pathophysiologic mechanism connecting atherosclerotic risk factors with this thrombotic disorder. Central RtVT is a common cause of visual loss and is second only to diabetic retinopathy as the most common cause of retinal vascular disease. RtVT leads to retinal venous hypertension, macular edema, and then visual loss. If severe, retinal ischemia can lead to neovascularization and subsequent vitreous hemorrhage or glaucoma.

Treatment can be quite complicated and requires the expertise of ophthalmologic surgery, including lowering of intraocular pressure, topical corticosteroids, cyclocryotherapy, and photocoagulation. Additional therapy includes aggressive management of the underlying medical disease. Because of the risk of vitreous hemorrhage, anticoagulants are rarely used.

Ovarian Vein Thrombosis

Ovarian vein thrombosis (OVT) is a rare but often serious complication of the postpartum state. This suppurative pelvic thrombophlebitis involves the right ovarian vein much more frequently than the left, which has been explained by the length, tortuosity, multiple incompetent valves, and antegrade flow of the right ovarian vein compared with the left. Complications of OVT are rare but have included PE, thrombus extension into the left renal vein or IVC, and ureteral obstruction. OVT has historically been diagnosed clinically during the postpartum period in the setting of fever unresponsive to antibiotics or at laparotomy. With the advancement of cross-sectional imaging, understanding of the incidence and clinical spectrum of OVT has evolved. OVT is therefore more frequently found incidentally, often as an asymptomatic complication of pelvic malignancy or pelvic surgeries. CT is currently recognized as the diagnostic modality of choice, whereas the sensitivity and specificity of MRI and ultrasonography are less certain.

Although not substantiated by prospective randomized clinical trial data, the current clinical practice is to provide a brief (7-10–day) course of heparin and antibiotics for postpartum OVT. Recommendations regarding anticoagulation vary greatly, however, and therapeutic management for OVT in non-pregnant patients remains unclear. In the absence of a neoplasm however, the clinical course is quite favorable with excellent long-term survival and a low rate of recurrent thrombosis or thromboembolic complications.

Upper Extremity Venous Thrombosis

With the increasing use of central venous catheters, permanent pacemakers, and defibrillators, the incidence of upper extremity venous thrombosis is likewise increasing. In hospitalized patients, particularly those in the intensive care setting, the prevalence of asymptomatic venous thrombosis associated with central lines approaches 50%. In non-hospitalized patients with idiopathic venous thrombosis of the upper extremity, complications of thoracic outlet syndrome must be considered. Malignancy and congenital and acquired thrombophilic disorders should also be considered in the evaluation of these patients. Complications from venous thrombosis of the upper extremity are less prevalent compared with thrombosis of lower limb venous segments. For example, the rate of PE from the axillosubclavian system is between 10% and 20%, compared with 30% to 50% for iliofemoral segments. Furthermore, death from PE is infrequent from these emboli, presumably because of smaller thrombus volumes.

Diagnosis of upper extremity venous thrombosis can be made readily with duplex ultrasonography, CT, or MRI. Confusion can arise, however, in correctly distinguishing the true deep venous segment from a large venous collateral that may have formed after central venous occlusion. This distinction can be made by ensuring that the identified deep venous segment is adjacent to a named artery. In contrast, collateral veins do not have an arterial accompaniment.

Treatment guidelines are not well established by randomized controlled trials. In general, idiopathic DVTs in the setting of thoracic outlet syndrome should be treated with catheter-directed thrombolysis and anticoagulation therapy, followed by surgical outlet decompression after convalescence. In contrast, line-associated DVTs can be managed more conservatively by simply removing the involved catheter and initiating anticoagulant therapy. Severe postphlebitic syndrome of the upper extremity is unusual largely owing to the robust venous collateral development potential of the upper extremity venous system.

- The rate of PE from the axillosubclavian system is 10%-20% vs 30%-50% for iliofemoral segments
- Line-associated DVTs can be managed by removing the catheter and initiating anticoagulant therapy
- Severe postphlebitic syndrome of the upper extremity is unusual, owing to the robust venous collateral development of upper extremity venous systems

Questions

1. Which of the following statements is true regarding VTE?
   a. Morbidity and mortality rates are relatively low.
   b. Recurrent VTE is rare after an initial event.
   c. Most cases occur in the 3rd to 5th decades owing to trauma, pregnancy, and oral contraception use.
   d. Clinical presentation always involves painful swelling of a limb.
   e. Twenty-four–hour mortality may be as high as 30%.

2. Which of the following variables is not associated with an increased risk of VTE?
   a. Total knee arthroplasty
   b. Hip fracture
   c. Alcoholic cirrhosis
   d. Breast cancer
   e. Stroke with left hemiparesis

3. Which of the following statements is true regarding fibrin D-dimer testing?
   a. A strongly positive test confirms the diagnosis of VTE with a high positive predictive value.
   b. Testing cannot be accurately performed in the presence of therapeutic heparin.
   c. A negative test excludes the diagnosis of VTE with a high negative predictive value.
   d. This test can be particularly helpful in postoperative patients if instability precludes transfer for definitive diagnostic imaging.

4. Which of the following has been shown to improve morbidity and mortality in patients with acute DVT?
   a. Unfractionated heparin
   b. Low-molecular-weight heparin
   c. Warfarin
   d. Recombinant tissue plasminogen activator
   e. IVC filters
   f. a, b, and c
   g. All of the above

5. What are the current indications for IVC filter placement?
   a. Massive bilateral PE
   b. Gastrointestinal tract bleeding requiring transfusions
   c. Recurrent PE despite therapeutic anticoagulants
   d. Massive bilateral DVT in the setting of metastatic colon cancer
   e. b and c
   f. All of the above

6. Which of the following is not true regarding postphlebitic syndrome?
   a. Incidence is decreased by 50% with the use of proper compression stockings
   b. Results from proximal deep venous obstruction
   c. Results from valvular incompetence
   d. Occurs in most patients with DVT
   e. May result in skin ulceration and chronic limb swelling

Suggested Readings

Brandjes DP, Büller HR, Heijboer H, et al. Randomised trial of effect of compression stockings in patients with symptomatic proximal-vein thrombosis. Lancet. 1997;349:759-62.

Büller HR, Agnelli G, Hull RD, et al. Antithrombotic therapy for venous thromboembolic disease: the Seventh ACCP Conference on Antithrombotic and Thrombolytic Therapy. Chest. 2004;126 Suppl:401S-28S. Erratum in: Chest. 2005;127:416.

Geerts WH, Pineo GF, Heit JA, et al. Prevention of venous thromboembolism: the Seventh ACCP Conference on Antithrombotic and Thrombolytic Therapy. Chest. 2004;126 Suppl:338S-400S.

Heit JA, O'Fallon WM, Petterson TM, et al. Relative impact of risk factors for deep vein thrombosis and pulmonary embolism: a population-based study. Arch Intern Med. 2002;162:1245-8.

Heit JA, Silverstein MD, Mohr DN, et al. Risk factors for deep vein thrombosis and pulmonary embolism: a population-based case-control study. Arch Intern Med. 2000;160:809-15.

Prandoni P, Lensing AW, Cogo A, et al. The long-term clinical course of acute deep venous thrombosis. Ann Intern Med. 1996;125:1-7.

Silverstein MD, Heit JA, Mohr DN, et al. Trends in the incidence of deep vein thrombosis and pulmonary embolism: a 25-year population-based study. Arch Intern Med. 1998;158:585-93.

7 Arterial Testing in the Vascular Laboratory

R. Eugene Zierler, MD

Introduction

The testing methods of the vascular laboratory have been developed to bridge the gap between the subjective clinical assessment of vascular disorders and assessment by invasive contrast studies. Many of the early non-invasive tests used continuous-wave (CW) Doppler ultrasonography to detect blood flow or used plethysmographic techniques to measure changes in limb volume. These tests were called "indirect" because they relied on the detection of major changes in pressure or flow produced by arterial disease. Only hemodynamically significant lesions could be reliably identified. Indirect tests included the periorbital Doppler examination for extracranial carotid artery disease and segmental arterial blood pressure measurement in the extremities. Some of these tests are still useful in the clinical setting, but many have given way to the direct approach of ultrasonographic duplex scanning, which combines B-mode imaging and pulsed-wave (PW) Doppler detection of blood flow. The main advantage of duplex scanning is that it obtains both anatomic and physiologic information directly from sites of vascular disease.

- Physiologic testing relies on alterations in blood pressure, flow, and other physiologic parameters to indirectly assess the severity of arterial disease
- The direct approach of duplex scanning combines B-mode imaging and PW Doppler detection of blood flow to obtain diagnostic information directly from sites of arterial disease

Vascular Ultrasonography

Principles

Ultrasound is produced by a transducer that converts electrical energy into mechanical energy or high-frequency sound waves that can be transmitted into tissue. The transducer can also be used to detect sound waves that are reflected from tissue, converting mechanical energy back into electrical energy. These returning sound waves can be processed to detect the Doppler frequency shift, or they can be used to create B-mode or color-flow images. In dedicated Doppler instruments, the transducers are mounted in a probe, whereas in more sophisticated imaging devices the transducers are contained within a scan head. The purpose of the scan head is to steer and focus the ultrasound beam.

Doppler Ultrasonography

The Doppler effect refers to the shift in frequency that is produced when sound waves are reflected from a moving object. In medical applications, Doppler frequency shifts occur when ultrasound waves encounter moving red blood cells, which are the principal sound reflectors in blood vessels. The Doppler shift in vascular diagnosis varies from a few hundred to several thousand cycles per second (Hz), and this signal can be amplified to provide an audible signal with a frequency (or pitch) that is directly proportional to blood velocity. The transmitting frequency of Doppler instruments used for arterial examinations is in the range of 2 to 10 MHz. Because the tissue depth to which the ultrasound beam penetrates is inversely proportional to the transmitting frequency, lower frequencies are best suited for examining deeply located vessels, such as those in the abdomen and thighs.

The Doppler shift is defined by the equation

$$\Delta f = (2f V \cos\theta)/C$$

where Δf is the difference between the frequency of the transmitted and reflected ultrasound waves (Doppler-shifted frequency), f is the frequency of the transmitted ultrasound waves, V is the velocity of the blood cells, θ is the angle between the incident ultrasound beam and the direction of blood cell motion (Doppler angle), and C is the speed of sound in tissue (≈1,540 m/s). The constant "2" in this equation accounts for the round trip path traveled by the sound waves from the source to the reflectors and back to the source.

Continuous-Wave and Pulsed-Wave Doppler

In CW Doppler, separate transmitting and receiving transducers operate simultaneously. Because a single transducer cannot transmit and receive at the same time, a CW Doppler instrument must have two transducers. The simplest Doppler instruments used in vascular diagnosis are CW devices that provide an audio output of the frequency shift through earphones or a loudspeaker. These are satisfactory for most arterial physiologic tests, but a direction-sensing Doppler instrument is necessary for more sophisticated testing. Although some CW instruments have directional capabilities, they cannot identify flow at a specific depth or site in tissue. A CW Doppler signal can actually represent a combination of signals obtained from flow at various points along the path of the ultrasound beam. Interpretation of these Doppler signals can be difficult if vessels are superimposed within the ultrasound beam or if complex flow disturbances are present within a single vessel. These disadvantages have been overcome by the development of PW Doppler systems and more sophisticated techniques for Doppler signal analysis.

With PW ultrasonography, flow can be detected at discrete points along the ultrasound beam, eliminating the problem of superimposed signals. In a PW Doppler system, a single transducer alternates between transmitting and receiving functions. A short burst or pulse of ultrasound is transmitted into the tissue and, after waiting for the return of the reflected signal from a specific depth, the receiver is activated. The speed of sound in tissue determines the time required for a round trip to a particular depth, and the region in which flow can be detected is called the sample volume. The size of the sample volume can be adjusted to suit a particular application, and it can be electronically positioned at any point along the ultrasound beam. A sample volume that is small relative to the vessel diameter allows the most detailed assessment of the flow pattern; a very large sample volume provides a signal similar to that from a CW Doppler system. As in directional CW Doppler systems, PW Doppler can distinguish between flow toward and away from the transducer.

To be certain that flow is sampled from only one depth, the reflected signal from each ultrasound pulse must be received before transmission of the next pulse. This limits the rate at which pulses can be transmitted. The maximum pulse repetition frequency (PRF) is defined as

$$PRF_{max} = C/2d$$

where C is the speed of sound in tissue and d is the distance between the transducer and the site of flow detection.

- In a CW Doppler instrument, separate transmitting and receiving transducers operate simultaneously
- CW Doppler instruments cannot identify flow at a specific depth in tissue; this makes interpretation of signals difficult when vessels are superimposed within the ultrasound beam
- A PW Doppler system uses a single transducer that alternates between transmitting and receiving functions; flow can be detected at discrete points along the ultrasound beam
- The region in which flow can be detected with PW Doppler is called the sample volume

Spectral Waveform Analysis

Spectral analysis is a signal processing technique that displays the complete frequency and amplitude content of the Doppler signal. As indicated by the Doppler equation, the Doppler-shifted frequency is directly proportional to blood cell velocity. The amplitude (or power) of the signal depends on the number of blood cells moving through the Doppler sample volume. As the number of blood cells producing the Doppler frequency shift increases, the signal amplitude becomes stronger.

The most common approach to spectral analysis is a mathematical method called Fourier analysis. The device used for this purpose in ultrasonography instruments is a fast Fourier transform analyzer, which works by processing short (1- to 5-millisecond) time segments of the Doppler signal and separating each segment into its component frequencies. Spectral information is presented graphically, with Doppler frequency (or blood flow velocity) on the y-axis, time on the x-axis, and amplitude indicated by shades of gray.

An adequate PRF is required for accurate display of Doppler-shifted frequencies by a PW Doppler system. With higher PRF values, more ultrasound pulses are available to sample flow, and a better representation of the Doppler signal is obtained. However, the PRF must be high enough to obtain at least two samples from each cycle of the Doppler signal. Therefore, the highest Dop-

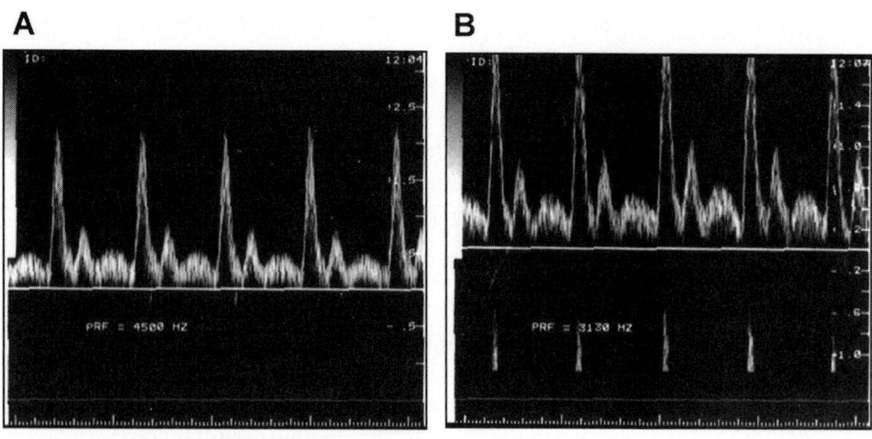

Fig. 7.1 Aliasing in spectral waveforms. *A*, Waveform taken with a pulse repetition frequency (PRF) of 4,500 Hz does not show aliasing. *B*, Waveform taken from the same vessel with a PRF of 3,130 Hz, and aliasing is present. The peaks of the aliased waveforms are "cut off" and appear below the zero-flow baseline.

pler frequency that can be accurately displayed is one-half the PRF, called the Nyquist limit. For example, if a PW Doppler system is operating with a PRF of 10 kHz, the Nyquist limit is 5 kHz.

If the Nyquist limit is exceeded, fewer than two samples are obtained per cycle of the PW Doppler signal, and the phenomenon of aliasing is observed (Fig. 7.1). A spectral waveform with aliasing appears to be "cut off" at the Nyquist limit, and the missing portion of the waveform "wraps around" and appears as flow below the baseline in the opposite direction. Aliasing is most likely to occur if blood flow velocity is increased, such as in a high-velocity jet associated with severe stenosis. The low PRF values that must be used to detect flow in deep vessels also lower the Nyquist limit and tend to produce aliasing. Aliasing does not represent actual flow but is an artifact of the PW Doppler sampling process. Because CW Doppler instruments do not sample the Doppler signal at discrete intervals, they are not subject to aliasing.

Spectral Waveforms and Flow Patterns

The flow pattern in a normal artery is uniform or laminar, and a spectral waveform taken with the PW Doppler sample volume in the center of the lumen shows a relatively narrow band of frequencies. Stenoses and other arterial wall abnormalities disrupt this normal pattern and produce flow disturbances that are apparent in spectral waveforms as a wider range of frequencies and amplitudes (Fig. 7.2). This increase in the width of the frequency band is referred to as spectral broadening. Severe stenoses that produce high-velocity jets are associated with an abnor-

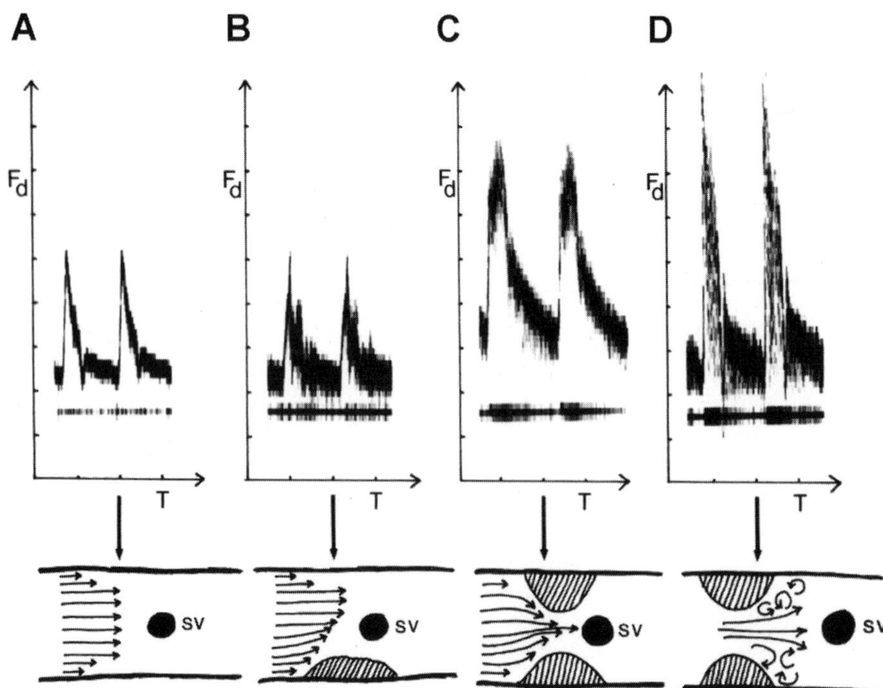

Fig. 7.2 Spectral waveforms associated with arterial disease. *A*, Normal center stream arterial flow is shown with a narrow band of frequencies. *B*, A minor lesion produces spectral broadening without any increase in peak systolic frequency or velocity. *C*, High-velocity jet and increased peak systolic frequencies associated with a severe stenosis. *D*, The high-velocity jet and spectral broadening found distal to a severe stenosis. F_d, Doppler-shifted frequency; SV, pulsed-wave Doppler sample volume; T, time.

mal increase in the peak systolic frequency. End-diastolic frequency is also increased in very severe stenoses. These spectral waveform features have been used to define criteria for classification of disease severity at various arterial sites. However, changes in both Doppler-shifted frequency and spectral width can result from artifacts or errors in examination technique. For example, if the PW Doppler sample volume is placed near the arterial wall instead of in the center of the flow stream, spectral broadening is produced by the velocity gradients that are normally present at that site; if this situation is not recognized, the severity of disease can be overestimated. Similarly, a sample volume that is large in relation to the vessel being examined will detect velocity gradients near the arterial wall even if it is correctly positioned in the center stream. In most clinical applications, a small sample volume provides the most reliable information.

- The flow pattern in a normal artery is laminar; a spectral waveform taken with the PW Doppler sample volume in the center of the lumen shows a relatively narrow band of frequencies
- Stenoses disrupt the normal flow pattern and produce spectral waveforms with a wider range of amplitudes and frequencies, called spectral broadening
- Severe stenoses that produce high-velocity jets are associated with an abnormal increase in the peak systolic frequency
- Aliasing of a spectral waveform is an artifact that results from an inadequate sampling rate (PRF is too low)

B-Mode Ultrasonography

When an ultrasound beam encounters an interface formed by two tissues with different acoustic properties, part of the incident beam is reflected and part is transmitted. The reflected portion travels back to the transducer and can be detected as an echo, the amplitude of which is proportional to the difference between the acoustic impedances of the tissues. Acoustic impedance can be defined as the speed of sound in a particular tissue multiplied by its density. Air-filled tissue such as lung has very low acoustic impedance, whereas dense tissue such as bone has extremely high acoustic impedance. However, for most other tissues, the range of acoustic impedances is relatively narrow.

In brightness ("B-mode") ultrasonography, the amplitudes of ultrasound echoes are represented by the brightness of individual pixels on a display screen. By assigning a gray-scale value to each location that corresponds to the position of the appropriate tissue interface, a two-dimensional gray-scale tissue image is created. Real-time B-mode images are obtained by rapidly sweeping a pulsed ultrasound beam over the site of interest to provide a continuous display of anatomic structures. Vessel walls and surrounding tissues produce relatively strong or bright echoes and appear as shades of gray; flowing blood appears relatively dark. Calcium deposits in atherosclerotic plaques result in very strong echoes that are associated with acoustic shadowing.

The attenuation of ultrasound as it travels through tissue is directly proportional to the transmitting frequency, so lower frequencies can penetrate to greater depths than higher frequencies. Therefore, lower ultrasound frequencies (2-3 MHz) are required for evaluating deep structures such as those in the abdomen, whereas relatively superficial vessels such as those in the neck can be examined with higher frequencies (5-10 MHz). The linear resolution of an ultrasonographic image depends on the ability to focus the beam. Sound beams emanating from high-frequency transducers can be focused more precisely than those from low-frequency transducers and thus provide clearer B-mode images of more superficial structures. For example, because the carotid artery is superficial, higher-frequency transducers can be used to provide much clearer B-mode images than are possible with deeper vessels such as the aorta or iliac arteries.

Duplex Scanning

Principles

Early experience with real-time B-mode imaging indicated that some thrombus and plaque had acoustic properties similar to blood, making it difficult to characterize arterial lesions by B-mode imaging alone. A logical solution to this problem was the addition of a Doppler device to detect blood flow in the imaged vessels. This led to the combining of real-time B-mode imaging and PW Doppler flow detection—"duplex scanning"—to obtain both anatomic and physiologic information on the status of blood vessels. In addition to the real-time B-mode imaging and PW Doppler systems, a duplex scanning instrument includes a spectrum analyzer for displaying pulsed Doppler waveforms and a selection of scan heads that contain the ultrasound transducers. The position of the Doppler beam and the PW Doppler sample volume are indicated by a line and a cursor, respectively, superimposed on the B-mode image.

A prototype duplex scanner, constructed at the University of Washington in the early 70s, was used to evaluate patients with extracranial carotid artery disease. The relatively high prevalence of carotid disease and the superficial location of the carotid arteries made this an ideal first clinical application. This approach has been extended to the lower extremity arteries, aortoiliac segments, and visceral arteries as a result of numerous technical advances that have occurred over the past 30 years. Such advances include major improvements in B-mode image resolution; better low-frequency scan heads that permit deeper penetration of the ultrasound beam; improvements in computer-based hardware and software; and addition of color-flow imaging. Three-dimensional duplex ultrasonography systems are currently in development, but their clinical utility remains to be demonstrated.

Color Flow

Color-flow imaging is an alternative to spectral waveform analysis for displaying the Doppler information obtained by duplex scanning. Within certain technical limitations, the color-flow image permits visualization of moving blood in the plane of the B-mode image, which is helpful for identifying vessels, particularly those that are small, deep, or anatomically complex. Color flow decreases the time required to perform a scan and is essential for duplex examination of vessels such as the renal and tibial arteries.

In contrast to spectral waveform analysis, which evaluates the entire frequency and amplitude content of the Doppler signal at a selected sample volume site, color-flow imaging provides a single estimate of the mean Doppler-shifted frequency for each site within the B-mode image. Consequently, the peak frequencies or velocities shown by spectral waveforms are generally higher than the frequencies or velocities indicated by color-flow imaging, and it is difficult to classify disease severity on the basis of the color-flow image alone. Even when color-flow imaging is used, spectral waveforms are still necessary for accurate disease classification. Color flow serves primarily as a guide in locating the vessels of interest and selecting specific sites for examination with PW Doppler.

- Color-flow imaging is an alternative to spectral waveform analysis for displaying Doppler information
- Color-flow imaging provides a single estimate of the mean Doppler-shifted frequency for each site within the B-mode image
- A color-flow image is produced by assigning colors to Doppler shifts

A color-flow image is produced by assigning colors to Doppler shifts. Returning echoes that are not Doppler shifted are used to create the B-mode image. The result is the depiction of flow as color superimposed on a gray-scale image. The hue and intensity of the color are determined by the direction and magnitude of the Doppler shifts. Varying shades of red and blue are typically used to distinguish flow away from or toward the transducer. By convention, most examiners assign red to arterial flow and blue to venous flow. Because color flow is based on PW Doppler, it is subject to the same limitations and artifacts as spectral waveform analysis. If the Doppler angle is 90°, there is no Doppler shift and no color assignment is made. Aliasing can also occur and is recognized on a color-flow image as a mosaic pattern that includes a "wrapping around" of the color scale. As with PW Doppler, color aliasing can be decreased by increasing the PRF.

Indirect Arterial Testing

Unlike duplex scanning, which characterizes arterial disease directly, the indirect tests rely on alterations in blood pressure, blood flow, and other physiologic parameters to assess the location and severity of arterial lesions. Because of this, the indirect tests are often referred to as "physiologic." However, duplex scanning is also a physiologic test because spectral waveforms and color flow clearly provide physiologic information. Contrast arteriography is generally regarded as the standard method for evaluating the arterial system, but it has limitations, particularly for estimating the hemodynamic significance of stenoses. In addition, the frequent presence of occlusive disease at multiple levels makes it difficult to predict which segment is most responsible for ischemic symptoms by using direct imaging methods alone. Because of the limitations and invasiveness of contrast arteriography, non-invasive physiologic methods have been developed for studying the arterial circulation.

Plethysmography

Plethysmographic methods rely on the detection and measurement of volume changes in the extremities. Because these changes result primarily from alterations in blood volume, plethysmographic measurements can be used to assess blood flow parameters such as arterial pulsations and limb blood pressure. Most plethysmographs used in the vascular laboratory measure volume indirectly on the basis of changes in limb circumference, electrical impedance, or reflectivity of infrared light.

- Plethysmographic methods rely on measurement of volume changes in the extremities caused primarily by alterations in blood volume
- Most plethysmographs measure volume indirectly based on changes in limb circumference, electrical impedance, or reflectivity of infrared light

Air-filled plethysmographs use pneumatic cuffs that are placed around the limb and inflated to a pressure of 10 to 65 mm Hg. Enlargement of the enclosed limb segment with each arterial pulse compresses the air in the cuff, and the resulting increase in cuff pressure is recorded by a pressure transducer. Strain-gauge plethysmography uses small silicone rubber tubes filled with mercury or a liquid-metal alloy. This gauge is wrapped around a digit or limb; the length of the strain gauge changes as the encircled body part expands or contracts. Because the electrical resistance of the gauge is proportional to its length, changes in circumference cause corresponding changes in the voltage decrease across the gauge. Assuming that the body part is cylindrical, changes in circumference can be used to calculate changes in volume.

Impedance plethysmography is based on changes in blood volume within a limb being reflected by changes in electrical impedance. The instrumentation usually includes four electrodes: an outer pair to send a weak current through the limb and an inner pair to sense the voltage decrease. This technique has been one of the most popular indirect methods for the non-invasive diagnosis of lower extremity deep vein thrombosis. However, it has not been widely used for arterial testing.

Photoelectric plethysmography (PPG) uses a sensor containing an infrared light–emitting diode and a phototransistor. When this sensor is placed on a body part, the infrared light is transmitted into the superficial layers of the skin, and the reflected light is received by the phototransistor. The resulting signal is proportional to the quantity of red blood cells in the cutaneous circulation. Although this method does not measure an actual volume change, the waveforms obtained resemble those acquired with strain-gauge plethysmography. The most common application of PPG in arterial testing is for the detection of arterial pulsations in the terminal portions of the digits, something that is especially difficult with Doppler or the other plethysmographic techniques.

Ankle-Brachial Index

The systolic pressure at any level in the lower extremity can be determined by using a pneumatic cuff placed at the desired site and measuring the Doppler flow signal in an artery distal to the cuff. In general, any patent distal artery can be used for flow detection, but the posterior tibial and dorsalis pedis arteries are usually most convenient. The cuff is inflated to greater than systolic pressure and the arterial flow signal disappears. As the cuff pressure is gradually decreased to slightly less than systolic pressure, the flow signal reappears, and the pressure at which flow resumes is recorded as the systolic pressure at the level of the cuff.

In the arterial circulation, systolic pressure increases as the pulse wave progresses down the lower limb due to reflected waves originating from the high peripheral resistance and differences in compliance between the central and peripheral arteries. The diastolic and mean pressures gradually decrease as the pulse wave moves distally. Because of this, the systolic pressure measured at the ankle is normally higher than that in the upper arm. Determination of systolic blood pressure is the most reliable pressure parameter for diagnosis of proximal arterial stenosis. Changes in diastolic and mean pressure are smaller in magnitude and more difficult to measure.

The measurement of ankle systolic pressure is the single most valuable physiologic test for assessing the arterial circulation in the lower limb. If the pressure measured by a cuff placed just above the malleoli is less than that in the upper arm, occlusive disease in the arteries of the lower limb is almost always present. Furthermore, the degree of reduction in the ankle systolic pressure is proportional to the severity of arterial obstruction. Patients with severe arterial occlusive disease and ischemic rest pain usually have ankle systolic pressures less than 40 mm Hg. However, occlusive lesions in the small arteries distal to the ankle cannot be detected by this method.

Because the ankle systolic pressure varies with the systemic blood pressure, it is useful to compare each ankle pressure measurement to the simultaneous systemic pressure. Assuming that the subclavian and axillary arteries are normal, the brachial systolic pressure as measured by Doppler and an upper arm cuff is essentially equal to systemic pressure. The ratio of ankle systolic pressure to brachial systolic pressure is called the ankle-brachial index (ABI; also called the ankle-pressure index or ankle-arm index). This index compensates for variations in systemic pressure and allows comparison of serial tests. In the absence of hemodynamically significant proximal arterial occlusive disease, the ABI is greater than 1.0, with a mean value of 1.11±0.10. However, because of variability related to the pressure measurement technique, values greater than 0.90 are typically interpreted as normal. Although the ABI does not discriminate among occlusions at various levels, in general, limbs with single-level occlusions have ABIs greater than 0.5 and limbs with lesions at multiple levels have ABIs less than 0.5.

- The measurement of ankle systolic pressure is the most valuable physiologic test for assessing the arterial circulation in the lower limb
- Systolic pressure measured at the ankle is normally higher than that in the arm
- The ABI is the ratio of ankle systolic pressure to brachial systolic pressure; it compensates for variations in systemic pressure
- Changes in the ABI must be ≥0.15 to be considered clinically significant
- Medial calcification can cause incompressibility and the recording of falsely high ankle systolic pressures; patients with diabetes mellitus are especially prone to medial calcification

The ABI provides a general guide to the degree of functional disability in the lower extremity. In limbs with intermittent claudication, the ABI ranges from about 0.2 to 1.0, with a mean value of 0.59±0.15. The ABI in limbs with ischemic rest pain ranges from 0 to 0.65, with a mean of 0.26±0.13. Limbs with impending gangrene tend to have the lowest ankle pressures, with a mean ABI of 0.05±0.08. Although the ABI can be used to assess the overall severity of arterial occlusive disease in the lower extremity, considerable overlap in values exists among patients with different clinical presentations. Therefore, this measurement should be combined with other clinical information to determine the physiologic and functional status of the patient.

Variability in measurements of arterial pressure results from biologic and technical factors. The ABI accounts for changes in systemic pressure, thus avoiding a major source of biologic variation. Because of variability related to technique, changes in ABI must be 0.15 or greater to be considered clinically significant. Accurate measurement of arterial pressure using pneumatic cuffs requires that cuff pressure be transmitted through the arterial wall to the bloodstream. Medial calcification in the arterial wall leads to varying degrees of incompressibility and the recording of falsely high systolic pressures. Patients with diabetes mellitus are especially prone to medial calcification, and artifactual elevation of ankle pressures must always be considered in this group. Occasionally, the distal flow signal cannot be eliminated, even with maximal cuff inflation pressures, and ankle pressures cannot be measured in approximately 5% to 10% of diabetic patients. In this situation, toe pressure measurement is a more reliable method for assessing the severity of arterial occlusive disease because the digital vessels are not usually affected by medial calcification.

In limbs with severe arterial occlusive disease and very low flow rates, Doppler signals can be difficult to obtain, even when the arteries are patent. Plethysmographic techniques can often provide diagnostic information in these cases. If weak Doppler signals are detected, it may be difficult to distinguish between arterial and venous flow based on the audible signal alone, and a direction-sensing Doppler device is useful. Venous signals are augmented by distal limb compression.

Segmental Limb Pressures

Although the ABI provides valuable information on the overall status of the lower extremity arteries, it does not indicate the location or relative severity of arterial lesions. However, some of this information can be obtained by measuring the systolic pressure at multiple levels in the lower extremity. One common technique uses four 11-cm-wide pneumatic cuffs placed at the upper thigh, above-knee, below-knee, and ankle levels. Systolic pressure is determined at each level using the Doppler technique described for the ABI. The Doppler probe can be placed over the posterior tibial or dorsalis pedis arteries for all measurements.

The systolic pressure in the proximal thigh, as measured by the four-cuff method, normally exceeds brachial systolic pressure by 30 to 40 mm Hg. Direct intra-arterial pressure measurements show that pressures in the brachial and common femoral arteries are equal in normal persons. However, the use of a relatively small cuff on the thigh results in a significant cuff artifact. The ratio of upper thigh systolic pressure to brachial systolic pressure (thigh-brachial index) is normally greater than 1.2. An index between 0.8 and 1.2 suggests aortoiliac stenosis, whereas an index less than 0.8 is consistent with complete iliac occlusion. Although patients with decreased thigh-brachial indices would be expected to have significant aortoiliac disease, the presence of superficial femoral and profunda femoris artery disease can also cause a decreased thigh-brachial index, even if the aortoiliac segment is hemodynamically normal.

The difference in systolic pressure between any two adjacent levels in the same leg should be less than 20 mm Hg in normal persons. Pressure gradients of more than 20 mm Hg usually indicate hemodynamically significant occlusive disease in the intervening arterial segment. In addition to vertical gradients down a single leg, horizontal gradients between corresponding levels in the two legs also suggest occlusive lesions. Systolic pressures measured at the same level in both legs normally should not differ by more than 20 mm Hg. Segmental pressure gradients provide only a general assessment of the location and hemodynamic significance of arterial occlusive lesions. If more specific anatomic detail is required for clinical decision making, direct imaging techniques such as duplex scanning must be used.

Cuff Artifacts and Sources of Error

For accurate indirect pressure measurement, the width of the pneumatic cuff should be at least 50% greater than the corresponding limb diameter. The use of smaller cuffs results in falsely elevated pressure readings, particularly in obese patients. However, in most patients, the magnitude of the cuff artifact can be anticipated, and relatively narrow cuffs can be successfully used to measure segmental pressure gradients, as described previously for the upper thigh pressure.

The pressure gradients between adjacent limb segments may be increased in severely hypertensive patients. On the other extreme, segmental pressure gradients can be decreased if cardiac output is very low. If the collateral vessels bypassing an arterial obstruction are unusually large, the corresponding resting segmental pressure gradient may be normal. If this is the case, a substantial gradient should become apparent after treadmill exercise.

Toe Pressures

Measurement of toe pressure can be used to identify occlusive disease involving the pedal and digital arteries which does not produce changes in ankle systolic pressure. Toe pressure measurement is also valuable if the ankle pressure is found to be falsely high because of arterial calcification. Because of the small size and low flow rates of digital arteries, Doppler methods are difficult to use, and a PPG sensor is necessary to detect flow.

The ratio of toe systolic pressure to brachial systolic pressure (toe-brachial index) ranges from 0.80 to 0.90 in normal persons. The mean toe-brachial index is 0.35±0.15 in patients with intermittent claudication and 0.11±0.10 in patients with rest pain or ischemic ulceration. No significant differences have been observed in mean toe-brachial indices between diabetic and non-diabetic patients.

Pulse Volume Recording

In addition to segmental pressure measurements, segmental plethysmographic waveforms have also been used to assess the lower extremity arteries. This approach is based on air plethysmography and is generally referred to as pulse volume recording. Pneumatic cuffs are applied at the upper thigh, calf, and ankle levels, with larger cuffs (18×36 cm) for the thigh and smaller cuffs (12×23 cm) for the distal sites. The cuffs are inflated to about 65 mm Hg, and waveforms are recorded from each site. These recordings can also be repeated after treadmill exercise.

The normal segmental volume pulse contour is characterized by a steep upstroke, a sharp systolic peak, a downslope that bows toward the baseline, and a prominent dicrotic wave (which represents the reverse-flow phase of the arterial flow pulse) approximately in the middle of the downslope (Fig. 7.3). Significant occlusive disease in the arteries proximal to the recording cuff is excluded by the presence of a dicrotic wave; however, the absence of a dicrotic wave has less diagnostic value. Distal to an arterial obstruction, the upslope is more gradual, the peak becomes delayed and rounded, the downslope bows away from the baseline, and the dicrotic wave disappears. As the proximal disease becomes more severe, the rise and fall times become more nearly equal, and the pulse amplitude decreases. Waveforms that become more distinctly abnormal after exercise indicate the presence of significant proximal obstruction.

- The normal segmental volume pulse is characterized by a steep upstroke, a sharp systolic peak, a downslope that bows toward the baseline, and a prominent dicrotic wave in the middle of the downslope
- Distal to an arterial obstruction, the upslope is more gradual, the peak becomes delayed and rounded, the downslope bows away from the baseline, and the dicrotic wave disappears

Although the actual volume change that occurs during each pulse is greater in the thigh than in the calf, the chart deflection at calf level normally exceeds that at the thigh by 25% or more. This "augmentation" is an important diagnostic criterion. If arterial disease is confined to the aortoiliac segment, the pulse contours at all levels are abnormal, but the amplitude of the calf pulse still exceeds that of the thigh pulse. Pulse contours are also abnormal at all levels in combined aortoiliac and superficial femoral artery disease, but the amplitude of the calf pulse is less than that of the thigh pulse. In limbs with isolated superficial femoral artery disease, the thigh volume pulse is normal but the calf and ankle pulses are abnormal.

Digital Plethysmography

Although digital plethysmography is a form of segmental plethysmography, volume pulses obtained from the tips of the toes or fingers have particular diagnostic significance. Because the waveforms are taken from the most distal portions of the limb, they reflect the physiologic status of the arteries from the aorta to the arterioles. Therefore, they are sensitive to both fixed occlusive lesions and vasospasm. Strain-gauge plethysmography or PPG is usually used for this application. Although PPG does not provide quanti-

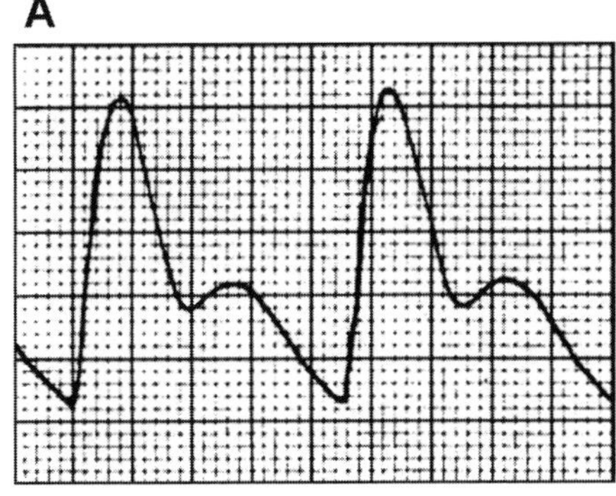

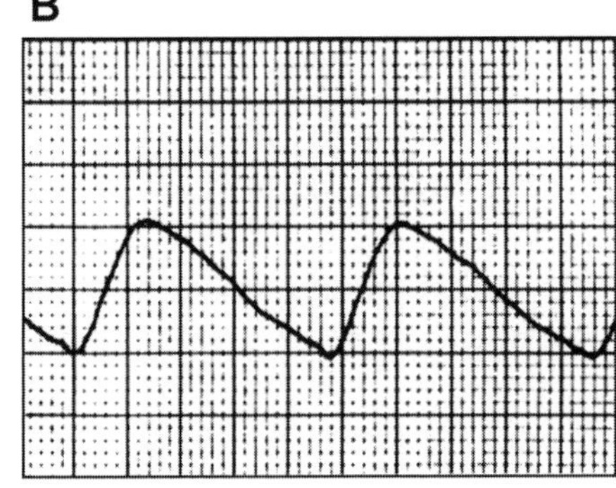

Fig. 7.3 Normal and abnormal pulse volume recording waveforms. *A*, A normal waveform shows a rapid systolic upstroke and sharp peak, with a downslope that bows toward baseline and contains a prominent dicrotic wave. *B*, The upstroke of an abnormal waveform is less steep, and the peak is delayed and rounded; the downslope bows away from baseline, and the dicrotic wave is absent.

tative data, it is the easiest technique and is preferred by many laboratories. These studies should be performed in a warm room to avoid vasospasm.

The contour of the digital volume pulse resembles that of the segmental pulses obtained more proximally in the limb. A normal toe pulse contour is good evidence that all segments from the heart to the digital arteries are widely patent. An obstructive pulse contour indicates one or more significant sites of obstruction in that limb. Because pedal or digital artery disease cannot be detected by recording ankle and segmental pressures or plethysmographic waveforms, digital pulses are especially valuable in the assessment of forefoot and toe ischemia. This is important in patients with diabetes mellitus who are prone to incompressible tibial arteries and lesions in the pedal arteries.

Stress Testing

Lower extremity exercise and reactive hyperemia both increase limb blood flow by causing vasodilatation of peripheral resistance vessels. In limbs with normal arteries, this increased flow occurs with little or no decrease in ankle systolic pressure. If occlusive arterial lesions are present in the lower limb, blood is diverted through high-resistance collateral pathways. Although the collateral circulation may provide adequate flow to the resting extremity with only a slight decrease in ankle pressure, the capability of collateral vessels to increase flow during exercise is limited. Pressure gradients that are minimal at rest can therefore be increased when flow rates are increased by exercise. Thus, stress testing provides a method for detecting less severe degrees of functionally significant arterial disease.

Treadmill Exercise

Walking on a treadmill is a simple way to stress the lower limb circulation. The main advantage of treadmill exercise testing is that it reproduces the patient's symptoms and determines the degree of disability under controlled conditions. It also permits an assessment of non-vascular factors that can affect walking ability, such as musculoskeletal or cardiopulmonary disease. A typical treadmill exercise protocol involves walking at 2 miles per hour on a 12% grade for 5 minutes or until symptoms occur and the patient is forced to stop. In general, longer walking times do not increase diagnostic accuracy. The walking time and nature of any symptoms are recorded, and the ankle and arm systolic pressures are measured before and immediately after exercise. Two components of the response to exercise are important: the magnitude of the immediate decrease in ankle systolic pressure, and the time for recovery to resting pressure. Changes in both these parameters are proportional to the severity of arterial occlusive disease.

- Lower extremity exercise and reactive hyperemia increase limb blood flow by causing vasodilatation of peripheral resistance vessels
- A typical treadmill exercise protocol involves walking at 2 mph on a 12% grade for 5 minutes or until symptoms occur and the patient must stop
- Two components of the response to exercise are important: the magnitude of the immediate decrease in ankle systolic pressure and the time for recovery to resting pressure

A normal response to treadmill exercise is a slight increase or no change in the ankle systolic pressure compared with the resting value. If the ankle pressure is decreased immediately after exercise, the test is considered positive, and repeated measurements are taken at 1- to 2-minute intervals for up to 10 minutes, or until the pressure returns to pre-exercise levels. If a patient is forced to stop walking because of symptomatic arterial occlusive disease, the ankle systolic pressure in the affected limb is usually less than 60 mm Hg. If symptoms occur without a pronounced decrease in the ankle pressure, a non-vascular cause of leg pain must be considered.

Reactive Hyperemia

Reactive hyperemia testing is an alternate method for stressing the peripheral circulation. Inflating a pneumatic cuff at thigh level to above systolic pressure for 3 to 5 minutes produces ischemia and vasodilatation distal to the cuff. The changes in ankle pressure that occur on release of cuff occlusion are similar to those observed in the treadmill exercise test. Although normal limbs do not show a decrease in ankle systolic pressure after treadmill exercise, a transient decrease of 17% to 34% occurs with reactive hyperemia. In patients with arterial disease, the maximum pressure decrease with reactive hyperemia and with treadmill exercise correlate well. However, considerable overlap may exist in the ankle pressure response to reactive hyperemia among normal subjects and patients with arterial disease. Patients with single-level arterial disease show less than a 50% decrease in ankle pressure with reactive hyperemia, whereas patients with multiple-level arterial disease show a pressure decrease greater than 50%. Reactive hyperemia testing is useful for patients who cannot walk on the treadmill because of amputations or other physical disabilities. Treadmill exercise is generally preferred over reactive hyperemia testing, because the former produces a physiologic stress that accurately reproduces a patient's ischemic symptoms.

Transcutaneous Oxygen Measurements

The transcutaneous oxygen tension ($TcPO_2$), or amount of oxygen diffusing through the skin from the capillaries, can be measured with an electrode applied to the skin surface. This method has been used for assessing skin blood flow to predict wound healing and the most appropriate level for amputation. Although $TcPO_2$ measurements are reliable for predicting healing at a particular level of the limb, this approach is less reliable for identifying sites that will fail to heal. In one study, successful healing of below-knee amputations occurred in 96% of patients with a calf $TcPO_2$ greater than 20 mm Hg but in only 50% of patients with a calf $TcPO_2$ less than 20 mm Hg. Modifications of this technique, such as use of a critical PO_2 index (calf-to-brachial $TcPO_2$ ratio or foot-to-chest $TcPO_2$ ratio) or breathing supplemental oxygen, may improve the overall predictive value.

- The $TcPO_2$ can be measured with an electrode applied to the skin surface
- This method has been used for assessing skin blood flow to predict wound healing and the most appropriate level for amputation

Penile Blood Flow

The penis is supplied by three paired arteries: the dorsal penile, the cavernosal (deep corporal), and the urethral (spongiosal) arteries. These arteries are terminal branches of the internal pudendal artery, which originates from the internal iliac artery. The cavernosal artery is most important for erectile function, and obstruction of any of the arteries leading to the corpora cavernosa, including the common iliac artery or terminal aorta, can be responsible for vasculogenic impotence.

Measurement of penile blood pressure is performed with a 2.5-cm-wide pneumatic cuff applied to the base of the penis. Return of blood flow as the cuff is deflated can be detected by a strain-gauge plethysmograph, PPG, or a Doppler flow detector. Because the penile blood supply is paired and obstruction can be limited to only one side, it has been recommended that pressures be measured on both sides of the penis. In normal men younger than 40 years, the penile-brachial index (penile pressure divided by brachial systolic pressure) is 0.99±0.15, indicating that the penile and brachial pressures are normally equivalent. Older men without symptoms of impotence tend to have lower indices, and penile-brachial indices greater than about 0.75 are considered compatible with normal erectile function. An index less than 0.60 is consistent with vasculogenic impotence.

Duplex Scanning

Carotid Duplex Scanning

Duplex Criteria

The primary goal of non-invasive testing for extracranial carotid artery disease is to identify patients who are at risk for stroke. A secondary goal is to document progressive or recurrent disease in patients already known to be at risk. Unlike arteriography, which can be interpreted in terms of a specific percentage of diameter reduction, duplex scanning classifies arterial lesions into categories that include ranges of stenosis severity. The criteria listed in Table 7.1 were developed at the University of Washington for classifying the severity of internal carotid artery (ICA) disease. These criteria have been validated by a series of comparisons with independently interpreted contrast arteriograms; they can distinguish between normal and diseased ICAs with a specificity of 84% and a sensitivity of 99%. The accuracy for detecting 50% to 99% diameter stenosis or occlusion is 93%.

To standardize the results of carotid artery duplex scanning, it is recommended that examinations be conducted

Table 7.1 Duplex Criteria for Classification of Internal Carotid Artery Disease

Arteriographic diameter reduction*	Peak systolic velocity, cm/s†	End-diastolic velocity, cm/s†	Spectral waveform characteristics
0% (Normal)	<125	...	Minimal or no spectral broadening; boundary layer separation present in the carotid bulb
1%-15%	<125	...	Spectral broadening during deceleration phase of systole only
16%-49%	<125	...	Spectral broadening throughout systole
50%-79%	≥125	<140	Marked spectral broadening
80%-99%	≥125	≥140	Marked spectral broadening
100% (Occlusion)	...	...	No flow signal in the internal carotid artery; decreased diastolic flow in the ipsilateral common carotid artery

*Diameter reduction is based on arteriographic methods that compared the residual internal carotid artery lumen diameter to the estimated diameter of the carotid bulb.

†Velocity criteria are based on the angle-adjusted velocity using a Doppler angle of 60° or less.

using a Doppler angle as close as possible to 60°. At this angle, errors in velocity calculations secondary to angle effects are relatively small; when the Doppler angle exceeds about 70°, these errors become much more pronounced. Small errors in determining the Doppler angle when the angle of insonation is 60° or less have little overall effect on the velocity calculation, and Doppler angles between 45° and 60° are acceptable for most clinical studies. An angle of 60° is readily obtained in most carotid artery duplex examinations. In the evaluation of other vessels, such as the renal arteries, it can be much more difficult to obtain a 60° angle.

All diagnostic tests must be reevaluated periodically to remain relevant to current clinical practice. The results of randomized trials of carotid endarterectomy in the 80s and 90s established "threshold" levels of ICA stenosis that, in appropriately selected patients, are best treated with carotid endarterectomy. Consequently, these results have also affected the interpreting and reporting of carotid duplex examinations. The North American Symptomatic Carotid Endarterectomy Trial (NASCET) established that symptomatic ICA stenosis of 70% to 99% is best treated by a combination of carotid endarterectomy and optimal medical management. A lesser benefit was obtained from surgical treatment of symptomatic ICA stenosis of 50% to 69%. The Asymptomatic Carotid Atherosclerosis Study (ACAS) found benefit for carotid endarterectomy in patients with asymptomatic ICA stenosis of 60% to 99%.

In the ACAS and NASCET studies, the percentage of ICA stenosis was determined by comparing the residual lumen diameter at the most stenotic site with that of the normal distal cervical ICA. Both measurements were obtained by contrast arteriography. The University of Washington criteria were also obtained by comparing duplex results with contrast carotid arteriography; however, arteriographic stenosis was calculated by comparing the narrowest residual lumen with the estimated diameter of the carotid bulb. Because the bulb is normally wider than the distal cervical ICA, calculations of stenosis using the distal ICA as the reference vessel result in lower calculated stenosis percentages than calculations of stenosis using the bulb as the reference site. In a review of 1,001 ICAs studied with arteriography, 34% of the ICAs in the study, using the bulb as the reference vessel, were classified as having 70% to 99% stenosis. However, when the distal cervical ICA was used as the reference site, only 16% of the ICAs were classified as having 70% to 99% stenosis.

The University of Washington duplex criteria for classification of ICA stenosis were based on comparison with carotid arteriograms using the bulb as the reference site. Furthermore, these criteria do not contain specific categories for the 60% and 70% threshold levels of ICA stenosis identified by the ACAS and NASCET trials, respectively. To ensure that carotid artery duplex scanning remained clinically relevant, additional duplex criteria were developed for 60% to 99% and 70% to 99% ICA stenosis using the distal ICA as the reference site.

The NASCET data indicated that carotid endarterectomy was the preferred treatment for 70% to 99% symptomatic ICA stenosis. However, the risk of major stroke or death at 2 years (about 28%) was not high enough to justify subjecting patients with less than 70% stenosis to diagnostic angiography or carotid endarterectomy. Therefore, duplex criteria with a high overall accuracy for detecting a 70% to 99% ICA stenosis should be used.

Duplex criteria for specific threshold levels of ICA stenosis are also important for identifying stenosis in patients with asymptomatic carotid artery disease (Table 7.1). For most surgeons, 80% to 99% ICA stenosis is the level of disease severity that would benefit from prophylactic carotid endarterectomy. This level was first suggested by the University of Washington group based on both natural history studies of 80% to 99% carotid stenosis and retrospective surgical series. The ACAS study showed that patients with 60% to 99% asymptomatic ICA stenosis benefited from carotid endarterectomy; however, the results were not nearly as striking as those of the NASCET study. To avoid performing unnecessary, potentially harmful operations on asymptomatic patients, the criteria used to screen for 60% or greater ICA stenosis should have a very high accuracy and positive predictive value.

Because of confusion regarding the many possible criteria for grading carotid artery stenosis, the Society of Radiologists in Ultrasound sponsored a consensus conference on this issue in 2003. A set of suggested criteria were developed for quantification of carotid stenosis using the distal ICA as the reference vessel in calculations of ICA stenosis. These criteria are summarized below and were derived from analysis of numerous studies. They have not been subject to retrospective or prospective evaluation, and they do not represent the results of any one laboratory or study. Duplex measurements of ICA peak systolic velocity (PSV) and end-diastolic velocity (EDV), and the ratio of ICA to common carotid artery (CCA) PSV (ICA:CCA ratio), are used for these criteria.

- The ICA is considered normal if the PSV is less than 125 cm/s with no visible plaque or intimal thickening. The consensus was that such arteries would also have an ICA:CCA ratio less than 2.0 and an ICA EDV less than 40 cm/s.
- Less than 50% ICA stenosis is present if the PSV is less than 125 cm/s with visible plaque or intimal thickening. Such arteries may also have an ICA:CCA ratio less than 2.0 and an ICA EDV less than 40 cm/s.
- 50% to 69% ICA stenosis is present if the PSV is 125 to 230 cm/s with visible plaque. Such arteries would prob-

ably also have an ICA:CCA ratio of 2.0 to 4.0 and an ICA EDV of 40 to 100 cm/s.

– 70% or greater ICA stenosis, but less than near occlusion of the ICA, is present if the PSV is greater than 230 cm/s along with visible plaque and lumen narrowing with gray-scale and color Doppler imaging. (The higher the PSV, the greater the likelihood of severe disease.) Such arteries are likely to also have an ICA:CCA ratio greater than 4 and an ICA EDV greater than 100 cm/s.

– In cases of near occlusion of the ICA, the velocity parameters may not apply. "Preocclusive" lesions can be associated with high, low, or undetectable velocity measurements. The diagnosis of near occlusion is therefore established primarily by the demonstration of a markedly narrowed lumen on color Doppler.

– Total occlusion of the ICA is diagnosed if no patent lumen is detectable by gray-scale and no flow is seen with spectral and color Doppler or power Doppler. The panel agreed that near-occlusive lesions can be misdiagnosed as total occlusions if only gray-scale and spectral Doppler are used. In some near-occlusive lesions, color Doppler can distinguish between near and total occlusion, demonstrating a thin wisp of color traversing the lesion.

Carotid Endarterectomy Without Arteriography

The high accuracy and reliability of carotid duplex scanning, along with increasing demands to minimize the costs and risks of medical care, have prompted many surgeons to perform carotid endarterectomy on the basis of the clinical evaluation and results of duplex scanning alone. If arteriography is performed routinely before carotid endarterectomy, the risks of arteriography must be combined with the risks of operation to reflect the overall risks of surgical treatment. The stroke rate from arteriography in the ACAS study was 1.2%, accounting for nearly half of the 2.3% stroke rate in the surgical treatment group. Clearly, a definitive approach to decreasing the morbidity and mortality of carotid endarterectomy is to eliminate the need for preoperative arteriography.

In a prospective study of the decision-making process in 94 cases considered for carotid endarterectomy, 87 patients (93%) had a duplex scan that was technically adequate and showed a surgically accessible lesion confined to the carotid bulb. Of the 7 remaining cases, lesions were not limited to the carotid bulb in 4, duplex assessment was technically incomplete in 1, and ICA occlusion could not be distinguished from high-grade stenosis in 2. The results of arteriography affected clinical decision making in only 1 case in which a technically satisfactory duplex scan showed a localized carotid stenosis; the patient, with combined extracranial and intracranial carotid disease, did not undergo endarterectomy and died of a stroke 5 months later.

On the basis of this experience, preoperative arteriography is not necessary in most patients being evaluated for carotid endarterectomy. Furthermore, the need for arteriography should be apparent from the clinical presentation and duplex scan results. Indications for selective use of preoperative arteriography include 1) undocumented reliability of the non-invasive vascular laboratory performing the tests; 2) a technically inadequate duplex scan; 3) presence of a lesion not limited to the carotid bulb; and 4) unusual carotid anatomy (aneurysms, kinks, or coils). The incidence of carotid surgery without routine preoperative arteriography will increase with further improvements in the technology of duplex scanning and other non-invasive imaging methods.

Transcranial Doppler/Duplex Scanning

Transcranial Doppler (TCD), introduced in 1982, uses a very low frequency (2 MHz) PW Doppler device to insonate the basal cerebral arteries through the skull. Early TCD instruments were based on PW Doppler only, but current instruments also use B-mode and color-flow imaging. TCD can be used to evaluate for intracranial arterial stenoses, vasospasm, and emboli and for monitoring during and after carotid or coronary artery interventions. Recently, the technique has also been used with thrombolytic therapy to assess clearing of middle cerebral artery emboli or thrombi in patients with acute ischemic stroke.

In TCD, the mean blood flow velocity is recorded rather than angle-corrected PSV. Mean velocity determinations are less angle dependent, and the early TCD devices lacked imaging capability, so the Doppler angle was unknown. Even though modern TCD devices include B-mode and color-flow imaging, the use of mean velocity remains standard. Normal mean blood flow velocities in the middle cerebral artery (MCA) are 30 to 80 cm/s. A mean velocity greater than 120 cm/s correlates with vasospasm or MCA stenosis. A hemispheric ratio calculated by comparing MCA mean velocity with the velocity in the distal extracranial ICA can help distinguish hyperemia from vasospasm when the MCA velocity is elevated. An increase in mean MCA velocity of approximately 100% or more identifies patients at risk for post–carotid endarterectomy hyperperfusion syndrome.

Visceral Artery Duplex Scanning

Duplex scanning can serve as a screening test for mesenteric arterial disease in patients with suspected chronic mesenteric ischemia and for follow-up of visceral artery reconstructions. Although lesions in the celiac, superior mesenteric, or inferior mesenteric arteries are relatively common in patients with widespread atherosclerosis, the collateral blood supply to the mesenteric circulation is remarkably efficient, and the clinical syndrome of chronic mesenteric ischemia develops in relatively few patients. Most patients with the typical symptoms of postprandial pain and weight loss are found to have significant occlusive disease in at least two of the three major mesenteric arteries. Because they are large, anterior, unpaired, and constant in location, the celiac and superior mesenteric arteries are relatively easy to evaluate by ultrasonography. Arteriographic confirmation of high-grade stenoses or occlusion is necessary for planning of interventions.

The arteries supplying the liver and spleen have a low resistance flow pattern that is typical of organs with relatively high and constant metabolic requirements. Therefore, celiac artery flow waveforms are normally monophasic with relatively high EDVs. In contrast, the normal fasting superior mesenteric artery (SMA) waveform is triphasic, reflecting the high vascular resistance of the intestinal tract at rest. Changes in the arterial waveforms in response to feeding are different in the celiac artery and SMA. Because the liver and spleen have fixed metabolic demands, celiac artery flow does not change substantially after eating. However, blood flow in the SMA increases markedly after a meal, reflecting a decrease in the vascular resistance in the small intestinal circulation. These postprandial waveform changes in the SMA include a near doubling of PSV, tripling of EDV, and loss of the end-systolic reverse-flow component. These changes are maximal about 45 minutes after ingestion of a meal and depend on the composition of the meal ingested. Mixed-composition meals produce the greatest increase in SMA flow when compared with equal caloric meals composed solely of fat, glucose, or protein.

Quantitative duplex criteria for stenoses in the SMA and celiac artery were first developed and validated at Oregon Health & Science University. In a prospective study of 100 patients who underwent mesenteric artery duplex scanning and lateral aortography, a PSV in the SMA of 275 cm/s or higher indicated a stenosis of 70% or greater with a sensitivity of 92%, a specificity of 96%, a positive predictive value of 80%, a negative predictive value of 99%, and an accuracy of 96%. A PSV of 200 cm/s or higher identified an arteriographic celiac artery stenosis of 70% or greater with a sensitivity of 87%, a specificity of 80%, a positive predictive value of 63%, a negative predictive value of 94%, and an accuracy of 82%. Other duplex criteria for mesenteric artery stenoses have also been described and validated. An SMA EDV greater than 45 cm/s correlates with a 50% or greater stenosis with a specificity of 92% and a sensitivity of 100%, whereas a celiac artery EDV of 55 cm/s or greater predicts a 50% or greater stenosis with a sensitivity of 93%, specificity of 100%, and accuracy of 95%.

- The celiac artery and SMA are relatively easy to evaluate by ultrasonography
- A PSV of ≥275 cm/s in the SMA indicates a ≥70% stenosis with a sensitivity of 92%, specificity of 96%, and accuracy of 96%
- A PSV of ≥200 cm/s in the celiac artery identifies a ≥70% stenosis with a sensitivity of 87%, specificity of 80%, and accuracy of 82%

Renal Artery Duplex Scanning

The goal of screening for renal artery disease is to identify patients who may have renovascular hypertension or renal failure secondary to chronic renal ischemia. Although it is technically demanding and time consuming, duplex scanning can serve as a non-invasive screening test for renal artery stenosis. The incidence of unsatisfactory examinations is 5% to 12%, usually secondary to obesity or bowel gas. In addition, accessory or polar renal arteries can be missed with duplex scanning. Once a renal artery stenosis has been identified, its functional significance must still be assessed.

Interpretation of Renal Duplex

Classification of renal artery disease by duplex scanning is based on spectral waveforms from the renal artery and adjacent abdominal aorta (Fig. 7.4). Because a normal kidney has low vascular resistance, the normal renal artery spectral waveform is monophasic with forward flow throughout the cardiac cycle, similar to that found in the celiac artery and ICA. The PSV associated with a significant renal artery stenosis increases relative to aortic PSV, and the ratio of velocities in the renal artery and aorta can be used to identify severe renal artery stenoses. This is referred to as the renal-aortic ratio (RAR). Renal artery occlusion is diagnosed if the artery is visualized but no flow signal can be detected in the proximal segment. The criteria developed at the University of Washington for classification of renal artery disease are shown in Table 7.2. In a prospective study of 58 renal arteries in 29 patients, an RAR of 3.5 or greater had a sensitivity of 84% and a specificity of 97% for the detection of 60% or greater renal artery stenosis. The same criteria have been successfully applied to the evaluation of renal artery interventions (angioplasty, stents, and bypass grafts).

- The PSV associated with significant renal artery stenosis increases relative to aortic PSV; the RAR can be used to identify severe renal artery stenoses

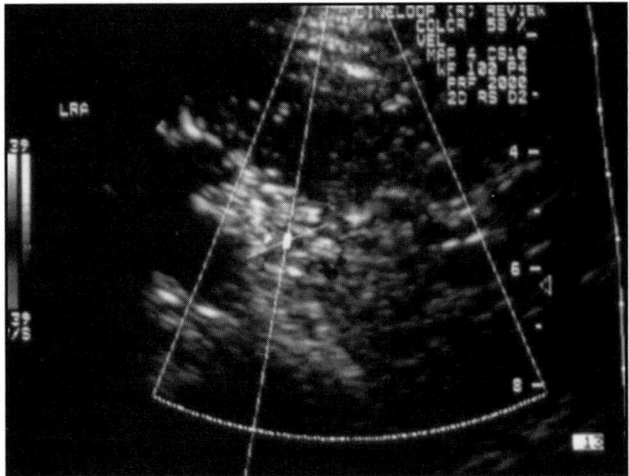

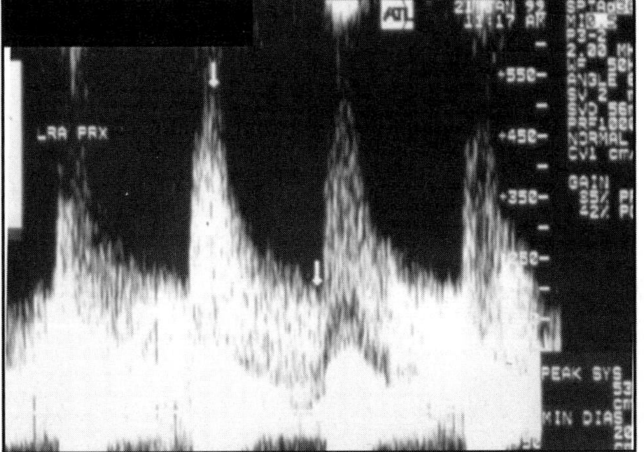

Fig. 7.4 Doppler ultrasonography of a left renal artery stenosis. The B-mode and color-flow image (*top*) and corresponding spectral waveform (*bottom*) are shown. The renal artery peak systolic velocity is ≈530 cm/s. Based on an aortic peak systolic velocity of 75 cm/s, the renal-aortic ratio is 7.1, indicating ≥60% stenosis.

Table 7.2 Duplex Criteria for Classification of Renal Artery Disease

Renal artery diameter reduction	Renal artery PSV	RAR
Normal	<180 cm/s	<3.5
<60%	≥180 cm/s	<3.5
≥60%	...	≥3.5
Occlusion (100%)	No signal	No signal

PSV, peak systolic velocity; RAR, renal-aortic ratio (ratio of the maximum PSV in the renal artery to the PSV in the adjacent normal abdominal aorta).

- RAR ≥3.5 has a sensitivity of 84% and a specificity of 97% for the detection of ≥60% renal artery stenosis
- Decreased renal parenchymal EDV can serve as a marker for parenchymal disease and correlates with clinical failure of renal artery interventions

Predicting Success of Renal Artery Interventions

Kidneys with parenchymal disease tend to have increased resistance to blood flow, which results in decreased EDV compared with normal kidneys. Therefore, decreased parenchymal EDV can serve as a marker for renal parenchymal disease. Because 20% to 40% of patients undergoing renal artery interventions do not show improvements in blood pressure or renal function, parenchymal resistance has been suggested as a possible predictor of clinical outcome after renal artery interventions. A renal resistive index (RRI) has been defined as (PSV–EDV)/PSV, with all velocities obtained from the renal parenchyma. Experience suggests that an RRI of 80 or more is abnormal and correlates with clinical failure of a renal artery intervention; patients with RRI values less than 80 generally have favorable outcomes. The RRI can also be of value in assessing the risk of early rejection of transplanted kidneys.

Lower Extremity Artery Duplex Scanning

The major application of lower extremity arterial duplex scanning is to determine candidates for intervention. Duplex scanning is particularly helpful for examining the aorta and the iliac segments, which are difficult to assess by the indirect non-invasive methods. However, it is not necessary to obtain a duplex scan for every patient being evaluated for peripheral arterial disease. The indirect tests are sufficient for the initial assessment of most patients, and those who do not require intervention can be followed up with ankle pressure measurements and treadmill exercise testing.

Duplex scanning often suggests which type of arterial intervention is most appropriate. Whether a patient is suitable for an endovascular procedure or direct arterial surgery depends on the specific characteristics of the arterial lesions. For example, focal stenoses or short occlusions in the iliac or superficial femoral arteries are usually amenable to catheter-based approaches, whereas arterial segments with very long stenotic lesions or extensive occlusions are better treated by direct arterial reconstruction. It is also essential to assess the status of the inflow to the diseased arterial segment and the quality of the distal runoff. Duplex scanning provides an effective method for obtaining this information without resorting to arteriography.

The systolic velocities observed in normal volunteers for segments proximal to the tibial arteries are summarized in Table 7.3. The velocities decrease in the more peripheral arterial segments; this observation also extends to the tibial arteries. Tibial artery flow velocities have been measured in normal volunteers and in patients with occlusive disease involving the aortoiliac segments, femoropopliteal arteries, and multiple levels. The data indicate

Table 7.3 Arterial Velocities Measured by Duplex Scanning

Artery	Mean±SD PSV, cm/s
External iliac	119.3±21.7
Common femoral	114.1±24.9
Superior femoral	90.8±13.6
Popliteal	68.8±13.5

PSV, peak systolic velocity.

that proximal occlusive disease decreases peak velocities in the tibial arteries. No significant differences in PSV are seen between the three tibial/peroneal arteries, and PSV decreases very little from proximal to distal in a continuously patent tibial artery.

Patients should be examined after an overnight fast to decrease interference from bowel gas during scanning of the abdominal vessels. A complete lower extremity duplex study begins with the upper abdominal aorta and proceeds distally. B-mode images and PW Doppler spectral waveforms are recorded from any areas where increased velocities or other flow disturbances are noted (Fig. 7.5). It is particularly important to sample the flow patterns at closely spaced intervals along the arteries, because the flow disturbances produced by arterial lesions are only propagated downstream for a short distance. Recordings are generally made from the proximal and distal abdominal aorta, the common and external iliac arteries, the common and deep femoral arteries, the proximal, middle, and distal superficial femoral arteries, and the popliteal arteries. If the status of the tibial and peroneal arteries is of clinical interest, recordings should also be made from these vessels.

The spectral waveform criteria for classification of lower extremity arterial stenoses are summarized in Table 7.4. Based on these criteria, stenoses that produce a significant pressure gradient or a diameter reduction of more than 50% at the time of arteriography can be identified by duplex scanning with a sensitivity of 82%, specificity of 92%, positive predictive value of 80%, and negative predictive value of 93%. The correlation is especially good for the iliac artery segment, in which significant stenoses were detected with a sensitivity of 89% and a specificity of 90%. In general, a PSV greater than 200 cm/s in a lower extremity artery is indicative of at least a 50% arteriographic stenosis.

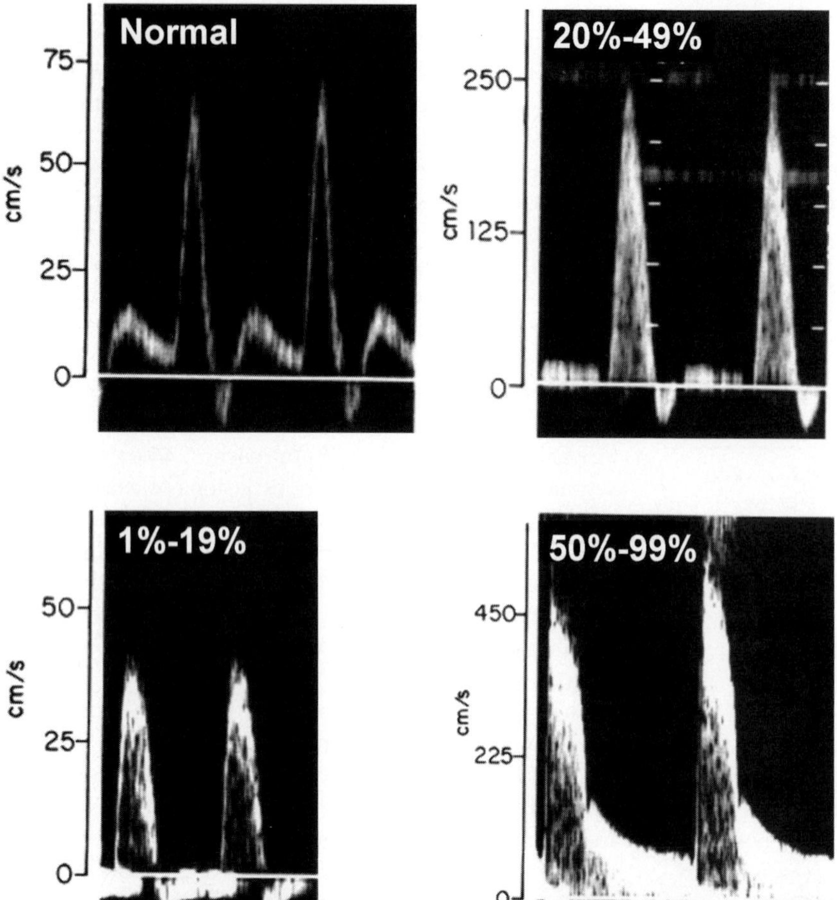

Fig. 7.5 Lower extremity spectral waveforms. These are typical waveforms for each of the stenosis categories described in Table 7.4.

Table 7.4 Duplex Criteria for Classification of Lower Extremity Arterial Lesions

Diameter reduction, %	Criteria
0 (Normal)	Triphasic waveform, no spectral broadening
1-19	Triphasic waveform with minimal spectral broadening only, PSV increased <30% relative to the adjacent proximal segment, proximal and distal waveforms remain normal
20-49	Triphasic waveform usually maintained, although reverse-flow component might be diminished, spectral broadening is prominent with filling-in of the clear area under the systolic peak, PSV increased from 30%-100% relative to the adjacent proximal segment, proximal and distal waveforms remain normal
50-99	Monophasic waveform with loss of the reverse-flow component and forward flow throughout the cardiac cycle, extensive spectral broadening, PSV increased >100% relative to the adjacent proximal segment, distal waveform is monophasic with reduced systolic velocity
100 (Occlusion)	No flow detected within the imaged arterial segment, preocclusive "thump" can be heard just proximal to the site of occlusion, distal waveforms are monophasic with reduced systolic velocities

PSV, peak systolic velocity.

- Duplex scanning often suggests which type of lower extremity arterial intervention is most appropriate
- Duplex techniques can also be used for intraoperative assessment and follow-up after endovascular or surgical interventions
- Velocities normally decrease as blood flows from the heart to the peripheral arterial segments
- In general, a PSV of >200 cm/s in a lower extremity artery is indicative of 50% arteriographic stenosis

Duplex techniques can also be used for intraoperative assessment and follow-up after endovascular or surgical interventions. Duplex scanning has been especially valuable in monitoring the function of bypass grafts in the leg, because clinical follow-up or use of ankle pressure measurements alone are not reliable for identifying grafts that are at risk for thrombosis. A wide range of blood flow velocities has been observed in infrainguinal vein grafts, but in most normally functioning grafts, PSVs in the middle and distal graft segments exceed 40 to 45 cm/s. The principal criterion for identifying a stenotic lesion in a vein graft is a high-velocity jet or localized increase in PSV associated with spectral broadening. In general, routine graft surveillance by duplex scanning and appropriate intervention results in a 20% to 25% increase in long-term graft patency.

Questions

1. What is the principal advantage of PW Doppler over CW Doppler?
   - **a.** Only PW Doppler can display direction of flow relative to the transducer.
   - **b.** PW Doppler devices are generally less expensive and easier to use.
   - **c.** Only PW Doppler can detect flow at discrete sites in tissue.
   - **d.** PW Doppler provides better depth penetration in tissue.

2. Why is the normal ABI greater than 1.0?
   - **a.** The systolic pressure increases as the pulse moves distally in the lower limb.
   - **b.** The tibial arteries are more compressible than the brachial arteries.
   - **c.** The mean arterial pressure increases as the pulse moves distally in the lower limb.
   - **d.** There is a significant cuff artifact at the ankle, resulting in higher pressures.

3. Which of the following statements regarding measurement of toe pressure and the toe-brachial index is true?
   - **a.** Toe pressures are difficult to measure when the tibial arteries are calcified.
   - **b.** There are no significant differences between diabetic and non-diabetic patients.
   - **c.** A normal toe-brachial index is in the range of 0.5 to 0.7.
   - **d.** For this test, a Doppler flow detector is easier to use than a PPG.

4. Which of the following features of a segmental plethysmographic waveform is most consistent with normal proximal arteries?
   - **a.** A downslope that bows away from the baseline
   - **b.** Equal rise and fall times
   - **c.** A decrease in amplitude after treadmill exercise
   - **d.** The presence of a dicrotic wave on the downslope

5. Which of the following statements regarding the treadmill exercise test is true?
   - **a.** The maximum change in ankle pressure occurs 5 to 10 minutes after exercise.
   - **b.** A slight increase in ankle pressure after exercise is abnormal.
   - **c.** It can identify occlusive arterial disease that is not functionally significant at rest.
   - **d.** If no leg symptoms occur after 5 minutes, another 5 minutes of walking time should be added.

Suggested Readings

Baker JD, Dix DE. Variability of Doppler ankle pressures with arterial occlusive disease: an evaluation of ankle index and brachial-ankle pressure gradient. Surgery. 1981;89:134-7.

Dawson DL, Zierler RE, Strandness DE Jr, et al. The role of duplex scanning and arteriography before carotid endarterectomy: a prospective study. J Vasc Surg. 1993;18:673-80.

Grant EG, Benson CB, Moneta GL, et al. Carotid artery stenosis: gray-scale and Doppler US diagnosis: Society of Radiologists in Ultrasound Consensus Conference. Radiology. 2003 Nov;229:340-6. Epub 2003 Sep 18.

Keagy BA, Pharr WF, Thomas D, et al. Comparison of reactive hyperemia and treadmill tests in the evaluation of peripheral vascular disease. Am J Surg. 1981;142:158-61.

Kram HB, Appel PL, Shoemaker WC. Multisensor transcutaneous oximetric mapping to predict below-knee amputation wound healing: use of a critical PO_2. J Vasc Surg. 1989;9:796-800.

Moneta GL, Edwards JM, Chitwood RW, et al. Correlation of North American Symptomatic Carotid Endarterectomy Trial (NASCET) angiographic definition of 70% to 99% internal carotid artery stenosis with duplex scanning. J Vasc Surg. 1993;17:152-7.

Moneta GL, Edwards JM, Papanicolaou G, et al. Screening for asymptomatic internal carotid artery stenosis: duplex criteria for discriminating 60% to 99% stenosis. J Vasc Surg. 1995;21:989-94.

Moneta GL, Yeager RA, Dalman R, et al. Duplex ultrasound criteria for diagnosis of splanchnic artery stenosis or occlusion. J Vasc Surg. 1991;14:511-8.

Moneta GL, Yeager RA, Lee RW, et al. Noninvasive localization of arterial occlusive disease: a comparison of segmental Doppler pressures and arterial duplex mapping. J Vasc Surg. 1993;17:578-82.

Olin JW, Piedmonte MR, Young JR, et al. The utility of duplex ultrasound scanning of the renal arteries for diagnosing significant renal artery stenosis. Ann Intern Med. 1995;122:833-8.

Ramsey DE, Manke DA, Sumner DS. Toe blood pressure: a valuable adjunct to ankle pressure measurement for assessing peripheral arterial disease. J Cardiovasc Surg (Torino). 1983;24:43-8.

Strandness DE Jr. Duplex scanning in vascular disorders. 3rd ed. Philadelphia: Lippincott Williams & Wilkins; 2002. p. 3-19.

Zagzebski JA. Essentials of ultrasound physics. St. Louis: Mosby; 1996. p. 46-68.

8 Venous Testing in the Vascular Laboratory*

Brenda K. Zierler, PhD
Gregory L. Moneta, MD

Vascular laboratory testing for venous disease uses physiologic and ultrasound-based techniques and can evaluate acute and chronic venous disorders. Ultrasonographic tests currently are used most frequently for evaluation of acute and chronic venous disease. Physiologic testing relies on detecting alterations in blood pressure, blood flow, and other physiologic parameters to assess the location and severity of venous lesions. Physiologic venous tests have some role in the evaluation of chronic venous disorders but are rarely used today to evaluate for acute deep vein thrombosis (DVT).

Acute Deep Vein Thrombosis

Venous thromboembolism consists of two related conditions: pulmonary embolism (PE) and DVT. Objective testing for venous thromboembolism is crucial because the clinical diagnosis is non-specific and insensitive. Originally, vascular laboratory techniques for diagnosis of DVT were based on plethysmography. These older techniques have been supplanted by ultrasound-based techniques. This discussion of vascular laboratory techniques for diagnosis of acute DVT will therefore focus on the utility of venous ultrasonography as the foundation for diagnosis of acute lower extremity DVT.

- Physiologic venous tests have some role in the evaluation of chronic venous disorders but are rarely used today to evaluate for acute DVT
- Objective testing for venous thromboembolism is crucial because the clinical diagnosis is non-specific and insensitive

*Portions of this chapter have been previously published in Zierler BK. Ultrasonography and diagnosis of venous thromboembolism. Circulation. 2004;109 Suppl 1:I9-14. Used with permission.

Impedance Plethysmography

Before the use of venous duplex scanning became common, impedance plethysmography (IPG) was the preferred non-invasive test for suspected acute DVT. Plethysmographic methods detect and measure volume changes in the extremities resulting primarily from alterations in blood volume. Most plethysmographs used in the vascular laboratory measure volume indirectly by detecting changes in limb circumference, electrical impedance, or reflectivity of infrared light. IPG is a reasonably sensitive (87%) and specific (up to 100%) test for proximal lower extremity DVT in symptomatic patients. Lower sensitivities for proximal DVT (65%) are reported in studies that only compare IPG with venography. IPG can miss non-occlusive proximal DVT and occlusive proximal DVT present in parallel venous systems (such as duplicated femoral or popliteal veins), and it does not detect DVT isolated to the calf. The limitations of IPG now make it a substandard examination for routine assessment for DVT.

Venous Ultrasonography

Duplex ultrasonography is the primary method for assessment of DVT, according to the standards of the Intersocietal Commission for the Accreditation of Vascular Laboratories. Secondary instrumentation such as IPG and continuous-wave Doppler are still used to supplement duplex ultrasonography but are not primary diagnostic methods.

The several types of venous ultrasonography include compression ultrasonography alone with B-mode imaging, duplex ultrasonography (B-mode imaging combined with Doppler waveform analysis), and color Doppler. The sensitivities and specificities of these methods for detecting acute DVT differ; different veins are best evaluated with different techniques. For example, compression ultrasonography is most useful for the proximal deep veins, specifically the common femoral, femoral, and popliteal veins. A combination of duplex and color Doppler are used to interrogate the calf and iliac veins.

Accuracy of Venous Ultrasonography

Traditionally, diagnostic strategies for acute DVT have been evaluated with accuracy studies in which the new test (e.g., venous ultrasonography) is compared with the gold standard (e.g., venography). The accuracy of venous ultrasonography compared with venography is well established. The weighted mean sensitivity and specificity of venous ultrasonography (including all types) for the diagnosis of proximal DVT are 97% and 94%, respectively. The high specificity allows treatment of DVT to be initiated without additional confirmatory tests; the high sensitivity permits withholding treatment if results are negative. If the examination is technically limited, serial examinations may be required. Contrast venography or computed tomography (CT) or magnetic resonance (MR) venography may also be indicated to supplement an incomplete ultrasonographic examination, especially if serial studies are not possible.

- The sensitivity and specificity of venous ultrasonography for the diagnosis of proximal DVT are 97% and 94%, respectively

Venous Ultrasonography as a Stand-Alone Diagnostic Test

Although most evaluations of venous ultrasonography are accuracy studies, management studies (in which patients are followed up to determine the safety of managing patients according to the results of the test) are also important and are currently of more interest. Such studies help in determining how to incorporate venous ultrasonographic testing most efficiently into clinical practice.

One management study used compression ultrasonography as a stand-alone examination in patients suspected of a first episode of proximal DVT. The trial involved 405 consecutive symptomatic outpatients and tested the safety of withholding anticoagulation in patients with normal compression ultrasonographic examinations of the proximal veins both at presentation and at a follow-up test 5 to 7 days later. Patients with initially abnormal ultrasonographic studies were treated with anticoagulation, whereas those with normal studies underwent repeat ultrasonography. Anticoagulation was withheld from patients with negative compression ultrasonography results. Patients were then followed up for 3 months. DVT developed in only two of 335 patients (0.6%) with initially normal studies. No deaths were reported in patients managed according to this protocol. An initial negative examination that includes both proximal veins and calf veins appears to be sufficient to withhold anticoagulation and to preclude the need for routine follow-up studies in patients without clinical suspicion of PE.

Many vascular laboratories still do not include ultrasonographic evaluation of calf veins as part of their routine evaluation for DVT, even in symptomatic patients, because ultrasonography is mistakenly believed to be inaccurate for evaluation for isolated calf vein DVT. However, ultrasonography, using a combination of B-mode, Doppler waveform analysis, and color Doppler, can now image calf veins in the large majority of patients. A well-trained technologist can interrogate these veins in 80% to 98% of cases. In technically adequate studies, the sensitivity and specificity of color-flow duplex scanning in isolated calf veins have exceeded 90%. Other studies have shown similar results.

Isolated calf vein (distal) thrombosis accounts for 20% of symptomatic DVT; treatment is recommended both for symptomatic distal DVT and for proximal DVT. If anticoagulation cannot be administered or is contraindicated, serial studies should be performed 10 to 14 days after presentation to assess for proximal progression of calf vein thrombus because approximately one-fourth of untreated symptomatic calf vein thrombi extend proximally within 1 to 2 weeks. (Calf vein thrombi are not readily detected by CT or MR venography.) Serial duplex scans are also indicated for patients who present with symptoms of possible DVT and who 1) have a negative venous ultrasonographic examination of the proximal veins, 2) do not or cannot have the calf veins adequately imaged, and 3) did not have contrast venography. These recommendations require an examination with excellent sensitivity and specificity for diagnosis of both above-knee and below-knee DVT. Color-flow duplex scanning is the most practical and cost-effective method.

- Isolated calf vein thrombosis accounts for 20% of symptomatic DVT
- Approximately one-fourth of untreated symptomatic calf vein thrombi extend proximally within 1 to 2 weeks

Limitations

Venous ultrasonographic examinations are not standardized and range from compression of as few as two deep veins to a complete duplex and color Doppler evaluation of the entire lower extremity. Stand-alone limited ultrasonographic examinations are incompatible with the recommendations of the American College of Chest Physicians and the American Thoracic Society. Examination of specific venous segments can be limited by factors such as morbid obesity, lower extremity edema or tenderness, or the presence of immobilization devices and bandages. Despite these limitations, complete venous duplex and color Doppler examination has become the standard for assessment of lower extremity DVT.

Negative Ultrasonography Studies

Of the 1 million patients per year who undergo ultrasonographic examination for suspected DVT, only 12% to 25% have positive results. Because of the cost associated with negative and, in some cases after-hours, examinations, strategies to decrease the number of negative examinations have been developed. The most commonly investigated alternatives to immediate duplex evaluation for suspected DVT are clinical prediction models and measurement of D-dimer levels.

- Complete venous duplex and color Doppler examination has become the standard for assessment of lower extremity DVT
- Of the 1 million patients per year who undergo ultrasonographic examination for suspected DVT, only 12% to 25% have positive results

Combined Approaches in the Diagnosis of DVT

Algorithmic approaches using a combination of clinical assessment, D-dimer measurements, and ultrasonography are being developed with the goals of standardizing the diagnostic approach to DVT and decreasing the number of negative ultrasonographic examinations. The utility of algorithms depends on the availability of diagnostic testing, the patient population, the cost of and reimbursement for different tests, and the interpretation of the results.

A strategy that is feasible for one institution may not be so for another—for example, a strategy that uses venography is useless if venography is not available. Potential approaches to limiting the use of ultrasonographic examinations for evaluation of possible DVT must therefore be specific to the organization. Although cohort studies have incorporated algorithms that use clinical pretest probability in combination with ultrasonography or D-dimer testing, Level 1 evidence on the validity and safety of these algorithms for the diagnosis of DVT is lacking.

Clinical Assessment Combined With Venous Ultrasonography

Some clinical presentations are more likely than others to be associated with DVT. In one model developed to assess the clinical likelihood of DVT in outpatients in whom it is suspected, patients are stratified into three risk categories—low, moderate, and high—on the basis of thrombotic risk factors, clinical signs and symptoms, and the possibility of alternative diagnoses. Patients with at least one risk factor and classic symptoms of unilateral pain and swelling have an 85% probability of DVT. Outpatients who present with no identifiable risk factors and with no typical features of DVT have about a 5% probability of having DVT (Table 8.1).

One study evaluated the accuracy of pretest probability assessment before compression ultrasonography in 593 patients with possible DVT. Those with low pretest probability underwent a single ultrasonographic test of the proximal veins. A negative ultrasonographic result was considered to exclude acute DVT. Positive studies were confirmed by venography. More than half the patients had 0 or fewer pretest points and were classified as having a "low" pretest probability of DVT. One-third had 1 or 2 points and thus a "moderate" probability, and 14% had at least 3 or more points and were assessed as having "high" probability of DVT. The incidence of positive venous ultrasonographic studies in the low, moderate, and high probability groups was 3%, 17%, and 75%, respectively.

A pretest probability model in conjunction with D-dimer testing has also been evaluated. D-dimer testing is controversial, and its precise role as an adjunct to ultrasonographic examination for DVT has not been definitively established. D-dimer measurements have a lower sensitivity for isolated calf vein thrombi. The negative predictive value of D-dimer testing varies with the pretest probability of disease. The negative predictive value is exceptionally good in low-risk patients but is unacceptable in high-risk patients. Results are variable and depend on thrombus location, size, interpretation of the results, and other factors. Results from one study using D-dimer as-

Table 8.1 Clinical Model for Predicting Pretest Probability of Acute DVT*

Clinical features/risk factors	Score
Active cancer within 6 months (ongoing treatment or palliative)	1
Immobilization by paralysis or plaster dressings	1
Recent surgery (within 4 weeks) or bed rest longer than 3 days	1
Localized tenderness along distribution of the deep venous system	1
Calf swelling (>3 cm increase in calf circumference vs asymptomatic leg) measured 10 cm below tibial tuberosity	1
Thigh and calf swelling (entire leg swollen)	1
Pitting edema confined to symptomatic leg†	1
Collateral superficial veins (non-varicose)	1
Alternative diagnosis as likely as or more likely than DVT	−2

DVT, deep vein thrombosis.
*Pretest probability calculated as the total score: low risk, ≤0; moderate risk, 1 or 2; high risk, ≥3. Alternatively, in the newer scoring system, the probability of having DVT is "likely" for a score ≥2, and a score <2 indicates that the probability of acute DVT is "unlikely."
†The more symptomatic leg is used if patients have symptoms in both legs.
From Zierler BK. Ultrasonography and diagnosis of venous thromboembolism. Circulation. 2004;109 Suppl 1:I9-14. Used with permission.

says cannot be extrapolated to other studies because the several different assays for D-dimer vary in sensitivity and specificity.

Several studies have shown the utility of D-dimer testing in combination with clinical assessment in the initial investigation of outpatients with suspected DVT. In one study, 1,096 consecutive outpatients suspected of having DVT were scored according to the clinical likelihood of thrombosis. They were then randomly assigned to undergo ultrasonographic imaging alone, or to undergo D-dimer testing followed by ultrasonographic imaging (unless the D-dimer test was negative and the patient was considered unlikely to have DVT). Only 0.4% of patients in whom DVT was ruled out by D-dimer testing eventually had DVT. The authors concluded that DVT could be excluded in a patient in whom it was clinically unlikely and who had a negative D-dimer test. They also concluded that ultrasonography could be safely omitted in outpatients with a negative D-dimer result and a low clinical likelihood of DVT.

- Several studies have shown the utility of D-dimer testing in combination with clinical assessment in the initial investigation of outpatients with suspected DVT
- Ultrasonography can be safely omitted in outpatients with a negative D-dimer result and a low clinical likelihood of DVT

Standardizing Protocols

Clinical models for standardizing the assessment of patients presenting with suspected DVT have been used in research settings and in some dedicated thrombosis centers in Canada and Europe. These models are not well accepted, however, and are infrequently used in clinical practice. Reasons for their infrequent use include the complexity of the algorithms, medicolegal concerns (should a DVT be missed because the algorithm did not require further evaluation), and because a negative venous duplex ultrasonographic result allows the evaluating physician to immediately consider alternative diagnoses.

Venous Ultrasonography in the Diagnosis of PE

The diagnosis of PE cannot be established without objective testing. Several studies have evaluated the utility of venous duplex scanning in patients suspected of having PE. These studies, often using ultrasonography of only the proximal veins and nuclear medicine–based ventilation perfusion scanning, have little relevance to modern practice; complete ultrasonographic examinations are now often routine, and CT or MR pulmonary angiography has supplanted ventilation perfusion scanning.

- The diagnosis of PE cannot be established without objective testing

The rationale for using lower extremity venous ultrasonography in patients who present with symptoms of PE is that a DVT diagnosis may suggest the diagnosis of PE, and further investigation to exclude PE may not be necessary if there is also an ultrasonographic diagnosis of DVT. This approach has several important limitations. First, venous duplex ultrasonography does not give a definitive diagnosis of PE. Even if DVT is present, patients can have pulmonary symptoms or hemodynamic instability from causes other than PE. Second, normal venous ultrasonographic scans do not rule out PE. Even if PE is definitely present, DVT of the proximal lower extremity veins is detectable by compression ultrasonography in only 50% of patients. If an objectively confirmed PE is diagnosed, and there is no evidence of lower extremity DVT, the PE could have originated from pelvic or arm veins or possibly embolized completely from a lower extremity vein. An objective diagnostic test for PE, such as CT pulmonary angiography, is indicated in most cases. A diagnostic algorithm for PE that does not include CT pulmonary angiography seems untenable in modern practice, despite the lack of Level 1 evidence to support it in the diagnosis of PE. The use of MR pulmonary angiography is increasing but also requires further validation in clinical trials.

Chronic Venous Insufficiency

Photoplethysmography

Photoplethysmography (PPG) uses a light-emitting diode and measurement of back-scattered light in combination with provocative limb maneuvers (calf muscle contraction) to assess the venous system. Measurements are made of venous refill time (VRT)—the time required for the PPG tracing to return to 90% of baseline after cessation of calf contraction. Much shorter VRTs are present in limbs with chronic venous insufficiency than in normal limbs. However, VRTs vary with technique and placement of the photosensor. Normal limbs generally have VRTs greater than 18 seconds, and abnormal limbs have VRTs less than 18 seconds. PPG-derived VRTs, however, do not adequately distinguish between varying severities of chronic venous insufficiency. PPG has fallen out of favor in many vascular laboratories as a means of assessing chronic venous insufficiency.

Air Plethysmography

Air plethysmography uses a low-pressure, air-filled cuff

applied to the lower leg from knee to ankle. The technique measures volume changes in the cuff in response to provocative maneuvers. A baseline volume is obtained with the patient resting and supine, after which the patient is asked to stand. The volume tracing gradually increases until it reaches a plateau. A single calf-contraction/tiptoe maneuver is performed and the volume change recorded. Next, the patient performs 10 tiptoe maneuvers to maximally empty the limb of blood. A tourniquet applied to the thigh isolates the deep from the superficial venous system. Information derived from air plethysmography theoretically allows assessment of reflux, calf muscle pump function, and overall venous function of the extremity.

Duplex Ultrasonography

Duplex ultrasonography can provide important physiologic and anatomic information on patients with possible chronic venous insufficiency, including the sites of reflux or venous obstruction. In patients with valve incompetence, reflux can be stimulated and then detected with duplex using a Valsalva maneuver, manual compression proximal to the transducer, or release of compression distal to the transducer.

The examination has been standardized using rapid inflation and deflation of a series of pneumatic cuffs at specific sites on the leg (with the leg under examination not bearing weight). In the upright position, reflux stimulated by cuff deflation that lasts more than 0.5 second is indicative of pathologic reflux. The technique allows localization of reflux to specific venous segments and can serve as a valuable preoperative planning tool to target specific venous segments for removal or reconstruction. It has a sensitivity of 82% and specificity of 100% for the identification of competent and incompetent perforating veins. Duplex determination of reflux sites and sites of venous occlusion has not been established as a means of assessing overall venous hemodynamics.

Questions

1. What is the primary ultrasonographic method for assessing for patency of the deep veins between the knee and the inguinal ligament?
   a. Color-flow ultrasonography
   b. Compressive B-mode ultrasonography
   c. Pulsed Doppler
   d. Gated pulse Doppler
   e. Fast Fourier transform analysis

2. If a technically adequate examination is possible, what is the sensitivity of color-flow duplex scanning to detect venous thrombosis isolated to the calf veins in symptomatic patients?
   a. About 50%
   b. About 60%
   c. About 70%
   d. About 80%
   e. About 90%

3. Which of the following sites is most difficult to examine with compressive B-mode ultrasonography?
   a. Common femoral vein
   b. Femoral vein proximal in the thigh
   c. Femoral vein in mid thigh
   d. Femoral vein at the adductor canal
   e. Popliteal vein

4. When assessing for lower extremity venous reflux using ultrasonography and the cuff deflation technique, what duration of reflux can be considered normal?
   a. <0.5 s
   b. <1.5 s
   c. <2.5 s
   d. <3.5 s
   e. <4.5 s

5. Which vascular laboratory test can provide information on the efficacy of the calf muscle pump?
   a. Compressive B-mode duplex ultrasonography
   b. Impedance plethysmography
   c. Photoplethysmography
   d. Air plethysmography
   e. Strain-gauge plethysmography

Suggested Readings

Anderson DR, Kovacs MJ, Kovacs G, et al. Combined use of clinical assessment and D-dimer to improve the management of patients presenting to the emergency department with suspected deep vein thrombosis (the EDITED Study). J Thromb Haemost. 2003;1:645-51.

Birdwell BG, Raskob GE, Whitsett TL, et al. The clinical validity of normal compression ultrasonography in outpatients suspected of having deep venous thrombosis. Ann Intern Med. 1998;128:1-7.

Christopoulos DG, Nicolaides AN, Szendro G, et al. Air-plethysmography and the effect of elastic compression on venous hemodynamics of the leg. J Vasc Surg. 1987;5:148-59.

Fedullo PF, Tapson VF. The evaluation of suspected pulmonary embolism. N Engl J Med. 2003;349:1247-56.

ICAVL: Essentials and standards for accreditation in noninvasive vascular testing. Part II. Vascular laboratory operations: peripheral venous testing. Columbia (MD): Intersocietal Commission for the Accreditation of Vascular Laboratories; 2000. p. 1-8.

Tick LW, Ton E, van Voorthuizen T, et al. Practical diagnostic management of patients with clinically suspected deep vein thrombosis by clinical probability test, compression ultrasonography, and D-dimer test. Am J Med. 2002;113:630-5.

van Bemmelen PS, Bedford G, Beach K, et al. Quantitative segmental evaluation of venous valvular reflux with duplex ultrasound scanning. J Vasc Surg. 1989;10:425-31.

Wells PS, Anderson DR, Bormanis J, et al. SimpliRED D-dimer can reduce the diagnostic tests in suspected deep vein thrombosis. Lancet. 1998;351:1405-6.

Wells PS, Anderson DR, Rodger M, et al. Evaluation of D-dimer in the diagnosis of suspected deep-vein thrombosis. N Engl J Med. 2003;349:1227-35.

9 Perioperative Management of Vascular Surgery

Joshua A. Beckman, MD
Mark A. Creager, MD

Introduction

Each year, approximately 6 million non-cardiac surgical procedures are performed in the United States. About 25% of these are major intra-abdominal, thoracic, vascular, and orthopedic procedures. Patients undergoing vascular operations, such as aortic reconstruction, infrarenal bypass, and carotid endarterectomy, frequently have coexisting coronary and cerebral atherosclerosis. Therefore, they are at increased risk for adverse perioperative cardiovascular events, including myocardial infarction, stroke, and death. This chapter highlights the clinical features and diagnostic tests used to assess cardiovascular risk in patients undergoing vascular surgery procedures and discusses the management of these patients during the perioperative period.

The recommendations in this chapter are derived from the ACC/AHA (American College of Cardiology/American Heart Association) Guideline Update on Perioperative Cardiovascular Evaluation for Noncardiac Surgery published in 2002. A quote from these guidelines underscores the importance of risk assessment: "The purpose of preoperative evaluation is not to give medical clearance but rather to perform an evaluation of the patient's current medical status; make recommendations concerning the ... risk of cardiac problems over the entire perioperative period; and provide a clinical risk profile that the patient, primary physician, anesthesiologist, and surgeon can use in making treatment decisions...."

Risk of Adverse Cardiovascular Events in Patients Undergoing Vascular Surgery

Vascular surgical operations are associated with the highest risk of adverse cardiovascular events among all major non-cardiac operations. In one study, the incidence of perioperative myocardial infarction for patients undergoing aortic surgery was approximately 6%, and for those undergoing infrainguinal bypass graft it was approximately 13%. An analysis of Medicare claims of patients undergoing vascular surgery showed the 30-day operative mortality rate to be 7.3% among patients undergoing aortic surgery and 5.8% among those undergoing infrainguinal bypass surgery. These outcomes reflect that many patients undergoing peripheral vascular surgical procedures have associated coronary artery disease. Therefore, it is extremely important to perform a careful history and physical examination to identify patients with coronary artery disease and to institute appropriate measures to decrease the risk of perioperative cardiovascular events.

- Vascular surgical operations are associated with the highest risk of adverse cardiovascular events among all major non-cardiac operations
- Many patients undergoing peripheral vascular surgical procedures have associated coronary artery disease

History and Physical Examination

The history should include queries to identify the presence of cardiac diseases, including coronary artery disease, congestive heart failure, valvular heart disease, and arrhythmias. Questions should be directed at symptoms of angina, exertional dyspnea and fatigue, palpitations, arrhythmias, prior myocardial infarction, prior cardiac surgery or percutaneous coronary interventions, and placement of a pacemaker or cardiac defibrillator. Questions about the patient's ability to perform common daily tasks and participation in sports or exercise programs should be used to assess functional capacity. In addition, queries should be directed at risk factors for atherosclerosis, including diabetes mellitus, hypercholesterolemia, cigarette smoking, hypertension, family history of premature coronary artery disease, and associated atherosclerotic conditions, including peripheral arterial disease and cerebrovascular disease. The presence of other comorbid conditions such as chronic pulmonary disease and renal insufficiency should be queried. Review of medications is important to ascertain the use of antihypertensive, antianginal, lipid-lowering, antiplatelet, and anticoagulant medications.

The cardiovascular examination includes measurement of heart rate, jugular venous pressure, and blood pressure in both arms; palpation and auscultation of the carotid pulses; percussion and auscultation of the lungs; and cardiac inspection, palpation, and auscultation to seek evidence of arrhythmias, valvular heart disease, and congestive heart failure. The abdomen should be palpated for aortic aneurysms, masses, and hepatosplenomegaly and auscultated for bruits. The extremities should be examined for edema and the presence of peripheral arterial disease.

Fundamental ancillary studies include electrocardiography (ECG), blood count, basic chemistries (to assess for diabetes mellitus, renal insufficiency, and liver abnormalities), and a coagulation profile (prothrombin time, partial thromboplastin time).

Important findings that increase the risk of perioperative events can be identified by a careful clinical evaluation. These include coronary artery disease, valvular heart disease (e.g., aortic stenosis) congestive heart failure, diabetes mellitus, and renal insufficiency.

Table 9.1 Clinical Predictors of Increased Perioperative Cardiovascular Risk (MI, Heart Failure, or Death)

Major
Unstable coronary syndromes
Acute or recent MI with evidence of important ischemic risk by clinical symptoms or non-invasive study
Unstable or severe angina (CCS class III or IV)
Decompensated heart failure
Significant arrhythmias
High-grade atrioventricular block
Symptomatic ventricular arrhythmias in the presence of underlying heart disease
Supraventricular arrhythmias with uncontrolled ventricular rate
Severe valvular disease
Intermediate
Mild angina pectoris (CCS class I or II)
Previous MI by history or pathologic Q waves
Compensated or prior heart failure
Diabetes mellitus (particularly insulin-dependent)
Renal insufficiency
Minor
Advanced age
Abnormal ECG results (left ventricular hypertrophy, left bundle branch block, ST-T segment abnormalities)
Rhythm other than sinus (e.g., atrial fibrillation)
Low functional capacity (e.g., inability to climb one flight of stairs with a bag of groceries)
History of stroke
Uncontrolled systemic hypertension

CCS, Canadian Cardiovascular Society; ECG, electrocardiography; MI, myocardial infarction.

Clinical Predictors

General Predictors

In general, the indications for further cardiac testing and treatment are the same as those that would guide management in the non-operative setting. The timing and use of these tests in patients undergoing vascular surgery is dependent on the urgency of the operation, the patient's risk factors, and the specific surgical procedure. Recommendations for coronary revascularization before vascular surgery (so the patient can "get through" the vascular operation) are appropriate for only a small subset of patients, as discussed later.

The ACC/AHA practice guidelines have characterized clinical predictors of increased perioperative cardiovascular risk (myocardial infarction, congestive heart failure, and death) (Table 9.1). The predictors are divided into major, intermediate, and minor. Major predictors include acute coronary syndromes, decompensated congestive heart failure, significant arrhythmias, and severe valvular heart disease. Major predictors mandate intensive management that could cause delay or cancellation of surgery unless it is urgent. Intermediate predictors are validated markers of enhanced risk of perioperative cardiovascular events which require careful assessment of the patient's status. These include other evidence of coronary artery disease such as angina or prior myocardial infarction, prior or treated congestive heart failure, diabetes mellitus, or renal insufficiency. Minor predictors are markers of cardiovascular disease that, independently, may not increase perioperative risk. Minor predictors include advanced age, rhythm other than sinus, abnormal ECG results, low functional capacity, and uncontrolled hypertension.

Surgery-specific risk is also characterized as high, intermediate, and low, depending on the type of surgery. High-risk procedures include aortic reconstruction and infrainguinal bypass surgery. These are associated with a 5% or greater risk of cardiac death or non-fatal myocardial infarction. Intermediate-risk procedures, such as carotid endarterectomy, are associated with a risk of death or non-fatal myocardial infarction between 1% and 5%. Low-risk procedures, such as saphenous vein ligation, are generally associated with a cardiac risk of less than 1%. Risk stratifi-

Table 9.2 Cardiac Risk Stratification for Non-Cardiac Surgical Procedures*

High risk
(Reported cardiac risk often greater than 5%)
- Emergent major operations, particularly in the elderly
- Aortic and other major vascular surgery
- Peripheral vascular surgery
- Anticipated prolonged surgical procedures associated with large fluid shifts or blood loss

Intermediate risk
(Reported cardiac risk generally less than 5%)
- Carotid endarterectomy
- Head and neck surgery
- Intraperitoneal and intrathoracic surgery
- Orthopedic surgery
- Prostate surgery

Low risk†
(Reported cardiac risk generally less than 1%)
- Endoscopic procedures
- Superficial procedure
- Cataract surgery
- Breast surgery

*Cardiac risk defined as combined incidence of cardiac death and non-fatal myocardial infarction.
†Do not generally require further preoperative cardiac testing.

cation for surgical procedures (Table 9.2) is adapted from the ACC/AHA guidelines.

Algorithm for Perioperative Cardiovascular Risk Assessment

A sequential approach is recommended to assist in making decisions regarding diagnostic testing and treatment for patients before undertaking vascular surgery. The first step is to consider the urgency of the vascular operation. In the case of urgent procedures, such as for ruptured abdominal aortic aneurysm or acute limb ischemia, there is insufficient time for an intensive preoperative cardiovascular risk evaluation. These patients should proceed to life- or limb-saving procedures. Selective postoperative risk stratification and therapies can be recommended after completion of the operation. The next step is to determine whether a patient has undergone a recent cardiovascular evaluation or had a coronary revascularization procedure. In patients who have undergone coronary revascularization procedures within the past 5 years, who have had no interval event, and whose clinical status has remained stable, the likelihood of perioperative cardiovascular events is low. In these patients, additional cardiac testing is usually not indicated. Similarly, if patients have undergone a recent cardiovascular evaluation, particularly in the preceding 2 years, and if this evaluation has included either non-invasive or invasive measures, repeat testing usually is not necessary for risk assessment.

Elective vascular surgery should be postponed in patients who have major clinical risk predictors such as acute coronary syndrome, decompensated congestive heart failure, severe valvular heart disease, or significant arrhythmias. These problems require further evaluation, and most require treatment before elective vascular surgery. The surgery-specific risk should also be taken into account when determining the need for preoperative cardiovascular testing. As noted above, aortic and infrainguinal bypass operations are deemed to have high surgery-specific risk, and carotid endarterectomy is an intermediate surgery-specific risk.

For patients with intermediate clinical risk predictors such as stable angina, prior myocardial infarction, treated congestive heart failure, diabetes mellitus, or renal insufficiency, additional diagnostic studies may be considered to refine the cardiovascular risk assessment and determine whether additional cardiac tests and intervention should be undertaken before vascular surgery. Among the most important considerations for assessing cardiovascular risk in patients with intermediate clinical predictors is functional status. Patients who are capable of exercising with a functional capacity of 10 metabolic equivalents (METs) generally have decreased risk of an adverse cardiovascular event. The Duke Activity Status Index includes questions that can be used to assess a patient's functional capacity and assess MET levels. Participation in strenuous sports exceeding 10 METs, such as singles tennis, swimming, and ice skating, is indicative of excellent functional capacity. The energy expenditures for activities such as playing golf, dancing, and scrubbing floors range between 4 and 10 METs. The energy expenditures for eating, dressing, walking around the house, and dishwashing range from 1 to 4 METs. Patients who are unable to perform at the level of 4 METs have poor functional capacity.

Patients with intermediate clinical risk predictors who have poor functional capacity (<4 METs) should undergo non-invasive testing to further assess cardiovascular risk before vascular surgery. In addition, patients with intermediate clinical predictors, yet with moderate-to-excellent functional capacity, who are undergoing high-risk surgical procedures such as aortic reconstruction or infrainguinal bypass surgery, should also be considered for non-invasive testing to assess risk. Patients with intermediate clinical risk predictors and moderate-to-excellent functional capacity who are undergoing an intermediate-risk procedure such as carotid endarterectomy can often proceed to the procedure with no additional risk stratification imposed by non-invasive testing. Opinions differ, however, regarding the need for non-invasive testing in patients with intermediate clinical predictors undergoing carotid endarterectomy. Patients with intermediate clinical predictors undergoing a low-risk surgical procedure, such as varicose vein stripping, do not require non-invasive testing before surgery.

- In patients who have undergone coronary revascularization procedures within the past 5 years, additional cardiac testing is usually not indicated
- Patients who are capable of exercising with a functional capacity of 10 METs generally have decreased risk of an adverse cardiovascular event
- Patients with intermediate clinical risk predictors who have poor functional capacity (<4 METs) should undergo non-invasive testing to further assess cardiovascular risk before vascular surgery

Interpretation and Utilization of Non-Invasive Testing

Various non-invasive tests can be used to assess a patient's exercise capacity, seek evidence of myocardial ischemia, assess cardiac function, and evaluate valvular heart disease. These include the standard treadmill exercise tolerance test, transthoracic echocardiography, nuclear myocardial perfusion imaging, and stress echocardiography.

Echocardiography

Echocardiography is useful for assessing left ventricular function and evaluating patients with suspected valvular heart disease. However, it should not be used as a routine preoperative test in patients who have no prior history or evidence of heart failure and no clinical suspicion of valvular heart disease. Echocardiography is not used to predict perioperative ischemic events. It is indicated, however, in patients with congestive heart failure to predict postoperative heart failure. The greatest risk of postoperative heart failure is in patients with a resting left ventricular ejection fraction less than 35%. Echocardiography is useful to assess aortic stenosis, aortic regurgitation, mitral stenosis, mitral regurgitation, and prosthetic heart valves; transthoracic echocardiography should be considered as a preoperative test if any of these conditions are known or suspected. Echocardiography can also be a helpful adjunctive test for many other less common, but important, cardiac conditions, including pulmonary hypertension and intracardiac shunts.

- Echocardiography is indicated in patients with congestive heart failure to predict postoperative heart failure

Treadmill Exercise Tolerance Testing

Standard treadmill exercise tolerance testing with ECG monitoring is one of the most useful means to assess a patient's functional capacity and evaluate for myocardial ischemia. This test, however, cannot be used in patients unable to walk because of severe claudication, critical limb ischemia, or other comorbid conditions such as arthritis of the hips or knees or obstructive lung disease (respiratory insufficiency can limit exercise capacity). Interpretation of ECG changes during exercise is limited in patients with left bundle branch block, left ventricular hypertrophy, or baseline ST-T segment abnormalities.

Treadmill exercise testing can be performed safely in patients with abdominal aortic aneurysm. In one series of more than 250 patients with aneurysms 4 cm in diameter or larger, the aneurysm ruptured in only one patient 12 hours after testing. The mean sensitivity and specificity of treadmill exercise testing for patients with coronary artery disease are 68% and 77%, respectively. In multivessel coronary artery disease, the sensitivity is 81% and the specificity is 66%.

The risk of an adverse cardiovascular event in the perioperative period is greatest in patients with a markedly abnormal exercise test—e.g., ST segment depression greater than 2 mm occurring at low work loads. In patients with adequate treadmill exercise tests that are negative for myocardial ischemia, the negative predictive value for an adverse cardiac event is very high, exceeding 90%.

Nuclear Myocardial Perfusion Imaging

Perfusion imaging can be accomplished with the use of different radioisotopes, including technetium Tc 99m or sestamibi. Imaging can be used as an ancillary measure of myocardial ischemia in patients undergoing treadmill testing. In patients unable to exercise, pharmacologic agents can be used to provoke myocardial ischemia, including intravenous dipyridamole, adenosine, or dobutamine. In addition, myocardial perfusion can be assessed with positron emission tomography using isotopes such as rubidium Rb 82.

Nuclear myocardial perfusion imaging is approximately 88% sensitive and 77% specific. A normal myocardial perfusion study has a negative predictive value exceeding 96%. An abnormal test has a positive predictive value that ranges from 4% to 20%, depending on the study. One study advised caution in using a dipyridamole thallium test as a routine screening study of all patients before vascular surgery. This study indicated that the presence of coronary disease and age greater than 65 years were better predictors of complications than was the perfusion imaging study. The risk of an adverse cardiovascular event in the perioperative period is greatest in those with the most significant perfusion abnormalities, typically a defect that is greater than 20% to 25% of the left ventricular mass.

Dobutamine Stress Echocardiography

Evaluation of left ventricular function and wall motion abnormalities by echocardiography during dobutamine administration is another method to assess patients for the presence of coronary artery disease. The sensitivity of this technique is 76% and the specificity is 88%. A new wall motion abnormality during dobutamine administration is interpreted as a positive test. Negative predictive values range from 98% to 100%; positive predictive values are 14% to 24%.

Additional Diagnostic Testing and Treatment

A decision to recommend cardiac catheterization or to perform coronary revascularization in patients with abnormal exercise tolerance tests or nuclear imaging studies must be made on an individual basis. Recent studies, however, suggest that medical management, particularly with β-adrenergic receptor blockers (β-blockers), is an effective means to substantially decrease adverse cardiovascular events in the perioperative period for most patients.

Several randomized trials have studied the effect of perioperative β-blockers on adverse cardiovascular events in the perioperative period. One study compared bisoprolol with placebo in patients at high risk based on abnormal dobutamine stress echocardiography. The rates of cardiac death and non-fatal myocardial infarction were substantially lower in patients randomly assigned to bisoprolol than in those assigned to placebo (3.4% vs 34%). However, patients with marked abnormalities on dobutamine stress echocardiography were excluded.

- Medical management, particularly with β-blockers, is an effective means to substantially decrease adverse cardiovascular events in the perioperative period

These findings were extended in a randomized trial that analyzed a total cohort of 1,351 consecutive patients. Among patients with a low risk of cardiac complications, β-blockers decreased the risk of cardiovascular events versus placebo (0.8% vs 2.3%). Even in patients with three or more risk factors and abnormal dobutamine stress echocardiography showing four or fewer segments with new wall motion abnormalities, β-blockers decreased the incidence of adverse cardiovascular complications in the perioperative period (2.3% vs 10.6% with placebo). In patients with the most extensive ischemia on dobutamine stress echocardiography (affecting five or more segments), β-blockers did not decrease the incidence of cardiac events. Another study examined the effect of intravenous atenolol followed by oral atenolol versus placebo in patients undergoing vascular surgery. No difference was found in the risk of perioperative myocardial infarction or death in this study, but incidence of these cardiac events was significantly decreased by 6 months after surgery (1% vs 10%).

The results of these studies indicate that most patients undergoing vascular surgery should be treated with β-blockers to decrease the risk of perioperative vascular complications. Whether additional diagnostic testing, such as cardiac catheterization, should be performed to decrease this risk further is unclear. However, those with the most severe abnormalities on non-invasive testing remain at high risk for adverse events. This risk may not be sufficiently reduced by β-adrenergic blockade.

The risk of cardiovascular events is lower in patients who have previously undergone coronary revascularization procedures. In the Coronary Artery Surgery Study (CASS), the risk of postoperative myocardial infarction and death was significantly lower among patients who had undergone prior coronary artery bypass grafting than among those who had not. This statistic, however, does not account for the risk of myocardial infarction and death associated with the cardiac surgery procedure.

The results of the Coronary Artery Revascularization Prophylaxis (CARP) trial are useful in determining which patients should be referred for cardiac catheterization and which should proceed to surgery with effective medical management. This study evaluated 5,859 patients undergoing vascular operations at 18 Veterans Affairs Medical Centers; 510 of these patients were randomly assigned to preoperative coronary artery revascularization (either percutaneous coronary intervention or coronary artery bypass grafting) or no revascularization. More than 90% of the patients scheduled for vascular surgery were excluded because of insufficient cardiac risk, an urgent need for vascular surgery, prior coronary revascularization, severe coexisting illness, inability or refusal to participate, or non-obstructive coronary artery disease at the time of cardiac catheterization. Patients with left main coronary artery stenosis of 50% or greater, left ventricular ejection fraction less than 20%, and severe aortic stenosis were also excluded.

Postoperative myocardial infarction within 30 days was similar in the revascularization (12%) and no revascularization groups (14%). Death occurred within 30 days in 3% of each group; mortality rates were also similar in the two groups after 2.7 years (23% vs 22%). On the basis of these findings, it is reasonable to infer that most patients scheduled for vascular surgery, including those with evidence of myocardial ischemia by stress testing and myocardial perfusion studies do not require coronary revascularization before vascular surgery. In this study, however, patients with significant left main coronary artery stenosis, severe left ventricular dysfunction, and severe aortic stenosis were excluded. Thus, if preoperative examination and non-invasive testing indicate the potential presence of any of these, cardiac catheterization for confirmation should still be considered appropriate before vascular surgery.

Coronary revascularization before vascular surgery should be recommended for most patients with left main stenosis, patients with three-vessel coronary artery disease and left ventricular dysfunction, and patients with intractable angina despite medical therapy. Coronary artery revascularization should also be considered in patients with three-vessel coronary artery disease that includes a stenosis of the proximal portion of the left anterior descending coronary artery.

It is important to recognize that percutaneous coronary interventions using stents will delay vascular surgery. These patients require treatment with dual antiplatelet therapy, including aspirin and clopidogrel, for a prolonged period. In patients who receive bare metal stents, at least 1 month of dual antiplatelet therapy is recommended; in patients who receive drug-eluting stents, up to 12 months of treatment may be recommended. Many surgeons are reluctant to perform operations in patients taking clopidogrel because of potential bleeding complications. Also, studies have reported an excessive risk of stent thrombosis, myocardial infarction, and death in patients who underwent surgery within several weeks of receiving a coronary stent.

- Coronary revascularization before vascular surgery should be recommended for most patients with left main stenosis, patients with three-vessel coronary artery disease and left ventricular dysfunction, and patients with intractable angina despite medical therapy

Preoperative Evaluation and Management of Comorbid Conditions

Hypertension

Many patients undergoing vascular surgery procedures have hypertension. In most cases, treated hypertension is not associated with an increased risk of perioperative cardiovascular events, and it is not necessary to delay surgery. Optimal control of high blood pressure is to treat patients to a target blood pressure of no higher than 140/90 mm Hg, unless they have diabetes mellitus or renal insufficiency, in which case the target should be no more than 130/80 mm Hg. In patients with stage 2 hypertension (≥160/100 mm Hg), particularly those with severe stage 2 hypertension (≥180/110 mm Hg), blood pressure should be controlled before surgery. This can usually be accomplished within several days to weeks. As noted above, β-blockers have beneficial effects in patients undergoing vascular surgery and should be considered as first-line agents to control hypertension.

Congestive Heart Failure

Patients with congestive heart failure preoperatively are at increased risk for congestive heart failure and pulmonary edema in the postoperative period. Patients with congestive heart failure based on symptoms, physical examination, chest radiography, and ancillary studies should be treated before vascular surgery. Treatment options include diuretics, angiotensin-converting enzyme inhibitors, angiotensin-receptor blockers, β-blockers (carvedilol or metoprolol), and spironolactone, depending on the severity of heart failure and the response to therapy.

Valvular Heart Disease

Severe aortic stenosis can substantially increase the risk for adverse cardiovascular events in the postoperative period; the mortality risk is approximately 10%. These patients should be evaluated and treated as if they were not undergoing vascular surgery. Patients with symptomatic aortic stenosis (e.g., congestive heart failure, angina, or syncope) should be evaluated and undergo aortic valve replacement before elective vascular surgery. It is not known whether patients with asymptomatic but severe aortic stenosis should undergo aortic valve replacement before vascular surgery. These patients are at increased risk for cardiac complications, including death, but it remains to be established whether aortic valve replacement before vascular surgery, taking into consideration the risk of cardiac surgery, decreases overall risk in patients undergoing vascular surgery.

- Severe aortic stenosis can substantially increase the risk for adverse cardiovascular events in the postoperative period; the mortality risk is approximately 10%

Patients with other valvular disorders such as aortic and mitral regurgitation should be approached as if they were not undergoing vascular surgery. In those who are not eligible for valve repair or replacement, preoperative attention to volume control and afterload reduction is recommended. Patients with valvular heart disease should be treated with appropriate antibiotic prophylaxis for bacterial endocarditis during the perioperative period. For patients with prosthetic heart valves and other conditions requiring anticoagulant therapy, perioperative heparin therapy is recommended. Warfarin can be discontinued approximately 4 days before scheduled surgery and replaced with unfractionated heparin or low-molecular-weight heparin before surgery. Anticoagulation with heparin is then resumed as soon as safe and possible in the postoperative period.

Arrhythmias

Most asymptomatic ventricular arrhythmias are not associated with perioperative cardiovascular complications. However, in patients with ventricular arrhythmias, evaluation for underlying cardiac disease is recommended in the preoperative period. β-Adrenergic blockade may be used to decrease the risk of a perioperative ventricular arrhythmia. In the absence of advanced atrioventricular block or history of syncope, patients with intraventricular conduction delays, right bundle branch block, left anterior or posterior hemiblock, left bundle branch block, or first-degree atrioventricular block do not require temporary pacemaker implantation. However, temporary or permanent pacing should be considered preoperatively in patients with high-grade conduction abnormalities such as complete atrioventricular block. Additional pharmacotherapy, catheter-based therapy, or insertion of devices may be required in patients with symptomatic or hemodynamically significant arrhythmias. Pacemakers and implantable cardioverter-defibrillators should be evaluated before the vascular surgery procedure to avoid inadvertent discharge during surgery. Cardioverter-defibrillators should be turned off before surgery and turned back on in the postoperative period.

Hemodynamic Monitoring

Most patients undergoing vascular surgery do not require placement of a pulmonary artery catheter to monitor cardiac hemodynamic function in the perioperative period. Several studies have found no differences in complications or outcomes between patients who were monitored with pulmonary artery catheters and those who were not. The decision to use a pulmonary artery catheter must also take into consideration the risk of complications from insertion and the skills of the health care team in using information derived from the catheter. Perioperative use of pulmonary artery catheters should be restricted to patients at risk for major hemodynamic disturbances, particularly those with congestive heart failure who are undergoing a procedure likely to cause substantial hemodynamic changes. Pulmonary artery catheter placement is not recommended for assisting in the management of myocardial ischemia or for patients with no, or minimal, risks of hemodynamic disturbances.

- Several studies have found no differences in complications or outcomes between patients who were monitored perioperatively with pulmonary artery catheters and those who were not

Surveillance for Postoperative Myocardial Infarction

Several studies have examined the importance of cardiac enzyme measurement in the postoperative period for assessing long-term outcome. Perioperative myocardial infarction has prognostic implications for subsequent myocardial infarction and coronary revascularization. In one study, cardiac troponin T levels were measured in patients who underwent non-cardiac procedures without major cardiovascular complication. In patients with elevated cardiac troponin T values, the relative risk of cardiac events in the 6-month follow-up period was 5.4. Patients undergoing vascular surgery with known or suspected coronary artery disease should have ECG preoperatively, immediately after the surgical procedure, and daily for the first 2 days after surgery. In addition, cardiac troponin should be measured 24 hours postoperatively and on the day of hospital discharge or on day 4 (whichever comes first) to detect perioperative myocardial infarction. ECG and cardiac enzyme measurements should also be performed for any patient in whom chest discomfort or hemodynamic instability develops in the postoperative period. Patients with a perioperative myocardial infarction require further clinical evaluation and institution of the appropriate medical and revascularization therapies defined in the recent ACC/AHA guidelines.

- Patients undergoing vascular surgery with known or suspected coronary artery disease should have ECG preoperatively, immediately after the surgical procedure, and daily for the first 2 days after surgery
- Cardiac troponin should be measured 24 hours postoperatively and on the day of hospital discharge or on day 4 (whichever comes first)
- ECG and cardiac enzyme measurements should also be performed for any patient in whom chest discomfort or hemodynamic instability develops in the postoperative period

Questions

1. A 64-year-old man with type 2 diabetes mellitus is scheduled to undergo a femoral-tibial artery bypass operation for severe claudication. He has no history of coronary artery disease and no symptoms of angina. ECG results are normal. Stress echocardiography shows a new inferior wall motion abnormality during the

dobutamine infusion. Which of the following should be recommended?
a. Cardiac catheterization to define coronary anatomy and revascularization of coronary artery stenoses
b. Dipyridamole-thallium scan to assess the severity of myocardial ischemia
c. Initiation of β-adrenergic blockade followed by vascular surgery
d. Cancellation of vascular surgery

2. A 78-year-old man with a history of myocardial infarction and congestive heart failure reports the acute onset of periumbilical abdominal pain. Abdominal examination is notable for a tender, pulsatile mass. Abdominal computed tomography shows a 6.6-cm abdominal aortic aneurysm. How should his case be managed?
a. Proceed urgently to surgical repair of the abdominal aortic aneurysm.
b. Perform emergent cardiac catheterization and percutaneous coronary intervention of any significant stenoses before proceeding to abdominal surgery.
c. Order adenosine-sestamibi nuclear scan and echocardiography to determine his risk for vascular surgery.
d. Begin metoprolol and nitroprusside and monitor the patient in the intensive care unit.

3. Preoperative evaluation is requested for a 58-year-old woman who presents with transient right-sided weakness. Carotid ultrasonography indicates a >80% left internal carotid artery stenosis. The vascular surgeon plans carotid endarterectomy. The patient has no history of coronary artery disease. She has hypertension that is treated with atenolol. She has hypercholesterolemia and was recently prescribed atorvastatin. She is an exercise enthusiast and swims one mile four times per week. ECG shows left ventricular hypertrophy and mild ST-T wave abnormalities. Aspirin therapy is initiated. Which of the following should be recommended?
a. Exercise tolerance test to assess the risk of a perioperative cardiovascular event
b. Dobutamine stress echocardiography to assess the risk of a perioperative cardiovascular event
c. Cardiac catheterization to assess coronary anatomy before carotid endarterectomy
d. Proceed with carotid endarterectomy

4. A 70-year-old man is scheduled to undergo repair of a 2.5-cm popliteal artery aneurysm. He had a myocardial infarction 4 years earlier. For the past 2 months, chest discomfort has occurred when he mowed the lawn or carried out the trash. His medications include metoprolol, simvastatin, and aspirin. An adenosine-sestamibi scan showed a fixed inferior perfusion defect and large reversible perfusion defects of the anterior and lateral segments. Left ventricular ejection fraction by gated single-photon emission computed tomography was 35%. Which of the following should be recommended?
a. Perform cardiac catheterization to identify coronary anatomy and coronary revascularization before vascular surgery.
b. Increase the dose of metoprolol and proceed with vascular surgery.
c. Increase the dose of metoprolol, add nitrates, and cancel vascular surgery.
d. Perform an exercise tolerance test to assess functional capacity before vascular surgery.

5. A 63-year-old woman with diabetes mellitus reports for a preoperative risk assessment before planned left lower extremity surgical revascularization for severe claudication and rest pain at night. She reports feeling well, although the leg pain prevents her from walking farther than across the room. She reports two episodes of syncope in the prior 6 months, the most recent 5 weeks before the visit. Physical examination indicates a 3/6 crescendo-decrescendo murmur in the right upper sternal border that radiates to the base of the neck. Echocardiography shows preserved left ventricular ejection fraction but moderate aortic valvular stenosis with an estimated valve area of 1.2 cm^2. Which of the following should be recommended?
a. Surgical referral for aortic valve replacement
b. Initiation of β-blockers followed by vascular surgery
c. Adenosine-sestamibi evaulation of the coronary arteries
d. Transesophageal echocardiography to confirm the aortic valvular stenosis

Suggested Readings

ACC/AHA guidelines for the management of patients with valvular heart disease: a report of the American College of Cardiology/American Heart Association. Task Force on Practice Guidelines (Committee on Management of Patients with Valvular Heart Disease). J Am Coll Cardiol. 1998;32:1486-588.

Ansell J, Hirsh J, Poller L, et al. The pharmacology and management of the vitamin K antagonists: the Seventh ACCP Conference on Antithrombotic and Thrombolytic Therapy. Chest. 2004;126 Suppl:204S-33S. Erratum in: Chest. 2005;127:415-6.

Antman EM, Anbe DT, Armstrong PW, et al. ACC/AHA guidelines for the management of patients with ST-elevation myocardial infarction: a report of the American College of Cardiology/American Heart Association Task Force on Practice Guidelines (Committee to Revise the 1999 Guidelines for the Management of Patients with Acute Myocardial Infarction). J Am Coll Cardiol. 2004;44:E1-E211.

Baron JF, Mundler O, Bertrand M, et al. Dipyridamole-thallium scintigraphy and gated radionuclide angiography to assess cardiac risk before abdominal aortic surgery. N Engl J Med. 1994;330:663-9.

Berlauk JF, Abrams JH, Gilmour IJ, et al. Preoperative optimization of cardiovascular hemodynamics improves outcome in peripheral vascular surgery: a prospective, randomized clinical trial. Ann Surg. 1991;214:289-97.

Best PJ, Tajik AJ, Gibbons RJ, et al. The safety of treadmill exercise stress testing in patients with abdominal aortic aneurysms. Ann Intern Med. 1998;129:628-31.

Boersma E, Poldermans D, Bax JJ, et al, DECREASE Study Group (Dutch Echocardiographic Cardiac Risk Evaluation Applying Stress Echocardiography). Predictors of cardiac events after major vascular surgery: role of clinical characteristics, dobutamine echocardiography, and beta-blocker therapy. JAMA. 2001;285:1865-73.

Braunwald E, Antman EM, Beasley JW, et al, American College of Cardiology, American Heart Association. ACC/AHA 2002 guideline update for the management of patients with unstable angina and non-ST-segment elevation myocardial infarction—summary article: a report of the American College of Cardiology/American Heart Association task force on practice guidelines (Committee on the Management of Patients With Unstable Angina). J Am Coll Cardiol. 2002;40:1366-74.

Detrano R, Gianrossi R, Mulvihill D, et al. Exercise-induced ST segment depression in the diagnosis of multivessel coronary disease: a meta analysis. J Am Coll Cardiol. 1989;14:1501-8.

Dormandy JA, Rutherford RB, TASC Working Group (TransAtlantic Inter-Society Consensus). Management of peripheral arterial disease (PAD). J Vasc Surg. 2000;31:S1-S296.

Eagle KA, Berger PB, Calkins H, et al, American College of Cardiology; American Heart Association. ACC/AHA guideline update for perioperative cardiovascular evaluation for noncardiac surgery—executive summary: a report of the American College of Cardiology/American Heart Association Task Force on Practice Guidelines (Committee to Update the 1996 Guidelines on Perioperative Cardiovascular Evaluation for Noncardiac Surgery). J Am Coll Cardiol. 2002;39:542-53. Erratum in: J Am Coll Cardiol. 2006;47:2356.

Eagle KA, Rihal CS, Mickel MC, et al, CASS Investigators and University of Michigan Heart Care Program. Cardiac risk of noncardiac surgery: influence of coronary disease and type of surgery in 3368 operations. Coronary Artery Surgery Study. Circulation. 1997;96:1882-7.

Fleisher LA, Eagle KA, Shaffer T, et al. Perioperative- and long-term mortality rates after major vascular surgery: the relationship to preoperative testing in the Medicare population. Anesth Analg. 1999;89:849-55.

Garber AM, Solomon NA. Cost-effectiveness of alternative test strategies for the diagnosis of coronary artery disease. Ann Intern Med. 1999;130:719-28.

Gianrossi R, Detrano R, Mulvihill D, et al. Exercise-induced ST depression in the diagnosis of coronary artery disease: a meta-analysis. Circulation. 1989;80:87-98.

Hlatky MA, Boineau RE, Higginbotham MB, et al. A brief self-administered questionnaire to determine functional capacity (the Duke Activity Status Index). Am J Cardiol. 1989;64:651-4.

Kaluza GL, Joseph J, Lee JR, et al. Catastrophic outcomes of noncardiac surgery soon after coronary stenting. J Am Coll Cardiol. 2000;35:1288-94.

L'Italien GJ, Cambria RP, Cutler BS, et al. Comparative early and late cardiac morbidity among patients requiring different vascular surgery procedures. J Vasc Surg. 1995;21:935-44.

Lopez-Jimenez F, Goldman L, Sacks DB, et al. Prognostic value of cardiac troponin T after noncardiac surgery: 6-month follow-up data. J Am Coll Cardiol. 1997;29:1241-5.

Mangano DT, Layug EL, Wallace A, et al, Multicenter Study of Perioperative Ischemia Research Group. Effect of atenolol on mortality and cardiovascular morbidity after noncardiac surgery. N Engl J Med. 1996;335:1713-20. Erratum in: N Engl J Med. 1997;336:1039.

McFadden EP, Stabile E, Regar E, et al. Late thrombosis in drug-eluting coronary stents after discontinuation of antiplatelet therapy. Lancet. 2004;364:1519-21.

McFarlane R, McCredie RJ, Bonney MA, et al. Angiotensin converting enzyme inhibition and arterial endothelial function in adults with type 1 diabetes mellitus. Diabet Med. 1999;16:62-6.

Nelson CL, Herndon JE, Mark DB, et al. Relation of clinical and angiographic factors to functional capacity as measured by the Duke Activity Status Index. Am J Cardiol. 1991;68:973-5.

Poldermans D, Boersma E, Bax JJ, et al, Dutch Echocardiographic Cardiac Risk Evaluation Applying Stress Echocardiography Study Group. The effect of bisoprolol on perioperative mortality and myocardial infarction in high-risk patients undergoing vascular surgery. N Engl J Med. 1999;341:1789-94.

Popma JJ, Ohman EM, Weitz J, et al. Antithrombotic therapy in patients undergoing percutaneous coronary intervention. Chest. 2001;119 Suppl:321S-36S.

Reilly DF, McNeely MJ, Doerner D, et al. Self-reported exercise tolerance and the risk of serious perioperative complications. Arch Intern Med. 1999;159:2185-92.

Smith SC Jr, Dove JT, Jacobs AK, et al, American College of Cardiology; American Heart Association Task Force on Practice Guidelines. ACC/AHA guidelines of percutaneous coronary interventions (revision of the 1993 PTCA guidelines)—executive summary: a report of the American College of Cardiology/American Heart Association Task Force on Practice Guidelines (committee to revise the 1993 guidelines for percutaneous transluminal coronary angioplasty). J Am Coll Cardiol. 2001;37:2215-39.

Stone GW, Ellis SG, Cox DA, et al, TAXUS-IV Investigators. One-year clinical results with the slow-release, polymer-based, paclitaxel-eluting TAXUS stent: the TAXUS-IV trial. Circulation. 2004 Apr 27;109:1942-7. Epub 2004 Apr 12.

Torsher LC, Shub C, Rettke SR, et al. Risk of patients with severe aortic stenosis undergoing noncardiac surgery. Am J Cardiol. 1998;81:448-52.

Wilson SH, Fasseas P, Orford JL, et al. Clinical outcome of patients undergoing non-cardiac surgery in the two months following coronary stenting. J Am Coll Cardiol. 2003;42:234-40.

Yeager RA, Moneta GL, Edwards JM, et al. Late survival after perioperative myocardial infarction complicating vascular surgery. J Vasc Surg. 1994;20:598-604.

Ziegler DW, Wright JG, Choban PS, et al. A prospective randomized trial of preoperative "optimization" of cardiac function in patients undergoing elective peripheral vascular surgery. Surgery. 1997;122:584-92.

10 Unusual Vascular Diseases

John R. Bartholomew, MD

The vascular medicine physician must be familiar with many uncommon disorders. Many of these disorders mimic more common diseases and cause confusion in the diagnosis and management of patients. These entities can be grouped as thermal or environmental disorders, non-inflammatory vascular diseases, vascular anomalies (tumors and malformations), vascular neoplasms and tumors, and syndromes associated with vascular lesions.

Thermal or Environmental Disorders

Erythromelalgia

Erythromelalgia is an uncommon disorder that generally affects middle-aged women, adolescents, and children. It is associated with a decreased quality of life and increased mortality. A triad of clinical findings that include erythema, increased warmth, and burning pain of the extremities (usually symmetric) is characteristic of the disease. The feet and hands are most commonly involved, although the knees, elbows, ears, and face can be affected. Ulceration and gangrene can occur in secondary forms. Attacks may last hours to days and are aggravated by drinking alcohol, warm rooms, exercise, summer heat, and wearing shoes and socks.

Erythromelalgia Characteristics

- Painful or burning, red, warm extremities
- Feet and hands most commonly affected
- Symmetric involvement
- Females affected more often than males

Erythromelalgia is classified as primary or secondary. The primary form is generally idiopathic, although a hereditary (autosomal dominant) form has been described; secondary erythromelalgia can be caused by several different diseases (Table 10.1). The diagnosis is based on the history and physical examination (results are normal unless the patient is examined during an attack). Peripheral pulses may be abnormal in some of the secondary forms. No objective laboratory tests can confirm the diagnosis, although some of the studies listed in Table 10.2 may be helpful. The differential diagnosis includes peripheral neuropathy, complex regional pain syndrome, cellulitis, dermatitis, osteomyelitis, Raynaud syndrome, chronic venous insufficiency, lipodermatosclerosis, and arterial insufficiency.

The underlying cause of erythromelalgia in most patients is believed to be a small-fiber neuropathy and a vasculopathy (defined as intermittent increased blood flow

Table 10.1 Causes of Erythromelalgia

Primary erythromelalgia
Idiopathic
Hereditary
Secondary erythromelalgia
Myeloproliferative disorders
Polycythemia vera
Essential thrombocythemia
Chronic myelogenous leukemia
Multiple sclerosis
Spinal cord disease
Connective tissue disorders
Systemic lupus erythematosus
Rheumatoid arthritis
Viral infections
Human immunodeficiency virus
Hepatitis B
Drugs
Calcium-channel blockers
Bromocriptine, pergolide
Cyclosporine

Table 10.2 Diagnostic Tests for Erythromelalgia

Clinical evaluation:
History and physical examination

Vascular evaluation:
Color change
Skin temperature
Blood flow (laser Doppler flowmetry)
Oxygen saturation (transcutaneous oximetry)
Ankle-brachial index

Neurologic evaluation:
Electromyography
Autonomic reflex screen
Quantitative sudomotor axon reflex test
Heart rate response to deep breathing and Valsalva ratio (cardiovagal function)
Adrenergic function testing
Consultation with a neurologist

From Davis MDP, Sandroni P, Rooke TW, et al. Erythromelalgia: vasculopathy, neuropathy, or both? A prospective study of vascular and neurophysiologic studies in erythromelalgia. Arch Dermatol. 2003;139:1337-43. Used with permission.

and shunting). The cause is generally unknown, but recent studies indicate that primary erythromelalgia is a neuropathic disorder of sodium channel function, involving a mutation of the gene encoding the $Na_v1.7$ sodium channel (located on 2q). Disorders of these channels, known as hereditary channelopathies, are also known to cause epilepsy, periodic paralysis, and certain arrhythmias.

Medications aimed at treatment of both the neuropathy and vasculopathy have been tried with varying degrees of success. Vasodilators (sodium nitroprusside and nitroglycerin), β-blockers, tricyclic antidepressants, intravenous prostaglandins, oral mexiletine, capsaicin, clonidine, narcotics, biofeedback, and sympathetic nerve block all have been shown to be beneficial in some patients. Aspirin or nonsteroidal antiinflammatory drugs can help in patients with an underlying myeloproliferative disorder. Recently, the lidocaine patch (a sodium-channel blocker) has been found useful in relieving pain in some patients. Patients must be taught to avoid aggravating conditions and to cool their extremities without causing tissue damage. Patients often require counseling because this is a particularly difficult condition to treat.

Pernio

Pernio (also called chilblain) is a localized vascular disorder most commonly seen in young females but also found in other age groups including children and older adults. Patients present with purple, erythematous, or cyanotic skin lesions that commonly affect toes or fingers. The skin may have a yellowish or brownish discoloration and can peel or ulcerate. Less commonly, the nose, cheeks, ears, and thighs are involved. Lesions are generally bilateral and females are more likely to be affected than males. Patients with pernio report intense itching or a burning pain that usually begins in late fall or early winter (in cold or damp climates) and disappears in the spring or early summer. Excessive cold exposure and parental neglect have led to pernio in children; in adolescents, pernio has been reported in association with thin body habitus.

Historically, pernio was quite common during wartime conditions in northern Europe. Pernio is now less common but can be found in the temperate and humid climates of northwestern Europe and the northern United States. It generally develops in susceptible persons who are exposed to non-freezing cold.

Pernio Characteristics

- Purple, erythematous, or cyanotic skin lesions
- Toes and fingers most often involved (symmetric)
- Intense itching or burning pain
- More pronounced in late fall or early winter (cold, damp climates)
- Develops in susceptible persons in response to moderate or non-freezing cold

Pernio can be classified as acute or chronic (Table 10.3). Acute pernio develops shortly after exposure to cold and disappears within a few weeks after the precipitating cause is removed. Intense itching or burning may occur. Chronic pernio develops after repeated episodes of cold exposure. It begins in the late fall or early winter and lasts

Table 10.3 Classification of Pernio

Characteristic	Acute	Chronic
Time of development	Develops within hours (12-24) after cold exposure	Develops after repeated exposures to cold or damp climates
Type of lesions	Erythematous-purplish edematous lesions, normal arterial examination	Brown plaques, or violet/yellow blisters
Previous history	No	Yes
Development of chronic occlusive disease	No (self-limited condition)	Yes

Table 10.4 Classification of Frostbite

Superficial	Deep
Affects skin and subcutaneous tissue	Affects bone, joints, and tendons
Pallor, edema, and blisters are seen	Anesthesia followed by hyperesthesia with burning, throbbing, aching; "block of wood sensation"
Transient stinging, burning, throbbing, and aching	Skin necrosis, blisters are hemorrhagic (violaceous), little edema
Blisters are clear	

until spring. Patients with chronic pernio have a history of similar episodes during previous winters; this can eventually lead to occlusive vascular disease. A form of chronic pernio has been described in patients with conditions such as anorexia nervosa, dysproteinemias, systemic lupus erythematosus, cold agglutinin or cryoglobulin disorders, and chronic myelomonocytic leukemia.

The diagnosis of pernio is made by performing a thorough history and physical examination and by excluding other disorders. Patients may have a vasospastic response to immersion in cold water. Physicians often lack familiarity with pernio. It is important to distinguish it from Raynaud syndrome, frostbite, atheroembolism, vasculitis, atherosclerosis with injury, and embolic events.

Pernio is believed to be caused by vasospasm induced by cold exposure or cold-induced trauma. It can eventually lead to structural changes in the skin due to vascular damage from tissue anoxemia and secondary inflammatory reactions. Histologically, perivascular lymphocytic infiltration of the arterioles and venules of the dermis, thickening and edema of the blood vessel walls, fat necrosis, chronic inflammatory reactions, and occasional giant cells are seen.

In treating patients with pernio, instructing them to avoid cold exposure is imperative. Calcium-channel blockers or selective $\alpha 1$-blockers may be helpful in alleviating symptoms. After pernio is recognized, patients should be instructed to dress warmly before going outside. Lesions generally resolve over several weeks if this approach is followed.

Frostbite

Frostbite is a local cold-induced injury that occurs when persons are exposed to temperatures below the freezing point of intact skin. It was once almost exclusively seen in military personnel but is now seen in persons engaged in outdoor winter sports (climbing, skiing), in homeless people, in patients with psychiatric illness, in association with excess drug or alcohol consumption, and after vehicular trauma. Men outnumber women approximately 10:1. The extremities (hands and feet) account for approximately 90% of injuries, although the ears, nose, and cheeks may be involved.

Patients generally report numbness in the affected area and clumsiness or a lack of fine motor coordination if the hands are involved. In rare cases, frostbite can develop in the absence of exposure to cold—for example, inhalation of freon-containing aerosols causing frostbite of the oropharynx in inhalant abusers. Patients with peripheral arterial disease appear to be at an increased risk for frostbite.

Frostbite Characteristics

- Hands and feet most often affected
- Commonly affects participants in winter sports, those with psychiatric illness, drug or alcohol abusers, and patients with peripheral arterial disease
- Men outnumber women 10:1

The diagnosis of frostbite is made by the history and physical examination. The severity of frostbite (superficial or deep, Table 10.4) appears to be related to the duration of exposure. Injury ranges from reversible to irreversible cellular destruction. Several factors can increase a person's susceptibility to cold-induced injury (Table 10.5).

Proper recognition of frostbite and uninterrupted rewarming is essential to treatment. Local rewarming should begin only if refreezing will not occur while the patient is being transferred to a hospital. Rapid rewarming in a water bath between 40°C and 42°C for 15 to 30 minutes may help minimize tissue loss. Splinting and elevation of the affected limb can help minimize edema and promote tissue perfusion. Wet clothing must be removed if it is non-adherent. It is generally advised that blisters not be removed, but if they rupture, the area should be

Table 10.5 Factors That Increase the Likelihood of Frostbite

General: advanced age, infancy, exhaustion
Drug use: alcohol, sedatives, clonidine, neuroleptics
Endocrine system: hypoglycemia, hypothyroidism, adrenal insufficiency, diabetes mellitus
Cardiovascular system: peripheral arterial disease, nicotine use
Neurologic system: peripheral neuropathy, spinal cord damage
Trauma: falls with head or spinal injury, fractures causing immobility
Infection: sepsis

debrided and covered with a topical antibiotic. Rubbing affected areas is not advised, and patients should receive tetanus toxoid and analgesics.

Treatment of Frostbite

- Proper rewarming is essential
- Remove wet clothing if it is non-adherent
- Administer tetanus toxoid and proper amounts of analgesics

Trench Foot

Trench foot, a condition that clinically resembles frostbite, is usually associated with damp and cold settings and is also known as "immersion foot," "sea-boat foot," or "foxhole foot." It was first described in the Napoleonic Wars but was commonly seen in soldiers of World War I who stood for days wearing tight boots in wet and cold trenches. It is caused by prolonged exposure of the foot to a non-freezing, moist environment and is made worse by high altitude, prolonged immobility, and dependency of the limbs. Smoking and underlying vascular problems can aggravate this condition. A warm-water variety was described during the Vietnam War, and more recently this condition has been recognized in elderly patients and homeless persons who have prolonged exposure to cold, damp conditions.

Acrocyanosis

Acrocyanosis is a bluish discoloration and coolness of the hands (and less commonly the feet) that persists in both cool and warm environments. The forehead, nose, cheeks, earlobes, elbows, and knees are rarely involved. It is more prevalent in those aged 20 to 50 years and affects men and women equally. Although acrocyanosis is rare, two types have been described: primary (seen in young women and reported in patients with anorexia nervosa, malignancies, infectious mononucleosis, and spinal cord injuries) and secondary (associated with connective tissue disorders). Acrocyanosis must be distinguished from peripheral cyanosis, Raynaud syndrome, and erythromelalgia.

Acrocyanosis Characteristics

- Affects hands most commonly but occasionally the feet
- Persistent bluish discoloration
- Primary and secondary forms

Several theories exist for the cause of acrocyanosis, including vasospasm, decreased capillary blood flow, and increased levels of (or an exaggerated response to) endothelin-1 occurring in response to cold stimulation. No pharmacologic treatment is necessary for acrocyanosis; patients should dress warmly and be given reassurance. In patients who are bothered by the physical appearance, low doses of guanethidine or reserpine have been used.

Livedo Reticularis

Livedo reticularis is a red, violet, or blue mottled discoloration (fishnet pattern) of the extremities or trunk. It has also been called cutis marmorata, livedo racemosa, and livedo annularis. It can be primary or secondary. Primary (idiopathic) livedo reticularis is commonly found in women during their 20s through 50s. It is aggravated by cold exposure and disappears with warming. Primary livedo reticularis with ulceration is also known as livedoid vasculitis. Patients present with purpuric macular lesions or cutaneous nodules that progress to painful ulcers on the calves, ankles, and feet. Secondary livedo reticularis is seen with vasculitis, atheromatous embolization, antiphospholipid antibody syndrome, Sneddon syndrome, myeloproliferative disorders, dysproteinemias, arterial disease, and infections.

Two secondary forms of livedo reticularis are important to recognize. Atheromatous embolization is a frequently misdiagnosed and unrecognized condition and is a major cause of morbidity and mortality. It is a complication often seen after surgical procedures of the aorta or after cardiac catheterization, percutaneous coronary intervention, or any angiographic procedure (renal, mesenteric, extremities). This is not a benign form of livedo reticularis and requires aggressive evaluation and treatment. Livedo reticularis secondary to antiphospholipid antibody syndrome is reported to occur in as many as 25% to 40% of patients with this condition. These patients are at increased risk for arterial or venous thrombosis or obstetric complications.

Primary livedo reticularis does not require treatment. Livedo reticularis with non-healing ulcers may respond to antiplatelet agents, anticoagulants, or thrombolytic therapy (tissue plasminogen activator), but it is often refractory to standard therapy. Treatment of the underlying disorder is important for the treatment of secondary forms.

Erythema Ab Igne

Erythema ab igne is a hyperpigmented skin condition that results from repeated exposure to a hot pad, space heater, or electric heating pad that is not warm enough to result in a burn. It can also result from repeated application of a hot water bottle to treat pain. It was once a common condition resulting from sitting too close to a fire but may be seen in persons who sit too close to space heaters, wood burning stoves, or car heaters. Erythema ab igne is an occupational hazard for persons who work in bakeries, foundries, or kitchens whose arms are repeatedly exposed to fire. The skin discoloration is a reticular, erythematous, hyperpigmented (brownish) pattern caused by chronic exposure to moderate levels of infrared radiation. Dysplastic changes can develop, predisposing the patient to actinic keratoses and squamous cell carcinomas. Patients generally have no symptoms, although some report a slight burning sensation. Removing the offending heat source is required for treatment.

Erythema Ab Igne Characteristics

- Reticular red-brownish skin discoloration
- Caused by chronic exposure to infrared radiation
- Treated by removing the causative heat source

Non-Inflammatory Vascular Disorders

Fibromuscular Dysplasia

Fibromuscular dysplasia (FMD) is a non-atherosclerotic, non-inflammatory vascular disease that affects small to medium-sized vessels. The renal and internal carotid arteries are the predominant sites of involvement, but FMD may affect any artery. Clinical findings of the different types of FMD are shown in Table 10.6. It is seen in young to middle-aged (generally white) women and can lead to aneurysm formation and dissection.

The cause of FMD is unknown, although environment, hormonal effects on smooth muscle, mechanical stress on vessel walls, and genetic factors have all been implicated. Most cases are sporadic, but inherited forms of FMD have been described. Cigarette smoking and hypertension are associated with an increased risk for this disease.

Renal FMD

FMD of the renal artery is classified by the arterial layer affected—intima, media, or adventitia—and accounts for approximately 10% of all cases of renovascular hypertension (Table 10.7). It has been suggested that renal

Table 10.6 Clinical Findings of Fibromuscular Dysplasia

Type	Characteristics
Renal	Hypertension Commonly affects women aged 15-50 y
Cerebrovascular	Headache, tinnitus, vertigo, syncope, TIA, CVA, cervical bruit, intracranial aneurysms May be asymptomatic
Visceral	Abdominal pain, weight loss, epigastric bruit
Extremity	Intermittent claudication, critical limb ischemia, or evidence of embolization

CVA, cerebrovascular accident; TIA, transient ischemic attack.

Table 10.7 FMD Characteristics by Arterial Layer Affected

Type of FMD	Characteristic
Medial fibroplasia	Most common form (75%-80%); string of beads; beads larger than the artery
Perimedial fibroplasia	In young girls; focal stenoses and constrictions; beads smaller than artery
Intimal fibroplasia	Incidence, <10%; mimics Takayasu or temporal arteritis; long smooth narrowing of vessels
Medial hyperplasia	Incidence, 1%-2%; often looks angiographically like intimal fibroplasia
Adventitial (periarterial) hyperplasia	Rarest form

FMD, fibromuscular dysplasia.

FMD may be more common in the elderly population than previously reported. Renal FMD can be diagnosed by performing duplex scanning of the renal arteries (elevated blood flow velocities are seen distally). Computed tomography (CT) angiography and magnetic resonance angiography (MRA) are less helpful than catheter-based angiography. The differential diagnosis for FMD includes atherosclerosis and vasculitis. Several syndromes are associated with FMD, including Ehlers-Danlos (type IV), Alport syndrome, pheochromocytoma, Marfan syndrome, and Takayasu arteritis.

The basis of treatment of renal FMD is medical management for hypertension. In patients with blood pressure that is difficult to control, persons who are non-compliant with taking medication, or those for whom the goal is to cure hypertension, percutaneous transluminal angioplasty is the best option. In a meta-analysis of 206 patients, technical success rates of 88% to 100% were reported. Angioplasty can also be indicated in patients who have lost renal volume as a result of ischemic nephropathy.

Cerebrovascular FMD

The clinical findings of cerebrovascular FMD include headache, syncope, Horner syndrome, amaurosis fugax, transient ischemic attack or stroke, and cranial nerve palsies. Symptoms may be a result of stenoses or occlusion of arteries, intravascular thrombi originating from stenotic areas, or rupture of an intracranial aneurysm.

A cervical bruit may be the only clue to cerebrovascular FMD. The diagnosis can be made by duplex ultrasonography (lower sensitivity than angiography) if irregular patterns of stenoses or aneurysms are seen. Diagnosis by duplex may be difficult, however, because FMD generally affects the middle and distal portions of the carotid and vertebral arteries where it is difficult to obtain images with ultrasonography. Angiography remains the diagnostic method of choice. Experience with CT angiography and MRA for diagnosis of FMD has been minimal, although

MRA should be performed to rule out the presence of intracranial aneurysms in patients with cerebrovascular FMD.

The treatment of cerebrovascular FMD consists of the use of antiplatelet agents in asymptomatic patients; angioplasty should be reserved for symptomatic patients. If aneurysms are found, they should be treated surgically.

FMD Characteristics

- Renal and cerebrovascular FMD are the most common types
- Consider FMD in a young person with new-onset hypertension or central nervous system symptoms
- Can lead to aneurysm formation or dissection
- Cause is unknown

Popliteal Artery Entrapment Syndrome

Popliteal artery entrapment syndrome (PAES) is a rare condition that is frequently misdiagnosed and overlooked. It is a potentially serious cause of disability in young adults, and males are more frequently affected than females (15:1 ratio). PAES occurs more often in athletic young men with no risk factors for atherosclerosis. It presents clinically as exercise-induced intermittent claudication (generally in the calf muscles) and may be reproduced only when the individual is walking, not running. Standing on the tips of the toes may be painful, or patients may report nocturnal cramps, numbness, or paresthesias. Rarely, a patient with PAES presents with acute limb-threatening ischemia. Because PAES is frequently symmetric, the contralateral limb should always be checked.

PAES Characteristics

- Occurs in young athletic males
- Presents as exercise-induced intermittent claudication
- May be symmetric
- Unusual cause of acute limb ischemia

The differential diagnosis for PAES includes a thrombosed popliteal artery aneurysm, atherosclerosis, and cystic adventitial arterial disease. The diagnosis of PAES should be considered in any young person presenting with intermittent claudication-type symptoms. The pulses are normal at rest unless the patient is examined with passive dorsiflexion of the foot or plantar flexion against active resistance that results in disappearance of the pedal pulse. Pulse volume recordings performed in the supine position, followed by flexion maneuvers, may help make the diagnosis. Stress testing with walking also can be useful. Arteriography performed in the neutral position, as well as with the foot in either dorsiflexion or plantar flexion (to elicit compression), will usually confirm the diagnosis. Medial deviation of the popliteal artery is often observed, and poststenotic or aneurysmal dilatation is also highly suggestive of PAES. Popliteal artery occlusion also may be seen. Duplex imaging may show stenosis, and increased velocities are seen with flexion maneuvers. CT or magnetic resonance imaging (MRI) to delineate soft tissue, vascular, and bony structures provides additional anatomic information.

Diagnosis of PAES

- Examine pulses with passive dorsiflexion or active plantar flexion of the foot
- Medial deviation of the popliteal artery is demonstrated angiographically
- Poststenotic dilatation, occlusion, or aneurysm formation may be seen

PAES is considered congenital, although iatrogenic entrapment after bypass surgery has been reported. It is characterized by extrinsic compression of the popliteal artery by the medial head of the gastrocnemius muscle (less commonly by the popliteal muscle). Repetitive trauma to the area can result in stenotic artery degeneration, complete artery occlusion, or aneurysm formation. Surgical treatment is recommended to relieve the entrapment. A vein graft is generally used to bypass the affected portion of the popliteal artery. In patients presenting with acute limb ischemia, thrombolysis may be necessary.

Cystic Adventitial Disease

Cystic adventitial disease is a rare cause of arterial insufficiency, representing only 0.1% of vascular disease. Patients present with unilateral intermittent claudication that may wax and wane over several months. Cystic adventitial disease occurs when mucin-containing cysts form within the adventitia of an arterial wall. Symptoms develop due to accumulation of gelatinous fluid within the arterial wall cysts, which can lead to stenosis or occlusion of an artery by direct pressure on the vessel lumen. Cystic adventitial disease affects young to middle-aged persons in an approximate 5:1 male:female ratio. Patients are usually nonsmokers without evidence of atherosclerosis.

Cystic adventitial disease was first identified in the external iliac artery but has been reported in the common femoral, ulnar, and radial arteries. It is most commonly found in the popliteal artery (85% of all cases). Possible causes of cystic adventitial disease include myxomatous degeneration due to systemic disease, trauma, cysts arising from synovial ganglia that migrate into the artery, or cysts arising from mucin-producing mesenchymal cells that become incorporated into the vessel wall during development.

Cystic Adventitial Disease Characteristics

- Most often seen in young to middle-aged men (5:1 male: female ratio)
- Chief complaint is intermittent claudication that may wax and wane over months
- Usually unilateral presentation
- Ishikawa sign; scimitar sign or hourglass appearance on angiography

The differential diagnosis for cystic adventitial disease includes PAES, Baker cyst, or an embolic event. The diagnosis should be suspected in any young person (especially male) who has decreased pedal pulses. A systolic bruit over the popliteal artery may be heard, or the classic finding of obliteration of the pedal pulse on flexion of the knee (Ishikawa sign) may be demonstrated. Duplex ultrasonography may indicate arterial stenosis with surrounding cysts, which contain no flow. MRI provides information on the cysts (hyperintense) and the amount of compression present. Angiography may show smooth, gradually tapering stenosis (scimitar sign or hourglass appearance) without poststenotic dilatation or evidence of atherosclerosis. Intravascular ultrasonography shows a normal muscular arterial wall and a sharply bordered, hypoechoic cyst located within the adventitia of the arterial wall. The cyst displaces the media centrally, and the arterial lumen is narrowed.

Ultrasonography or CT-guided needle aspiration of the cysts is one form of treatment; however, the cysts can reappear with time. Balloon angioplasty does not appear beneficial because it does not affect the cystic compression of the artery. Intra-arterial thrombolytic therapy can be useful if the artery is acutely occluded. Surgical therapy (evacuation of the cyst) is the preferred treatment.

Vascular Anomalies

Vascular anomalies are a heterogeneous group of lesions that often confuse physicians. Part of this confusion is caused by the nomenclature and classification systems. For many years, authors have used terms such as congenital vascular malformations, birthmarks (strawberry hemangioma, cherry angioma, port-wine stain, or salmon patch), angiomas, or benign vascular tumors to distinguish these lesions. By agreement of the International Society for Vascular Anomalies in 1996, the term now accepted is "vascular anomalies." The two major categories of vascular anomalies are vascular tumors (mainly hemangiomas) and vascular malformations (Table 10.8).

Vascular Tumors

Hemangiomas

Hemangiomas are proliferative lesions characterized by increased endothelial cell turnover. Approximately 50% of all hemangiomas are present at birth, and girls are affected more often than boys. The skin (cervicofacial region most

Table 10.8 Distinguishing Features of Vascular Anomalies

Feature	Vascular tumors	Vascular malformations
Presentation	Not normally present at birth; most seen within first few weeks after birth	Most present at birth but not always obvious
Female:male ratio	3:1 to 5:1	1:1
Incidence	10%-12% at 1 y	0.3%-0.5%
Natural history	Rapid growth for 10-12 mo, then progressive involution over 10-12 y	Do not involute, grow proportionately with the patient; can rapidly enlarge due to hormonal changes, puberty, pregnancy, trauma, or infection
Pathophysiology	Increased endothelial cell turnover	Normal cell turnover
Treatment	Most undergo involution; laser, cryotherapy, corticosteroids, interferon, embolization, or excision can be used if necessary	Do not respond to radiation or chemotherapy; may respond to hormonal modulation, sclerosis, or embolization
Examples	Hemangiomas (GLUT-1 positive) Superficial Deep (cavernous hemangioma) Compound or mixed Others (see Table 10.9)	Simple malformation Capillary (port-wine stain) (low-flow) Venous (low-flow) Lymphatic (low-flow) Arteriovenous malformation (high-flow) Combined malformation Capillary-lymphatic (KTS) Capillary venous (mild cases of KTS) Capillary venous with shunting (port-wine stain)

KTS, Klippel-Trénaunay syndrome.

common), liver, gastrointestinal tract, and brain are the most frequent sites of involvement, and hemangiomas are usually superficial, deep within the dermis, or visceral. They are crimson (if superficial) or pale blue or a purple mass (if deep) and are not obvious on physical examination if visceral.

- Hemangiomas are proliferative lesions characterized by increased endothelial cell turnover

Complications and clinical manifestations of hemangiomas include ulcers, located in the lips and genital areas; impairment or loss of vision; airway obstruction due to intranasal or subglottic lesions; auditory canal obstruction due to parotid gland lesions; and congestive heart failure due to hepatic lesions creating arteriovenous fistulas and cardiac decompensation.

Although most hemangiomas can be diagnosed clinically, CT, MRI, arteriography, and ultrasonography can be helpful to demonstrate visceral involvement, plan surgical excision, or assess treatment efficacy. MRI generally shows a lobulated soft tissue mass with flow voids, whereas CT reveals a distinctive soft tissue mass that enhances with contrast. Arteriography is usually reserved for questionable cases and therapeutic embolization, and duplex ultrasonography can be used to demonstrate the high-flow nature of these tumors.

Hemangiomas contain increased markers of angiogenesis, including basic fibroblast growth factor, vascular endothelial cell growth factor, matrix metalloproteases, proliferating cell nuclear antigen, the endothelial cellular adhesion molecule E-selectin, and type IV collagenase. Hemangiomas share common antigenicity with placental tissue, including glucose transporter isoform-1 (GLUT-1) immunoreactivity. The presence of GLUT-1 distinguishes hemangiomas from vascular malformations and is now used for histopathologic differentiation of vascular anomalies.

Treatment is aimed at confirming the correct diagnosis, because most hemangiomas undergo involution (if left alone) by age 5 to 7 years. Treatment may be indicated to prevent functional disturbances (loss of vision, airway obstruction) or psychological harm due to appearance. Treatment options include local excision, laser therapy, cryotherapy, corticosteroids, interferon, and antiproliferative agents (chemotherapy, radiation). Embolization for lesions associated with life-threatening coagulopathy, congestive heart failure, or airway obstruction may be needed in more severe cases.

Superficial (Capillary) Hemangiomas

The most familiar superficial hemangioma has been called capillary hemangioma in the past. Most grow slowly with the growth of the person. One type (formerly known as "strawberry hemangioma") grows rapidly during the first few months of life and then regresses (80% regress completely by 5 years). Most patients have solitary lesions, but 20% have two or more lesions. Superficial hemangiomas are usually found on the skin and mucous membranes of the head and neck. They are small (<1 cm) red cutaneous spots or blue plaques or nodules that blanch with pressure. They are more common in white infants, and girls are affected two to five times as often as boys. Treatment can be avoided in most patients (spontaneous regression). Other vascular tumors are described in Table 10.9.

- 80% of "strawberry hemangiomas" regress completely by 5 years of age

Table 10.9 Comparison of Other Vascular Tumors

	Vascular tumor			
Characteristic	**Tufted angioma**	**Kaposiform hemangioendothelioma**	**Cherry (capillary) angioma**	**Pyogenic granuloma**
Age group	Children	Infants	Adults	Any age, but usually older children and young adults
Appearance	Red-brown	Purplish, indurated	Red papule	Red papules or polyps; sessile or pedunculated
Location	Upper body	Trunk, lower extremities, and retroperitoneum	Trunk and upper extremities	Fingers, head, and neck; cheeks, lips, and face of pregnant women
Presentation	Seen in association with Kasabach-Merritt phenomenon	Kasabach-Merritt phenomenon accompanies this tumor	Cosmetic concern	...
Treatment	Spontaneous regression unusual; excision, laser	Corticosteroids, chemotherapy, embolization; poor prognosis for retroperitoneal tumors	Surgery or electrocoagulation	Excision, silver nitrate sticks, antibiotics if secondary infection develops

Glomus Tumors

Glomus tumors are benign vascular tumors that are most common between the ages of 20 and 50 years; males and females are affected equally. Glomus tumors are found most commonly in the subcutaneous tissue of the extremities, but are also reported in the stomach, cervix, vagina, and nose. They appear as small red-to-blue nodules and are derived from modified smooth muscle cells of the glomus body, a specialized arteriovenous anastomosis important in thermal regulation.

Bacillary (Epithelioid) Angiomatosis

Bacillary angiomatosis is a result of a reactive process that simulates a neoplasm. It occurs in immunocompromised hosts (e.g., patients with human immunodeficiency virus) and is infectious in origin, caused by *Bartonella henselae* (cause of cat-scratch fever) or *B quintana* (responsible for trench fever). Clinically, multiple pink-to-red nodules involving the skin, soft tissue, and subcutaneous tissue are seen. The lesions are friable and prone to ulceration and bleeding. Bacillary angiomatosis can resemble Kaposi sarcoma and must be considered in the differential diagnosis of this disorder. The lesions are reported to respond to antibiotics (erythromycin) or antiretroviral therapy.

Intravascular Papillary Endothelial Hyperplasia

Papillary endothelial hyperplasia is also known as Masson pseudoangiosarcoma, vegetant intravascular hemangioendothelioma, or intravascular angiomatosis. The lesion is generally intravascular and can develop in any vessel, including the vascular channels of a hemangioma, vascular malformation, or pyogenic granuloma. It has been rarely reported to occur extravascularly in the thyroid gland, intracranially, in association with an adrenal cyst, as a mass in the shoulder, or cutaneously. Its cause is unknown. Clinically it is no more than an unusually prolific organizing thrombus that presents as a mass (commonly in veins on the head, neck, hands, and feet). There may be a slight female preponderance, and the lesions appear as slowly enlarging red-blue papules or nodules.

Vascular Malformations

Many physicians continue to use terms such as "cavernous hemangioma" for venous malformation and "port-wine stain" for capillary malformation. Malformations are the result of errors in morphogenesis and are divided into capillary, venous, arterial, lymphatic, and combined forms. These malformations are also classified according to their flow characteristics: high-flow lesions include arteriovenous malformations and arteriovenous fistulas, and low-flow lesions include capillary, lymphatic, and venous malformations. The cells involved have normal turnover, unlike those in hemangiomas.

Port-Wine Stain

These benign vascular tumors are present from birth and may grow proportionately with the child. They are often unsightly and demonstrate no tendency to fade. They are associated with Sturge-Weber syndrome, Klippel-Trénaunay syndrome, and Parkes Weber syndrome. Their cause is unclear.

Cavernous Hemangiomas

Cavernous hemangiomas are most commonly found during childhood. They are located in the upper portions of the body and the viscera. Their appearance differs from the hemangiomas (paler than capillary hemangiomas), and they form a soft, spongy mass that may reach 2 to 3 cm in size. Cavernous hemangiomas grow slowly and can exert pressure on adjacent structures, sometimes becoming locally destructive. They are less likely to regress and may require surgical intervention if they become invasive. Kasabach-Merritt syndrome, Maffucci syndrome, and blue rubber bleb nevus syndrome are associated with cavernous hemangiomas.

Vascular Neoplasms and Tumors

Vascular tumors can lead to substantial morbidity and mortality. A vascular tumor is generally an unanticipated finding during physical examination, surgery, or autopsy. Patients may present with non-specific and vague symptoms including fever, nausea, malaise, or fatigue; obstruction of an artery or vein; or embolization. These tumors can also be found unexpectedly during diagnostic procedures such as arteriography, venography, CT, ultrasonography, MRI, or radiography.

Vascular Neoplasms Involving Major Veins

Sarcomas

Sarcomas are rare tumors that are accompanied by diverse symptoms related to the size of the tumor and the degree of obstruction of the involved vessel. Sarcomas are further classified as leiomyosarcomas, angiosarcomas, or intimal sarcomas.

Leiomyosarcomas usually involve the vena cava and pulmonary artery and grow into the lumen, obstructing the vessel or eroding through the vein wall. The most common sites include the inferior vena cava (IVC), followed by the iliac, femoral, or saphenous veins. In the arterial circulation, the pulmonary artery is the most commonly involved site.

- Leiomyosarcomas usually involve the vena cava and pulmonary artery

Approximately 80% to 90% of patients with leiomyosarcoma are women. Symptoms depend on the location of the tumor and include lower extremity edema, right upper quadrant pain, Budd-Chiari syndrome, renal insufficiency, renal or hepatic vein thrombosis, right ventricle failure, cardiac arrhythmia, and cardiac arrest. The clinical presentation of leiomyosarcoma is related to the segment of the IVC involved. A suprahepatic location is characterized by cardiac arrhythmias, syncope, and pulmonary embolism. Leiomyosarcomas in the suprarenal IVC are associated with Budd-Chiari syndrome, ascites, abdominal pain, renal insufficiency, and nephrotic syndrome, whereas pain, dilated veins, and lower extremity edema can accompany an infrarenal IVC lesion.

A leiomyosarcoma of the lower extremity veins usually appears as a mass, and edema is the most common clinical finding. The diagnosis is often made post mortem, although CT or MRI can be helpful. Treatment is surgical if the tumor is localized, otherwise the prognosis is generally poor.

Sarcomas involving the pulmonary arteries are rare, and both intimal sarcomas and leiomyosarcomas have been reported. These sarcomas typically arise during adulthood (40s or 50s), and there is no predilection for either sex. Patients may present with syncope, palpitations, dyspnea, chest pain, cough, hemoptysis, or overt right ventricular failure.

Sarcomas of the pulmonary artery are so uncommon that the diagnosis is not usually considered until the tumor is found during surgery or autopsy. The patient is often incorrectly treated for acute pulmonary embolism; the diagnosis of pulmonary artery sarcoma should be considered if the patient does not respond to standard treatment for embolism. Ventilation perfusion scanning can show perfusion defects, and filling defects are typically seen on pulmonary angiography. An MRI with gadolinium enhancement can help distinguish tumor from thrombus, but definitive diagnosis requires biopsy.

Vascular Neoplasms and Tumors Involving Major Arteries

Primary tumors of large arteries are rare. The aorta is the most common site, although tumors have been reported in the iliac, subclavian, carotid, renal, and popliteal arteries. Primary aortic tumors are classified as intimal or mural. Intimal tumors grow along the endothelial surface of the vessel and lead to large artery occlusion, whereas mural tumors grow outward and surround structures. Common arterial tumors include sarcomas, malignant fibrous histiocytomas, angiosarcomas, leiomyosarcomas, fibrosarcomas, myxomas, and hemangioendotheliomas.

The diagnosis of arterial blood vessel tumor is often delayed because clinical findings are non-specific (weight loss, fatigue, and nausea). Patients may present with signs of embolization such as blue toe syndrome, an acutely ischemic limb, or mesenteric ischemia. These tumors are often mistaken for an atherosclerotic lesion, aortic aneurysm, or dissection.

Sarcomas of the Aorta

Most sarcomas of the aorta occur in the abdominal aorta or descending thoracic aorta and are usually intimal sarcomas or leiomyosarcomas. Aortic sarcomas may resemble thrombi, although they can also be mistaken for aneurysm. The clinical findings are related to embolic events or obstruction by the tumor. Claudication, back and abdominal pain, and shock from rupture are reported. Most patients are in their 60s, and there is no sex predilection. Metastases to the kidney, thyroid gland, pancreas, and brain have been reported. Generally the correct diagnosis is only made by histologic examination.

Intimal Sarcomas

Intimal sarcomas are rare tumors that originate in the major arteries. Their distinctive feature is their growth—both within the lumen and along the surface of the blood vessel. Intimal sarcomas closely resemble thrombi when they are luminal. They can cause thinning and aneurysmal dilatation of the vessel wall and may be mistaken for aneurysm. Most intimal sarcomas arise in the abdominal aorta. Symptoms can include intermittent claudication, abdominal pain, bowel ischemia, or renal infarction. Middle-aged to elderly men are at greatest risk. These tumors metastasize to bone, peritoneum, and liver. MRI using gadolinium or multidetector-row CT can help make the diagnosis.

Hemangioendothelioma

Hemangioendotheliomas are considered low-grade malignant vascular tumors. They occur over a wide age range but are unusual in childhood. Both sexes appear to be equally affected. They are found mainly in soft tissue and muscle, although they can occur in the head, neck, liver, lung, and bone. Many of the tumors in this classification have been described only recently. Epithelioid hemangioendothelioma, once considered a benign tumor, has been found to metastasize at a substantial rate and is now considered malignant. It is the most frequent of the hemangioendotheliomas and may be identified as a solitary, painful subcutaneous mass, or may be recognized because of clinical findings consistent with obstructive vascular symptoms such as claudication or peripheral edema.

Cardiac Myxomas

Cardiac myxomas are the most common intracardiac tumors. They occur in people of all ages, may be familial, and are found more often in women younger than 50 years. Myxomas are most commonly located in the left atrium, followed by the right atrium and either ventricle. Symptoms and laboratory results common to left atrial cardiac myxomas are shown in Table 10.10.

Two-dimensional echocardiography and transesophageal echocardiography are the most useful procedures for diagnosing cardiac myxoma. The differential diagnosis for myxoma includes systemic illness such as a collagen vascular disease, malignancy, endocarditis, or antiphospholipid antibody syndrome. An unusual form of myxoma, referred to as Carney complex or Carney syndrome, is characterized by spotty pigmentation, atrial myxomas, and endocrine hyperactivity (pituitary adenoma, adrenocortical disease, or testicular tumors). This complex is familial and occurs primarily in young people.

- Cardiac myxomas are the most common intracardiac tumors
- Myxomas are most commonly located in the left atrium

Paragangliomas

Paragangliomas arise in association with major blood vessels and include the carotid body paragangliomas and aortic body tumors (jugulotympanic and mediastinal paragangliomas). Tumors originating from the ear and jugular vein are commonly referred to as glomus jugulare or glomus tympanicum tumors.

Table 10.10 Characteristics of Left Atrial Myxoma

Symptoms	Laboratory findings
Intracardiac obstruction secondary to tumor	Hemolytic anemia
	Elevated white blood cell count
Central or peripheral embolism	Thrombocytopenia
Constitutional symptoms: fever, weight loss, cachexia, fatigue, malaise, arthralgias, Raynaud syndrome, dizziness, heart failure	Elevated erythrocyte sedimentation rate
	Positive C-reactive protein
	Abnormal serum γ-globulins

Carotid Body Tumors

Carotid body tumors (paragangliomas), also known as chemodectoma, arise in association with the carotid body and are found on the posterior aspect of the bifurcation of the common carotid artery. These highly vascular tumors are the most common extra-adrenal paragangliomas. They are more common in patients living at altitudes higher than 6,000 feet and in patients with cyanotic heart disease or chronic obstructive pulmonary disease.

Carotid body tumors are usually benign, may be bilateral, and present in men and women aged 40 to 60 years. There may be a familial predilection (autosomal dominant), and in this setting the incidence of bilateral tumors is higher. Patients may notice a slowly enlarging, painless, pulsatile mass in their neck, or a carotid bruit may be heard on physical examination. Symptoms include ear or neck pain, dysphagia, tongue weakness, hoarseness due to vocal cord paralysis, tinnitus, headache, syncope, Horner syndrome, and hypertensive crises. Disability and death (due to asphyxia or intracranial extension of the tumor) are reported. Secondary tumors are common in patients with carotid body tumors, including pheochromocytomas.

- Carotid body tumors are usually benign, may be bilateral, and present in men and women aged 40 to 60 years
- Treatment of carotid body tumor is usually surgical, although selective intravascular embolization or radiation therapy may be tried in patients who are not acceptable surgical candidates

The diagnosis is made using Doppler color-flow ultrasonography, which indicates a highly vascularized, well-delineated mass at the carotid bifurcation. Arteriography shows intensive blushing and a hypervascular mass in the crotch of the carotid bifurcation. MRI and CT can also help in distinguishing between aneurysms and neoplasms. Plasma and urine catecholamine levels may be elevated, but this finding is extremely rare, and screening studies for these metabolites in the absence of hypertension are not warranted. The differential diagnosis includes tuberculosis lymphadenitis, brachial cleft cyst, carotid artery aneurysm, schwannoma, metastatic carcinoma, and lymphoma.

Treatment is usually surgical, although selective intravascular embolization or radiation therapy may be tried in patients who are not acceptable surgical candidates.

Aortic Body Tumors

Aortic body tumors (mediastinal paragangliomas) are paragangliomas that originate in the pulmonary artery and aortic arch. They often present as an asymptomatic mass (incidental finding on chest radiography), although symptoms may include pressure and hoarseness. Only 6% of these tumors metastasize, although up to 40% of patients die from local invasion. The diagnosis can be confirmed by angiography revealing a highly vascular tumor. Surgical excision is recommended.

Vascular Neoplasms and Tumors Presenting as Tumor-Thrombi

In addition to the IVC tumors mentioned above, several other tumors invade the blood vessels and can be confused with thromboembolic disease. These can include pheochromocytoma and germ cell tumors (such as embryonal teratocarcinoma) in addition to the tumors discussed below.

Renal Cell Carcinoma

As many as 10% to 15% of renal cell carcinomas will show invasion of the veins in the renal pelvis at the time they are discovered. Renal cell carcinoma represents 3% of all adult malignancies and 95% of kidney cancers. It is well known to invade adjacent blood vessels such as the IVC and can extend up the IVC into the right side of the heart. Renal carcinomas can be hereditary or non-hereditary, and an association with structural alterations of 3p has been noted.

Renal cell carcinoma affects patients older than 40 years. The classic presentation triad of flank pain, gross hematuria, and a palpable mass is highly suggestive of this disease, although most tumors are not detected by physical examination. CT, MRI, venacavography, and echocardiography are all useful in the diagnosis and management.

- As many as 10% to 15% of renal cell carcinomas will show invasion of the veins in the renal pelvis at the time they are discovered

Adrenocortical Carcinoma

Adrenocortical tumors are rare. They can cause Cushing syndrome, virilization, or hyperaldosteronism or can present with hypertension or an abdominal mass. They can also be asymptomatic and discovered incidentally. Although adrenocortical tumors can develop at any age, the age distribution is bimodal with disease peaks before the age of 5 years and in the 40s and 50s. The level of aggressiveness and pace of disease progression is more rapid in adults than in children. A female predominance and metastasis to the IVC and right atrium have been reported.

Endometrial Stromal Cell Sarcoma of the Uterus

Endometrial stromal sarcomas are tumors of proliferating endometrium. They characteristically invade the myometrium, but also invade lymphatic and vascular channels. Patients may present with a uterine mass or with an occlusive process of the pelvic veins extending into the IVC. Swelling of the lower extremities or abnormal vaginal bleeding may be seen, and intracardiac invasion has been reported. Patients may report fatigue, palpitations, dizziness, arrhythmias, and conduction defects. Sudden cardiac death can occur.

Leiomyomatosis of the Uterus

Leiomyoma of the uterus is a common benign tumor that involves the myometrium. Rarely, this tumor grows into the pelvic veins, IVC, hepatic veins, right side of the heart, and even the pulmonary vasculature. In this setting, some authors prefer the term "intravenous leiomyomatosis." Patients may have a pelvic mass and present with vaginal bleeding or pelvic pain, dyspnea, generalized weakness, syncope from cardiac obstruction, lower extremity swelling, ascites, or Budd-Chiari syndrome. It occurs most commonly in postmenopausal women. The diagnosis is usually made during surgery, although CT, MRI, and ultrasonography may show a mass; venacavography or transesophageal echocardiography can be helpful. Unless the tumor is in a surgically inaccessible location, excision should be curative.

Testicular Neoplasms

Testicular neoplasms comprise the most common solid malignancies affecting males between the ages of 15 and 35 years, although they represent only about 1% of all solid tumors in men. The two main categories of testicular tumors are germ cell tumors and sex cord–stromal tumors. Germ cell tumors can metastasize to the IVC (embryonal and teratocarcinoma), and reports of right heart involvement have been noted.

Vascular Neoplasms and Tumors Presenting as Soft Tissue Masses

Kaposi Sarcoma

Kaposi sarcoma is a vascular tumor of endothelial origin. Histologically, the two important features are the presence of spindle cells and vascular proliferation. Patients generally present with a solitary nodule or papule localized to the feet or ankles. These lesions vary in size and coalesce into plaques, nodules, ulcerations, or even polypoid

Table 10.11 Clinical or Epidemiologic Forms of Kaposi Sarcoma

Type	Characteristics
Classic or sporadic (European-endemic)	A disease of elderly men, found between 5th and 7th decades. Predilection for Eastern European, Mediterranean, and Ashkenazi Jewish males. Found on lower extremities. Has a benign course.
African or endemic (two forms identified)	First found in Central Africa in younger children with lymph node involvement (lymphadenopathy). Also affects the lower extremities, gastrointestinal tract, or bones. The course is fatal. Second form found in sub-Saharan Africa in young adults, with predilection for extremities.
AIDS-related (epidemic)	Found in homosexual and bisexual men. Lesions are brown-red and may be elevated as plaques or nodules. Lesions can involve multiple skin sites, lymph nodes, mucocutaneous areas, and visceral organs. An aggressive disease.
Immunosuppressive therapy– or transfusion-related	Found mainly in renal (and other organ) transplant recipients who receive immunosuppressive agents. A cutaneous and lymph node–based disease.

AIDS, acquired immunodeficiency syndrome.

growths. Almost 90% of all cases involve men, and there is an increased association with secondary malignancies including lymphomas, leukemia, Hodgkin disease, melanoma, and myeloma. Several different forms have been identified (Table 10.11).

The causes of Kaposi sarcoma are multifactorial. Genetic, geographic, and viral factors all have a role, as does the immunocompetence of the host. The herpesvirus-like DNA sequence found in acquired immunodeficiency syndrome (AIDS)-associated Kaposi sarcoma was identified in 1994 and has been designated human herpesvirus 8, although it is not specific for Kaposi sarcoma. Treatment of Kaposi sarcoma depends on the form identified. The classic form usually has an indolent course, and a conservative approach is used. In other forms, a wide range of chemotherapeutic agents have been tried. Treatment of the immunosuppressive form relies on discontinuing the drugs responsible. For AIDS-related Kaposi sarcoma, interferon therapy is advocated. Local therapy (liquid nitrogen cryotherapy and intralesional vincristine) may be helpful. Patients usually die from wasting, cachexia, or opportunistic infections.

Angiosarcomas

Angiosarcomas are rare, malignant vascular tumors of endothelial cells. Five types of angiosarcoma have been identified and are described in Table 10.12. Angiosarcomas can arise at any age but are most often seen in persons older than 50 years. They are most commonly found on the skin but also are found in breast, bone, and liver. Angiosarcomas are the most common primary malignant tumor of the heart.

Lymphangiosarcomas

Lymphangiosarcoma (lymphedema-associated angiosarcoma) is a highly aggressive tumor and generally arises

Table 10.12 Types of Angiosarcoma

	Angiosarcoma				
Characteristic	Idiopathic	Lymphedema-associated (lymphangiosarcoma)	Radiation-induced	Soft tissue	Breast
Age	Elderly	5th-7th decades	...	Older males	Reproductive age women (3rd-4th decade)
Appearance	Bruise-like, firm or ulcerated lesion	Solitary or multiple lesions; purplish red to bluish red macules, nodules, or palpable purpura; ulceration or necrosis may be seen	...	Associated with Maffucci or Klippel-Trénaunay syndrome	Rapidly growing mass causes diffuse breast enlargement, blue-purple discoloration
Location	Scalp or neck	Mostly arm, rarely lower extremity (Stewart-Treves syndrome), in the setting of postmastectomy lymphedema	Skin of the breast after radiation therapy	Lower limbs or abdominal cavity	Breast
Treatment	Mohs surgery	Surgery, chemotherapy, or radiation	...	...	...
Prognosis	Poor	Poor	Poor	...	Poor

in the setting of chronic lymphedema. Most cases develop after surgery for breast cancer, usually 10 years after mastectomy. They can also be found in the lower extremities and in areas without lymphedema. Their cause is multifactorial and appears related to persistent lymphedema after radical mastectomy, radiation therapy, and local defects in cellular immunity. Lymphangiosarcomas can be confused initially with an ecchymosis or cellulitis. They spread proximally and distally and eventually metastasize to the lungs, pleura, chest wall, shoulder, liver, or bone. They are associated with a poor prognosis, although amputation, including shoulder disarticulation and hindquarter or forequarter amputation, offers the best option to prevent disease spread.

- Angiosarcomas are the most common primary malignant tumor of the heart
- Lymphangiosarcoma is a highly aggressive tumor and generally arises in the setting of chronic lymphedema
- Most cases of lymphangiosarcoma develop after surgery for breast cancer, usually 10 years after mastectomy

Syndromes Associated With Vascular Anomalies

Several diverse syndromes are associated with vascular anomalies, as compared in Table 10.13 and discussed below.

PHACES Syndrome

PHACES syndrome is associated with cervicofacial hemangiomas. The name is derived from the main characteristics of the syndrome: **p**osterior cranial fossa malformation, **h**emangioma, **a**rterial anomalies, **c**ardiac anomalies, **e**ye anomalies, and **s**ternal cleft. The cause of PHACES syndrome is unknown, but it occurs at 8 to 10 weeks of gestation. Anomalies include the Dandy-Walker malformation (absence of carotid/vertebral vessels) and a bifid or cleft sternum. The vast majority of affected patients are girls (9:1 ratio), who are especially prone to occlusive cerebrovascular accidents at an early age.

- PHACES syndrome is associated with cervicofacial hemangiomas

Klippel-Trénaunay Syndrome

Three features characterize Klippel-Trénaunay syndrome: hemangioma, atypical varicosities or venous malformations, and bony or soft tissue hypertrophy (usually affecting one extremity). The diagnosis can be made if two of these features are present. A port-wine stain that ranges from very light in color to deep maroon is common. These lesions may be prone to skin breakdown, bleeding, and infection. The hemangioma may lighten over time, but in some patients dark (deep blue to black) 1- to 2-mm nodules develop on top of the hemangioma. Patients with this syndrome are particularly prone to cellulitis.

- Three features characterize Klippel-Trénaunay syndrome:
  - Hemangioma
  - Atypical varicosities or venous malformations
  - Bony or soft tissue hypertrophy

Venous involvement is usually superficial and can range from subtle abnormalities to massive varicosities. Some patients also have deep venous abnormalities. Bone hypertrophy commonly involves the lower extremity, although the upper extremity is affected in as many as one-fourth of all patients. Some patients have soft tissue hypertrophy involving the chest, back, arm, or leg. Klippel-Trénaunay syndrome must be distinguished from Parkes Weber syndrome. In the latter, arteriovenous fistulas are clinically apparent, whereas in Klippel-Trénaunay syndrome, any arteriovenous fistulas are microscopic.

Table 10.13 Syndromes Associated With Vascular Anomalies

Syndrome/disease	Characteristics
PHACES syndrome	Arterial anomalies and cerebrovascular accidents
Klippel-Trénaunay syndrome	Capillary malformations (port-wine stain), venous varicosities, and bony or soft tissue hypertrophy
Parkes Weber syndrome	Port-wine stain and clinically apparent arteriovenous malformations
Hereditary hemorrhagic telangiectasia	Cutaneous telangiectasia and visceral arteriovenous malformations, prone to bleeding
Sturge-Weber syndrome	Port-wine stain associated with meningeal angioma
von Hippel-Lindau disease	Hemangioblastoma and hemangiomas of the liver
Maffucci syndrome	Multiple hemangiomas of the soft tissue and skin
Kasabach-Merritt syndrome	Cavernous hemangioma with thrombocytopenia, now thought to be associated with vascular tumors: kaposiform hemangioendothelioma and tufted angioma
Fabry disease	Lysosomal storage disease, Raynaud syndrome, reactive angiokeratomas, appearance similar to cherry angiomas
Blue rubber bleb nevus syndrome	Cutaneous and gastrointestinal venous malformations
POEMS syndrome	Cutaneous angiomas

Therapy consists of both non-operative and surgical approaches. Elastic support hose, heel lifts, and antibiotics may be all that is necessary for a patient with a difference in limb length, varicosities, or recurrent infection. Surgical options include ligation and stripping of the varicose veins, laser therapy, debulking procedures, amputations, and epiphysiodesis.

Hereditary Hemorrhagic Telangiectasia

Hereditary hemorrhagic telangiectasia (HHT) is also known as Rendu-Osler-Weber disease. It is autosomal dominant and characterized by epistaxis, cutaneous telangiectasia, and visceral arteriovenous malformations. Telangiectasia is the characteristic lesion of this syndrome.

The diagnosis is based on a combination of the following: spontaneous, recurrent epistaxis; telangiectases often seen on the lips, oral cavity, fingers, or nose; visceral lesions including gastrointestinal telangiectasia, as well as pulmonary, hepatic, cerebral, or spinal arteriovenous malformations; and family history. Endoscopy is helpful in diagnosing HHT of the gastrointestinal tract. Chest radiography, helical CT, or angiography help diagnose lung involvement, and CT, MRI, MRA, and angiography may be required for liver or central nervous system and spinal cord involvement.

Treatment of HHT includes nose packing, humidification, laser therapy, septal dermoplasty, and therapeutic embolization for nose involvement. Skin lesions may respond to topical agents and laser therapy, whereas iron supplementation, transfusion, estrogen/progesterone therapy, and laser therapy can be helpful for treatment of the gastrointestinal tract. Therapeutic embolization may be necessary for lung, liver, or central nervous system involvement, and liver transplantation and stereotactic radiosurgery have been used.

Sturge-Weber Syndrome

Sturge-Weber syndrome is a neurocutaneous syndrome associated with port-wine stain in the distribution of the ophthalmic branch of the trigeminal nerve. Seizures, hemiplegia, and secondary mental retardation may develop. This syndrome typically occurs in the first year of life and rarely after the age of 40 years. Central nervous system malformations (ipsilateral meningeal angioma) may occur.

von Hippel-Lindau Disease

von Hippel-Lindau disease is an inherited, autosomal dominant syndrome that presents with benign and malignant tumors. The von Hippel-Lindau tumor suppressor gene (*VHL*) was identified in 1996; defects in this gene appear to be responsible for approximately 60% of all clear renal cell cancers. Initial clinical manifestations may present in childhood or adolescence. Tumors seen include hemangioblastomas of the cerebellum and spinal cord and renal cell carcinomas. Affected persons can have angiomatous or cystic lesions of the kidneys, pancreas, and epididymis, as well as adrenal pheochromocytomas. Retinal angiomas with blindness have been reported.

- Sturge-Weber syndrome is a neurocutaneous syndrome associated with port-wine stain in the distribution of the ophthalmic branch of the trigeminal nerve
  - Seizures, hemiplegia, and secondary mental retardation may develop
- von Hippel-Lindau disease is an inherited, autosomal dominant syndrome that presents with benign and malignant tumors

Maffucci Syndrome

Maffucci syndrome consists of multiple hemangiomas of the soft tissue, and multiple enchondromas, most often in the phalanges and long bones. Bone and vascular lesions are present at birth or occur during childhood. Maffucci syndrome can be associated with benign or malignant tumors (goiter, parathyroid adenoma, pituitary adenoma, adrenal tumor, breast cancer, and astrocytoma).

Kasabach-Merritt Syndrome

Kasabach-Merritt syndrome was initially described as a large (cavernous) hemangioma associated with a coagulopathy (thrombocytopenia). More recently, this syndrome has been reported to be associated not with common hemangiomas but with other vascular tumors such as kaposiform hemangioendothelioma and tufted angioma.

Fabry Disease

Fabry disease should be suspected in patients with Raynaud syndrome, acroparesthesias, angiokeratomas, left ventricular hypertrophy, corneal opacities, and lenticular lesions. It is a lysosomal storage disease caused by an absence of a-galactosidase. The reactive angiokeratomas have a clinical appearance similar to cherry angiomas.

Blue Rubber Bleb Nevus Syndrome

Blue rubber bleb nevus syndrome is a rare disorder characterized by cutaneous and gastrointestinal venous malformations. Skin lesions appear as multiple, raised, bluish-black lesions. They number from a few to hundreds, are usually present at birth, and tend to increase in size and number with age, but they rarely bleed. The lesions can be found from the mouth to the anus, but are most commonly found in the small intestine. They can lead to massive (or occult) gastrointestinal hemorrhage in the form of hematemesis or melena. The lesions may also cause abdominal pain, volvulus, intramural hemorrhage, or infarction. Iron deficiency anemia results from the recurrent bleeding episodes.

POEMS Syndrome

POEMS syndrome consists of **p**olyneuropathy, **o**rganomegaly, **e**ndocrinopathy, **M** protein, and **s**kin changes, combined with multicentric Castleman disease. Glomeruloid hemangiomas—reactive ectatic vascular spaces filled with capillary aggregations and reminiscent of renal glomeruli—can be seen. Patients present with numerous cutaneous angiomas; some cases of arterial occlusion have been reported. In one series of 20 patients, 4 patients had recurrent thrombotic events leading to successive amputations or death. Three of the patients had no known risk factors for atherosclerosis, and POEMS syndrome was believed to be a major contributing factor.

- POEMS syndrome consists of **p**olyneuropathy, **o**rganomegaly, **e**ndocrinopathy, **M** protein, and **s**kin changes, combined with multicentric Castleman disease

Questions

1. What are the most common clinical characteristics of erythromelalgia?
  a. Increased warmth, erythema, and burning feet
  b. Intense itching and burning pain in the feet
  c. Occurs most often in late fall
  d. Occurs more commonly in elderly patients with peripheral arterial disease

2. What are the most common clinical characteristics of frostbite?
  a. Purple, erythematous, or cyanotic skin lesions
  b. Painful, burning extremities
  c. Numbness or clumsiness in affected areas
  d. Females more likely to be affected than males

3. Which statement is true regarding PAES?
  a. It is most commonly seen from age 50 to 70 years.
  b. Popliteal artery aneurysm may be the presenting feature.
  c. Angiography may be normal in the resting position.
  d. It is most common in young persons with no risk factors for atherosclerosis.

4. Which statement is true regarding cystic adventitial disease?
  a. It is best treated by aspiration of the cystic contents using ultrasonography or CT guidance.
  b. It is most common in the radial artery.
  c. It generally occurs bilaterally.
  d. It is most often seen in young to middle-aged men.

5. Which statement is true regarding Kaposi sarcoma?
  a. It is a disease of men, generally presenting between age 30 and 50 years.
  b. It is more common in Ashkenazi Jewish males and affects the upper extremities.
  c. It is generally benign if found on the lower extremities of elderly males.
  d. It is never found in younger children.

6. Which statement is true regarding Klippel-Trénaunay syndrome?
  a. It is characterized by arteriovenous malformation, port-wine stain, and soft tissue or bony hypertrophy.
  b. It is characterized by port-wine stain, soft tissue or bony hypertrophy, and venous varicosities.
  c. It is characterized by thrombocytopenia, a consumption coagulopathy, and cavernous hemangioma.
  d. It is characterized by port-wine stain, mental retardation, and seizures.

7. What are the most common clinical characteristics of pernio?
  a. Intense itching and burning pain more commonly seen in females
  b. Stasis ulceration that recurs in late fall and winter
  c. Edema and burning pain that occurs in late spring and summer
  d. Commonly results in amputation if not recognized

Suggested Readings

Arzimanoglou AA, Andermann F, Aicardi J, et al. Sturge-Weber syndrome: indications and results of surgery in 20 patients. Neurology. 2000;55:1472-9.

Biem J, Koehncke N, Classen D, et al. Out of the cold: management of hypothermia and frostbite. CMAJ. 2003;168:305-11.

Blei F. Basic science and clinical aspects of vascular anomalies. Curr Opin Pediatr. 2005;17:501-9.

Boultwood J. Ataxia telangiectasia gene mutations in leukaemia and lymphoma. J Clin Pathol. 2001;54:512-6.

Couch V, Lindor NM, Karnes PS, et al. von Hippel-Lindau disease. Mayo Clin Proc. 2000;75:265-72.

Curti BD. Renal cell carcinoma. JAMA. 2004;292:97-100.

Davis MDP, O'Fallon WM, Rogers RS III, et al. Natural history of erythromelalgia: presentation and outcome in 168 patients. Arch Dermatol. 2000;136:330-6.

Davis MDP, Sandroni P, Rooke TW, et al. Erythromelalgia: vasculopathy, neuropathy, or both? A prospective study of vascular and neurophysiologic studies in erythromelalgia. Arch Dermatol. 2003;139:1337-43.

Ertem D, Acar Y, Kotiloglu E, et al. Blue rubber bleb nevus syndrome. Pediatrics. 2001;107:418-20.

Espiritu JD, Creer MH, Miklos AZ, et al. Fatal tumor thrombosis due to an inferior vena cava leiomyosarcoma in a patient with antiphospholipid antibody syndrome. Mayo Clin Proc. 2002;77:595-9.

Fuchizaki U, Miyamori H, Kitagawa S, et al. Hereditary haemorrhagic telangiectasia (Rendu-Osler-Weber disease). Lancet. 2003;362:1490-4.

Gampper TJ, Morgan RF. Vascular anomalies: hemangiomas. Plast Reconstr Surg. 2002;110:572-86.

Granter SR, Longtine JA. Neoplastic and non-neoplastic vascular tumors. In: Creager MA, editor. Vascular disease. St. Louis: Mosby; 1996. p. 256-68.

Jacob AG, Driscoll DJ, Shaughnessy WJ, et al. Klippel-Trenaunay syndrome: spectrum and management. Mayo Clin Proc. 1998;73:28-36.

Jermann M, Eid K, Pfammatter T, et al. Maffucci's syndrome. Circulation. 2001;104:1693.

Kottke-Marchant K, Bartholomew JR. Vascular tumors. In: Young JR, Olin JW, Bartholomew JR, editors. Peripheral vascular diseases. 2nd ed. St Louis: Mosby; 1996. p. 621-36.

Lambert AW, Wilkins DC. Popliteal artery entrapment syndrome. Br J Surg. 1999;86:1365-70.

Muhm M, Polterauer P, Gstottner W, et al. Diagnostic and therapeutic approaches to carotid body tumors: review of 24 patients. Arch Surg. 1997;132:279-84.

O'Hara CD, Nascimento AG. Endothelial lesions of soft tissues: a review of reactive and neoplastic entities with emphasis on low-grade malignant ("borderline") vascular tumors. Adv Anat Pathol. 2003;10:69-87.

Oumeish OY, Parish LC. Marching in the army: common cutaneous disorders of the feet. Clin Dermatol. 2002;20:445-51.

Percell RL Jr, Henning RJ, Siddique Patel M. Atrial myxoma: case report and a review of the literature. Heart Dis. 2003;5:224-30.

Powell J. Update on hemangiomas and vascular malformations. Curr Opin Pediatr. 1999;11:457-63.

Simon TD, Soep JB, Hollister JR. Pernio in pediatrics. Pediatrics. 2005;116:e472-5.

Simpson WL Jr, Mendelson DS. Pulmonary artery and aortic sarcomas: cross-sectional imaging. J Thorac Imaging. 2000;15:290-4.

Slovut DP, Olin JW. Fibromuscular dysplasia. N Engl J Med. 2004;350:1862-71.

Tegtmeyer CJ, Matsumoto AH, Johnson AM. Renal angioplasty. In: Baum S, Pentecost MJ, editors. Abrams' angiography: interventional radiology. Vol 3. Boston: Little, Brown and Company; 1997. p. 294-325.

Viguier M, Pinquier L, Cavelier-Balloy B, et al. Clinical and histopathologic features and immunologic variables in patients with severe chilblains: a study of the relationship to lupus erythematosus. Medicine (Baltimore). 2001;80:180-8.

Vos LD, Tielbeek AV, Vroegindeweij D, et al. Cystic adventitial disease of the popliteal artery demonstrated with intravascular US. J Vasc Interv Radiol. 1996;7:583-6.

Waxman SG, Dib-Hajj SD. Erythromelalgia: a hereditary pain syndrome enters the molecular era. Ann Neurol. 2005;57:785-8.

Wright LB, Matchett WJ, Cruz CP, et al. Popliteal artery disease: diagnosis and treatment. Radiographics. 2004;24:467-79.

11 Leg Ulcerations

Mark D. P. Davis, MD

Introduction

Leg ulcerations are a common clinical problem with significant attendant morbidity. They are a source of great discomfort and can substantially affect quality of life. Treatment can be difficult and a cure can be elusive.

Significant strides have been made in wound healing in recent years. For example, foot ulcers due to diabetic neuropathy are more likely to heal today than 10 years ago. The primary reason for this improvement is that patients are seeking care early, when wounds are most easily treated, so success is more likely.

Epidemiology

Although incidence and prevalence rates have not been well established for most forms of leg ulceration, leg ulcerations are a common clinical problem. Most leg ulcers (70%-80%) are due to "venous" disorders. Venous leg ulcers are common among those aged 65 years and older, with a prevalence of 1.69%. The overall incidence rate for men is 0.76 per 100 person-years and for women, 1.42 per 100 person-years. Each year in the United States alone, more than 50,000 patients require amputation for osteomyelitis, which in most cases began as diabetic foot ulcers.

Etiology

A summary of factors that cause and perpetuate ulcerations is provided in Table 11.1. The most common causes of leg ulcerations are vascular (venous, arterial, small-vessel disease) or neuropathic. However, it is also important to recognize other causes such as trauma, infection, inflammation, connective tissue disease, coagulopathy, malignancy, hematologic, drug-induced, metabolic, or pyoderma gangrenosum. All of these possible causes must be considered, because appropriate therapy depends on an accurate diagnosis of the ulcer origin.

- 70%-80% of leg ulcers are due to venous disorders; venous leg ulcers are common in the elderly
- The possible causes of a leg ulceration include vascular (venous, arterial, small-vessel disease), neuropathic, infection, inflammation, collagen vascular disease, coagulopathy, malignancy, hematologic, drug-induced, metabolic, and pyoderma gangrenosum

Diagnosis

Ulcer diagnosis requires an adequate history, physical examination, and appropriate investigations, keeping in mind that the cause of ulcerations may be multifactorial.

History

Factors important in the diagnosis of leg ulcers are outlined in Table 11.2. Details about how the ulceration started, how it progressed, the speed of development, duration of the ulceration, associated pain, medical and surgical history, medications, family history, social history, and review of systems are all important clues that may help to identify the cause, course, and treatment options for the ulcer.

Physical Examination

Key elements of the ulcer examination are outlined in Table 11.3. The description of an ulceration should include location, size, pattern, base, edges, surrounding skin, pulses, vascular status (venous, arterial, presence or absence of

Table 11.1 Causes of Leg Ulcerations

I. Venous

II. Ischemic
A. Atherosclerosis
B. Atherosclerosis with superimposed trauma
C. Atheroemboli (cholesterol emboli)
D. Arteriolar
E. Vasculitis (leukocytoclastic vasculitis)
F. Vascular occlusion
  1. Coagulopathy
  2. Livedoid vasculopathy

III. Neuropathic
A. Diabetes mellitus
B. Tabes dorsalis (syphilis)
C. Spinal cord lesions
D. Any condition associated with decreased sensation

IV. Non-vascular
A. Trauma
  1. Pressure
  2. Injury (external, self-induced/factitial)
  3. Burns (chemical, thermal, radiation)
  4. Cold (frostbite)
  5. Spider bite (brown recluse spider)

IV. Non-vascular (continued)
B. Infection
  1. Bacterial
  2. Fungal or deep-fungal
    a. Blastomycosis
    b. Cryptococcosis
    c. Coccidioidomycosis
    d. Histoplasmosis
  3. Viral (herpes simplex virus)
  4. Mycobacterial
  5. Parasitic (leishmaniasis)
  6. Spirochetal
  7. Osteomyelitis
C. Inflammation
  1. Connective tissue disease
    a. Lupus erythematosus
    b. Polyarteritis nodosa
    c. Rheumatoid arthritis
    d. Wegener granulomatosis
  2. Panniculitis
    a. Infectious
    b. Non-infectious
      i. Necrobiosis lipoidica
      ii. Pancreatic fat necrosis (malignancy pancreas)
      iii. α1 antitrypsin panniculitis

IV. Non-vascular (continued)
D. Malignancy
  1. Squamous cell carcinoma
  2. Basal cell carcinoma
  3. Melanoma
  4. Lymphoma
  5. Metastatic
  6. Sarcoma
    a. Kaposi
    b. Angiosarcoma
E. Metabolic
  1. Diabetes mellitus
  2. Gout
  3. α1 antitrypsin deficiency
  4. Calciphylaxis
F. Hematologic
  1. Sickle cell anemia
  2. Thalassemia
  3. Coagulopathy
  4. Cryoglobulinemia
G. Drug-induced (hydroxyurea)
H. Pyoderma gangrenosum
  1. Ulcerative
  2. Bullous
  3. Pustular
  4. Vegetative
I. Multifactorial—any combination of causes

Table 11.2 Features of Patient History Important in Diagnosis of Ulcerations

I. Pain
  A. Pain is usually severe when associated with ischemic ulcers, pyoderma gangrenosum, calciphylaxis, or hydroxyurea-induced ulcerations
  B. Pain associated with venous ulcers is less severe
II. Speed of onset (rapid vs slow)—ulcerations of pyoderma gangrenosum are rapidly progressive
III. Duration of ulcer—ulcerations of longer duration are slower to heal
IV. Prior therapy
V. Medical/surgical history
  A. History of ulcers—predictive of future ulcers
  B. Venous disease, arterial disease, lymphedema
  C. Neurologic disease
  D. Diabetes mellitus
  E. Hematologic disease—sickle cell anemia, thalassemia, coagulopathy
  F. Gastrointestinal disease—inflammatory disease may underlie pyoderma gangrenosum
  G. Renal disease—calciphylaxis
  H. Rheumatologic disease—connective tissue disease
  I. Skin disease
  J. Psychiatric disease
VI. Medications—hydroxyurea
VII. Family history
  A. Ulcerations
  B. Metabolic disorders
  C. Coagulopathy
VIII. Social history
  A. History of picking at skin
  B. Psychologic or psychiatric factors that may be contributing
  C. Smoking exacerbates ischemic ulcerations

varicose veins), and neurologic assessment (presence or absence of neuropathy [large or small fiber]).

The location provides diagnostic information. For example, the diagnosis of a venous leg ulcer is usually made in patients with a chronic wound in the "gaiter area" of the lower extremity (between the lower third of the calf and 1 inch below the malleolus) and with other clinical signs compatible with venous abnormalities (e.g., varicose veins, venous blush, lipodermatosclerosis) in persons with adequate arterial circulation.

Diagnostic Testing

Diagnostic testing (Table 11.4) can include, as appropriate, assessment of blood, vascular status (first non-invasive, then invasive, if appropriate), and neurologic status. A tissue biopsy specimen may be taken for histologic studies and for culture (a wound swab is less desirable; its use is controversial). Radiologic evaluations may be used to investigate osteomyelitis, if appropriate. The best means of diagnosing osteomyelitis is controversial, although many believe that magnetic resonance imaging is most reliable.

Pathogenesis of Chronic Ulcerations

Normal wound healing is a complex, dynamic, and integrated process and requires the interaction of factors in-

Table 11.3 Physical Examination Features Important in Diagnosis and Prognosis of Leg Ulceration

I. Location
A. Ulcerations in the "gaiter" area of the lower extremity (between the lower third of the calf and 1 inch below the malleolus) are characteristic of venous disease
B. Lateral malleolus, bony prominences, and distal ulcerations are more characteristic of arterial disease
C. Pressure points on feet (e.g., metatarsal head or heel) are more characteristic of neuropathic ulcerations
D. Thigh ulcerations are more characteristic of polyarteritis nodosa, calciphylaxis, or factitial ulcerations

II. Size
A. Larger ulcerations are slower to heal
B. Smaller ulcerations (<1.5 cm) are more likely to heal within 20 weeks

III. Pattern—linear ulcerations are likely to be factitial

IV. Base
A. Color
  1. Beefy red appearance—better prognosis
  2. Necrotic yellow/brown fibrinous slough or debris inhibits wound healing
  3. Dusky red base is unhealthy
B. Depth
  1. Superficial—more likely to heal
  2. Muscle/bone—ulceration is deep, more difficult to heal
  3. Bone—suspect osteomyelitis
  4. Undermining—pockets of undermining may be nidus for recurrence of ulceration, infection of ulcer ("dead space")
C. Moist/dry/wet
  1. Moist environment preferred for healing
  2. Dry or wet wounds are less likely to heal
    a. Desiccation of tissue with dry wounds
    b. Maceration of tissue with wet wounds
D. Exudate
  1. Clear—edema
  2. Yellow—infection

IV. Base (continued)
E. Odor—infection; fishy odor likely *Pseudomonas*

V. Edges of ulcer
A. Sloping—characteristic of venous ulcer
B. Vertical—characteristic of arterial ulcer
C. Rolled—characteristic of basal cell carcinoma
D. Undermined, violaceous—characteristic of pyoderma gangrenosum
E. Stellate—livedoid vasculopathy

VI. Surrounding skin
A. Normal
B. Skin disease
  1. Psoriasis
  2. Dermatitis
  3. Dry skin (asteatosis/xerosis)
  4. Panniculitis
  5. Other rash
C. Color
  1. Pale—ischemic disease
  2. Hyperpigmented—postinflammatory hyperpigmentation
  3. Yellow plaques—necrobiosis lipoidica
D. Edema
  1. Venous disease
  2. Lymphedema
  3. Systemic (cardiac/pulmonary/renal) disease
E. Induration—lipodermatosclerosis
F. Patterned
  1. Livedo reticularis, polyarteritis nodosa
  2. Livedoid vasculopathy

VII. Pulses—diminished indicates large-vessel disease

VIII. Varicose veins—predispose to ulceration

IX. Sensation/motor function—impaired indicates neurologic disease

volved in the four phases of wound healing: hemostasis, inflammation, proliferation, and remodeling. In ulcers that don't heal, the wounds seem to be "stuck" in the inflammatory or proliferative phase. However, problems in any of the phases of wound healing can lead to chronic ulceration.

In some chronic ulcers, certain cells such as fibroblasts appear almost senescent; they are odd-shaped and dysfunctional. Recent evidence has shown excesses of growth factors and metalloproteases, which are associated with a state of ongoing destruction within the wound. Biofilms—communities of microorganisms adhering to environmental surfaces, encased in a polysaccharide capsule—can colonize the wound; the polysaccharide capsules are difficult for antibiotics to penetrate. These biofilms may have a role in delaying wound healing. Old age, nutritional deficiency, chronic illness, chronic immunosuppression, hypoxia, vasculopathy, and infection can all contribute to chronic ulceration.

Often, ulcerations are multifactorial, with several contributing factors. For example, a "diabetic" foot ulcer may be due to a combination of lower-limb arterial insufficiency, lower-limb diabetic neuropathy, and local trauma. The primary factor for about 20% of diabetic patients with foot ulcers is inadequate arterial blood flow, for approximately 50% it is diabetic neuropathy, and approximately 30% have both conditions. Foot ulcers in patients with diabetes mellitus who lack protective sensation and have adequate arterial blood flow to the foot are termed "diabetic neuropathic foot ulcers." Diabetes mellitus is a significant risk factor for foot ulcerations: whereas only 4% of the population has diabetes mellitus, 46% of those admitted to a hospital with a foot ulcer have diabetes, and half of all lower extremity amputations in hospitalized patients occur in diabetic patients.

Ulcerations are less likely to heal in older persons; in nutritional deficiency (protein, calorie, vitamins A or C, trace metals such as zinc or copper); in a setting of chronic

Table 11.4 Investigations of Leg Ulcerations (Use if Clinically Indicated)

I. Arterial studies
  A. ABI
  B. PVR/SBP/Doppler
  C. Exercise ABI
  D. Arterial DUS
  E. MRA
  F. CTA
  G. Angiography
  H. Transcutaneous oximetry measurements ($TcPO_2$)
  I. Laser Doppler flowmetry
II. Venous studies
  A. Duplex ultrasonography—to rule out DVT
  B. Venography—contrast venography
  C. Functional testing—plethysmography
III. Lymphatic studies
  A. Lymphangiography
  B. Lymphoscintigraphy
  C. Abdominal/pelvic CT/MRI
IV. Neurologic studies
  A. Electromyography
  B. Small-fiber nerve testing—autonomic reflexes (Valsalva, table tilting, QSART)
V. Blood tests
  A. Complete blood count
  B. Erythrocyte sedimentation rate, C-reactive protein
  C. Blood chemistry (liver, kidney, thyroid function tests)
  D. Protein electrophoresis
  E. Special coagulation profile (including antiphospholipid antibody screening)
  F. Rheumatologic investigations—antinuclear factor, antineutrophil cytoplasmic antibodies
  G. Special coagulation studies—factor V Leiden, cryofibrinogens, proteins C and S, cryoglobulins, anticardiolipin antibody
VI. Wound swab
  A. Staining—Gram, fungal, acid-fast, *Nocardia* smear
  B. Culture/PCR—virus, bacteria, mycobacteria, fungi
VII. Biopsy of the edge of ulceration—elliptical incisional biopsy preferred to punch biopsy; include edge of the ulceration to depth of subcutaneous fat
  A. Routine histology (hematoxylin and eosin staining)
  B. Special staining (Gram, methenamine silver, Fite) to detect microorganisms
  C. Culture in appropriate medium for bacteria, fungi, mycobacteria
VIII. Radiologic studies—to rule out osteomyelitis
  A. Radiography of underlying bone
  B. MRI
  C. Bone scan

ABI, ankle-brachial index; CT, computed tomography; CTA, computed tomography angiography; DUS, duplex ultrasonography; DVT, deep vein thrombosis; MRA, magnetic resonance angiography; MRI, magnetic resonance imaging; PCR, polymerase chain reaction; PVR, pulse-volume recording; QSART, quantitative sudomotor axon reflex testing; SBP, systolic blood pressure.

illness; with use of some medications such as immunosuppressive drugs (corticosteroids, cyclosporine, azathioprine, penicillamine), antineoplastic drugs, anticoagulants (aspirin, warfarin, heparin), and nonsteroidal antiinflammatory drugs; in hypoxic states (oxygen is required for bacterial phagocytosis, and hypoxia allows contamination with normally subinfective levels of bacteria); if normal blood flow is interrupted due to coagulopathy or arterial, venous, or lymphatic insufficiency; in a setting of infection; or with an excess of metalloproteases.

Therapy

Appropriate management of leg ulcer wounds is essential both to optimize the chances of healing and minimize the need for amputation, and to minimize associated pain and morbidity and improve quality of life.

General Principles

The general principles of wound healing include recognizing, treating, and managing the underlying cause of the wound (Table 11.5). An accurate diagnosis is essential. Numerous materials are available to optimize wound treatments, but if the diagnosis of the underlying problem is not correct, a wound will not heal. For example, if the ulceration is due to a deep fungal infection, the infection must be treated in addition to the ulcer itself. If multiple factors are involved, all must be treated.

The basic tenets of good wound care include maintenance of a moist and clean healing environment. Infection should be treated appropriately, devitalized tissue should be debrided, and dressings appropriate to maintain a moist environment should be used. Pain should be managed aggressively to minimize morbidity.

A schema for the management of ulcerations is summarized in Table 11.6. The techniques used, many of which have not changed in the past century, must be individualized to the wound type. For example, compression remains the cornerstone of venous ulcer management. Methods of compression vary but may include stockings, multilayered bandages, high-pressure compression boots, intermittent pneumatic compression, and Unna boots. In general, the higher the level of compression obtained, the greater the chance of healing, regardless of method. Com-

Table 11.5 Principles of Leg Ulceration Management

Recognize and treat underlying disease
Treat arterial disease with revascularization, venous disease with compression, neuropathic disease with off-loading, and infectious disease with appropriate antimicrobial drugs
Debride devitalized tissue
Maintain a moist, clean environment for healing
Minimize pain
For ulcerations of prolonged duration and large size (recalcitrant to the above measures), consider adjunctive methods, perhaps in the setting of a wound healing center

Table 11.6 Management of Leg Ulcerations

I. *Ischemic ulcerations: in general do not debride before revascularization*
A. Large vessel: revascularize
B. Atheroemboli: find source of embolus, treat
C. Vasculitis: treat underlying disease; consider immunosuppressive drugs, corticosteroids
D. Coagulopathy: identify exact cause; use aspirin, anticoagulants

II. *Venous ulcerations/lymphedema ulcerations*
A. Compression therapy (standard treatment)
B. Medical
  1. Edema reduction—leg elevation
  2. Pumps—intermittent pneumatic compression postulated to mainly improve calf pump function
  3. Massage (MLD, CDT)
C. Surgical/endovascular
  1. PTA/stents/bypass (for venous obstruction)
  2. Venous valve repair/transplant
  3. Vein stripping
  4. Catheter-based vein ablation
  5. Sclerotherapy
D. Prevention/chronic management
  1. Skin care
  2. Stockings

III. *Neuropathic*
A. Off-loading the foot
B. Orthotics
C. Platelet-derived growth factor, recombinant (becaplermin)
D. Skin graft, tissue-engineered skin
E. Amputation

IV. *Non-vascular causes: treat as appropriate (diabetes mellitus, infection, connective tissue disease, drug induced)*

CDT, complete decongestive therapy; MLD, manual lymph drainage; PTA, percutaneous transluminal angioplasty.

pression therapy at 30 to 40 mm Hg is generally recommended for venous ulcerations.

Other types of ulcers require specific therapy. Ischemic ulcerations must be revascularized, ulcers due to coagulopathy require anticoagulant or antiplatelet therapy, and infection requires antimicrobial medications. Diabetic neuropathic ulcers must be off-loaded (taking pressure off the area) to maximize the chance of healing. These basic techniques (wound off-loading, debridement, and compression) are inexpensive, remain the mainstays of therapy, and can heal most wounds. Advanced techniques can be used for recalcitrant ulcerations.

Several important advances recently have been made in the management of recalcitrant lower extremity wounds. Adjunctive techniques include recombinant growth factors, tissue-engineered skin, vacuum-assisted closure techniques, hyperbaric oxygen, and other interventions that are the subject of ongoing investigations. All are expensive; some require expertise to use. Wound healing centers have become central resources for these techniques.

Prognostic Indices

Generally, standard measures are used to treat most ulcers, and adjunctive measures are reserved for ulcers recalcitrant to standard care. However, some factors may be used to determine which ulcers will not respond to standard care. Some studies have demonstrated that the longer venous leg ulcers are present and the bigger they are, the more resistant they will be to healing. These factors can be used to distinguish between patients who would respond well with standard limb compression therapy and those who would not.

Treat Infection

Systemic antibiotic therapy should be used if there is evidence of frank wound infection such as cellulitis; the choice of antibiotic must be geared toward the suspected organism. Empiric therapy is appropriate early in the course of care; regimens might include cephalexin, clindamycin, and the fluoroquinolones. Tissue biopsies are necessary to determine the organism responsible for the infection. Swab cultures are not especially useful because organisms other than those responsible for the infection might also colonize the wound.

Principles of Management of Infection in Leg Ulcerations

- Systemic antibiotic therapy should be used for frank wound infection such as cellulitis
- Choice of antibiotic must be directed against the suspected organism
- Use of antibiotics without clear evidence of infection is controversial

If there is no clear evidence of infection, such as cellulitis, the use of antibiotics is controversial. Empiric use of systemic antibiotics has not been shown to decrease wound bioburden (colonization) or to decrease the progression of ulceration to amputation. Studies have also shown that topical antibiotics do not improve the probability of treatment success and that topical antiseptic solutions are generally ineffective for treating infection and can damage granulation tissue. Yet antiseptic solutions are frequently used in the care of leg ulcerations; in recent years, interest has been renewed in antimicrobial dressings that use slow-release iodine and silver.

Debride Devitalized Tissue

It is generally agreed that devitalized tissue is an impediment to wound healing and is best removed, except in the context of ischemic ulcers. Debridement is thought to stimulate the underlying granulation tissue and might assist in removal of biofilms. Types of debridement include surgical, mechanical, autolytic, enzymatic, and maggot debridement.

Apply Appropriate Dressings

A broad array of topical medications is available on the market. The general recommendation is to keep the wound moist but avoid maceration of the surrounding tissue. Dressings can do more than provide a moist environment; they can help debride, change the bacterial flora, and change the biochemical environment of the wound. Dressing classes available include gauze (may be impregnated with petrolatum or other agent), hydrocolloids, transparent films, hydrogels, foams, alginates, antimicrobials (iodine, silver, alcohols, biguanides, chlorine), and collagen. Different classes are combined in commercially available forms, such as silver combined with alginate or collagen combined with hydrocolloid. The best combinations for exudative wounds are alginates, foams, and dry gauze. The best for dry wounds are hydrogels, hydrocolloids, and impregnated gauze.

Skin Grafts and Flaps, Tissue-Engineered Skin

Skin grafts and flaps have long been used for the management of chronic ulcerations. They should be applied only to clean, uninfected ulceration with an adequate vascular supply. The grafts and flaps cover the wound, often relieving pain. It has been suggested that the benefit of skin grafts is the transplanted cells, which can secrete growth factors and other products that may enhance healing.

Studies have compared cultured keratinocyte allografts with standard dressings, but a pooled analysis did not demonstrate a significant benefit of allografts over control dressings. These trials were all small and may have been underpowered.

There is increased interest in tissue-engineered skin. Different approaches to artificial skin have been used. One type is a bilayered skin equivalent that includes dermal and epidermal components and is manufactured by harvesting neonatal foreskin and extracting both keratinocytes and fibroblasts that are then cultured separately to create the epidermal and dermal components. A second type of artifical skin is composed of human fibroblasts on a bioabsorbable scaffold. The US Food and Drug Administration (FDA) has approved both these products for management of diabetic neurotrophic ulcers. The bilayered skin also has approval for use on venous ulcerations. One study compared tissue-engineered skin with split-thickness allograft but failed to show that either treatment had any significant benefit. Graft classes available include full thickness, partial thickness, allogeneic (cultured), and artificial (tissue-engineered skin).

Advanced Wound Care Techniques Being Investigated

Topical Negative Pressure Therapy (Vacuum-Assisted Closure)

Vacuum-assisted closure involves applying open-cell foam to a wound, adding a seal of adhesive drape, and then applying subatmospheric pressure to the wound in a controlled way, either intermittently or continuously. This method is said to remove exudate, decrease bacteria in the wound, exert mechanical stress causing granulation tissue formation and angiogenesis, and encourage migration of keratinocytes across wound defects. Encouraging results in rates of healing have been reported in the literature, but few randomized controlled trials with statistical significance are available to substantiate the findings. Vacuum-assisted closure is also costly.

Hyperbaric Oxygen

Hyperbaric oxygen is an intermittent inhalation therapy in which the patient breathes oxygen at pressure greater than 1 atm. This requires placing the patient into a sealed vessel (chamber) that is capable of withstanding pressurization. It can be used for diabetic, venous, arterial, and pressure ulcers. Advocates say that its clinical application is to improve tissue oxygenation when wound hypoxia interferes with healing. It typically is used as an adjunct to other techniques for improving wound oxygenation, particularly when angioplasty or revascularization is not feasible.

Use of hyperbaric oxygen is controversial. A systematic review of randomized controlled trials involving the use of hyperbaric oxygen for chronic wounds suggested that this technique decreases the risk of major amputation in hypoxic, problematic, diabetic foot wounds from 45% to 19% and somewhat improves wound healing (from 48% to 76%). Data are lacking for venous, arterial, or pressure ulcers. Hyperbaric oxygen treatments are expensive—about $400-$500 per session. Angiogenesis and infection control are said to be achieved with 14 to 21 treatments. In osteomyelitis, as many as 60 treatments may be necessary.

Growth Factors

Animal models of chronic wounds have shown that growth factors can be used to improve wound healing. Overall, clinical trials using growth factors to accelerate wound healing have been disappointing. The FDA has approved only one, recombinant platelet-derived growth factor (PDGF)-BB (becaplermin), for use in diabetic neuropathic foot ulcers. Efficacy studies have demonstrated a modest benefit of becaplermin for these ulcers when added to standard care alone (off-loading and twice-daily dressing changes). The percentage of wounds healed at 20 weeks increased by an absolute margin of 10% to 20%.

Autologous platelet releasate has been studied as an ulcer therapy. The releasate is derived by drawing a patient's blood and exposing it to a plastic that encourages platelet degranulation—forming a platelet "soup," in large part PDGF—which is then injected into the patient's wound. No well-designed controlled trial has demonstrated the efficacy of this approach, but one study showed a modest beneficial effect. The most severe wounds were most likely to benefit.

Granulocyte colony-stimulating factor (GCSF) is a growth factor that has also been studied. It induces the release of neutrophils from the bone marrow. A recombinant GCSF product (filgrastim) has been produced and studied for infected diabetic foot ulcers. It seemed to work as a subcutaneous agent, and fewer amputations were necessary in the treatment arm.

Management of Ulceration Pain

In general, pain management is an often-neglected aspect of wound care. Recent interest in the inadequacy of prevalent pain management protocols has revived research in this area, but there remain no evidence-based studies of pain management for chronic wounds. Much of the research in this area is in the nursing literature. Many leg ulcerations are associated with disabling pain and consequent impingement on the activities of daily living and sleeping at night. Because chronic wounds persist for months to years, a chronic pain syndrome can develop. In patients with venous ulcerations, quality-of-life measures such as bodily pain, mental health, and social functioning are decreased when compared with age-equivalent controls. Both systemic and local measures should be taken to control pain.

Wound Care Centers

With recalcitrant wounds, considerable benefit can be gained by referring a patient to a multispecialty wound care/wound healing center staffed by specialists in the field and with many specialized tools available.

Questions

1. Most chronic wounds seem to be "stuck" in the stage of:
a. Hemostasis
b. Inflammation
c. Proliferation
d. Remodeling
e. Inflammation or proliferation

2. Ulcerations occurring on pressure points such as the head of the metatarsal or heel are most characteristic of:
a. Venous disease
b. Arterial disease
c. Polyarteritis nodosa
d. Neuropathy
e. Factitial disease

3. For a very exudative wound, what is the most effective absorbent dressing class?
a. Gauze
b. Transparent films
c. Hydrocolloids
d. Alginates
e. Collagen

4. For a dry wound, what it is the most appropriate class of dressing to apply?
a. Gauze
b. Foam
c. Alginates
d. Silver
e. Hydrogel

5. What is an effective class of antimicrobial dressings for infected ulcerations?
a. Transparent film
b. Foam
c. Alginates
d. Silver-containing dressing
e. Hydrogel

6. What environment is thought to be most effective for wound healing?
a. Dry
b. Wet
c. Open to the air
d. Covered
e. Moist

7. When should antibiotics be used in management of wounds?
a. When a thick crust with purulence is noted on the wound
b. When there is surrounding cellulitis
c. When swab culture of the wound demonstrates *Staphylococcus*, *Streptococcus*, or *Pseudomonas*

d. When a substantial amount of devitalized tissue is associated with the wound

e. Antibiotics should be used in all wounds

Suggested Readings

Alvarez OM, Childs EJ. Pressure ulcers: physical, supportive, and local aspects of management. Clin Podiatr Med Surg. 1991;8:869-90.

Boyce ST, Warden GD, Holder IA. Cytotoxicity testing of topical antimicrobial agents on human keratinocytes and fibroblasts for cultured skin grafts. J Burn Care Rehabil. 1995;16:97-103.

Chantelau E, Tanudjaja T, Altenhofer F, et al. Antibiotic treatment for uncomplicated neuropathic forefoot ulcers in diabetes: a controlled trial. Diabet Med. 1996;13:156-9.

Charles H. Does leg ulcer treatment improve patients' quality of life? J Wound Care. 2004;13:209-13.

Davis MD. Lidocaine patch helpful in managing the chronic pain of leg ulceration. J Am Acad Dermatol. 2003;49:964.

de Lalla F, Pellizzer G, Strazzabosco M, et al. Randomized prospective controlled trial of recombinant granulocyte colony-stimulating factor as adjunctive therapy for limb-threatening diabetic foot infection. Antimicrob Agents Chemother. 2001;45:1094-8.

Edmonds M, Bates M, Doxford M, et al. New treatments in ulcer healing and wound infection. Diabetes Metab Res Rev. 2000;16 Suppl 1:S51-4.

Emflorgo CA. The assessment and treatment of wound pain. J Wound Care. 1999;8:384-5.

Falabella AF, Kirsner RS, editors. Wound healing. Boca Raton (FL): Taylor & Francis Group; 2005.

Gough A, Clapperton M, Rolando N, et al. Randomised placebo-controlled trial of granulocyte-colony stimulating factor in diabetic foot infection. Lancet. 1997;350:855-9.

Gould D. Wound management and pain control. Nurs Stand. 1999;14:47-54.

Heinen MM, van Achterberg T, op Reimer WS, et al. Venous leg ulcer patients: a review of the literature on lifestyle and pain-related interventions. J Clin Nurs. 2004;13:355-66.

Kantor J, Margolis DJ. Management of leg ulcers. Semin Cutan Med Surg. 2003;22:212-21.

Lambert KV, Hayes P, McCarthy M. Vacuum assisted closure: a review of development and current applications. Eur J Vasc Endovasc Surg. 2005;29:219-26.

Larkin JM, Moylan JA. The role of prophylactic antibiotics in burn care. Am Surg. 1976;42:247-50.

Leaper DJ. Prophylactic and therapeutic role of antibiotics in wound care. Am J Surg. 1994;167:15S-19S.

Lipsky BA, Berendt AR. Principles and practice of antibiotic therapy of diabetic foot infections. Diabetes Metab Res Rev. 2000;16 Suppl 1:S42-6.

Margolis DJ, Allen-Taylor L, Hoffstad O, et al. Diabetic neuropathic foot ulcers: the association of wound size, wound duration, and wound grade on healing. Diabetes Care. 2002;25:1835-9.

Margolis DJ, Allen-Taylor L, Hoffstad O, et al. The accuracy of venous leg ulcer prognostic models in a wound care system. Wound Repair Regen. 2004;12:163-8.

Margolis DJ, Allen-Taylor L, Hoffstad O, et al. Healing diabetic neuropathic foot ulcers: are we getting better? Diabet Med. 2005;22:172-6.

Margolis DJ, Berlin JA, Strom BL. Which venous leg ulcers will heal with limb compression bandages? Am J Med. 2000;109:15-9.

Margolis DJ, Bilker W, Santanna J, et al. Venous leg ulcer: incidence and prevalence in the elderly. J Am Acad Dermatol. 2002;46:381-6.

Margolis DJ, Kantor J, Santanna J, et al. Effectiveness of platelet releasate for the treatment of diabetic neuropathic foot ulcers. Diabetes Care. 2001;24:483-8.

Mol MA, Nanninga PB, van Eendenburg JP, et al. Grafting of venous leg ulcers: an intraindividual comparison between cultured skin equivalents and full-thickness skin punch grafts. J Am Acad Dermatol. 1991;24:77-82.

National Diabetes Data Group. Diabetes in America. 2nd ed. Bethesda (MD): National Institutes of Health, National Institute of Diabetes and Digestive and Kidney Diseases; 1995. (NIH) 95-1468.

Persoon A, Heinen MM, van der Vleuten CJ, et al. Leg ulcers: a review of their impact on daily life. J Clin Nurs. 2004;13:341-54.

Reiber GE. The epidemiology of diabetic foot problems. Diabet Med. 1996;13 Suppl 1:S6-11.

Roeckl-Wiedmann I, Bennett M, Kranke P. Systematic review of hyperbaric oxygen in the management of chronic wounds. Br J Surg. 2005;92:24-32.

Rook JL. Wound care pain management. Nurse Pract. 1997;22:122-6.

Senecal SJ. Pain management of wound care. Nurs Clin North Am. 1999;34:847-60.

Shai A, Maibach HI. Wound healing and ulcers of the skin: diagnosis and therapy—the practical approach. Berlin: Springer-Verlag; 2005.

Strauss MB. Hyperbaric oxygen as an intervention for managing wound hypoxia: its role and usefulness in diabetic foot wounds. Foot Ankle Int. 2005;26:15-8.

12 Clinical Evaluation of Peripheral Arterial Disease—Lower Extremity

Paul W. Wennberg, MD

Clinical evaluation of peripheral arterial disease (PAD) of the lower extremity involves a thorough history and physical examination. This chapter discusses practical techniques that may be used to make a diagnosis of PAD.

Patient History

Pain

Pain is the most important factor in the diagnosis of PAD. Although pain is common in PAD, the discomfort felt by the patient may be only partly due to or not at all due to arterial disease (Table 12.1). Claudication (leg pain or weakness with walking) is due to a lack of blood flow. Therefore, activities that require more blood flow make the pain worse, and those that require less make it better. A careful evaluation of pain must be made using a systematic approach, asking specific questions, and pushing for specific answers. If the questions are left open ended, little useful information may be gained.

Location

Several important questions regarding pain include: "Where is the discomfort?" "Is it in the muscle or the joint?" "Does it move or travel anywhere?" "Is it present on both sides, and if so, is it with the same severity?" Claudication is rarely symmetric. If pain is located in a joint, it is unlikely to be due to arterial insufficiency. If it shoots down the leg it is more likely to originate from the nervous system. If fatigue or cramp progresses into adjacent muscle groups, arterial insufficiency is more likely.

Table 12.1 Causes of Lower Extremity Discomfort

Arterial
Atherosclerosis
Fibromuscular dysplasia
Cystic adventitial disease
Popliteal artery entrapment syndrome
Compartment syndrome
Thromboangiitis obliterans
Takayasu arteritis
Iliac endofibrosis (in cyclists)
Embolism
Thrombosis in situ
Retroperitoneal fibrosis
Venous
Venous incompetence
Venous obstruction
May-Thurner syndrome
Neurotrophic
Pseudoclaudication
Spinal stenosis or cauda equina syndrome
Sciatica
Piriformis syndrome
Restless legs syndrome
Autonomic neuropathy
Diabetic neuropathy
Musculoskeletal
Degenerative joint disease
Back
Hip
Knee
Foot/ankle
Fracture
Myositis
Fasciitis
Baker cyst
Other
Cellulitis

Duration

"When did the pain first start?" "How long does it last?" True claudication has an insidious onset. It is often recognized only in retrospect, for example if a patient suddenly remembers an event in which he or she felt pain or fatigue or "just couldn't keep up." It may have been on a tour, hunting, or trying to play with grandchildren. An event that was passed over initially may be uncovered later with the right question.

Severity

Questions addressing pain severity may not help to diagnose PAD, but they are valuable for determining its impact or aim for treatment. Possible questions include: "Does the pain prevent you from finishing tasks, and if so which tasks?" "Have you changed your activities or given up anything because of the pain?" If a patient has stopped going grocery shopping or cannot walk from the parking lot and must be let off at the front door, a significant lifestyle change has occurred. Similarly, if a 50-year-old can no longer hunt because of leg pain, there has been a lifestyle change.

Quality

"What does the pain feel like? Describe it for me." Patients often have difficulty with this question. They may ask what the pain is *supposed* to feel like. However, some may offer very detailed descriptions. If the description can be reduced to "crampy or fatigued sensation" versus "joint pain or shooting pain" versus "constant burning or prickly pain," these distinctions can be helpful in making the diagnosis.

Exacerbation

"What brings on the pain?" "What makes it worse?" "Is it present as soon as you stand?" Any activity that increases the usual workload requires more energy and, therefore, more blood flow. Walking in snow or carrying something heavy will worsen arterial insufficiency by increasing oxygen need. Pain while standing at a counter (e.g., while doing dishes) suggests a non-arterial etiology such as spinal stenosis. Pain that occurs immediately with standing suggests orthopedic or musculoskeletal pain.

Relief

"What can you do to make the pain better?" "Do you have to sit?" "Have you needed pain medication?" What alleviates the pain is often clearer to patients than what makes it worse. By thinking in terms of reversing the anatomic or hemodynamic process, the etiology may become clear. Leg elevation for relief suggests orthopedic or venous etiology. Hanging the leg for relief, typical in ischemia, uses gravity to improve distal blood delivery but may also explain concurrent edema.

Consistency

"Is the pain the same every day?" "Once it comes and goes away, can you continue on?" "How far each time?" Arterial pain with walking should occur at essentially the same distance and in the same anatomic location each time. After a rest, it should be possible to reach the same distance again. Non-arterial pain is suggested if the distance walked or location of discomfort, its quality, and severity are all variable.

History Questions to Distinguish PAD From Non-PAD Etiology

- Where is the discomfort?
- How much can you do before it starts?
- What does the discomfort feel like?
- What makes it worse?
- What brings relief?
- Is it the same every time?

Other Aspects of Patient History

General health in patients with PAD may be quite good. Patients with claudication often state that if it weren't for the leg pain they would feel great. Unfortunately, claudication can limit exertion such that angina, dyspnea due to chronic obstructive pulmonary disease, or musculoskeletal symptoms are suppressed. Except in severe PAD with critical limb ischemia, appetite and weight should be stable. If severe fatigue or other constitutional symptoms are present, a systemic illness such as vasculitis should be considered. If severe ischemia is present in a limb, pain and tissue loss can produce anorexia.

Risk factors for PAD are the same as for coronary artery disease or carotid artery disease. These risk factors—hypertension, hypercholesterolemia, arterial disease in another location, tobacco use, diabetes mellitus, increasing age, and male sex—are discussed in other chapters.

Asymptomatic PAD is rarely detected unless a screening arterial test is performed and incidentally shows a low ankle-brachial index (ABI) or abnormal Doppler signal. Detection of asymptomatic PAD has become more common as abnormal ABIs are discovered at health fairs and screening clinics throughout the community. These lesions may be asymptomatic because they simply are not severe enough to cause symptoms, the patient does not exert to a level to bring on symptoms, the arterial supply is well supplemented by collateral vessels, or the leg muscle may have been trained to function with less blood supply. In any case, asymptomatic PAD stratifies the patient into a group that is at higher risk of cardiovascular events; secondary prevention measures should be implemented.

Table 12.2 Location of Symptoms Based on Site of Arterial Occlusion

Site of lesion	Site of symptoms
Infrapopliteal isolated	Foot or none
Popliteal artery	Foot and calf
Femoral artery	Foot, calf, knee
Iliac artery	Foot, calf, thigh; impotency common
Aortoiliac segment	Bilateral foot, calf, thigh, and buttock
Deep femoral artery	Thigh and knee
Internal iliac artery	Buttock and hip; impotency if bilateral

Claudication due to arterial insufficiency is pain within a muscle group, occurring at a predictable distance or workload, essentially unchanged from day to day or from session to session. Symptoms usually occur one joint lower than the site of vascular occlusion, in part due to the collateral vascular supply around major joints (Table 12.2). Common descriptions of the pain include cramping, fatigue, hard pain, or weakness. The discomfort is relieved by rest, such as standing, and a specific position is not needed to obtain relief.

It is not uncommon to have months or years of mild symptoms worsen "suddenly" after an illness or injury that forces sedentary status. It is also common to have an event such as a walking tour or a hunting trip bring on limiting symptoms that in usual situations could be ignored. Distance and limitations provided by the patient are of dubious quantitative value—the perceived distance is rarely accurate. Patients should undergo some form of quantifiable and reproducible testing for confirmation and so that improvement or deterioration can be followed.

Rest pain due to ischemia may present in many ways. In a patient with neuropathy, an ischemic limb may have little or no pain. In contrast, a patient with intact sensation can have unrelenting pain that produces interference with sleep, anorexia, and little regret if amputation is required for relief. The stereotypical "nervous" sensations of shooting, sharp, burning, or tingling pain or "pins and needles" may be present. Rest pain initially presents as pain with limb elevation or while supine. This awakens the patient at night, resulting in paradoxic "walking to get rid of the pain." Hanging the limb over the side of the bed or sleeping in a chair is often noted. However, using gravity to increase delivery of oxygen may result in edema that can be severe. An increased diffusion gradient caused by the edema further decreases oxygenation of the limb.

Ulceration and gangrene are the presenting symptoms in many patients with PAD or other types of vascular disease (Table 12.3). An ischemic ulcer may initially present as a fissure, nail loss, or ulcerated lesion. Uncomplicated ischemic ulcers are typically dry, moderately painful, and pale at the base. If edema or infection is present, the wound may be wet. Underlying abscess or osteomyelitis is likely if tracking is present or bone is palpable when probed with a sterile swab. History should seek a trauma as the precipitating event. The trauma can be as blatant as a horse stepping on the foot or as subtle as a new pair of stockings with a big seam at the toes. Patients with a marginal nutrient supply may have no problems for years until injury occurs.

Erectile dysfunction is common in men with PAD and should be routinely inquired about during screening. When present, impotence with claudication suggests aortoiliac disease (Leriche syndrome if occlusion is complete) or bilateral internal iliac disease. Revascularization may improve symptoms.

Progression of PAD Severity

- Asymptomatic PAD—typically found only by screening studies or incidentally on physical examination
- Claudication—classically starts distally within a muscle group and ascends with continued activity

Table 12.3 Recognition of Ulcers of Vascular Etiology

	Ulcer type			
Characteristic	Venous	Arterial	Neurotrophic	Arteriolar
Location	Above medial and lateral malleoli	Shins, toes, sites of injury	Plantar surface, pressure points	Shin, calf
Pain	No, unless infected	Yes	No	Extreme
Skin	Stasis pigmentation; thickening with lipodermatosclerosis	Shiny; pale, decreased hair; may see livedo	Callous; normal to changes of ischemia	Normal or "satellite" ulcers in various stages
Edges	Clean	Smooth	Trophic, calloused	Serpiginous
Base	Wet, weeping, healthy granulation	Dry, pale with eschar	Healthy to pale depending on ASO	Dry, punched out, pale, thin eschar
Cellulitis	Common	Often	Common	No
Treatment	Compression	Revascularize	Revascularize, relieve pressure	Treat underlying disease and pain

ASO, arteriosclerosis obliterans.

- Rest pain—present with leg supine or elevated initially and relieved paradoxically by walking (due to gravity effect on increased oxygen delivery)
- Ulceration and gangrene—tissue loss due to hypoxia (dry ulcer) or infection with hypoxia (wet ulcer)

Physical Examination

It is rare that the physical examination cannot define the location, severity, and etiology of the pathologic process and account for the symptoms obtained in the history. However, vascular disease is not an isolated process. If the concern is right great toe pain and only the right leg is examined, pertinent information from the left side, at the carotid or the aorta, will likely be missed. The physical examination is indispensable and should be based on all the senses.

Sight

Observation of gait can provide much information. In the ideal setting, watching the patient walk down the hall before entering the examining room is very helpful. Antalgic gait, posturing, limb stiffness, and unsteadiness are all immediately noted by simple observation. Noting any gait abnormalities is extremely important when a dressing or special footwear is required, because the forced change in mechanics may not be tolerated well and in some instances can even be unsafe.

Pallor with elevation and rubor during dependency of the limb should be timed to help quantify the severity of ischemia (Table 12.4). Venous refilling is determined by elevating the patient's legs (while in the supine position) to drain the veins. Once the veins are empty, the patient sits and the legs are allowed to hang loosely as the time for the foot veins to fill is then recorded for each leg (Table 12.4). However, this test is not accurate in the setting of varicose veins.

Table 12.4 Tests for Ischemia Severity

Test	Measure
Elevation pallor*	**Pallor onset**
Normal	None
Grade I	>60 s
Grade II	30-60 s
Grade III	<30 s
Grade IV	Without elevation
Venous refilling time†	**Refill time, s**
Normal	<15
Moderate deficiency	15-40
Severe deficiency	>40

*Feet held passively at 60° while supine.
†Upon sitting after elevation of legs.

Hair growth patterns are altered with severe PAD. Differences in patterns between the legs may be noticed, but differences in the need to shave the legs (frequency of shaving) should also be asked about.

All toes should be examined for the presence of wounds. The toes must be separated to exclude "kissing ulcers" hidden between the toes. This also allows for evaluation of cracking due to tinea pedis that can lead to cellulitis. Redness of the skin on the legs that does not go away when supine suggests cellulitis.

Telangiectasias are common in connective tissue diseases such as scleroderma and mixed connective tissue disease. The hands are frequently involved, on both the palmar and dorsal surfaces. If a connective tissue disease is suspected, the nail folds should be closely examined for edema or tenderness and the nails for pitting.

Splinter hemorrhages are a common finding in atheroembolism and septic embolism due to endocarditis. The clinical setting distinguishes which is more likely. If splinter hemorrhages are seen on one limb, all others should be inspected, as well as the skin of the trunk.

Livedo reticularis that is not relieved by warmth or activity, as with vasospasm, suggests atheroemboli. Again, the nails, trunk, and limbs should be thoroughly inspected. Defining the distribution of "downstream" involvement can help guide the clinician to the most likely source of the embolism.

Skin changes such as dryness, port wine staining, and surgical scars should be noted. It is not uncommon for a patient to forget to mention prior bypass surgery during the history. Skin fissures or cracking of the toes or the heel is an important finding, representing the earliest stage of wounds.

Petechiae and purpura are rarely caused by atherosclerotic disease. When they are present, vasculitis, platelet abnormalities, or infection must be considered.

Physical Examination: Sight

- Constant livedo is present with atheroembolism
- Dynamic livedo is more suggestive of vasospasm
- The feet must be thoroughly inspected, including between toes, to rule out ulceration

Touch

The vast majority of arteries are accessible to palpation. The only exceptions are the intrathoracic, intracranial, and mesenteric vessels. In the upper extremity, the radial arteries should be palpated simultaneously to rule out proximal coarctation, and the right radial and femoral arteries palpated to rule out distal coarctation. Palpating a radial artery during auscultation is helpful in locating soft bruits and timing the extension into diastole if present.

Most institutions have a pulse grading scale. The scale used at Mayo Clinic is from 0 to 5, with 0 being absent and 4 being normal. The American College of Cardiology and American Heart Association have recently proposed a 0 to 3 pulse grading scale (Table 12.5).

The aorta is palpable, with size estimation possible in thin to mildly obese patients. If the aorta is easily palpable in an obese patient, an aneurysm should be considered. The iliac vessels are not typically palpable except in very thin patients. If palpable in others, aneurysm is likely. The aorta is best examined with the patient relaxed, knees bent slightly, with slowly increasing pressure and depth of palpation on each exhalation. The examiner may use two hands, approaching from each side to "trap" the aorta, or the fingers on one side and thumb on the other to "pinch" the aorta for size estimation.

Popliteal vein palpation is difficult. Full examination involves palpation of the popliteal fossa proximally and distally, with the patient sitting and supine. If the popliteal artery is easily palpable or widened, ectasia, aneurysm, or a Baker cyst is likely. If widened bilaterally, aneurysm is highly likely and should be ruled out with duplex ultrasonography; the incidence of aortic aneurysm is high in the setting of a widened popliteal artery. Reexamination of the aorta and duplex ultrasonography may be appropriate.

The dorsalis pedis and posterior tibial arteries are fairly easily examined. Both can be trapped against bony structures and have minimal overlying tissue. Slow steady pressure and patience allow these arteries to be palpated and graded, even if pedal edema is present.

The temporal artery may be tender in the setting of giant cell arteritis. (Tenderness during palpation may be present in any inflamed artery.) Nodules can be felt unilaterally or bilaterally in acute giant cell arteritis. If giant cell arteritis or Takayasu arteritis is suspected and the artery is not palpable, the artery may be occluded more proximally. The best site for palpation is very proximal, just anterior and superior to the tragus, at the hollow formed at the junction with the pinnae. By sliding a finger down the tragus into the hollow, the artery usually lands under the finger pad. Even if the distal temporal artery has undergone biopsy, this segment usually has a palpable pulse.

The radial artery is easily palpable along much of its course. The ulnar artery, however, may be problematic to palpate. The ulnar artery is more frequently diseased than the radial, in part due to hypothenar hand syndrome—trauma to the ulnar artery near the hook of the hamate bone caused by using the hand as a hammer or using a tool that puts pressure on the hypothenar eminence. Examination is best done by coming from underneath the patient's hands, palms up, wrapping the fingers around the hook of the hamate. One finger is below the hamate, one directly over, and one or two distal. This allows the ulnar artery to be trapped, avoiding the rolling that usually occurs. It also allows both proximal and distal segments to be palpated at the same time, making assessment of ulnar aneurysm due to trauma much easier.

The Allen test is done by closing the hand tightly to exsanguinate the tissues, with the examiner's fingers occluding the radial artery, then relaxing the hand to open it "halfway," while maintaining occlusion of the radial artery. If the ulnar artery is occluded, the hand will remain pale (i.e., fail to "pink up"). The reverse Allen test is the same, except the ulnar artery is occluded; failure to pink up suggests radial artery occlusion. Note that the thumb may be spared because of its vascular supply coming high off the radial. If there is an incomplete palmar arch, one or two fingers on the ulnar or radial side might remain pale. This finding neither excludes nor confirms disease in the radial or ulnar distribution.

Skin changes may be more apparent by palpation than by sight. In an ischemic limb, temperature is usually decreased. This finding is non-specific, but if different from that in the opposite limb, it is of value.

Muscle mass and tissue loss can be present in chronic ischemia. Wounds are obvious. Loss of calf mass and volume is common. More common but frequently overlooked is loss of the fat pad at the heel. If present, heel breakdown is imminent.

Pain during examination is common in critical limb ischemia. However, if pain seems out of proportion to the ischemia, lasts the duration of the examination, or occurs in the setting of minor trauma, fracture should be considered. Pain to light touch suggests neuropathy.

Table 12.5 Pulse Grading Scales

Grade	Pulse
Mayo Clinic	
0	Absent
1	Present, cannot count pulse
2	Reduced, can count pulse
3	Reduced
4	Easily found, normal
5	Widened, ectatic, or aneurysmal
ACC/AHA	
0	Absent
1	Dampened
2	Normal
3	Bounding

ACC/AHA, American College of Cardiology/American Heart Association.

Physical Examination: Palpation

- Tender arteries suggest inflammation such as arteritis
- Temperature discrepancy between limbs is suggestive of severe PAD
- The Allen test is performed by occluding the radial artery, testing patency of the ulnar artery
- The reverse Allen test is performed by occluding the ulnar artery, testing patency of the radial artery

Hearing

Auscultation over the arterial course is indicated in all examinations. The bell is best for low-pitched sounds, the diaphragm for high. Ideally, both are used in each location. Sensitivity for soft bruits can be improved if systole is timed by palpating a pulse (radial is convenient in most situations) while auscultating. If a bruit is found, it should be tracked proximally to determine the origin. The higher the pitch, the tighter the stenosis. If the bruit extends into diastole (best determined by simultaneous palpation) it is most likely high grade.

Carotid bruits are found more easily when patients hold their breath in mid exhalation. If a patient cannot do so, examination is quite difficult. If found, the bruit should be traced proximally and distally to estimate its location. A change in pitch or intensity may suggest multiple lesions (e.g., in the innominate and the carotid). Accurately identifying a carotid lesion in the setting of aortic stenosis is very difficult; ultrasonography is usually required to ensure adequate assessment of the bruit.

Mesenteric bruits also must be tracked, usually distally, to estimate the origin. Renal bruits tend to radiate laterally, mesenteric bruits centrally, and iliac bruits inferiorly. Depending on body habitus, the bruit may be loud or subtle. Simultaneous palpation of a radial artery can greatly help in identifying the bruit and timing into systole, especially in the presence of active bowel sounds. A bruit that comes and goes with respiration is most likely due to arcuate ligament compression of the celiac artery.

Blood pressure should be taken bilaterally at the arms as part of the physical examination. If a discrepancy between the arms greater than 15 mm Hg is present after retaking the pressures, simultaneous pressures should be obtained.

All vascular physicians should be proficient in the use of handheld continuous-wave Doppler. When used along with a blood pressure cuff, the ABI is easily obtained.

Physical Examination: Auscultation

- The origin of a bruit can be predicted if it is tracked proximally to a source point
- Excluding a carotid bruit in the setting of aortic stenosis is difficult. Imaging is often required
- A dynamic bruit in the abdomen suggests arcuate artery compression of the celiac artery

Smell

Odor is often present with wounds. To the experienced examiner, specific bacteria can be suggested by the odor alone, which helps with choice of initial antibiotic coverage. A pungent, musty (manure-like) odor, especially in a diabetic patient with ischemia, suggests anaerobic bacteria, and appropriate antibiotic coverage should be selected.

History and Examination Pearls in the Differential Diagnosis of Claudication

Pseudoclaudication

- Relief of symptoms is possible only with a change of position that mechanically relieves the nerve compression.
- Pain may start proximally or distally but is rarely cramping in sensation.
- Patients frequently have both PAD and neurogenic claudication.

Cystic Adventitial Disease

- Consider this in young patients, especially males, with classic claudication and no other risk factors.

Popliteal Artery Entrapment

- Passive and active plantar flexion and dorsiflexion of the foot often result in a loss of pulse or Doppler signal.
- Both the dorsalis pedis and posterior tibial pulses should be examined.

Fibromuscular Dysplasia

- Consider this in a young woman with hypertension or acute onset of neck pain (carotidynia) with a carotid bruit.

Thromboangiitis Obliterans

- Consider this in men and women younger than 40 years with a history of ongoing or recent tobacco use.
- Ischemic ulceration of the upper or lower extremity with extreme pain is common.

- Cannabis has been reported to result in a similar disease even in non-tobacco smokers.

Takayasu Arteritis

- This should be considered in loss of pulses, discrepant blood pressures, or arm (less often leg) claudication in a young woman.
- Preceding history of malaise, fatigue, or viral syndrome is common.

Iliac Endofibrosis

- Functional testing should use cycling, not walking or running, as the stressor.

Retroperitoneal Fibrosis

- If affecting the aorta, the resting or post-exercise ABI can be decreased.
- The inferior vena cava may be affected, leading to a history of venous claudication or edema.

Embolism

- "Blue toe syndrome" is common with acute embolism after catheterization.
- This is commonly associated with fixed livedo.
- Findings on the plantar surface are best seen with elevation and may be present for months.

Venous Claudication

- A bursting or heavy feeling in the limb may occur after exercise if mild, during exercise if severe.
- Relief comes with elevation.
- Pulse examination is normal; varicose veins may be mild.

Peripheral Neuropathy

- Typical description is burning, jabbing, "pins and needles," numbness, or walking on marbles.
- It may be worse at night.
- Patients frequently have both PAD and peripheral neuropathy.

Questions

1. Which of the following best describes discomfort due to arterial insufficiency?
   a. Above the level of arterial occlusion or stenosis
   b. Within a joint upon weight bearing
   c. Within a muscle group
   d. Occurring at a shorter distance when walking on uneven surfaces or up a grade

2. Which of the following is true of pseudoclaudication?
   a. Discomfort is relieved by standing upright.
   b. Walking with a shopping cart is easier than without.
   c. It seldom involves hip or back discomfort.
   d. Patients seldom have PAD.

3. Which of the following is not suggestive of atheroembolism after coronary catheterization?
   a. Multiple blue toes on the side of the catheterization only
   b. Multiple blue toes on both feet
   c. Livedo reticularis that does not change with warming over the dorsal and plantar surfaces of the feet
   d. Raynaud syndrome with blue fingers and toes that resolves with warming

4. Which of the following is not a common site of an ischemic wound?
   a. The anterior shin
   b. The finger tips
   c. Between the toes
   d. The heel

5. A 70-year-old obese man presents with hypertension and a history of tobacco use. His body mass index is 38, and his waistline is 44 inches. Which of the following physical findings is most suggestive of an abdominal aortic aneurysm?
   a. A bruit over the umbilicus
   b. A wide, bounding pulse at the right popliteal artery with no pulses at the left popliteal, posterior tibial, or dorsalis pedis arteries
   c. Bilateral bruits at the femoral arteries with blue toes bilaterally
   d. A diastolic murmur of aortic insufficiency

Suggested Readings

Juergens JL, Spittell JA Jr, Fairbairn JF II, editors. Peripheral vascular diseases/Allen-Barker-Hines. 5th ed. Philadelphia: WB Saunders Company; 1980.

Rutherford RB, editor. Vascular surgery. 5th ed. Philadelphia: WB Saunders Company; 2000.

Young JR, Olin JW, Bartholomew JR, editors. Peripheral vascular diseases. 2nd ed. St. Louis (MO): Mosby; 1996.

13 Lower Extremity Peripheral Arterial Disease: Natural History, Epidemiology, and Prognosis

Mary M. McDermott, MD

Lower extremity peripheral arterial disease (PAD) affects 10% to 15% of community-dwelling older men and women. PAD affects 25% to 30% of men and women aged 50 years and older in primary care medical practices. PAD is likely to become even more common as the population survives longer with chronic disease. Intermittent claudication is the most classic symptom of PAD. However, many persons with PAD are asymptomatic or have exertional leg symptoms that are not typical of intermittent claudication. Thus, diagnosing PAD often requires screening with the ankle-brachial index (ABI), a non-invasive measure of the presence and severity of PAD. Clinicians should consider screening high-risk patients for PAD with the ABI.

Intermittent Claudication

The original Rose intermittent claudication questionnaire was developed in 1962 by epidemiologist Geoffrey Rose. The questionnaire was designed to assess the incidence and prevalence of intermittent claudication in large epidemiologic studies. Classic Rose intermittent claudication is defined as exertional calf pain that does not begin when at rest, does not resolve during walking, causes a patient to stop walking, and resolves within 10 minutes of rest (Table 13.1). Thus, classic symptoms of leg ischemia are comparable to classic symptoms of coronary ischemia (i.e., typical angina).

Symptoms of intermittent claudication are similar to symptoms of spinal stenosis, which is also associated with exertional leg discomfort relieved with rest in older patients. However, onset of spinal stenosis symptoms during walking can come and go or occur at variable walking distances. In contrast, intermittent claudication symptoms typically occur consistently at the same distance after onset of walking.

Table 13.1 Symptoms of Classic Intermittent Claudication

Calf pain caused by exertion that:
- Does not occur at rest
- Does not resolve during walking
- Stops the patient from continued walking
- Resolves within 10 minutes of rest

The incidence of classic Rose intermittent claudication in the Framingham Study was 5.3 per 1,000 among men aged 55 to 64 years and 5.4 per 1,000 among women aged 65 to 74 years. In other epidemiologic studies of community-dwelling men and women, the prevalence of intermittent claudication has typically ranged from 1% to 5% among patients aged 50 years and older, with higher prevalences observed among older populations. In addition to older age, risk factors for intermittent claudication generally are similar to those for PAD and include cigarette smoking, diabetes mellitus, hypertension, and hyperlipidemia.

The sensitivity of the Rose claudication questionnaire for PAD is low. Only 10% to 30% of patients with PAD have classic symptoms of intermittent claudication. Modifications of the original Rose claudication questionnaire have been developed in an effort to increase its sensitivity for PAD. For example, some patients with PAD have exertional leg symptoms that resolve during walking. The ABI is a much more sensitive measure of PAD than claudication questionnaires.

- Intermittent claudication is the most classic manifestation of PAD
- The prevalence of intermittent claudication is 1%-5% among community-dwelling men and women aged 50 years and older
- Risk factors for intermittent claudication include cigarette smoking, diabetes mellitus, hyperlipidemia, and hypertension

- The sensitivity of the Rose claudication questionnaire for PAD is approximately 10%-30%
- In contrast to spinal stenosis, onset of symptoms of claudication occur consistently at the same threshold of walking distance

Spectrum of Leg Symptoms in PAD

As described above, the Rose claudication questionnaire is relatively insensitive to the presence of PAD. Among persons with an ABI less than 0.90, the prevalence of classic symptoms of intermittent claudication ranges from 10% to 30%. The prevalence of asymptomatic PAD (defined as PAD without exertional leg symptoms) is 25% to 60%. However, a substantial proportion of patients with asymptomatic PAD have development of exertional leg symptoms during a 6-minute walk test, which suggests that for some patients, lack of physical activity contributes to the absence of exertional leg symptoms.

Populations with more severe PAD and patients with clinically recognized PAD have a higher percentage of intermittent claudication symptoms and a lower prevalence of asymptomatic PAD. In addition, patients with exertional leg symptoms other than intermittent claudication are more likely to have comorbid diseases such as lower extremity arthritis or spinal disk disease. Thus, comorbid conditions in elderly patients with PAD can contribute to exertional leg symptoms and make ischemic leg symptoms more difficult to recognize. Table 13.2 summarizes the prevalence of specific leg symptom categories in defined populations of patients with PAD.

- Among patients with PAD, 25%-60% are asymptomatic
- Classic intermittent claudication symptoms are more common in patients with severe PAD and with clinically recognized PAD
- Comorbid diseases contribute to atypical exertional leg symptoms in persons with PAD

ABI as a Measure of Presence and Severity of PAD

The ABI is calculated from Doppler-recorded systolic pressures in the ankle and the brachial arteries. The ABI is calculated as the ankle systolic pressure divided by the brachial artery pressure. Normally, systolic pressures increase with increasing distance from the heart. Thus, in a patient without lower extremity atherosclerosis, the ankle systolic pressure is higher than the arm systolic pressure. In the presence of PAD, the pressures at the ankle decrease. If the ankle pressure is at least 10% lower than the brachial pressure the ABI is less than 0.90, and this finding is highly sensitive and specific for the presence of PAD.

Among community-dwelling older men and women (65 years or older), the prevalence of PAD as measured by an ABI of less than 0.90 is approximately 10% to 15%. The prevalence of PAD increases significantly with older age. In the NHANES (National Health and Nutrition Examination Survey) study, the prevalence of PAD, defined by ABI less than 0.90, was approximately 1% among persons aged 40 to 49 years and 14% among those aged 70 years and older. Prevalences of low ABI values are higher in medical practice settings. In the PARTNERS (PAD Awareness, Risk, and Treatment: New Resources for Survival) study of nearly 7,000 adult patients of general medical practices across the United States, the prevalence of PAD among at-risk patients was 29%. Table 13.3 summarizes the prevalence of PAD in defined populations.

Although an ABI less than 0.90 is typically the threshold for diagnosing PAD, recent data show that patients with ABIs of 0.90 to 1.10 have an increased prevalence of subclinical atherosclerosis compared with patients with ABI values between 1.10 and 1.30. Mortality rates are also

Table 13.2 Prevalence of Specific Leg Symptom Categories in Patients With Lower Extremity PAD*

	Study†		
Symptom	Cardiovascular Health Study‡	PARTNERS§ Study (previous PAD diagnosis)	PARTNERS Study (new PAD diagnosis)
Classic intermittent claudication	9	13	5.5
Atypical exertional leg symptoms	32	61	46.5
Asymptomatic	59	26	48

PAD, peripheral arterial disease.
*PAD was defined as an ankle-brachial index <0.90.
†Values are percentage of patients with the symptom.
‡The Cardiovascular Health Study was a study of community-dwelling men and women aged 65 years and older.
§PARTNERS (PAD Awareness, Risk, and Treatment: New Resources for Survival) was a study of men and women aged 50 years and older identified from general medical practices.

Table 13.3 Prevalence of PAD in Defined Populations

Study	Age range, y	Population description	Prevalence of ABI <0.90, %*
NHANES	≥40	Representative sample of U.S. population	4.5
CHS	≥65	Community-dwelling men and women	12
PARTNERS	≥50	Men and women in primary care settings who were either aged ≥70 years or aged 50-69 years with history of diabetes mellitus or smoking	29
MESA	45-84	Community-dwelling men and women without clinically evident atherosclerotic disease	3.7

ABI, ankle-brachial index; CHS, Cardiovascular Health Study; MESA, Multi-Ethnic Study of Atherosclerosis; NHANES, National Health and Nutrition Examination Survey; PAD, peripheral arterial disease; PARTNERS, PAD Awareness, Risk, and Treatment: New Resources for Survival.
*ABI <0.90 is considered 95% sensitive and 99% specific for PAD.

higher in patients with PAD and an ABI of 0.90 to 1.10 than in those with ABIs of 1.10 to 1.40. Thus, ABI levels between 0.90 and 1.10 appear to indicate mild or subclinical PAD.

Among patients with PAD, lower ABI values indicate more severe disease. Thus, an ABI less than 0.40 indicates severe PAD whereas ABI values of 0.70 to 0.90 indicate relatively mild PAD.

- An ABI <0.90 is highly sensitive and specific for the presence of PAD
- Among community-dwelling older men and women, the prevalence of PAD is approximately 10%-15%
- The prevalence of PAD increases markedly with older age
- The prevalence of PAD is 25%-30% among high-risk persons identified from general medical practices

Risk Factors for Lower Extremity PAD

Traditional atherosclerotic disease risk factors (older age, hyperlipidemia, diabetes mellitus, cigarette smoking, and hypertension) are also risk factors for PAD. However, cigarette smoking and diabetes are particularly strong risk factors for PAD; it is approximately twice as common among patients with diabetes mellitus than those without and is approximately four times more common among current cigarette smokers than among non-smokers. Cigarette smoking appears to be more strongly associated with PAD than with coronary artery disease (CAD), whereas hyperlipidemia is a stronger risk factor for CAD than for PAD. Increasing age is also a risk factor for PAD. Although the overall prevalence of a low ABI was 12% among men and women aged 65 years and older participating in the Cardiovascular Health Study (CHS), the prevalence of low ABI was approximately 20% in those aged 75 to 79 years, 25% in those aged 80 to 84 years, and 30% in those aged 85 years and older.

No substantial difference is apparent in the prevalence of PAD between men and women. This has been shown in multiple cohorts, including the NHANES, MESA (Multi-Ethnic Study of Atherosclerosis), and the CHS. However, black Americans have an increased prevalence of intermittent claudication compared with whites. For example, in the NHANES study, non-Hispanic blacks had a 2.4-fold increased prevalence of PAD compared with whites, adjusting for differences in atherosclerotic risk factors between whites and blacks.

- Diabetes mellitus and cigarette smoking are particularly important risk factors for PAD
- The prevalence of PAD is approximately equal among men and women
- PAD prevalence is increased among black Americans

Hyperhomocysteinemia and PAD

Hyperhomocysteinemia is associated independently with an increased prevalence of atherosclerosis. Approximately 30% of patients with premature onset of PAD have increased levels of homocysteine. Increased levels of homocysteine may be more important for the development of PAD than for CAD. In a 1995 meta-analysis, the odds ratio for PAD associated with elevated homocysteine was 6.8. In comparison, odds ratios for CAD associated with elevated homocysteine levels were 1.6 for men and 1.8 for women.

- Elevated levels of homocysteine are associated with an increased prevalence of PAD
- Elevated levels of homocysteine may be more strongly associated with PAD than with CAD

Renal Disease and Lower Extremity PAD

Patients with renal disease have an increased prevalence of PAD compared with those without renal disease. PAD prevalence is increased among patients with end-stage renal disease and with chronic renal insufficiency. The relationship between PAD and renal disease is independent of diabetes mellitus, hypertension, race, and age. The mechanism of the association between PAD and renal disease is unclear, but hyperhomocysteinemia and inflammation are potential links between PAD and chronic renal disease. Among patients with PAD, those with renal disease have an increased prevalence of critical limb ischemia and mortality. Progressively lower creatinine clearance levels are associated with a higher prevalence of critical limb ischemia and a greater risk of total mortality.

- Patients with renal disease have an increased prevalence of PAD
- Among patients with PAD, progressively poorer renal function is associated with a higher prevalence of critical limb ischemia
- Among patients with PAD, lower renal function is associated with increased mortality

Inflammation and PAD

Inflammation is an integral component of atherosclerosis. Patients with PAD have increased levels of inflammatory blood factors such as high-sensitivity C-reactive protein (hsCRP) and interleukin-6. The converse is also true: increased levels of inflammatory blood factors (e.g., hsCRP and soluble intracellular adhesion molecule-1 [ICAM-1]) are associated with an increased incidence of PAD. Increased levels of inflammation in patients with PAD may reflect an increased burden of atherosclerosis, because patients without PAD but with a history of CAD have increased levels of inflammatory markers compared with patients without atherosclerosis. In addition, lower levels of physical activity are associated with increased levels of inflammation, and patients with PAD have significantly reduced physical activity levels versus those without PAD.

Among persons with PAD who undergo lower extremity revascularization, increased levels of hsCRP are associated with increased rates of cardiovascular events and restenosis. At least four studies have shown associations between higher baseline hsCRP levels and increased rates of restenosis after lower extremity angioplasty in persons with PAD. Inflammation promotes plaque rupture, vascular smooth muscle proliferation, and constrictive neointima formation. These associations may mediate relationships between increased hsCRP and restenosis after lower extremity angioplasty.

Increased levels of inflammation in patients with PAD also possibly contribute to PAD-associated functional impairment, because inflammatory states characterized by increased circulating levels of inflammatory cytokines appear to contribute to sarcopenia, an age-related decrease in muscle strength and mass. Reduced muscle strength and mass in turn contribute to functional impairment. Consistent with these hypotheses, a previous study showed that higher levels of hsCRP in PAD are associated with increased functional impairment. In addition, higher levels of inflammation, measured by several inflammatory blood markers, are associated with greater functional decline in persons with PAD.

- Patients with PAD have increased levels of inflammatory markers compared with those without PAD
- Higher levels of hsCRP and ICAM-1 are associated with an increased incidence of PAD
- Increased levels of inflammation in patients with PAD are associated with increased functional impairment
- Increased levels of hsCRP are associated with increased mortality and myocardial infarction after lower extremity revascularization
- Increased levels of hsCRP are associated with increased rates of restenosis after lower extremity angioplasty

Coexistence of CAD and Cerebrovascular Disease With PAD

Most patients with PAD have concomitant CAD. Between 1978 and 1981, all patients presenting to the Cleveland Clinic for elective vascular surgery (*N*=381) underwent coronary angiography. Only 10% of these patients had normal coronary arteries. Twenty-eight percent had severe three-vessel CAD that either required coronary revascularization or was inoperable. Similarly, PAD is more prevalent among those with clinically evident CAD than those without CAD. In one study, 33% of patients with CAD had concomitant PAD. Cerebrovascular disease is also prevalent among patients with PAD; carotid artery duplex studies show significant atherosclerosis in 25% to 50%. However, clinically evident CAD could be more common than clinically evident cerebrovascular disease.

- CAD and cerebrovascular disease frequently coexist with PAD
- Among patients with PAD, clinically evident CAD could be more common than clinically evident cerebrovascular disease

Cardiovascular Morbidity and Mortality in Patients With PAD

Patients with PAD have an increased risk (2.0- to 4.0-fold) of mortality compared with persons without. The association between PAD and increased cardiovascular death is observed in patients with and without classic symptoms of intermittent claudication. During 5 years of follow-up, the risk of mortality in patients with PAD is approximately 25%. Most of the excess risk of death in PAD is due to cardiovascular death (≈75% of deaths).

Risk factors for morbidity and mortality among patients with PAD include cigarette smoking, diabetes mellitus, and hypertension. Increased levels of inflammation, as measured by an increased leukocyte count or increased fibrinogen, are also associated with an increased risk of mortality in patients with PAD. However, the association between PAD and cardiovascular mortality is maintained even after adjustment for cigarette smoking, diabetes mellitus, hypertension, and other cardiovascular disease risk factors. Thus, there are currently other unidentified factors linking PAD with an increased risk of cardiovascular mortality. Intensive treatment of cardiovascular disease risk factors is important for preventing cardiovascular events in those with PAD.

- Patients with PAD have an increased risk of mortality from cardiovascular disease
- Most deaths in patients with PAD are secondary to cardiovascular causes
- Associations between PAD and cardiovascular mortality are maintained after accounting for the increased prevalence of diabetes mellitus, smoking, older age, and other cardiovascular disease risk factors
- Among patients with PAD, diabetes mellitus, smoking, hypertension, and inflammation are associated with increased risk of cardiovascular disease mortality

Associations Between ABI and Mortality

Consistent with the association between PAD and increased rates of cardiovascular events, persons with an ABI less than 0.90 have increased mortality compared with those with an ABI of 0.90 to 1.40. In addition, among patients with established PAD, lower ABI values are predictive of greater mortality. Thus, the ABI can be used as a prognostic tool to identify patients at increased risk of death.

Persons with an ABI of greater than 1.40 also have an increased risk of cardiovascular disease mortality compared with those with an ABI between 0.90 and 1.40. An ABI greater than 1.40 indicates non-compressible lower extremity arteries, which artificially elevate the ABI. Persons with such an elevated ABI have an increased prevalence of diabetes mellitus and renal disease and are typically older than those without non-compressible lower extremity arteries. Thus, both low and high levels of ABI are associated with an increased risk of total mortality. The ABI is a non-invasive, office screening tool that can identify patients who are at risk of increased cardiovascular morbidity and mortality.

- Among persons with PAD, lower ABI values (<0.30) indicate increased risk of mortality compared with higher ABI levels
- Elevated ABI values (>1.40) are typically observed in persons with history of renal disease or diabetes mellitus
- ABI values greater than 1.40 are also associated with increased mortality compared with normal ABI levels

Natural History of Lower Extremity PAD

In most people with PAD, critical limb ischemia does not develop, and they do not require amputation. Traditionally, among patients with intermittent claudication, less than 5% require amputation, and 75% report stabilization or improvement of their claudication symptoms over a 5-year period. Risk factors for critical limb ischemia or amputation among patients with intermittent claudication include cigarette smoking (smokers are more likely to require lower extremity revascularization or amputation) and diabetes mellitus (amputation and critical limb ischemia are more likely). Increasing restrictions on physical activity levels may explain the lack of symptom progression in most patients with PAD and claudication. For example, many patients with asymptomatic PAD have exertional leg symptoms during the 6-minute walk test, suggesting that leg symptoms reported by patients with PAD are influenced by the patient's physical activity level.

- Over 5 years of follow-up, most PAD patients with intermittent claudication report stabilization or improvement of claudication symptoms
- Improvement or stabilization of claudication in PAD patients may reflect increasingly restricted physical activity
- Over 5 years of follow-up, less than 5% of patients with PAD require amputation
- Diabetes mellitus and cigarette smoking are associated with an increased risk of requiring lower extremity revascularization or amputation

Functional Decline in Patients With PAD

Observational studies from the 1960s and 1970s suggested that the natural history of lower extremity disease in patients with PAD and intermittent claudication was benign because of the relatively small proportion of patients reporting symptomatic worsening over 5 to 10 years of follow-up. More recent data indicate that patients with PAD have greater annual decline in objective measures of functional performance at 2-year follow-up than those without PAD. Functional decline in patients with PAD appears to be greatest in measures of walking endurance, such as the 6-minute walk test. As described above, symptom stabilization or improvement in PAD patients with intermittent claudication could be due to progressively greater restriction in physical activity, thereby reducing leg symptoms caused by exertion.

The nature of leg symptoms reported by patients with PAD is associated with the degree of functional decline. For example, patients with exertional leg pain that sometimes begins at rest have increased rates of functional decline compared with other PAD patients. Marked functional decline is observed even in asymptomatic PAD patients compared with persons without PAD. Other patient characteristics associated with increased rates of functional decline in PAD include a body mass index greater than 30 kg/m^2, lack of walking exercise, history of pulmonary disease, and a history of spinal stenosis. Rates of functional decline among persons with PAD are similar between men and women and between blacks and whites. Although diabetes mellitus and cigarette smoking are associated with an increased risk of critical limb ischemia, these characteristics are not associated with increased rates of functional decline among persons with PAD.

- Stabilization or improvement in leg symptoms over time in patients with intermittent claudication appears to be due to progressive restriction in physical activity
- Patients with PAD have decreases in objectively measured lower extremity functioning at 2-year follow-up compared with persons without PAD
- Functional decline in patients with PAD appears to be greatest in measures of walking endurance
- Among patients with PAD, a body mass index greater than 30 kg/m^2, history of pulmonary disease, and history of spinal stenosis are associated with increased rates of functional decline
- Lack of walking exercise is associated with increased functional decline in patients with PAD
- Functional decline occurs even in PAD patients who are asymptomatic

Critical Limb Ischemia

Critical limb ischemia develops in approximately 1% of patients with claudication per year. Risk factors for development of critical limb ischemia are older age, cigarette smoking, and diabetes mellitus. Among cigarette smokers, risk increases with the number of cigarettes smoked per day. PAD patients with diabetes are approximately 10 times more likely to require amputation than those without. In addition, PAD patients with diabetes mellitus typically require amputation at younger ages than those without diabetes.

Patients with gangrene or ulcers are more likely to require lower extremity amputation than those with rest pain. The size and number of ulcers are less important determinants of amputation. Among patients with rest pain, ankle systolic pressure of less than 40 mm Hg is a risk factor for limb loss. However, ankle pressure is a less useful predictor of limb loss in patients with gangrene or ulcer.

- Critical limb ischemia develops in 1% of patients with PAD each year
- Among patients with PAD, risk factors for critical limb ischemia are diabetes and smoking
- Among patients with critical limb ischemia, those with gangrene or ulcers are more likely to undergo amputation than those with rest pain
- Among PAD patients with rest pain, ankle systolic pressure less than 40 mm Hg is an important predictor of limb loss

Questions

1. What are the most important risk factor(s) for PAD?
   - **a.** High levels of low-density lipoprotein (LDL)
   - **b.** Diabetes mellitus
   - **c.** Obesity
   - **d.** Cigarette smoking
   - **e.** Both diabetes mellitus and cigarette smoking

2. What is the most appropriate range of relative risk for cardiovascular mortality among patients with lower extremity PAD compared with those without PAD?
   - **a.** 1.5 to 2.5
   - **b.** 3.0 to 4.0
   - **c.** 5.0 to 6.0
   - **d.** 10.0 to 12.0

3. What is the most correct range for the sensitivity of intermittent claudication symptoms for the presence of lower extremity PAD?
   - **a.** 1% to 5%
   - **b.** 5% to 10%
   - **c.** 10% to 25%
   - **d.** 25% to 50%

4. What is the strongest risk factor for critical limb ischemia among patients with PAD?
   - **a.** Hypertension
   - **b.** Hyperlipidemia
   - **c.** Hyperhomocysteinemia
   - **d.** Cigarette smoking

5. Which of the following patients is least likely to undergo amputation?

a. A patient with PAD and multiple ischemic ulcers
b. A patient with PAD and rest pain
c. A patient with PAD and gangrene
d. A patient with PAD and an ischemic ulcer who does not smoke cigarettes

Suggested Readings

Boushey CJ, Beresford SA, Omenn GS, et al. A quantitative assessment of plasma homocysteine as a risk factor for vascular disease: probable benefits of increasing folic acid intakes. JAMA. 1995;274:1049-57.

Criqui MH, Fronek A, Klauber MR, et al. The sensitivity, specificity, and predictive value of traditional clinical evaluation of peripheral arterial disease: results from noninvasive testing in a defined population. Circulation. 1985;71:516-22.

Criqui MH, Langer RD, Fronek A, et al. Mortality over a period of 10 years in patients with peripheral arterial disease. N Engl J Med. 1992;326:381-6.

Hertzer NR, Beven EG, Young JR, et al. Coronary artery disease in peripheral vascular patients: a classification of 1000 coronary angiograms and results of surgical management. Ann Surg. 1984;199:223-33.

Hirsch AT, Criqui MH, Treat-Jacobson D, et al. Peripheral arterial disease detection, awareness, and treatment in primary care. JAMA. 2001;286:1317-24.

McDermott MM, Liu K, Greenland P, et al. Functional decline in peripheral arterial disease: associations with the ankle brachial index and leg symptoms. JAMA. 2004;292:453-61.

O'Hare AM, Glidden DV, Fox CS, et al. High prevalence of peripheral arterial disease in persons with renal insufficiency: results from the National Health and Nutrition Examination Survey 1999-2000. Circulation. 2004 Jan 27;109:320-3. Epub 2004 Jan 19.

Resnick HE, Lindsay RS, McDermott MM, et al. Relationship of high and low ankle brachial index to all-cause and cardiovascular disease mortality: the Strong Heart Study. Circulation. 2004;109:733-9.

Selvin E, Erlinger TP. Prevalence of and risk factors for peripheral arterial disease in the United States: results from the National Health and Nutrition Examination Survey, 1999-2000. Circulation. 2004 Aug 10;110:738-43. Epub 2004 Jul 19.

14 Medical Treatment of Peripheral Arterial Disease

William R. Hiatt, MD

Introduction

Peripheral arterial disease (PAD) of the lower extremities is one of the major manifestations of systemic atherosclerosis. The age-adjusted prevalence of PAD is approximately 12% (29% in a primary care clinic population), and the disorder affects men and women equally. The risk of PAD increases two- to threefold for every 10-year increase in age after 40 years and is highly associated with cardiovascular risk factors such as cigarette smoking, diabetes mellitus, hyperlipidemia, and hypertension. The two most important of these risk factors are diabetes mellitus and smoking, each being associated with a three- to fourfold increase in the risk for PAD.

PAD is highly associated with coronary and carotid artery diseases, which put these patients at a substantially increased risk of myocardial infarction, ischemic stroke, and vascular death. In patients with PAD, the adjusted all-cause mortality risk is increased threefold and cardiovascular mortality risk is increased sixfold. These risks are approximately equal in men and women and remain elevated even if the patient has no prior clinical evidence of cardiovascular disease. Therefore, a primary goal of therapy for PAD is to aggressively manage cardiovascular risk factors to prevent the progression of lower extremity arterial disease and to decrease the risk of ischemic events.

- Age-adjusted incidence of PAD is 12%, 29% in a primary care clinic population
- Risk of PAD increases two- to threefold for every 10-year increase in age after 40 years
- Associated risk factors:
  - Smoking: three- to fourfold increased risk for PAD
  - Diabetes mellitus: three- to fourfold increased risk for PAD
  - Hyperlipidemia
  - Hypertension
- PAD is highly associated with critical coronary and carotid artery disease
- For patients with PAD, all-cause mortality risk is increased threefold and cardiovascular mortality risk is increased sixfold

The limb manifestations of PAD fall mainly into the categories of chronic stable claudication, critical leg ischemia, and, rarely, acute limb ischemia. In a patient with claudication, the principal symptomatic medical treatments include supervised exercise therapy and the selected use of drugs to improve exercise tolerance and walking distance. Patients with critical leg ischemia require restoration of blood flow to heal wounds, relieve ischemic pain, and prevent limb loss.

Pharmacologic Modification of Ischemic Risk

A primary goal of therapy for PAD is to reduce cardiovascular risk factors. Pharmacologic therapy can be used to decrease the risk of ischemic events due to many of these risk factors.

Cigarette Smoking

Smoking cessation is a cornerstone of the management of PAD. Although advice to stop smoking is associated with modest quit rates, the combination of physician recommendation, a smoking cessation program, and nicotine replacement has shown benefit. With this intervention, treated subjects had a 5-year quit rate of 22% (compared with only 5% for usual care) and a survival advantage on long-term follow-up. Pharmacologic therapy can assist in smoking cessation, including nicotine replacement, antidepressant drug therapy, and varenicline (a partial nicotinic cholinergic receptor agonist and antagonist). Nicotine replacement can be achieved with a patch, gum, or spray and has been shown to increase quit rates. Certain classes of antidepressant drugs facilitate quitting in smokers who are also depressed, but the drug bupropion is effective in all smokers. Thus, a practical approach would be to combine behavior modification, nicotine replacement or varenicline therapy, and bupropion to achieve the best quit rates.

Although smoking cessation is beneficial for the treatment of PAD, its role in treating the symptoms of claudication is not as clear; studies have not consistently shown that smoking cessation is associated with improved walking distance. Therefore, patients should be encouraged to stop smoking primarily to decrease their systemic risk and their risk of progression to amputation, but they should not be promised improved symptoms immediately upon cessation.

Hyperlipidemia

Independent risk factors for PAD include increased levels of total cholesterol, low-density lipoprotein (LDL) cholesterol, triglycerides, and lipoprotein (a). Increases in high-density lipoprotein (HDL) cholesterol and apolipoprotein A1 are protective against PAD. Current recommendations for the management of lipid disorders in PAD are to achieve an LDL cholesterol level of less than 100 mg/dL and to modulate the increased triglyceride and low HDL pattern. However, these recommendations regarding PAD are based on small trials that focused on surrogate end points and extrapolations from large randomized trials in patients with coronary artery disease. Subgroup analyses of these large trials in patients with coronary artery disease also showed that aggressive lipid lowering was associated with a decreased risk of claudication or an absent femoral pulse.

Until recently, no direct evidence has shown mortality benefits for treating PAD with statin drugs. Data from the Heart Protection Study (HPS) help in understanding the importance of lowering LDL cholesterol levels in this population. The study enrolled more than 20,500 subjects at high risk for cardiovascular events, including 6,748 patients with PAD. Patients were randomly assigned (using a 2×2 factorial design) to receive simvastatin (40 mg), antioxidant vitamins (vitamin E, vitamin C, and β-carotene), a combination of the treatments, or placebo. Total follow-up in the study was 5 years.

In the HPS, simvastatin was associated with decreases in total mortality (12%), vascular mortality (17%), coronary events (24%), all strokes (27%), and non-coronary revascularizations (16%). Similar results were obtained in the PAD subgroup whether the patient had evidence of coronary disease at baseline or not. Furthermore, statin therapy was associated with benefit regardless of cholesterol value. In contrast, no benefit (or harm) was observed with the use of antioxidant vitamins to prevent ischemic events. Thus, the study showed that in patients with PAD (even in the absence of prior myocardial infarction or stroke), aggressive LDL lowering was associated with a marked decrease in cardiovascular events (myocardial infarction, stroke, and vascular death).

The HPS was the first large, randomized trial of statin therapy to show that aggressive lipid modification can improve outcomes in the PAD population by using a target LDL cholesterol level of less than 100 mg/dL. Patients with PAD typically also have disorders of HDL and triglyceride metabolism. The combination of extended-release niacin and a statin drug has favorable effects on levels of HDL cholesterol, LDL cholesterol, triglycerides, and lipoprotein (a). Clinical studies of this combination therapy showed slowing of the progression of atherosclerosis and suggested a mortality benefit.

Hypertension

Patients with PAD are in a high-risk group for cardiovascular events, and the treatment goal for these patients should be to decrease blood pressure to 130/80 mm Hg or less. β-Adrenergic receptor blocking drugs (β-blockers) previously were considered to be contraindicated in patients with PAD because of the possibility of worsening claudication symptoms. However, this concern has not been borne out by randomized trials. Thus, β-blockers can be used in patients with claudication. In particular, patients with PAD who have concomitant coronary disease and previous myocardial infarction have additional cardioprotection with β-blockers. Therefore, this should be considered an important class of drugs for these patients.

The angiotensin-converting enzyme (ACE) inhibitors have also shown benefit beyond blood pressure lowering in high-risk groups. Specific results from the HOPE (Heart Outcomes Prevention Evaluation) study of 4,046 patients with PAD showed a 22% reduction of risk in patients randomly assigned to receive ramipril compared with those receiving placebo. This reduction was independent of the lowering of blood pressure. On the basis of this finding, the US Food and Drug Administration (FDA) has now approved ramipril for its cardioprotective benefits in patients at high cardiovascular risk, including those with PAD. Thus, ACE inhibitors would certainly be recommended for these patients.

Diabetes Mellitus

Although diabetes mellitus is highly associated with peripheral atherosclerosis, the degree of glycemic control does not predict the severity of peripheral atherosclerosis. Studies have shown that the glycoprotein level is highly associated with PAD; every 1% increase in glycoprotein is associated with a 26% increase in PAD risk. These observations suggest that diabetes mellitus is a critical risk factor for PAD.

Several studies of both type 1 and type 2 diabetes mellitus have shown that aggressive blood sugar lowering can prevent microvascular complications (particularly retinopathy) but not cardiovascular disease, including PAD. Thus, although the current American Diabetes Association–recommended goal for treatment of diabetes is a hemoglobin A_{1c} level of 7% or less, it is unclear whether achieving this goal protects the peripheral circulation.

Hyperhomocysteinemia

Elevated plasma homocysteine levels are an independent risk factor for PAD. Although supplementation with B vitamins can decrease homocysteine levels, evidence of this treatment preventing cardiovascular events is lacking.

Inflammation

Markers of inflammation have been associated with the development of atherosclerosis and cardiovascular events. In particular, C-reactive protein (CRP) is independently associated with PAD, even in patients with normal lipid levels. In the Physicians' Health Study, an elevated CRP level was a risk factor for the development of symptomatic PAD and also a risk for peripheral revascularization. The measurement of CRP may also guide lipid therapy in that statin drugs lower CRP levels, which may be one reason for the benefits of these drugs. Recent studies have shown that monitoring CRP levels in patients with cardiovascular disease treated with statins independently predicts outcomes.

Hypercoagulable States

Alterations in coagulation are commonly associated with the development of venous thrombosis and thromboembolism. However, except for those associated with abnormal homocysteine metabolism, hypercoagulable states have been less well evaluated in patients with PAD. In one study, presence of the lupus anticoagulant and anticardiolipin antibodies was associated with peripheral atherosclerosis. Markers of platelet activation, such as increases in β-thromboglobulin levels, are also associated with PAD.

Antiplatelet drug therapy has been evaluated in patients with PAD. Aspirin is a well-recognized antiplatelet drug that has clear benefits in patients with cardiovascular diseases. Numerous publications from the Antithrombotic Trialists' Collaboration have concluded that patients with cardiovascular disease have a 25% odds reduction for subsequent cardiovascular events with the use of aspirin. A recent meta-analysis also clearly showed that low-dose aspirin (75-160 mg) is protective against cardiovascular events and is probably safer than higher doses of aspirin in terms of gastrointestinal tract bleeding. Thus, current recommendations strongly favor the use of aspirin at a dose of 81 mg in patients with cardiovascular diseases.

Remarkably, specific studies using aspirin in the PAD population have not shown a statistically significant decrease in cardiovascular events. When PAD data were combined from trials using not only aspirin but also more effective agents such as clopidogrel and picotamide, a significant 23% decrease in the odds of ischemic events was observed. Thus, although antiplatelet drugs are clearly indicated in the overall management of PAD, aspirin does not have FDA approval in this patient population.

In addition to aspirin, the thienopyridines are an important class of antiplatelet agents that has been well studied in patients with cardiovascular disease. Ticlopidine has been evaluated in several trials in patients with PAD; it has been shown to decrease the risk of myocardial infarction, stroke, and vascular death. However, the clinical usefulness of ticlopidine is limited by unacceptable adverse effects such as neutropenia and thrombocytopenia. In contrast, clopidogrel was studied in the CAPRIE (Clopidogrel Versus Aspirin in Patients at Risk of Ischaemic Events) trial and was shown to be highly effective in the PAD population. The overall benefit in this group was a 24% risk reduction over the use of aspirin, with an acceptable safety profile and only rare reports of thrombotic thrombocytopenic purpura. Thus, current consensus documents recommend clopidogrel as an important agent in the PAD population, which may be more effective than aspirin alone.

Recent publications regarding patients with acute coronary syndrome suggest that combination therapy with aspirin and clopidogrel is more effective than aspirin alone but has a higher risk of major bleeding. Whether combination therapy is more effective in the PAD population is not known.

Systemic Therapy for PAD

- Complete smoking cessation
- Blood pressure target of <130/80 mm Hg
- LDL cholesterol target of <100 mg/dL
- In patients with diabetes mellitus, a hemoglobin A_{1c} target of <7.0%

- Antiplatelet therapy for all patients with PAD: aspirin or clopidogrel for those with other forms of cardiovascular disease, clopidogrel for those without other forms of cardiovascular disease

Treatment of Lower Extremity Symptoms

Exercise Rehabilitation for Claudication

The use of a formal exercise program to treat claudication is the best studied and most effective non-surgical therapy. Numerous types of exercise programs have been devised, but the most successful are supervised programs in a cardiac rehabilitation environment that use repeated treadmill walking. The initial evaluation of the patient consists of a clinical assessment using several well-established questionnaires (e.g., Walking Impairment Questionnaire, Medical Outcomes SF-36). Patients should also undergo an exercise test to assess maximal claudication pain, which helps determine the initial training workload during the rehabilitation program. On completion of the exercise program, similar evaluations are performed to define improvements in treadmill walking distance and questionnaire end points.

A typical supervised exercise program lasts 60 minutes and is monitored by a skilled nurse or technician. Patients should be encouraged to walk primarily on a treadmill because this most closely reproduces walking in the community setting. The initial workload of the treadmill is set to a speed and grade that brings on claudication pain within 3 to 5 minutes. Patients walk at this work rate until claudication of moderate severity occurs. They then rest until the claudication abates and then resume exercise. Patients should be reassessed clinically every week as they are able to walk farther and farther at the chosen workload. The typical duration of an exercise program is 3 to 6 months. This intervention allows patients to walk 100% to 150% farther and improves quality of life. The mechanism of benefit for exercise training has been extensively reviewed.

Drug Therapy for Claudication

Vasodilators were an early class of agents used to treat claudication, but they have not been shown to have clinical efficacy. In 1984 pentoxifylline was approved for the treatment of claudication. In early controlled trials, the drug produced a 12% improvement in the maximal treadmill walking distance. A meta-analysis concluded that the drug produced modest increases over placebo in treadmill walking distance, but the overall clinical benefits were questionable.

Cilostazol is currently the most effective drug for claudication. Approved by the FDA in 1999, the primary action of cilostazol is to inhibit phosphodiesterase type 3, which results in vasodilation and inhibition of platelet aggregation, arterial thromboses, and vascular smooth muscle proliferation. A meta-analysis of six randomized, controlled trials showed an approximate 50% improvement in peak exercise performance compared with placebo, as well as improved quality of life. The most common adverse effects of cilostazol are headache, transient diarrhea, palpitations, and dizziness. Cilostazol should not be given to patients with claudication who also have congestive heart failure. Data from more than 2,700 patients treated for claudication with cilostazol (with up to 6 months' follow-up) have been evaluated. Total cardiovascular morbidity and all-cause mortality was similar for cilostazol (200 and 100 mg/d) and placebo (6.5%, 6.3%, and 7.7%, respectively). These data do not indicate an increased cardiovascular mortality risk with cilostazol. However, this drug still has an FDA black box warning stating that the drug should be avoided in patients with PAD who also have any clinical evidence of heart failure.

Treatment of Leg Symptoms

- Supervised exercise training recommended as first-line therapy
- Cilostazol is the only recommended claudication drug; it shows less benefit than exercise

Pharmacologic Issues With Revascularization

Revascularization may be necessary for patients who do not have an adequate response to exercise or drug therapy. However, after the limb has been revascularized there remains a role for medical therapy.

Good evidence is available that the use of antiplatelet drugs, particularly aspirin, prevents graft occlusion after peripheral vascular surgical procedures. In the Antithrombotic Trialists' Collaboration meta-analysis of 3,000 patients having peripheral artery procedures, the graft occlusion rate in the group receiving antiplatelet therapy (principally aspirin) was 16%, compared with 25% in the control group (P<.001). Similar to the findings for systemic risk reduction, low doses of aspirin (50-100 mg) were as effective as higher doses (900-1,000 mg).

Anticoagulation has also been recommended as an adjuvant to maintain surgical graft patency. The largest study of different treatment options was the Dutch Bypass Oral Anticoagulants or Aspirin Study, which compared aspirin with oral anticoagulation. The study included

2,690 patients undergoing infrainguinal bypass, half of whom were treated for claudication and half for critical leg ischemia; the distribution of graft composition (vein versus prosthetic material) was fairly even among the patients. The aspirin dose was 80 mg/d, and in patients randomly assigned to anticoagulation with warfarin, the international normalized ratio was maintained at 3.0 to 4.5. The primary end point of patency was equal between the groups after 21 months of follow-up. However, when the patients were divided into subgroups according to type of graft material, anticoagulation maintained vein graft patency better than aspirin but with a higher risk of bleeding complications. In contrast, aspirin maintained prosthetic graft patency better than anticoagulation. Although subgroup analyses should be interpreted with caution, these results suggest that patients receiving vein grafts should be preferentially treated with warfarin and those receiving prosthetic material, with aspirin.

In summary, antiplatelet therapy has a clear preventative role for patients undergoing revascularization. This treatment can decrease the risk of graft occlusion and systemic events such as myocardial infarction, stroke, and vascular death. Regarding the choice of antiplatelet drug, adequate trials have not been performed comparing aspirin, ticlopidine, and clopidogrel to determine which drug or combination of drugs is best for maintaining graft patency. In selecting between antiplatelet and anticoagulant therapy, aspirin may be favored for prosthetic grafts, and anticoagulation may be favored for vein grafts or in patients at higher risk for occlusion.

Conclusions

Although PAD is common, it is substantially under-recognized and undertreated. Given the systemic nature of atherosclerosis, all patients with PAD, whether they have a history of coronary artery disease or not, should be considered for secondary prevention strategies. This includes aggressive management of smoking, treatment of high LDL cholesterol (to <100 mg/dL), treatment of high blood pressure (to <130/80 mm Hg), and management of diabetes mellitus (to a glycohemoglobin level <7.0%). Drugs shown to have particular benefit in these patients include statins for LDL reduction, ACE inhibitors for blood pressure lowering, and β-blockers. In addition, all patients should be given an antiplatelet drug; clopidogrel shows more benefit than aspirin in the PAD population.

Once systemic risk has been adequately managed in PAD patients, those with symptomatic claudication should also be considered for further medical management. If an exercise program fails, the only approved drug with clinically relevant efficacy is cilostazol. A trial of this drug should be considered and continued for at least 3 months before a decision is made regarding efficacy. Cilostazol should be avoided in patients with heart failure. All patients undergoing revascularization should be treated with antiplatelet drugs to promote patency. Aspirin remains a mainstay of therapy, with newer agents or combinations of agents still under evaluation.

Questions

1. All patients with PAD should be treated with aggressive risk factor modification and antiplatelet therapies. Two approved drugs commonly used in this population are aspirin and clopidogrel. Which statement is true?
   a. Clopidogrel is more effective than aspirin in preventing cardiovascular events.
   b. Clopidogrel has similar efficacy to aspirin in preventing cardiovascular events.
   c. Aspirin is more effective than clopidogrel.

2. In a patient with PAD and diabetes mellitus, what is the optimal blood pressure?
   a. Less than 150/90 mm Hg
   b. Less than 140/90 mm Hg
   c. Less than 130/80 mm Hg
   d. Less than 125/75 mm Hg

3. In patients with PAD, what is the recommended target LDL cholesterol goal?
   a. Less than 130 mg/dL
   b. Less than 100 mg/dL
   c. Less than 70 mg/dL

4. A formal exercise program can improve treadmill exercise performance. In general, what is the expected degree of improvement in walking capacity on the treadmill in patients with claudication?
   a. 10%
   b. 50%
   c. 100%
   d. 1000%

5. Two drugs are approved in the United States for treatment of claudication: pentoxifylline and cilostazol. Which statement is true of cilostazol compared with pentoxifylline?
   a. It is less effective.
   b. It is similarly effective.
   c. It is more effective.

6. What is the expected percentage improvement in peak exercise performance in patients with claudication treated with cilostazol (compared with placebo)?
   a. 10%

b. 25%
c. 50%
d. 100%

7. Which drug(s) has(have) an FDA warning regarding use in patients with heart failure?
a. Cilostazol
b. Pentoxifylline
c. Both

Suggested Readings

Antithrombotic Trialists' Collaboration. Collaborative meta-analysis of randomised trials of antiplatelet therapy for prevention of death, myocardial infarction, and stroke in high risk patients. BMJ. 2002;324:71-86. Erratum in: BMJ. 2002;324:141.

CAPRIE Steering Committee. A randomised, blinded, trial of clopidogrel versus aspirin in patients at risk of ischaemic events (CAPRIE). Lancet. 1996;348:1329-39.

Criqui MH, Fronek A, Barrett-Connor E, et al. The prevalence of peripheral arterial disease in a defined population. Circulation. 1985;71:510-5.

Criqui MH, Langer RD, Fronek A, et al. Mortality over a period of 10 years in patients with peripheral arterial disease. N Engl J Med. 1992;326:381-6.

Dutch Bypass Oral Anticoagulants or Aspirin (BOA) Study Group. Efficacy of oral anticoagulants compared with aspirin after infrainguinal bypass surgery (The Dutch Bypass Oral Anticoagulants or Aspirin Study): a randomised trial. Lancet. 2000;355:346-51. Erratum in: Lancet. 2000;355:1104.

Gardner AW, Poehlman ET. Exercise rehabilitation programs for the treatment of claudication pain: a meta-analysis. JAMA. 1995;274:975-80.

Girolami B, Bernardi E, Prins MH, et al. Treatment of intermittent claudication with physical training, smoking cessation, pentoxifylline, or nafronyl: a meta-analysis. Arch Intern Med. 1999;159:337-45.

Heart Protection Study Collaborative Group. MRC/BHF Heart Protection Study of cholesterol lowering with simvastatin in 20,536 high-risk individuals: a randomised placebo-controlled trial. Lancet. 2002;360:7-22.

Hirsch AT, Criqui MH, Treat-Jacobson D, et al. Peripheral arterial disease detection, awareness, and treatment in primary care. JAMA. 2001;286:1317-24.

Muluk SC, Muluk VS, Kelley ME, et al. Outcome events in patients with claudication: A 15-year study in 2777 patients. J Vasc Surg. 2001;33:251-7.

Poldermans D, Boersma E, Bax JJ, et al, Dutch Echocardiographic Cardiac Risk Evaluation Applying Stress Echocardiography Study Group. The effect of bisoprolol on perioperative mortality and myocardial infarction in high-risk patients undergoing vascular surgery. N Engl J Med. 1999;341:1789-94.

Pratt CM. Analysis of the cilostazol safety database. Am J Cardiol. 2001;87:28D-33D.

Radack K, Deck C. Beta-adrenergic blocker therapy does not worsen intermittent claudication in subjects with peripheral arterial disease: a meta-analysis of randomized controlled trials. Arch Intern Med. 1991;151:1769-76.

Regensteiner JG, Ware JE Jr, McCarthy WJ, et al. Effect of cilostazol on treadmill walking, community-based walking ability, and health-related quality of life in patients with intermittent claudication due to peripheral arterial disease: meta-analysis of six randomized controlled trials. J Am Geriatr Soc. 2002;50:1939-46.

Ridker PM, Cannon CP, Morrow D, et al, Pravastatin or Atorvastatin Evaluation and Infection Therapy-Thrombolysis in Myocardial Infarction 22 (PROVE IT-TIMI 22) Investigators. C-reactive protein levels and outcomes after statin therapy. N Engl J Med. 2005;352:20-8.

Stewart KJ, Hiatt WR, Regensteiner JG, et al. Exercise training for claudication. N Engl J Med. 2002;347:1941-51.

Tangelder MJ, Lawson JA, Algra A, et al. Systematic review of randomized controlled trials of aspirin and oral anticoagulants in the prevention of graft occlusion and ischemic events after infrainguinal bypass surgery. J Vasc Surg. 1999;30:701-9.

Yusuf S, Sleight P, Pogue J, et al, The Heart Outcomes Prevention Evaluation Study Investigators. Effects of an angiotensin-converting-enzyme inhibitor, ramipril, on cardiovascular events in high-risk patients. N Engl J Med. 2000;342:145-53. Erratum in: N Engl J Med. 2000;342:1376. N Engl J Med. 2000;342:748.

15 Acute Arterial Disorders

Anthony J. Comerota, MD, FACS

Patients presenting with an acute arterial occlusion are some of the most challenging cases a physician will encounter. Time is of the essence to establish the correct diagnosis and to select the most appropriate therapy. The patient also may have had an acute myocardial infarction (MI) or the onset of a new cardiac arrhythmia, which compounds the challenge. In addition, ischemia in a limb or the mesenteric circulation may have triggered a cascade of systemic metabolic events that can be life threatening if not corrected expeditiously.

Acute Arterial Occlusion

Incidence

Unlike chronic limb ischemia, acute arterial occlusion has been the focus of few epidemiologic studies. Patients with acute limb ischemia may have a history of peripheral arterial disease and may have had prior vascular interventions, but most have no prior history. Available data from community studies in Sweden and Great Britain show an incidence of acute leg ischemia of about 1 per 6,000 persons per year. Newer and more sophisticated methods of vascular diagnosis and intervention do not appear to decrease the incidence or prevalence of acute arterial occlusion. Trends from recent studies suggest that the incidence is increasing, partly because of the increasing elderly population.

Pathophysiology

Ischemia and reperfusion injury represent the principal pathophysiologic events in patients with acute arterial occlusion and subsequent revascularization. The extent of tissue damage is determined by the duration and degree of ischemia and the sensitivity of the tissue to ischemia. In general, central nervous system tissue is thought to be the most sensitive—irreversible injury can occur within minutes. Skeletal muscle appears to be more tolerant—full recovery is possible even after several hours of profound ischemia. Aside from time and tissue sensitivity, the status of the collateral circulation also has a crucial role. If the arterial occlusion occurred in the presence of preexisting atherosclerotic disease, collateral circulatory pathways may have had time to develop, thus minimizing the amount of tissue at risk. Conversely, a limb without preexisting occlusive disease, and therefore fewer collaterals, will have more severe ischemia after acute occlusion. However, no single overriding factor, but rather the interplay of multiple factors, determines a patient's status, which necessitates specific diagnostic evaluation in each case.

At the cellular level (Table 15.1), ischemia develops when the ratio of oxygen delivery to demand falls below 2:1. At that point, the metabolic activity of most tissues becomes oxygen-delivery dependent—i.e., increased extraction can no longer compensate for decreased supply.

Although reperfusion of ischemic tissue is necessary for tissue survival and recovery, it can also cause or exacerbate tissue damage. This process has been termed "reperfusion injury" and encompasses several complex and incompletely understood mechanisms. Highly reactive, partially reduced oxygen species initiate the tissue injury; they are derived from purine metabolites and free fatty acid pathways, and their production is favored by decreased local tissue pH and high reperfusion oxygen tension. Once generated, the oxygen radicals interact with cellular lipids, proteins, and nucleic acids. Of all target mechanisms, lipid peroxidation may be the most immediately important: lipid peroxides migrate to the cell surface, impairing the fluidity and ultimately the functional integrity of the cell membrane.

Table 15.1 Pathophysiology of Ischemia and Reperfusion Injury

Cellular level changes	Microcirculation changes	Systemic effects
Anaerobic metabolism	Capillary sludging	Electrolyte and acid-base disturbances
Sodium-potassium ATPase pump failure	"No reflow" phenomenon	Cardiopulmonary dysfunction (hypotension, cardiac arrest)
Activation of calcium-dependent lytic enzyme cascades	Thrombus propagation	Pulmonary edema
Oxygen radical production	Loss of microcirculatory autoregulation	Renal impairment and failure
Lipid peroxidation		Systemic inflammatory response syndrome

At the microcirculatory level (Table 15.1), progressive cellular edema can lead to capillary obstruction, perpetuating the ischemic insult even if axial blood flow is restored. This "no reflow" phenomenon appears to worsen with prolonged or repeated periods of ischemia. Also, poor red cell plasticity from ATP depletion contributes to capillary sludging and stasis, thus promoting thrombosis.

The systemic effects of ischemia and reperfusion range from electrolyte and acid-base disturbances to impaired cardiopulmonary and renal function (Table 15.1). Abnormalities may be mild at first, but oliguria, tachypnea, and even cardiac arrest can occur early in the presentation. Once initiated, the inflammatory response may be difficult to control and can quickly lead to multisystem organ failure.

Etiology

Acute limb ischemia can have many different causes, as shown in Table 15.2. In general, the source of an arterial occlusion can be categorized as intrinsic or extrinsic to the native artery.

Intrinsic Occlusions

Intrinsic acute arterial occlusions are more common than extrinsic occlusions. An embolus is implicated as the cause in about 70% of cases and a thrombus in 30%. Of all peripheral arterial emboli, 80% originate from the heart. In the left atrium, thrombi form in areas of low flow or stasis resulting from atrial fibrillation, mitral valve disease, or both. Because rheumatic mitral valve disease is becoming less common, atrial fibrillation now accounts for about 80% of all cardiogenic emboli. In rare instances, atrial thromboemboli can originate from a left atrial myxoma. The left ventricle can be the embolic source after MI, ventricular aneurysms, arrhythmias, and in progressive congestive heart failure or cardiomyopathies (Fig. 15.1). Cardiac valves may be involved by thrombus formation on mechanical valve prostheses or in vegetative endocarditis.

Paradoxic embolism from a venous source may pass through an atrial or ventricular septal defect, or through a patent foramen ovale. Less than 10% of all arterial macroemboli arise from proximal ulcerated plaques or aneurysms in a process called arterio-arterial embolization. Although arteriogenic macroemboli can pose a threat to an entire limb, microemboli present with more limited pathology such as skin necrosis or digital ischemia. The occlusion of small digital arteries by microemboli has been termed "blue toe syndrome" or, more generally, atheromatous emboli syndrome and is managed differently from macroembolization. Finally, thromboemboli in the absence of cardiac or atherosclerotic disease may have such different

Table 15.2 Causes of Acute Limb Ischemia

Embolus
Cardiac
- Atrial fibrillation and other arrhythmias
- Acute myocardial infarction
- Valvular disease and prostheses
- Atrial myxoma
- Arterio-arterial embolization
- Aneurysm, ruptured plaque

Paradoxic
- Venous thromboembolism with patent foramen ovale or atrioseptal defect

Thrombus
Preocclusive atherosclerosis
Low-flow states
- Congestive heart failure, hypovolemia, shock

Thrombophilias
- Lupus anticoagulant, protein C and S deficiency, antithrombin deficiency, heparin-induced thrombocytopenia

Arteritis
Bypass graft occlusion
- Technical failure early after operation
- Atherosclerotic disease progression inflow or outflow distribution
- Intimal hyperplasia in proximal or distal graft

Trauma
Thromboembolization, intimal tear, direct disruption, external compression, dissection, occlusion by indwelling device, compartment syndrome
- Iatrogenic
- Accidental
- Spontaneous, acute vessel wall dissections

Other
Venous outflow occlusion in compartment syndrome or phlegmasia
Drug associated (therapeutic or inadvertent administration or abuse)

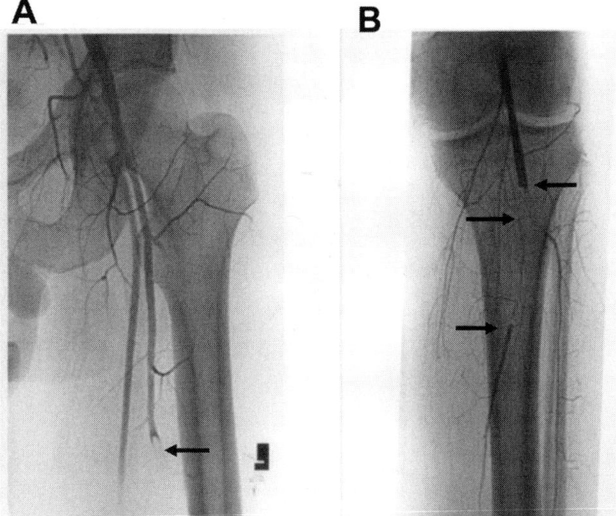

Fig. 15.1 Patient with viral cardiomyopathy and acute leg ischemia due to embolism from a left ventricular wall thrombus. Arteriography shows common radiographic features of embolic occlusion: meniscus sign, multiple occlusions, and intact vascular system proximal and distal to the occlusion. *A*, Left profunda femoris embolus (*arrow*). *B*, Thromboembolization to the left popliteal artery, the proximal anterior tibial artery, and the tibioperoneal trunk (*arrows*).

causes as hypercoagulable states, including those associated with malignancy, the "white clot syndrome" associated with heparin-induced thrombocytopenia or vessel wall compression, and damage from cervical ribs.

- An embolus is implicated in 70% of intrinsic acute arterial occlusions and a thrombus in 30%
  - 80% of all peripheral arterial emboli originate from the heart
- Paradoxic embolism from a venous source through a patent foramen ovale should be considered particularly in younger patients
- Less than 10% of all arterial macroemboli arise from proximal ulcerated plaques or aneurysms (arterio-arterial embolization)

Arterial emboli usually lodge at or proximal to arterial bifurcations and predominantly affect the lower extremities. About three-fourths of all cases occur between the aortic and popliteal bifurcation; the rest affect the upper limbs and the cerebral and visceral circulations. In the lower extremities, obstruction of the common femoral artery is most common. The propensity of emboli to lodge proximal to major bifurcations further exacerbates ischemia, preventing possible alternate arterial supply through collateral circulation.

Acute arterial thrombosis, the other common cause of intrinsic acute arterial ischemia, occurs most frequently in patients with peripheral arterial disease (Table 15.2). Because atherosclerosis progresses gradually, collateral circulation may have had time to develop in these patients. Thrombosis can therefore present more insidiously and less dramatically than an acute embolus. However, propagation of the thrombus may ultimately lead to profound ischemia requiring immediate intervention. Frequently, acute arterial thrombosis occurs in conjunction with low-flow states such as congestive heart failure, hypovolemia, or hypotension. Restoration of cardiac output should be managed first, followed by specific interventions directed at the ischemic limb. Improving cardiac hemodynamics also can identify and significantly help the occasional patient in whom progressive heart failure has worsened preexisting ischemic symptoms, which mimics acute thrombosis. Other causes such as popliteal, iliac, aortic, or upper extremity aneurysms and thrombophilias can be associated with acute arterial thrombosis, thrombus extension, and thromboembolism.

Vascular bypass graft failure represents a special category of thrombosis (Table 15.2). If thrombosis occurs early after the revascularization procedure, it is usually related to a technical problem. If grafts fail years later, it is most commonly because of disease progression. The propensity of an arterial bypass graft to fail depends on several factors, including the nature of the conduit (autogenous or prosthetic), length of the graft, and the quality of inflow and outflow. Anticoagulation, platelet inhibition, and duplex ultrasonographic surveillance all extend the patency of bypass grafts. The presentation of graft failure varies, depending on the initial surgical indication, timing, disease progression, and whether the thrombus in the graft extends into the native arterial circulation. Symptoms can be similar to those of native artery thrombosis.

An embolic versus thrombotic cause of acute arterial occlusion may be difficult to determine; in at least 20% to 25% of cases, embolism cannot be distinguished from thrombosis purely on clinical grounds (Table 15.3). However, the two diagnoses have very different therapeutic implications. Removing an acute embolus from a relatively disease-free arterial tree restores adequate flow—in the absence of new emboli—under most clinical circumstances. After embolectomy, ongoing anticoagulation is commonly necessary to decrease the risk of recurrent embolization. In contrast, thromboembolectomy in acute thrombosis, without definitive correction of the diseased artery through endovascular intervention or bypass grafting, often leads to rethrombosis and ultimate limb loss.

Extrinsic Occlusions

Extrinsic causes of acute arterial ischemia include those from penetrating, blunt, or iatrogenic trauma, acute spontaneous dissections, or external compression (Table 15.2).

Table 15.3 Characteristic Features of Embolic Versus Thrombotic Occlusion

	Source of occlusion	
Feature	**Embolus**	**Thrombus**
Onset of extremity symptoms	Sudden, rapid	Insidious, slower
Prior symptoms	Rare	Frequent
Common clinical association	Recent heart disease: arrhythmias, acute myocardial infarction	PAD
Stigmata of PAD	Possible	Common
Examination of opposite limb	Usually normal	Often abnormal
Arteriography	Crescent/meniscus sign, multiple sites, and vessel bifurcations	Blurred demarcations, prominent collaterals, atherosclerosis
Treatment strategy	Thromboembolectomy, thrombolysis; detect and eliminate embolic source	Thrombolysis, thrombectomy; correct/bypass underlying vascular disease
Long-term pharmacologic therapy	Anticoagulation (if cardiac source)	Platelet inhibition (add anticoagulation if indicated)
Comparative morbidity and mortality	Threat to life; cardiac disease	Threat to limb; generalized atherosclerosis (coronary, carotid, mesenteric, renal arteries)

PAD, peripheral arterial disease.
Modified from Comerota AJ, Harada RN. Acute arterial occlusion. In: Young JR, Olin JW, Bartholomew JR, editors. Peripheral vascular diseases. 2nd ed. St. Louis: Mosby; 1996. p. 273-87. Used with permission.

Traumatic arterial occlusions are usually apparent or at least suspected by a wound or fracture or after an invasive medical procedure. The injury can manifest as an intimal flap or disruption, a large and expanding hematoma, or an arterial transsection. If flow is not initially disrupted, occlusion often follows after secondary thrombosis or thromboembolism. These mechanisms are also involved when indwelling intraluminal medical devices such as radial artery lines or intra-aortic balloon pumps cause acute ischemia resulting from obstruction and intimal injury.

Acute aortic dissections may lead to acute occlusion of any aortic branch through a dissecting hematoma. The dissection is often characterized by tearing pain in the back, chest, or abdomen that began in the interscapular area. Extrinsic arterial compression may be secondary to a tight cast or an expanding traumatic hematoma. It can also result from reperfusion edema after restoration of blood flow following prolonged ischemia or from outflow venous obstruction such as in phlegmasia cerulea or alba dolens. In these clinical scenarios, pressure in the extremity compartments increases, and because the fascia surrounding the compartments limits volume expansion, a compartment syndrome may develop.

- Thromboembolectomy in acute thrombosis without definitive correction of the diseased artery through endovascular intervention or bypass grafting often leads to rethrombosis and ultimate limb loss
- Acute aortic dissections may lead to acute arterial occlusion of any aortic branch
- Conditions such as vasospasm, acute deep vein thrombosis, or acute compressive neuropathy may mimic the symptoms of acute limb ischemia

Differential Diagnosis

Conditions such as vasospasm, acute iliofemoral deep vein thrombosis (phlegmasia cerulea dolens), or acute compressive neuropathy can mimic the symptoms of acute limb ischemia due to acute arterial occlusion. These possible diagnoses are suggested by the presence of palpable pulses or biphasic or triphasic Doppler signals, pronounced edema, or a warm limb with immediate capillary refill. Vasospasm presents a diagnosis of exclusion but should be suspected with ergotism or intra-arterial drug injection. Generally, this diagnosis should be confirmed by arteriography because the clinical findings may be similar to those of acute thrombotic occlusion. Most extrinsic or graft-associated acute occlusions do not present a diagnostic dilemma and should lead to timely corrections.

Clinical Presentation and Evaluation

Patients with acute arterial occlusion frequently report pain, weakness, coldness, and paresthesias distal to the site of occlusion. They may remember the exact time of symptom onset or may describe a prolonged and progressive course over weeks or months with a rapid, recent deterioration. The status of the contralateral limb often provides a model of the affected limb before symptom onset. Chest pain, palpitations, abdominal pain, and pulsations are other key points of a clinical history that guide the initial evaluation. The medical history should be queried for preexisting cardiac conditions such as congestive heart failure, angina, arrhythmias, or MI; peripheral arterial occlusive disease, claudication, and previous vascular procedures; or cerebral or visceral embolic events.

The six cardinal signs of acute limb ischemia are pain, pallor, paralysis, paresthesias, poikilothermia, and pulselessness. The most common manifestation is pain, which is frequently severe and progressive and affects the most distal part of the extremity first. Early in the course of an acute occlusion, commonly during the first 8 hours, the extremity is pale as a result of initial hypoperfusion and perhaps vasospasm of the arterial tree. Vasodilatation and thrombosis from stagnant flow in the circulatory bed subsequently lead to mottling and cyanosis over the following 12 to 24 hours. The presence of blanching in the mottled areas denotes a potentially salvageable circulatory bed at this stage.

- The cardinal signs of acute limb ischemia are:
  - Pain
  - Pallor
  - Paralysis
  - Paresthesias
  - Poikilothermia
  - Pulselessness
- Weakness and paralysis generally imply a poor prognosis

Sensory deficits and paralysis usually occur later in the course of acute arterial occlusion. Absence of pain should always trigger a more detailed evaluation and not be interpreted immediately as a "good" sign. Proprioception is often lost before pressure, deep pain, and temperature sensation which are transmitted by large sensory fibers. Weakness and paralysis generally are associated with a poor prognosis. Unless reperfusion is restored swiftly, ischemia becomes irreversible, and even under optimal technical circumstances, the limb cannot be salvaged. In the absence of effective intervention, tender muscle eventually develops signs of rigor, signifying muscle death.

Bedside Doppler evaluation of the lower extremities is a natural extension of the physical examination. Triphasic, biphasic, or monophasic arterial signals suggest unimpeded, diminished, or severely compromised flow, respectively. In many patients with severe ischemia, arterial Doppler signals are absent. Venous flow typically changes with respiration but may be impaired, as indicated by an absence of respiratory variation or lack of augmentation upon distal compression. Doppler data help with disease localization, assessment of the severity of ischemia, and monitoring after intervention.

The physician should be aware of the pitfalls of Doppler examination, such as misinterpreting venous for arterial signals or obtaining false-negative results. An ankle-brachial index (ABI) should be obtained whenever a Doppler signal is present at the ankle. If a signal is not available, the ABI of the contralateral limb can be helpful to gain information about the patient's baseline vascular status. The ABI is calculated by dividing the highest systolic pressure at the ankle (dorsalis pedis or posterior tibial) by the higher of the two brachial systolic pressures.

Clinical Categories of Acute Limb Ischemia

Early in the patient evaluation, the severity of limb ischemia must be established to determine the urgency of intervention (Table 15.4). The commonly used categories of acute limb ischemia, advanced by the TransAtlantic Inter-Society Consensus Working Group for peripheral vascular disease, provide an objective framework and facilitate communication among physicians. The limb at risk should be described as "viable," "threatened viability," or "irreversible ischemia."

– Viable: the extremity is not immediately threatened. The patient does not have continuous ischemic pain or compromised neurologic function. Examination shows adequate skin capillary circulation and Doppler signals with arterial pulsatile flow.

– Threatened viability: implies reversible ischemia and the possibility of avoiding major amputation if flow is restored promptly. This category consists of patients with

Table 15.4 Clinical Categories of Acute Limb Ischemia

		Findings		Doppler examination	
Category	**Description/prognosis**	**Sensory loss**	**Muscle weakness**	**Arterial signals**	**Venous signals**
I. Viable	Not immediately threatened	None	None	Audible	Audible
II. Threatened viability					
a. Marginally	Salvageable if promptly treated	Minimal (toes, dorsum of foot) or none	None, mild	Inaudible (often)	Audible
b. Immediately	Salvageable with immediate revascularization	More than toes, associated with rest pain	Mild, moderate	Inaudible (usually)	Audible
III. Irreversible ischemia	Major tissue loss or permanent nerve damage inevitable	Profound, anesthetic	Profound, paralysis (rigor)	Inaudible	Inaudible

From Dormandy JA, Rutherford RB, TASC Working Group. Management of peripheral arterial disease (PAD). TransAtlantic Inter-Society Consensus (TASC). Section C: acute limb ischemia. J Vasc Surg. 2000;31(1 Pt 2):S143. Used with permission.

marginally or immediately threatened limbs. The limb lacks clearly audible arterial pedal Doppler signals even though venous signals, particularly with distal compression, may still be demonstrable. Patients with a marginally threatened extremity have only transient or minimal sensory loss restricted to the toes and do not have persistent pain. In contrast, those with an immediately threatened limb have continuous ischemic rest pain, sensory loss above the toes, and variable degrees of motor loss including paresis or paralysis.

– Irreversible ischemia: usually requires major amputation or results in significant permanent neuromuscular damage independent of therapy. Examination shows profound sensory loss, muscle paralysis extending above the foot, absence of arterial and venous pedal Doppler signals, or evidence of more advanced ischemia, including muscle rigor and skin marbling.

Clinical distinction between an immediately threatened and irreversibly ischemic limb may not be straightforward. However, in the absence of better markers of extremity ischemia, this classification scheme represents the best available practical guide. Furthermore, with the advent of new modalities such as thrombolysis or percutaneous mechanical clot extraction, these specific categories help decide for whom these interventions are indicated.

Initial Diagnosis

Laboratory Studies

Baseline laboratory studies that should be obtained on presentation include complete blood cell count, prothrombin time/international normalized ratio, activated partial thromboplastin time, electrolytes, renal chemistries, cardiac enzymes, and total creatine kinase. Electrocardiography and chest radiography should also be performed. Frequently, the test results help confirm or rule out an initial diagnostic impression such as advanced ischemia and sepsis or renal impairment.

Arteriography

The need for arteriography is largely determined by patient presentation. If the cause appears embolic, the limb severely ischemic, and the site of occlusion apparent and surgically accessible, no diagnostic procedures beyond the principal clinical evaluation are needed. If arteriography will not contribute significant additional information or affect the choice of therapy, it should not be performed. In addition, referral for arteriography may unduly delay needed surgical embolectomy if personnel and facilities for testing are not readily available. Similarly, in unstable multisystem trauma associated with limb ischemia, treatment priorities preclude detailed radiographic evaluation. In this case, "on-table" arteriography is performed in the operating room to delineate the site of injury and the extent of underlying pathology.

If the diagnosis is not clear-cut, such as in thrombotic or embolic occlusion, arteriography can help distinguish between them and provide information about multivessel atherosclerotic disease and location of the occlusion. Computed tomography angiography (CTA) and magnetic resonance angiography (MRA) with gadolinium can be performed rapidly and can help with intervention planning. After distal arterial patency is demonstrated, a surgical road map of inflow and outflow can be obtained should a bypass procedure be required. Unusual causes of acute ischemia, such as giant cell arteritis, dissecting aneurysms, and low-flow states, can be appropriately identified or excluded. Arteriography should be obtained if the cause of the acute ischemia is unclear or if the approach to treatment potentially may be altered by the radiographic findings.

Ultrasonography

Duplex ultrasonography can be helpful if the origin of the embolus is thought to be arterio-arterial, such as in an abdominal aortic, iliofemoral, or popliteal artery aneurysm. Duplex studies have been useful in evaluation of extremity trauma. Findings may include hematoma, intimal flaps, abnormal velocity patterns, pseudoaneurysms, arteriovenous fistula, or occlusion. Ultrasonographic findings may obviate the need for arteriography or may require further clarification by arteriography. As for any test, unreasonable delay is unacceptable in any patient with an ischemic limb.

Management

Initial management of acute arterial occlusion emphasizes systemic stabilization by addressing cardiac, pulmonary, and renal function. Intravenous access is obtained, resuscitation with appropriate intravenous fluids started, and cardiac support and monitoring provided, including pulmonary artery catheter placement if indicated by the clinical history and status. Anticoagulation is important and should be started early to prevent prograde and retrograde thrombus extension and to minimize the risk of additional embolic episodes and venous thrombosis. Depending on the degree of ischemia and the time to arteriography or surgery, a bolus of heparin (5,000-20,000 U) is administered intravenously. A continuous heparin infusion of 2,000 to 4,000 U/h is used for high-dose supratherapeutic anticoagulation, or a rate of 15 U/kg per hour is started and adjusted to maintain a therapeutic prothrombin time between 60 and 90 seconds. Available data suggest that supratherapeutic anticoagulation with heparin in the absence of comorbid conditions for bleeding is more effective than standard heparin therapy and does not increase the bleeding risk. Patients with contraindications to heparin use such as heparin-induced thrombocytopenia require alternative forms of anticoagulation.

If the acutely occluded limb is not immediately threatened, alternative methods such as catheter-directed thrombolysis or percutaneous aspiration thromboembolectomy can be considered. Furthermore, given the high risk for recurrent embolization (40% without anticoagulation), a concerted effort is made to determine the embolic source. A thorough history and physical examination and baseline electrocardiography often establish the cause. Echocardiography via a transthoracic or transesophageal approach is the next diagnostic test. If echocardiography is negative, CTA or MRA of the chest and abdomen should be performed. Most patients can be diagnosed with careful evaluation, but in 5% to 10% the embolic source cannot be determined.

In contrast to patients with acute arterial thrombosis, patients with embolic occlusion have a comparably greater threat to life than to the ischemic limb. The outcome is generally more favorable for those with atrial fibrillation as opposed to MI or heart failure as the embolic source. Overall, acute embolic arterial occlusion is associated with a 10% to 15% mortality rate and a 5% to 10% amputation rate in the perioperative period.

Arteriography and thrombolysis can establish the precise nature of lesions, collateral pathways, and runoff vessels in patients with acute thrombotic occlusion. This information helps in determining the most appropriate procedure for definitive therapy. Simple thrombectomy would be insufficient and would fail to address the underlying disease.

Clinical trials have established the benefit of catheter-directed thrombolysis, which has led to less extensive surgical procedures, improved limb salvage, and decreased early mortality in selected patients with acute symptoms of leg ischemia. However, the effectiveness of thrombolysis may be technically limited if the catheter cannot be properly positioned. In addition, thrombolysis may be contraindicated for patients with central nervous system disease (e.g., recent transient ischemic attack or stroke, head trauma, or neurosurgical procedures), recent gastrointestinal tract hemorrhage, or a bleeding diathesis. Generally, urgent surgical intervention is more appropriate than catheter-directed thrombolysis if the limb is immediately threatened. If irreversible ischemia has occurred, timely amputation can be lifesaving.

Compared with acute embolic arterial occlusion, thrombosis carries twice the risk of limb loss. Platelet inhibition and anticoagulation may be indicated and improve long-term outcome. Furthermore, patients with peripheral arterial occlusive disease should be routinely evaluated for coronary and carotid artery disease.

Macroscopic atheroemboli with the potential to occlude large extremity arteries can originate in virtually any vessel but are found more commonly in association with small aortic aneurysms and aortoiliac occlusive disease. Macroemboli are less frequent than microemboli. Atheroemboli as a cause of acute embolic arterial occlusion should be suspected if initial echocardiography results are negative. Arteriography is then the first localizing study. In contrast, thoracoabdominal contrast computed tomography (CT) is usually the best initial study to determine the source of microemboli. If results are negative, complete arteriography from the aortic arch distally is obtained to evaluate for an intraluminal source.

Associated Complications and Postoperative Care

Most patients with acute limb ischemia, independent of specific treatment, have the systemic effects of a cytokine-driven inflammatory response with an immediate and longer-term effect on almost all major organ systems. Patients with this inflammatory response are often critically ill; during their care, careful attention must be paid to oxygen delivery, correction of electrolyte disturbances, and management of volume status, possible renal failure, and pulmonary complications including acute respiratory distress syndrome. Specialized observation in the intensive care unit and monitoring of oxygenation, arterial blood gases, electrocardiograms, and pulmonary artery catheter parameters are usually indicated. Medications used for the supportive treatment of these patients are described in Table 15.5.

Because most of these patients have underlying cardiac disease, cardiac evaluation and consultation should be obtained early. Depending on the specific clinical circumstances, coronary vasodilators, inotropic support, cardiac catheterization, and even coronary revascularization may be appropriate interventions in addition to anticoagulation. The benefit of perioperative β-blockade in high-risk cardiac patients undergoing vascular surgery has been established recently in a large multicenter trial.

After restoration of blood flow, potassium released as a result of cell wall damage can lead to sudden and profound hyperkalemia, potentially resulting in cardiac arrhythmias, arrest, or MI. Emergent therapy includes administration of insulin and calcium gluconate followed by cation-exchange resins. Coexisting renal failure can exacerbate hyperkalemia, bring about volume overload, and require early hemodialysis. Similarly, anaerobic metabolism with release of lactate may lead to profound metabolic acidosis with subsequent myocardial depression, hypotension, and inadequate oxygen delivery. Acid-base management

Table 15.5 Medications of Potential Benefit for Acute Limb Ischemia

Drug	Rationale/indication	Dose	Major mechanism	Comments
Heparin	Decrease risk of recurrent embolization Prevent thrombus propagation and new thrombus formation	Bolus: 100 U/kg Infusion: 15 U/kg/h with aPTT at 1.5-2.0× control, or use high-dose therapy at 2,000-4,000 U/h	Potentiates antithrombin function; thus inactivates thrombin, tissue factor/VIIa complex, and clotting factors IX, X, and XI	Start heparin as early as possible Observe for HIT
Tissue plasminogen activator	Lyse thrombus to restore perfusion to entire arterial tree Decrease extent of subsequent revascularization procedure	Depends on catheter administration technique Bolus: 2-4 mg Infusion: 0.5-1.0 mg/h	Promotes conversion of plasminogen to plasmin & enhances proteolytic degradation of fibrin in thrombus (high fibrin specificity)	Consider if limb not immediately threatened & occlusion of <14 d Adjunct to thromboembolectomy, lyse surgically inaccessible clot
Low-molecular-weight heparin	Decrease risk of thrombosis (same as heparin)	Depends on specific product	Releases tissue factor pathway inhibitor Inhibits plasma factor Xa and IIa	Use mostly in postoperative period
Aspirin	Decrease risk of thrombosis by platelet inhibition	160-325 mg/d	Irreversibly acetylates platelet cyclooxygenase	Reduces risk of all cardiovascular events
Clopidogrel	Decrease risk of thrombosis by platelet inhibition	75 mg/d	Inhibits ADP-mediated platelet aggregation	Add to aspirin in patients with prior MI/coronary artery disease
Warfarin	Reduce risk of recurrent cardiac embolization Decrease risk of thrombosis	Titrate to maintain INR between 2.0-3.0 (therapeutic range)	Inhibits coagulation factors II, VII, IX, and X	Consider in distal extremity bypass, poor vein quality, marginal arterial runoff, prior failed bypass
Mannitol	Promote diuresis	12.5-25 mg IV	Osmotic diuretic Free radical scavenger	May prevent renal impairment, useful in myoglobinuria
Insulin, glucose, calcium gluconate	Reduce serum potassium Protect heart in hyperkalemia	12.5-25 g glucose, 5-10 U insulin 2.25-14 mEq IV, slow titration	Shifts potassium into cells Stabilizes cell membrane potential	Emergent hyperkalemia treatment Cardioprotection in hyperkalemia
Sodium bicarbonate	Ameliorate acidosis	Titrate to serum pH, base deficit, lactate	H^+ reduction	Use in severe metabolic acidosis Avoid fluid overload, hypernatremia
Alternative anticoagulants	Anticoagulation if heparin or warfarin cannot be given	Depends on specific product	Depends on specific product	Consider agents such as lepirudan, danaparoid, argatroban in HIT

ADP, adenosine diphosphate; aPTT, activated partial thromboplastin time; HIT, heparin-induced thrombocytopenia; INR, international normalized ratio; IV, intravenously; MI, myocardial infarction.

Modified from Quiñones-Baldrich WJ. Acute arterial and graft occlusion. In: Moore WS, editor. Vascular surgery: a comprehensive review. Philadelphia: WB Saunders Company; 1998. p. 667-89. Used with permisison.

may include judicious intravenous fluid administration, ventilatory support, and bicarbonate use.

The breakdown of muscle proteins leading to myoglobinuria after acute limb ischemia has been well described experimentally and clinically. Under conditions of low and even physiologic pH, myoglobin precipitates in the renal tubules, potentially leading to renal failure. Preventive therapy aims to maintain renal flow with a target urine output of 60 mL/h through administration of fluid and diuretics. Mannitol is the preferred diuretic because it also acts as a free-radical scavenger. Traditionally, bicarbonate has been added to intravenous fluids to alkalinize the urine and prevent tubular myoglobin precipitation. The benefit of bicarbonate infusion, however, is not as clearly established as that of fluid administration. Use of bicarbonate must consider its effect on the volume and electrolyte status and the ultimate need for CO_2 elimination.

Clinical and experimental studies also have shown the detrimental effect of the venous effluent from a revascularized extremity on the pulmonary circulation and respiratory function. Patients may have pulmonary dysfunction ranging from mild respiratory impairment to irreversible acute respiratory distress syndrome, which is mediated through cytokine release. Basic treatment remains supportive and includes careful fluid management (avoiding volume overload) and ventilatory support strategies to optimize oxygen delivery while minimizing oxygen toxicity and barotrauma.

Based on current understanding of the reperfusion syndrome and "no reflow" phenomenon, novel strategies have focused on oxygen radical scavengers (e.g., calcium-channel blockers, vitamins A and E, and glutathiones), initial drainage of venous effluent from a reperfused limb, gradual limb reperfusion, and hypothermia. To date, no convincing evidence supports the therapeutic superiority of any specific protocol. Prompt diagnosis, anticoagulation, restoration of blood flow, and supportive intensive care measures remain the basis of patient care.

Future Directions

The past four decades have seen remarkable progress in the treatment of patients with acute arterial occlusion, in part because of innovations such as routine anticoagulation, balloon thromboembolectomy catheters, percutaneous mechanical clot aspiration, catheter-directed thrombolysis, endovascular intervention, and bypass grafting techniques. Recent pharmacologic innovations have led to the development of drugs that directly dissolve clots and do not require plasminogen activators to generate plasmin. Two such drugs are alfimeprase and plasmin (both in clinical trials); the drugs are delivered into the thrombus, and early observations suggest rapid thrombus dissolution. The agents are rapidly bound by either α_2-macroglobulin (alfimeprase) or antiplasmins (plasmin) upon entry into the systemic circulation; therefore, distant bleeding complications are expected to be minimal.

The development of new catheters that incorporate segmental pharmacomechanical thrombolysis and ultrasound-accelerated thrombolysis offers potentially effective options to patients with more severe ischemia, who traditionally undergo surgical intervention. In addition, sophisticated intensive care monitoring and therapy have contributed to a marked decrease in mortality and morbidity. However, recent data from large clinical series still document 30-day mortality rates of 15% and amputation rates between 15% and 30% for patients presenting with acute arterial occlusion. In a recent European study of patients treated between 1985 and 1996, the 5-year survival was 17% for patients with acute embolic occlusion and 44% for those with acute thrombotic occlusion.

Atheromatous Embolization

Atheromatous embolization is caused by debris from atherosclerotic plaque that has fragmented and embolized to distal tissues, classically confirmed on pathologic microscopic examination by observing slits in tissues left by cholesterol crystals. The clinical spectrum can be broad, from asymptomatic and relatively clinically silent emboli to multiple cholesterol emboli leading to skin necrosis, multiple organ dysfunction, and death.

The clinical presentation of atheromatous emboli can be confused with thrombotic occlusion of small vessels. Conditions such as "blue toe syndrome" can result from either; however, the association with livedo reticularis and tenderness of calf muscles generally represents atheromatous embolism, whereas an isolated ischemic toe without other associated findings is more likely caused by a thrombotic embolus.

Prevalence

Most patients with clinical atheromatous embolization are men aged 60 years or older. Whites are more frequently affected than blacks for reasons that are unclear. Natural history studies of atheroembolism underestimate its prevalence in the present environment of endovascular procedures. Catheter manipulation in atherosclerotic central arteries frequently leads to atheroembolism, which is often underdiagnosed or missed completely.

An atherosclerotic aorta, with protruding plaque and often with fibrin-platelet thrombus attached to ulcerated endothelium, represents the underlying pathology. Aneurysmal disease of the aorta and popliteal and femoral arteries is also a recognized cause. In one study, 33% of patients with protruding atheromas in the thoracic aorta had embolic events to the brain, eye, kidney, bowel, or lower extremities. Because these lesions appear to change with time, forming additional mass and resolving mobile components, a dynamic process is suggested, with important therapeutic implications.

Etiology

Atheromatous embolism can have various causes. It can result after interventions such as catheter-based procedures, vascular surgery, or cardiovascular surgery with aortic clamping; after therapy with thrombolytics or warfarin anticoagulation; or from abdominal aortic aneurysms (spontaneous, ruptured, aneurysm repair surgery), popliteal aneurysm, or spontaneous atheroembolization. Most patients with clinically apparent atheroemboli present after catheter manipulation through atherosclerotic arteries (Fig. 15.2) or vascular surgical procedures. The pressure injection associated with arteriography produces catheter vibration and whipping of the catheter tip against the diseased vessel wall. Disruption of the fibrous cap of plaques containing lipomatous debris leads to showers of emboli. Frequently, this is observed immediately after the invasive procedure; however, such presentation also can be delayed by weeks to months after the procedure.

Causes of Atheromatous Embolism

- Catheter-based procedures
- Vascular surgery
- Cardiovascular surgery with aortic clamping
- Abdominal aortic aneurysms (spontaneous, ruptured, repair surgery)
- Popliteal aneurysm
- Thrombolytic therapy, warfarin anticoagulation
- Spontaneous

A

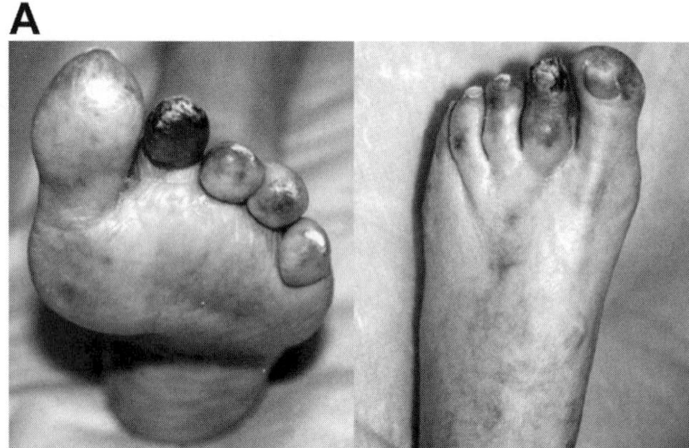

B

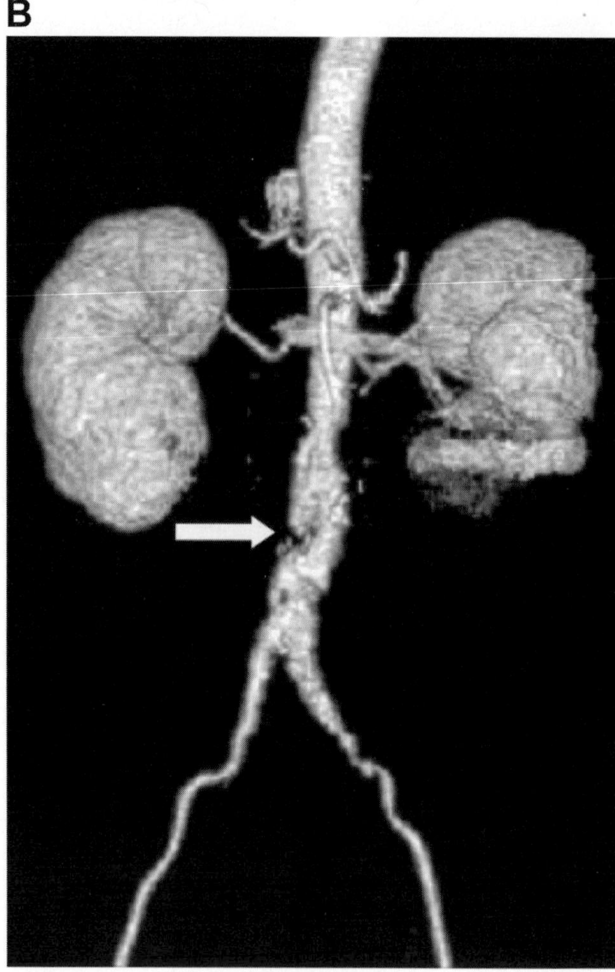

C

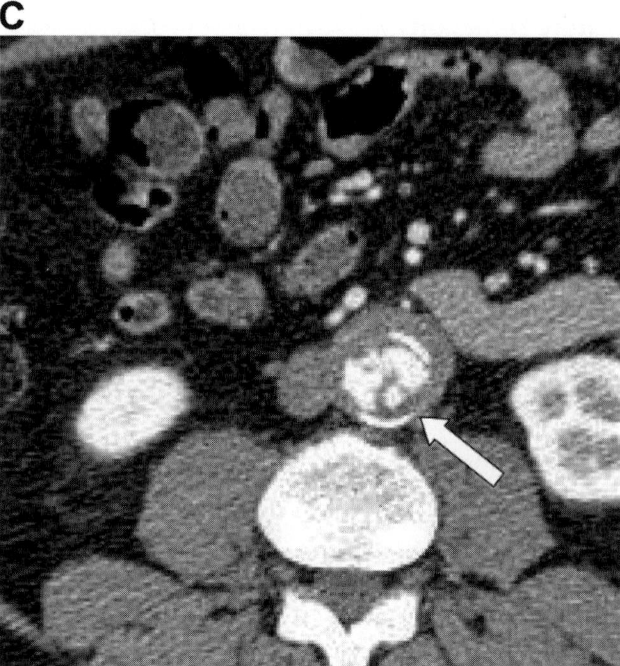

Fig. 15.2 *A*, Patient with painful ischemic toes and forefeet occurring 2 weeks after cardiac catheterization. *B*, Three-dimensional computed tomography (CT) shows plaque (*arrow*) in the infrarenal aorta. *C*, Cross-section of the CT image shows irregular, multilobular plaque (*arrow*) in the infrarenal aorta.

The likelihood of cholesterol emboli varies and is directly linked to the extent of disease within the blood vessels accessed. One of the highest rates of cholesterol emboli reported was a 25% incidence in the kidneys, found during autopsies of deceased patients who had had previous catheterization. Most series report a prevalence of cholesterol emboli of 1% or less.

Spontaneous emboli can occur after a sudden increase in intra-abdominal pressure, such as occurs with coughing, heavy lifting, tenesmus, and blunt abdominal injury. Although atheromatous emboli have been reported to occur with thrombolytic therapy and anticoagulation therapy for thrombotic disorders, ischemic events of embolization of thrombotic material must not be confused with true cholesterol embolization.

Clinical Presentation

Most patients with clinically recognizable atheromatous emboli syndrome present with skin manifestations. Approximately 35% of patients with atheromatous emboli have cutaneous manifestations, and livedo reticularis, involving the lower half of the body, accounts for about half of these manifestations. Frequently, the areas of involvement are scattered and can be unilateral or bilateral, depending on the artery containing the culprit lesion. If the feet and toes are involved, the lesions can be extremely painful. Ulcerations can result, with the formation of areas of erythema and multiple purpuric halos. Patients can also present with petechiae and raised skin plaques.

Palpable pulses are frequently observed throughout the extremity. However, if arterial thrombosis results from the embolic episode and the ensuing inflammatory response, more profound distal ischemia occurs. The kidneys are the most common organ involved with atheromatous emboli. Because of renal compensation, embolic episodes are clinically silent until renal function becomes impaired; consequently, many patients go undiagnosed.

- Most patients with clinically recognizable atheromatous emboli syndrome present with skin manifestations
- Livedo reticularis represents approximately half of all cutaneous manifestations (involves the lower half of the body)
- The kidneys are the organ most commonly involved with atheromatous emboli

Cholesterol emboli to the gastrointestinal tract can produce abdominal pain, nausea, vomiting, and distension. Severe forms of bowel ischemia have been reported, resulting in overt bowel infarction. Splenic infarction, cholecystitis, gangrene of the gall bladder, pancreatitis, and pancreatic necrosis have been reported. Carotid artery disease causing amaurosis fugax as a result of retinal ischemia presents with the physical findings of Hollenhorst plaques in the retina. If embolization occurs in the cerebral arteries, transient ischemic attacks or strokes result. Spinal cord infarction causing lower extremity paralysis has been described after intra-aortic balloon counterpulsation, with typical cholesterol emboli found in the distribution of the anterior spinal artery and sacral cord arteries. Painful hemorrhagic cystitis, prostatitis, and orchitis have also been reported. Myocardial ischemia with typical and atypical angina and infarction of cardiac muscle have been described. Hypertension is commonly associated with atheromatous emboli, especially in patients with kidney involvement. Patients with atheromatous emboli from a diffusely diseased aorta have a particularly poor outcome.

Pathologic Response to Cholesterol Embolization

Cholesterol emboli have been found in virtually all organs and tissues examined. The typical microscopic finding of atheromatous embolism is the cholesterol crystal, which is needle shaped and frequently surrounded by an inflammatory reaction. The crystals cause a foreign body response with giant cells, lymphocytes, and eosinophils. With time, the cholesterol crystals become surrounded by fibrous tissue, and the lumen of the embolized vessel occludes. Amorphous eosinophilic material, lipophages, and hyalinized foci of intimal thickening are observed.

Cholesterol crystals have been injected into the arteries of animals; panarteritis develops within 3 days, which includes eosinophils and giant cells surrounding the crystals, intimal hyperplasia, and leukocytes in the outer layers of the vessel wall. At 6 days, intimal fibrosis was observed, which persisted up to 5 months. When embolized into the lower extremities of animals, the cholesterol crystals acted as non-removable foreign bodies, leading to thrombosis of the embolized vessel.

Laboratory Studies

The laboratory findings in atheromatous embolization depend on the end organ involved and the severity of the embolic process. Because an inflammatory reaction is frequently stimulated, acute-phase reactants such as the erythrocyte sedimentation rate are often elevated. Thrombocytopenia and hypocomplementemia have also been observed. Patients with emboli to the gastrointestinal tract frequently present with anemia. In patients with renal atheroemboli, 80% have eosinophilia and 80% to 90% have eosinophiluria. Azotemia, proteinuria, and microscopic hematuria can also occur. In other patients, laboratory results may include increased blood urea nitrogen and creatinine levels.

If the upper gastrointestinal tract is involved, specifically the pancreas and liver, pancreatic enzymes and liver enzymes may be elevated. Cholesterol emboli to the coronary arteries can result in increases of the myocardial band of creatine kinase and troponins. However, for some patients, no laboratory abnormalities are found.

- Laboratory findings depend on the end organ involved and the severity of the embolic process
- Findings may include:
  - Eosinophilia
  - Eosinophiluria
  - Increased erythrocyte sedimentation rate
  - Thrombocytopenia
  - Anemia
  - Hypocomplementemia
  - Increased blood urea nitrogen and creatinine levels

Diagnosis

The definitive diagnosis of atheromatous embolization is made by the observation of cholesterol crystals (more precisely, the remaining space of cholesterol crystals) in tissue biopsy specimens. Skin biopsies have the highest yield in the areas suspected, namely those with livedo reticularis. Properly performed skin biopsy has a diagnostic yield of greater than 90%. To avoid false-negative results, it is important that the biopsy specimen be deep enough to include the dermal vessels. Muscle biopsies have a higher diagnostic yield than those from skin but are more invasive. For patients presenting with progressive renal dysfunction, a kidney biopsy is often diagnostic.

The clinical evaluation of patients should be thoughtful and direct. Cardiac causes such as arrhythmia, endocarditis, valvular heart disease, and ventricular aneurysm should be excluded. Abdominal aortic aneurysm and peripheral arterial aneurysm should be excluded. Transesophageal echocardiography provides a good view of the aortic arch and thoracic aorta. Standard arteriography is considered desirable by many physicians; however, unless a catheter-based intervention is planned, arteriography should be avoided because the risk of additional embolization is increased with catheter manipulation. Other imaging studies such as high-resolution CTA and MRA should be considered to evaluate for atherosclerotic disease of the aorta. These methods may be more sensitive than conventional arteriography for identifying the culprit lesion and avoid the likelihood of recurrent atheroemboli from catheter trauma (Fig. 15.3).

Other diagnoses that should be considered in patients who present with digital ischemia, extremity livedo reticularis, or both include vasculitis, endocarditis, malignancy, polycythemia, intracardiac thrombus, arrhythmia, polyarteritis nodosa, thrombocythemia, cryoglobulinemia and macroglobulinemia, valvular heart disease, malfunctioning prosthetic heart valves, circulating anticoagulants and antiphospholipid antibodies, calciphylaxis, and reactions to corticosteroids or β-blockers.

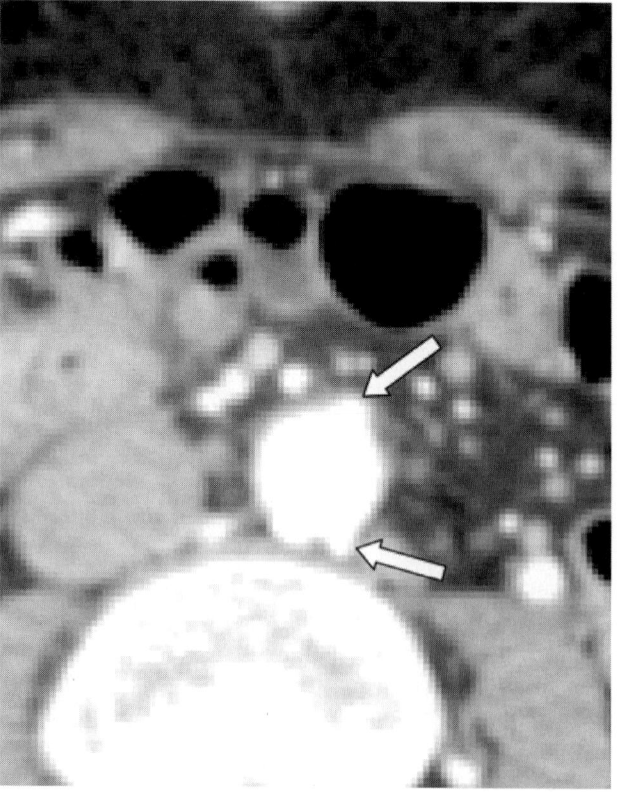

Fig. 15.3 Computed tomography angiography shows ulcerated atherosclerotic lesions (*arrows*) of the infrarenal aorta.

Management

The ultimate goal and the most effective treatment for patients with atheromatous embolism is to find and eliminate the embolic source, especially if the embolic event was spontaneous. If the embolic event was the result of mechanical intervention, the culprit lesion does not restrict blood flow, and embolism has not recurred, aggressive medical management and risk factor reduction are appropriate. Focal lesions of peripheral arteries can be well managed surgically or with endovascular procedures. Resection of an aneurysm, endarterectomy of a focal lesion, or balloon angioplasty and stenting of focal lesions generally are associated with good results.

In patients with adequate perfusion to the extremity but with painful ischemic digits, lumbar sympathectomy may be of benefit. Proper patient selection is important, and preoperative lumbar sympathetic block is helpful to identify patients who are likely to respond. Patients with a suprarenal atheroembolism have the poorest outcomes. Lesions in this location are the most difficult to treat. However, with the advent of thoracic stent grafts, the prognosis may change for these patients.

Optimal risk factor modification should be implemented in all patients with atheroembolism. Smoking cessation is essential, as is aggressive control of high blood pressure, with a target of less than 130/80 mm Hg. Patients with diabetes mellitus should have a hemoglobin A_{1c} value of less than 7% and a low-density lipoprotein cholesterol level less than 70 mg/dL. Statins are thought to be effective in patients with atheroembolism because of their plaque-stabilizing and antiinflammatory effects in addition to their lipid-lowering capabilities. Nevertheless, statins should be considered in all patients regardless of their lipid status because atheromatous embolization is direct evidence of atherosclerotic disease. Statin therapy has been shown to decrease recurrent embolic events in patients with plaques of 4 mm or greater in the thoracic aorta.

Platelet inhibition with aspirin, clopidogrel, or dipyridamole is thought to be important in the management of these patients. In patients with non-occlusive lesions and atheromatous emboli of the toes, one study showed a strong correlation of clinical improvement with platelet inhibition. Patients improved when platelet inhibitors were administered and deteriorated when platelet inhibitors were withheld.

- Pharmacotherapy with aspirin, clopidogrel, or anticoagulation has variable results
- The prognosis is poor for patients with cholesterol embolization in whom a focal source is not identified and corrected

Pentoxifylline may have some role in the management of these patients by increasing erythrocyte flexibility and improving microcirculatory perfusion. Cilostazol may also improve conditions in these patients because of its combined antiplatelet and vasodilatory effects. Prostacyclin analogs have improved outcomes in patients with small-vessel, microvascular disorders and may be of value in patients with severe atheromatous embolism. Improvement in digital ischemia and renal function has been shown in patients with atheroembolism treated with iloprost.

Corticosteroids may be an important therapy in patients with severe atheroembolism. Patients with recurrent episodes of atheroemboli, systemic evidence of inflammation, and severe mesenteric and lower extremity symptoms have been shown to benefit from corticosteroids.

Anticoagulation can be used to decrease secondary small vessel thrombosis resulting from thrombus propagation in vessels with atheromatous emboli. However, anticoagulation to treat the primary lesion may be ineffective, may result in further atheroembolization, and for the most part is not recommended, unless there is another pressing reason to use it (i.e., non-valvular atrial fibrillation).

The prognosis for patients with cholesterol embolization in whom a focal source is not identified and corrected is poor. A diffusely involved aorta and emboli to multiple organs is termed "malignant cholesterol emboli syndrome." Because the aorta is diseased above and below the diaphragm, this process is frequently not controllable, and many patients die within a year.

Aggressive supportive care has been reported to significantly improve survival. Because the major causes of mortality with widespread atheroembolism are recurrent events, heart failure, and cachexia, a treatment plan directed at these events is proposed. Preventing recurrence by eliminating anticoagulants, avoiding invasive procedures, aggressively treating heart failure, and providing nutritional support and hemodialysis is associated with significantly improved outcomes.

The reported mortality rate for patients with embolization after a catheterization procedure is 50% to 60%. However, patients in whom embolization stops spontaneously before organ failure occurs have a reasonably good prognosis.

Vascular Trauma

The diagnosis and timely repair of injuries are crucial for the successful management of vascular trauma. Upper extremity wounds account for more than one-third of peripheral vascular injuries; however, the more difficult and complex clinical problems occur with thoracic, abdominal, and lower extremity injuries. Common mechanisms of injury include blunt trauma, such as automobile accidents and falls, fracture dislocations, and penetrating injuries. Survival is threatened in patients with major thoracic and abdominal vascular injuries. Inadequate treatment of extremity injuries or severe extremity trauma often leaves patients with a painful or non-functioning limb. The diagnosis and management of vascular trauma has changed from a policy of mandatory exploration for all suspected and potential vascular injuries to one of selective evaluation and non-operative treatment of minimal injuries.

Thoracic Vascular Trauma

Patients involved in automobile accidents always should be considered for evaluation of major vascular trauma. A high index of suspicion is the most important factor in initiating a search for thoracic aortic disruption. Automobile accidents and falls can transfer considerable energy, leading to blunt injury to the aorta and its branches. Automobile deceleration injuries can be compared with the impact from an equivalent free fall (Table 15.6). Even in the absence of physical findings, falls from 30 feet or higher and automobile accidents at speeds of 40 miles per hour or more should generate a high degree of suspicion of thoracic vascular injury and lead to appropriate evaluation.

Symptoms of thoracic vascular injury include retrosternal or intrascapular pain, dyspnea, loss of consciousness, and hypotension. Only one-third of patients with blunt aortic trauma have physical evidence of thoracic injury at presentation. No single physical finding is diagnostic of acute thoracic aortic rupture; however, fracture of the first or second rib is a marker for severe blunt trauma, and a thorough evaluation should be initiated. Cephalic hypertension, discrepancy of upper and lower extremity pulses, a precordial or intrascapular systolic murmur, and acute voice change are physical findings highly suggestive of

Table 15.6 Impact Velocity and Injury Risk: a Comparison of Auto Deceleration and Equivalent Free Falls

Impact velocity, mph	Risk, % Morbidity	Risk, % Mortality	Impact velocity,mph	Equivalent free fall, ft
1-10	2.5	0.1	10	5
11-20	6.0	1.0	20	13
21-30	25.0	3.0	30	28
≥40	70.0	40.0	40	54
			50	84
			60	121

From Bongard F. Thoracic and abdominal vascular trauma. In: Rutherford RB, editor. Vascular surgery. Vol 1. 5th ed. Philadelphia: W.B. Saunders Company; 2000. p. 871-92. Used with permission.

thoracic aortic rupture. Expedient patient evaluation and accurate diagnosis are lifesaving.

The number of patients with traumatic aortic dissection continues to increase; aortic dissection is responsible for 10% to 15% of deaths from automobile accidents. Persons who are ejected from the vehicle have a 27% risk of aortic rupture, compared with 12% for those who are not. Only 10% to 20% of patients with acute thoracic disruptions survive the initial trauma: of these, 30% die within 6 hours, 40% within 24 hours, and 72% within the first week. If the injury is not repaired, 90% of the initial survivors will die within 10 weeks.

- The diagnosis and management of vascular trauma have changed from a policy of mandatory exploration for all suspected and potential vascular injuries to one of selective evaluation and non-operative treatment of minimal injuries
- Symptoms of thoracic vascular injury include:
  - Retrosternal or intrascapular pain
  - Dyspnea
  - Loss of consciousness
  - Hypotension
- Only one-third of patients with blunt aortic trauma have physical evidence of thoracic injury at presentation

Radiographic imaging is crucial for proper diagnosis. An erect chest radiograph that shows widening of the aortic arch should lead to CT and possibly transesophageal echocardiography to establish or exclude the diagnosis of aortic rupture. The newer, high-speed contrast CT techniques have shown excellent diagnostic sensitivity compared with arteriography, which has been the gold standard. Penetrating injuries in stable patients can be evaluated arteriographically and with other imaging techniques. In an unstable patient, thoracotomy is often required.

Abdominal Vascular Trauma

Blunt injuries to the abdomen are less common than penetrating abdominal vascular injuries. Rapid deceleration or compression produces sufficient shear stress to avulse mobile smaller vessels from their fixed mesenteric origins, especially with branches arising from the superior mesenteric artery and from the portal vein. Occlusion of the aorta by an intimal flap is found with the "seatbelt aorta" and with occlusion of the proximal renal arteries.

In patients presenting with penetrating abdominal trauma associated with hypotension, abdominal exploration is warranted. During resuscitation, if the patient is sufficiently stable, chest radiography and a one-shot intravenous pyelogram should be obtained. This provides important information about the kidneys and ureters, which is invaluable during intraoperative decision making.

Although surgical exploration and direct repair have been the mainstays of treating major vascular injury, percutaneous endovascular techniques are being applied with increasing frequency and success.

Carotid Artery Injuries

Most wounds of the cervical vessels are caused by penetrating trauma; however, blunt trauma can cause endothelial disruption, subintimal dissection, and occlusion. Although blunt trauma can be accompanied by bruises and cuts on the neck, approximately half of patients have no superficial evidence of trauma. In addition to the telltale bruises, clinical features raising the suspicion of blunt trauma to the carotid artery include bruits, Horner syndrome, transient ischemic attacks, and a lucid interval after injury followed by neurologic symptoms and limb paresis in an alert patient. Some patients have no neurologic symptoms even in the presence of severe carotid injury. Hyperextension neck injuries are particularly worrisome for causing an intimal disruption in the distal cervical internal carotid artery.

Penetrating wounds of the mid neck traditionally have been explored. In the absence of clear signs of vascular injury, the patient can be evaluated with arteriography and endoscopy in preference to mandatory exploration in all patients. Patients with injury at the base of the neck and the base of the skull preferentially should undergo arteriography.

- Clinical features raising the suspicion of blunt trauma to the carotid artery include:
  - Bruits
  - Horner syndrome
  - Transient ischemic attacks
  - Lucid interval after injury, followed by neurologic symptoms and limb paresis in an alert patient

All carotid artery injuries should be repaired if the vessel is patent. Those with occlusion of the internal carotid artery probably should not undergo attempted revascularization because complete thrombus removal cannot always be ensured at the time of reperfusion. The clinical condition of the patient is an important factor in determining the advisability of carotid artery repair. Surgical repair of all carotid injuries in patients with no or mild neurologic deficits is recommended, whereas patients with severe neurologic deficits associated with carotid occlusion are poor candidates for vascular reconstruction because of excessive mortality risk.

Vertebral Artery Injuries

Wounds of the vertebral arteries are much less common than those of the carotid artery. Preoperative arteriography is essential for proper diagnosis, assessing damage accurately, and evaluating the collateral circulation. Although direct repair is possible and should be considered in patients with a single dominant vertebral artery, most patients have a patent contralateral vertebral artery offering good collateral circulation. Therefore, catheter-based embolic occlusion is the preferred management.

Vascular Injury of the Extremities

The signs suggesting injury to the arteries supplying the extremities are shown in Table 15.7. The "hard signs" are nearly pathognomonic of an underlying arterial injury. The "soft signs" are less specific, are suggestive of vascular injury, and should be followed up with further investigation. Generally, hard signs of vascular injury mandate operative exploration. The urgency of operation depends on the number and severity of associated injuries, the amount of ongoing blood loss, the degree of distal ischemia, and the location of the injury.

The femoral arteries are among the most frequently injured vessels, comprising approximately 20% of all arterial injuries. Popliteal artery injuries are associated with significant morbidity if the injury is not repaired. Although penetrating injuries in the vicinity of blood vessels generally are evaluated with arteriography, blunt injury, especially posterior dislocation of the knee, may be associated with popliteal artery injury, which is often overlooked. In one report of 152 patients with knee dislocations, 28% had popliteal artery injury, with half of those patients eventually losing the limb. Observations such as these have led some to perform arteriography on all patients with a posterior knee dislocation, regardless of physical findings.

- The femoral arteries are among the most frequently injured vessels (≈20% of all arterial injuries)
- Popliteal artery injuries are associated with significant morbidity if not repaired

Table 15.7 Signs of Extremity Arterial Injury

Hard signs
Distal circulatory deficit
Ischemia
Pulses diminished or absent
Bruit
Expanding or pulsatile hematoma
Arterial bleeding
Soft signs
Small or moderate-sized stable hematoma
Adjacent nerve injury
Shock (unexplained by other injuries)
Proximity of penetrating wound to a major vascular structure
Ankle-brachial index <0.9

Patients with substantial blood loss should be resuscitated. Those with limb fractures should have the fracture stabilized. In an unstable patient with severe trauma, this is best accomplished in the operating room. Concomitant injuries of the common femoral vein and the popliteal vein should be repaired; ligation of these major veins is associated with extensive morbidity and significantly threatens the success of the arterial repair.

Patients who are stable or who do not have hard signs of vascular injury should undergo a thoughtful, non-invasive evaluation. Measurement of ABI and arterial duplex ultrasonographic examination can reliably evaluate these patients. The negative predictive value of an ABI greater than 0.9 is reported to be 99%, with excellent sensitivity of an abnormal ABI in predicting vascular injury. A normal arterial duplex scan associated with a normal ABI virtually excludes vascular injury.

Minimal Vascular Injury

Many small vascular injuries have been observed to heal spontaneously. In light of this, some authors have suggested that "minimal vascular injuries" can be observed, anticipating that spontaneous healing will occur. Such minimal injuries include intimal defects, small irregularities adjacent to the arterial wall; intimal flaps smaller than 3 mm; pseudoaneurysms less than 0.5 cm; minor arterial stenoses; and small arteriovenous fistulas. Although several series have reported good outcomes in patients with these minimal injuries, some patients have had additional problems. Pseudoaneurysms appear to have the greatest propensity to thrombose or enlarge; therefore, these require the closest follow-up if treated non-operatively.

Venous Injury

Most vascular surgeons agree that, if possible, venous injuries should be repaired rather than ligated. The beneficial results of repairing major venous injury include a higher likelihood of successful repair of a concomitant arterial injury, a decreased likelihood of postoperative venous insufficiency, and a decreased likelihood of compartment syndrome.

Generally, venous injuries should be repaired if there is an associated arterial injury. Acute ligation restricts venous outflow and has been shown to compromise the patency of associated arterial repairs. Animal studies have shown a decrease in arterial inflow that persists up to 3 days after venous ligation. Furthermore, clinical reports of combined arterial and venous injury have shown improved limb salvage in patients undergoing venous reconstruction. Even in patients with isolated popliteal vein injuries, repair is associated with decreased morbidity compared with ligation.

Compartment Syndrome

A frequent concern with revascularization after acute ischemia due to arterial injury, particularly in the lower legs, is acute compartment syndrome. It is especially common in patients with combined arterial and venous injury because of the added venous hypertension. The increased compartmental pressure is the result of reperfusion of ischemic tissues after arterial reconstruction, relative venous hypertension due to venous obstruction, and direct tissue injury. Patients presenting with prolonged ischemia (>6 hours), with combined arterial and venous injury, with severe soft tissue trauma, and with an already swollen limb should have fasciotomy at the time of vascular reconstruction.

Patients at risk for compartment syndrome who are being clinically evaluated and in whom the diagnosis is suspected should have measurement of the compartment pressure. Compartment pressures greater than 30 cm of water indicate the need for fasciotomy. Compartmental hypertension may be decreased by the infusion of hypertonic mannitol, which decreases the edema resulting from reperfusion of ischemic muscle. Patients requiring fasciotomy should have all four compartments (anterior, lateral, superficial posterior, and deep posterior) of the leg decompressed to avoid irreversible nerve and soft tissue injury; on rare occasions, fasciotomy of the thigh is required (Fig. 15.4). Adequate decompression can be accomplished only by long, bilateral skin incisions offering access to the four compartments, or by perifibular fasciotomy, which can be performed through a single anterolateral incision.

Questions

1. Which of the following statements is true regarding acute arterial occlusions?
- **a.** The most common form of acute arterial occlusion is a thrombosis.
- **b.** Most arterial emboli occur between the aortic and popliteal bifurcations.
- **c.** Compared with thrombotic arterial occlusions, embolic arterial occlusions carry twice the risk of limb loss.
- **d.** The most common patient presentation of acute arterial occlusion is a cold extremity.

2. Which of the following is not associated with an increased risk of atheromatous embolism?
- **a.** Abdominal aortic aneurysm
- **b.** Catheter-based procedures
- **c.** Anticoagulation therapy
- **d.** Black male older than 50 years
- **e.** Popliteal aneurysm

3. Which of the following are symptoms of thoracic vascular injury?
- **a.** Loss of consciousness
- **b.** Dyspnea
- **c.** Cephalic hypotension
- **d.** Retrosternal or intrascapular pain
- **e.** All of the above
- **f.** b, c, and d
- **g.** a, b, and d

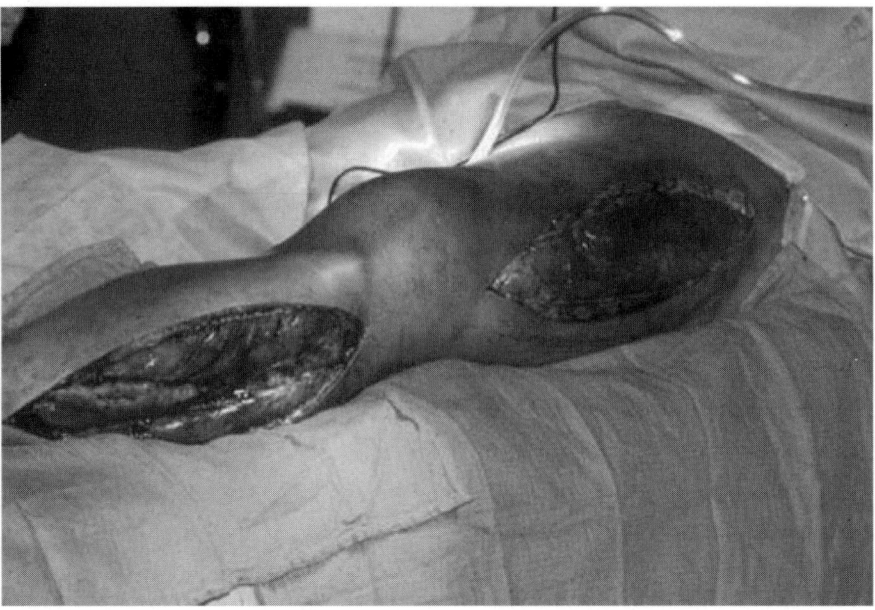

Fig. 15.4 Operative photograph of thigh and four-compartment leg fasciotomy after revascularization for profound left lower extremity ischemia due to acute iliofemoral arterial occlusion. Note extreme muscle edema and need for full-length skin incision for adequate decompression.

4. Which of the following statements is correct regarding acute compartment syndrome?
   a. Compartment pressures >20 cm of water indicate the need for fasciotomy.
   b. Combined arterial and venous injuries increase the risk of acute compartment syndrome.
   c. Acute compartment syndrome primarily occurs in patients for whom the ischemic limb has been revascularized too rapidly.
   d. Most cases of acute compartment syndrome are able to be treated with a fasciotomy of the thigh only.

Suggested Readings

Aune S, Trippestad A. Operative mortality and long-term survival of patients operated on for acute lower limb ischaemia. Eur J Vasc Endovasc Surg. 1998;15:143-6.

Belenfant X, Meyrier A, Jacquot C. Supportive treatment improves survival in multivisceral cholesterol crystal embolism. Am J Kidney Dis. 1999;33:840-50.

Coffman JD. Atheromatous embolism. Vasc Med. 1996;1:267-73.

Comerota AJ, Harada RN. Acute arterial occlusion. In: Young JR, Olin JW, Bartholomew JR, editors. Peripheral vascular diseases. 2nd ed. St. Louis: Mosby; 1996. p. 273-87.

Dormandy J, Heeck L, Vig S. Acute limb ischemia. Semin Vasc Surg. 1999;12:148-53.

Dormandy JA, Rutherford RB, TASC Working Group. Management of peripheral arterial disease (PAD). TransAtlantic Inter-Society Consensus (TASC). Section C: acute limb ischemia. J Vasc Surg. 2000;31:S135-67.

Fabbian F, Catalano C, Lambertini D, et al. A possible role of corticosteroids in cholesterol crystal embolization. Nephron. 1999;83:189-90.

Fine MJ, Kapoor W, Falanga V. Cholesterol crystal embolization: a review of 221 cases in the English literature. Angiology. 1987;38:769-84.

Frykberg ER, Dennis JW, Bishop K, et al. The reliability of physical examination in the evaluation of penetrating extremity trauma for vascular injury: results at one year. J Trauma. 1991;31:502-11.

Johansen K, Lynch K, Paun M, et al. Non-invasive vascular tests reliably exclude occult arterial trauma in injured extremities. J Trauma. 1991;31:515-9.

Keen RR, McCarthy WJ, Shireman PK, et al. Surgical management of atheroembolization. J Vasc Surg. 1995;21:773-80.

Lie JT. Cholesterol atheromatous embolism: the great masquerader revisited. Pathol Annu. 1992;27:17-50.

Phifer TJ, Gerlock AJ Jr, Vekovius WA, et al. Amputation risk factors in concomitant superficial femoral artery and vein injuries. Ann Surg. 1984;199:241-3.

Ramirez G, O'Neill WM Jr, Lambert R, et al. Cholesterol embolization: a complication of angiography. Arch Intern Med. 1978;138:1430-2.

Richardson JD, Vitale GC, Flint LM Jr. Penetrating arterial trauma: analysis of missed vascular injuries. Arch Surg. 1987;122:678-83.

Sirinek KR, Levine BA, Gaskill HV III, et al. Reassessment of the role of routine operative exploration in vascular trauma. J Trauma. 1981;21:339-44.

The STILE Investigators. Results of a prospective randomized trial evaluating surgery versus thrombolysis for ischemia of the lower extremity: the STILE trial. Ann Surg. 1994;220:251-66.

Working Party on Thrombolysis in the Management of Limb Ischemia. Thrombolysis in the management of lower limb peripheral arterial occlusion—a consensus document. Am J Cardiol. 1998;81:207-18.

16 Aortic Aneurysms

Joshua A. Beckman, MD
Mark A. Creager, MD

Introduction

An aneurysm is a pathologic expansion of all three layers of an artery. In the aorta, aneurysm formation may occur in any segment, from the aortic root to the bifurcation into the iliac arteries. The frequency of aneurysm formation and the prognostic implications vary considerably depending on the site of the aneurysm. Aortic aneurysms are associated with more than 15,000 deaths per year in the United States. This chapter highlights the natural history, epidemiology, pathophysiology, diagnosis, and treatment of aortic aneurysms.

Definition of Aortic Aneurysm

The definition of an aortic aneurysm includes two factors: absolute size and relative change. In normal adults, the aorta has a diameter of approximately 3 cm at the root, 2.5 cm in the mid portion of the descending aorta, and 2 cm in the infrarenal aorta. In the abdominal aorta, a diameter of 3 cm or more often is used to define an aneurysm. However, this primary definition does not account for the wide variation in body size, so a secondary definition may be applied when needed. For example, a 50% increase in size relative to the proximal normal segment also connotes an aneurysm. Aneurysms may be fusiform (expansion of the entire vessel circumference) or saccular (evagination of a segment of the circumference). Fusiform aneurysm formation is more common.

Pathophysiology of Aneurysm Formation

Formerly, aneurysm formation was thought to be a variant of the process of atherosclerosis. More recently, these processes have been separated histologically and physiologically. Atherosclerosis is a proliferative intimal and medial process, whereas aneurysm formation is characterized by the elimination of supporting structures in the medial and adventitial layers. Microscopic evaluation of an aortic aneurysm shows elastin and collagen destruction, a paucity of vascular smooth muscle, many inflammatory cells, and neovascularization. Aneurysm formation in patients with Marfan syndrome, bicuspid aortic valve, and other disease states predisposed to thoracic aneurysm formation manifest less inflammation, whereas abdominal aortic aneurysms (AAAs) usually do not contain cystic medial necrosis. Despite these differences, aneurysm formation in varying segments of the aorta is more similar than different.

Aneurysm formation is characterized by a weakened aortic wall resulting from the loss of the structural proteins elastin and collagen. Elastin provides the aorta the flexibility and resiliency to deform in response to the pulse of the heart and then return to its original conformation. Loss of elastin is the seminal event in aneurysm formation; this loss initially is compensated for by increased collagen production. Collagen provides tensile strength to the aorta but cannot accommodate the effects of pulsatile stretch; therefore, aortic expansion ensues. With collagen degradation, aneurysms form and the risk of rupture increases. The major pathophysiologic processes underlying breakdown of elastin and collagen are inflammation, proteolysis, and, in the abdominal aorta, changes in biomechanical wall stress.

Nearly all aneurysm specimens show signs of mild or moderate inflammation. The cellular constituents, including B and T lymphocytes and macrophages, are concentrated in the adventitia and media. These cells create an inflammatory environment with increased levels of inflammatory cytokines and increased expression of cellular adhesion molecules. The signal that initiates this process remains undefined. However, once activated, a mechanism important to the process of aneurysm formation is proteolysis. The structural components of the aorta are degraded by matrix metalloproteases (MMPs), which are increased in concentration. The most important MMPs for aneurysm formation are MMP2 and MMP9. Activation of MMPs may occur as a result of increased oxidative stress, increased expression of plasminogen activators (which regulate MMP activation), or inadequate expression of tissue inhibitors of MMPs to compensate for the increased concentration of MMPs.

The propensity for AAA formation may be attributable to structural variations among the segments of the aorta and flow disturbances specifically associated with the abdominal aorta. The abdominal aorta contains fewer elastic lamellae than the thoracic aorta, making it less able to accommodate decreases in elastin levels. Moreover, the vasa vasorum (nutritive vessel network) is less abundant in this segment of the aorta. Decreased perfusion is associated with increased vessel rigidity, decreased compliance, and decreased ability to accommodate pulsatile flow. Finally, the pattern of blood flow may predispose the abdominal segment to aneurysm formation. This section withstands the greatest level of oscillating blood flow and reflected pressure waves. Experimentally, decreases in this oscillation reduce aneurysm formation.

Compensatory mechanisms may inhibit further increases in aneurysm size. Increased production of elastin has been observed in aortic aneurysms, but the elastin is disorganized and does not add to the vessel's structural integrity. Intraluminal thrombus formation within the aneurysm may also decrease wall stress—up to 38% in some experimental studies. However, the thrombus also may be a source of proteolytic enzymes and enzyme activators, serving as a pathologic reservoir of elements destructive to the aortic wall.

- Aortic aneurysms are associated with more than 15,000 deaths per year in the United States
- Microscopic evaluation of an aortic aneurysm shows:
  - Elastin and collagen destruction
  - Few inflammatory cells
  - Neovascularization
- The structural components of the aorta are degraded by MMPs

Abdominal Aortic Aneurysm

Epidemiology

In the abdominal aorta, the upper limit of size is usually defined as 29 mm. Using this definition of an aneurysm (abdominal aorta diameter >29 mm), a series of 24,000 consecutive autopsies showed an aneurysm prevalence of 2%. In targeted populations of older men, the rate has ranged from 0.7% to 8.4%. The Aneurysm Detection and Management (ADAM) study, which screened more than 73,000 veterans aged 50 to 79 years, reported a prevalence of 4.0% for aneurysms 3.0 cm or larger and 1.4% for aneurysms 4.0 cm or larger. Aortic aneurysms are less likely to develop in women. In a subsequent report of the ADAM study that included more than 125,000 subjects (3,450 women), the prevalence of aneurysms 3.0 cm and larger was 1.0% for women and 4.3% for men.

Three risk factors are important for the development of AAAs: age, sex, and cigarette smoking. Every epidemiologic study has shown an effect of age on aneurysm formation, with little risk in persons younger than 50 years and a sharp increase beginning at age 60 years. In a Norwegian population-based study, the incidence increased from 0% among those aged 25 to 44 years to 18% for persons aged 75 to 84 years. Aneurysms are two to six times more likely to develop in men than in women. Perhaps the most important societal risk factor is cigarette smoking. The risk of aneurysm increases approximately threefold in smokers when compared with non-smokers and is associated with the number of cigarettes smoked, the duration of cigarette smoking, and the degree of cigarette filtration.

- The ADAM screening study of more than 73,000 veterans aged 50-79 years showed:
  - A prevalence of 4% for aneurysms ≥3 cm
  - A prevalence of 1.4% for aneurysms ≥4 cm
- Aortic aneurysms are less likely to develop in women

Some persons have a genetic predisposition for AAA formation. Patients with first-degree relatives with AAA are at much higher risk for AAA formation than are age- and sex-matched controls. Aneurysms develop earlier for patients with a family history of AAA, and their age at aneurysm rupture is nearly a decade younger than that of patients without a family history. Indeed, the risk of AAA is greater than 20% for men older than 50 years with a first-degree relative with an AAA. Although many studies confirm the importance of family history, no candidate gene has been identified that explains the pattern of inheritance.

- Three risk factors are important for the development of AAAs:
  - Age
  - Sex
  - Cigarette smoking
- Some patients have a genetic predisposition for AAA formation

Natural History

For nearly all patients, AAAs are asymptomatic. Over time, aneurysms expand and may rupture if untreated.

The rate of rupture increases markedly as the aortic diameter increases beyond 5 cm. The 1-year risk of rupture is 9.4% for aneurysms of 5 to 5.5 cm but is 32.5% for aneurysms greater than 7 cm in diameter. On the basis of these data, two large randomized trials were performed to determine the optimal time for intervention. Patients were enrolled if they had asymptomatic aneurysms larger than 4 cm but smaller than 5.5 cm. Patients were randomly assigned to early surgical repair or to monitoring with ultrasonography until the aneurysm reached 5.5 cm, at which time surgery was performed. Both studies showed no difference in survival between the two groups at 5 years. Although the total mortality rate was 20% to 25% in the two studies, aneurysm-related mortality, even in these high-risk patients, accounted for no more than 5% of total deaths. Cardiovascular disease was the most common cause of death in both studies. Cigarette smoking, high blood pressure, and female sex increased the risk of rapid expansion and aortic rupture.

- 1-year risk of aneurysm rupture:
  - 9.4% for aneurysms of 5-5.5 cm
  - 32.5% for aneurysms ≥7 cm
- The most common cause of mortality is cardiovascular disease

Presentation

Although nearly all patients with AAAs are asymptomatic, symptoms, when present, include abdominal or back pain, leg discomfort, groin pain, anorexia, nausea, vomiting, and constipation. Aneurysm expansion may compress adjacent structures, including the left iliac vein (causing leg swelling), the left ureter (causing hydronephrosis), and vertebrae and lumbar nerve roots (causing back pain). Frank rupture of AAAs typically results in hemodynamic collapse, back pain, and a pulsatile abdominal mass, although fewer than half of patients present with all three symptoms.

A pulsatile abdominal mass is the classic physical finding of an AAA. However, even with direct abdominal palpation, the sensitivity of physical examination for detection of an AAA is 30% to 50%. The factor most associated with failure to detect an aneurysm is large abdominal girth. After aneurysm rupture, patients most likely will have circulatory collapse with tachycardia, pallor, and hypotension.

Diagnostic Tests

Currently, diagnostic tests are performed only if an aneurysm is suspected clinically. Screening recently has been recommended by the United States Preventive Services Task Force for male smokers aged 65 to 75 years, although screening is not supported by any funding agency. In the Multicentre Aneurysm Screening Study, which included nearly 68,000 men aged 65 to 74 years, a 42% decrease in aneurysm-related mortality was observed in the screened population when compared with the control group. No significant decrease in total mortality was noted. Patients with an inherited disorder of connective tissue (e.g., Marfan syndrome or Ehlers-Danlos syndrome) or siblings of patients with an AAA should also undergo diagnostic tests.

Ultrasonography is the conventional test for AAA diagnosis and follow-up. The test is rapid and safe, does not use ionizing radiation, and is 100% sensitive for AAAs larger than 3 cm. Although several investigators have found that ultrasonography may underestimate AAA size by as much as 0.5 cm, two large trials comparing observation versus early surgery showed ultrasonography to be effective for aneurysm follow-up. After surgical repair, ultrasonography is an acceptable method for diagnosing anastomotic pseudoaneurysm formation and measuring perianeurysm aortic size. However, ultrasonography is not appropriate for follow-up evaluation after repair with an aortic endograft. Its ability to evaluate endoleaks, device migration, and device failure is limited.

Computed tomography (CT) is the preferred preoperative imaging modality. Multidetector-row CT angiography (CTA, currently with up to 64 rows) creates high-resolution images of the aorta that are used to determine aneurysm size with 0.2-mm resolution. CT can accurately define the proximal and distal extent of the AAA, the origins of major branch vessels, and the degree of branch vessel disease. CT is commonly used before and after aortic repair with endograft placement because it can show aortic angulation, iliac artery tortuosity, the presence of preexisting iliac artery atherosclerosis before placement, endoleaks, stent graft migration, and device failure after placement. Magnetic resonance imaging is equivalent to CT for characterization of aortic aneurysms and may be used for surgical planning and follow-up. Intra-arterial contrast angiography is used infrequently. Like CT and magnetic resonance imaging, it can define the location of the AAA relative to branch arteries (e.g., the renal arteries), but it cannot determine the size of an aneurysm. The invasive nature of the procedure and the nephrotoxicity of the contrast agent have limited the use of contrast angiography for evaluation of AAA.

- Ultrasonography is inappropriate for follow-up after endograft placement because of its limited ability to evaluate endoleaks, device migration, and device failure
- CT is the preferred preoperative imaging modality

Therapy

Data supporting specific medical therapy for aneurysms are limited. β-Adrenergic receptor blockers are commonly recommended for decreasing the rate of aneurysm growth. One trial showed a decrease in the growth rate of thoracic aortic aneurysms with the use of β-blockers in patients with Marfan syndrome, but this finding cannot necessarily be extrapolated to AAA. In one trial, β-blockers did not significantly change AAA growth rates or rates of surgery or mortality, but they made patients feel worse. β-Blockers, however, are appropriate for patients with AAA who also have hypertension or coronary artery disease.

Cigarette smoking is associated with more rapid aneurysm expansion rates and increases the risk of rupture. Thus, all patients should be encouraged to quit smoking. Doxycycline decreases MMP production and inhibits aneurysm expansion in experimental animal models, but it is not known whether doxycycline inhibits aneurysm growth in humans.

To decrease mortality rates in patients with aortic aneurysms, treatment should not focus solely on the aneurysm. In two small randomized AAA trials, cardiovascular morbidity and mortality were much greater than aneurysm-related mortality. AAA is associated with atherosclerosis and may be considered an equivalent risk factor for coronary heart disease, which should prompt risk factor modification.

- In small randomized AAA trials, cardiovascular morbidity and mortality were much greater than aneurysm-related mortality

Current indications for AAA repair were defined by two large trials—the United Kingdom Small Aneurysm Trial and the ADAM study. In both trials, sonographic surveillance (until the aneurysm diameter was 5.5 cm) was as safe as immediate repair for patients with AAAs between 4 and 5.5 cm. The general consensus is that all AAAs 5.5 cm in diameter or larger should be repaired to decrease the risk of rupture unless comorbid conditions preclude intervention or adversely affect the patient's long-term prognosis. Patients with chronic lung disease and renal dysfunction have the highest risk of death after surgery. Surgical approaches include a midline abdominal approach and a retroperitoneal approach. For both, the aneurysm is incised, and a graft is inserted between the two closest normal aortic segments or from the aneurysm site to the iliac arteries. The complications of surgery are primarily cardiac. The mortality rates range from 2% to 6% in published series. Other complications include distal embolization, visceral ischemia, and infection.

Recently, the US Food and Drug Administration approved endografting for AAA repair. The stent grafts are inserted via the femoral artery and self expand or are balloon expanded to exclude the aneurysm from active circulation. Recent randomized trials showed that percutaneous repair was associated with decreased morbidity at 30 days when compared with open repair, but mortality rates were similar at 2 years. Longer-term outcomes are not yet available, and the superior therapy has not been determined. Potential late outcomes with endografting include development of endoleaks and a higher rate of late failure than that for surgical repair. Approximately 30% of all patients treated with endografts will require another procedure within 5 years of the initial device placement. Also, endografting requires yearly CT examinations to monitor the device. Over time, the cost of the less-invasive procedure may not be less than that of the open procedure.

Thoracic Aortic Aneurysm

Thoracic aortic aneurysms (TAAs) are less common than AAAs. In Olmsted County, Minnesota, only 72 of approximately 45,000 residents (0.16%) received a diagnosis of TAA over a 30-year period. Similarly, in a CT screening program of middle-aged men and women in Japan, 11 of the 6,971 subjects (0.16%) had TAA. Thus, the frequency of this disease is low. An autopsy study of more than 44,000 subjects showed that 63 had died from a ruptured TAA.

Etiology

The causes of TAA include medial degeneration, aortic dissection, inherited abnormality of collagen, spondyloarthropathies, infection, aortitis, and trauma (Table 16.1). Idiopathic medial degeneration occurs in approximately 80% of cases. Many of the risk factors for TAA are similar to those for AAA. TAA occurs more often in older persons; the peak incidence occurs between 70 and 80 years. The risk of TAA development is two times higher in men than women. Among the segmental locations of TAA, the descending thoracic aorta is involved in more than half of TAAs, whereas the ascending aorta is involved in about one-third of cases.

Two well-described, inherited connective tissue disorders cause aortic aneurysm: Marfan syndrome and Ehlers-Danlos syndrome. For patients with Marfan syndrome, the abnormal synthesis of fibrillin adversely affects collagen production. Patients with Ehlers-Danlos syndrome have a defect of collagen synthesis. Up to 80% of patients with Ehlers-Danlos syndrome have a visceral or vascular rupture by the age of 40 years, which yields a mean survival of 48 years.

The presence of a bicuspid aortic valve increases the risk of an ascending TAA. The aortic abnormality is unrelated to the severity of valve dysfunction. The aortic wall

Table 16.1 Causes of Thoracic Aortic Aneurysms

Degenerative
Idiopathic
Associated with atherosclerosis
Cystic medial necrosis
Marfan syndrome
Ehlers-Danlos syndrome
Bicuspid aortic valve
Aortic dissection
Vasculitis
Takayasu arteritis
Giant cell arteritis
Behçet syndrome
Spondyloarthropathies
Ankylosing spondylitis
Reiter syndrome
Relapsing polychondritis
Infection
Mycotic (e.g., *Staphylococcus, Salmonella*)
Tuberculosis
Syphilis
Trauma

in patients with bicuspid aortic valves has less fibrillin-1, tends to be thicker than that of age-matched controls, and shows increased rates of vascular smooth muscle apoptosis. MMP2 and MMP9 also show increased expression. Patients with Turner syndrome are likely to have a bicuspid aortic valve and an increased prevalence of TAA.

Takayasu arteritis usually occurs in the teens through age 40 years. It most commonly causes occlusive disease (80%-95% of patients), but aortic aneurysm may occur in as many as 25% of patients with Takayasu arteritis. Aortic aneurysm formation is associated with worse outcome. Giant cell arteritis (temporal arteritis) typically affects the primary and secondary branches of the aorta and occurs in patients older than 50 years. Women are twice as likely as men to have giant cell arteritis. Between 1% and 20% of patients with giant cell arteritis will also have an aortic aneurysm, most commonly in the thoracic aorta. Behçet syndrome is a small vessel vasculitis that may also manifest in large vessels by affecting the vasa vasorum. Vascular lesions, including aneurysms, occur in as many as 38% of these patients and should be treated with corticosteroids.

- Inherited connective tissue disorders that cause aortic aneurysm:
  - Marfan syndrome
  - Ehlers-Danlos syndrome
- The presence of a bicuspid aortic valve increases the risk of an ascending TAA
- A TAA develops in 1%-20% of patients with giant cell arteritis
- Aneurysms occur in up to 38% of patients with Behçet syndrome

Spondyloarthropathies are a heterogenous group of diseases that commonly show spinal and sacroiliac inflammation, an association with HLA-B27, and the absence of rheumatoid factor. Each of the disorders, which include ankylosing spondylitis, Reiter syndrome, and relapsing polychondritis, is associated with TAA. Aortic root and valve disease is present in up to 80% of patients with ankylosing spondylitis. Aortic valvular regurgitation is noted in approximately half the patients.

Mycotic aneurysms are rare, with an incidence of 0.03% in a large autopsy series. The typical patient with a mycotic aneurysm is a man aged 60 to 70 years. Infection affects a vessel that is "at risk" because of prior disease or damage. Because only a portion of the vessel is infected, mycotic aneurysms often are saccular. The organisms most commonly involved include *Staphylococcus* and *Salmonella* species, which cause 40% and 20% of mycotic aneurysms, respectively. Rupture occurs in as many as 80% of mycotic aneurysms; therefore, surgical referral should be prompt. Historically, tuberculosis and syphilis were important causes of aortic aneurysms, but both are less common today. Tuberculosis affects the aorta after spreading from a contiguous infection originating in the spine or lung. Syphilitic aortitis occurs in as many as 10% of patients with tertiary stage disease. Luetic aneurysms typically affect the ascending aorta and are saccular. Involvement of the coronary artery ostia may cause angina. The diagnosis is suggested by linear calcification of the ascending aorta (determined by chest radiography).

- Ankylosing spondylitis, Reiter syndrome, and relapsing polychondritis are associated with TAA
- Mycotic aneurysms are commonly saccular; most are caused by *Staphylococcus* or *Salmonella* species
- Tuberculosis and syphilis previously were important causes of aortic aneurysms, although both are less common today

Patients who survive an aortic dissection are at risk for late development of an aortic aneurysm. Dissection is a preceding occurrence that leads to aneurysm dilatation in 15% to 20% of patients with TAA. The two most important factors that predict the requirement for aneurysm repair are a baseline aortic diameter exceeding 39 mm and a patent false lumen. Because of this late risk, patients with aortic dissection require follow-up with CT or magnetic resonance imaging at 3, 6, and 12 months after the sentinel dissection. Thereafter, yearly imaging should be performed.

Prognosis

The greatest risks associated with TAA are aneurysmal expansion and rupture. Survival rates range from 39% to 87% at 1 year and 13% to 46% at 5 years. The aneurysm diameter at diagnosis is predictive of rupture. In one study, patients with a TAA diameter 5 cm or larger had a 3-year survival rate of 60%; those with an aneurysm smaller than 5 cm had a 90% 3-year survival rate. The optimal diameter at which a TAA should be repaired is not well defined. Most studies suggest repair of an ascending aortic aneurysm at a diameter of 5.5 to 6.0 cm. For patients with Marfan syndrome, repair is recommended at a diameter of 4.5 to 5.0 cm. For patients with descending TAAs, repair should be considered at a diameter of 6.5 to 7.0 cm.

- Dissection precedes aneurysm dilatation in 15% to 20% of patients with TAA
- The optimal diameter for repair of TAA is not well defined
  - For an ascending aortic aneurysm: 5.5-6.0 cm
  - For patients with Marfan syndrome: 4.5-5.0 cm
  - For a descending TAA: 6.5-7.0 cm

Popliteal Artery Aneurysm

Peripheral artery aneurysms most commonly are located in the popliteal artery. The incidence of popliteal artery aneurysms is 0.1% to 0.3%. They occur in approximately 3% to 10% of patients with AAA. As with AAA, most patients are 65 years or older and are predominantly men. These aneurysms occur bilaterally for more than 50% of patients. Older age and hypertension are associated with aneurysm expansion. Popliteal aneurysms may be saccular or fusiform. Saccular aneurysms may cause symptoms of compression, whereas fusiform aneurysms are more likely to cause distal embolization or to thrombose. Both types may rupture, although rupture is rare.

The most common symptoms at presentation are ischemia (resulting from distal embolization), popliteal artery thrombosis, and peroneal nerve compression. Venous compression may occur if the aneurysm is larger than 2 cm. Popliteal artery aneurysm can be diagnosed by palpation in more than 90% of cases (if performed by an experienced clinician). However, approximately 75% of popliteal aneurysms will be undetected by general practitioners, even in symptomatic patients. Imaging of the popliteal artery should be performed for confirmation; duplex ultrasonography is 100% sensitive for the diagnosis of a popliteal aneurysm.

The threshold for repair of asymptomatic aneurysms is controversial. Some suggest repair when the diameter is 2 cm, whereas others recommend 3 cm. The risk of symptoms is approximately 25% at 1 year and 67% at 5 years. Symptomatic aneurysms require repair. The most common surgical repair includes ligation at the proximal and distal ends of the aneurysm and a saphenous vein bypass. Thrombolysis may be used occasionally to clear the runoff vessels and improve graft patency.

- Popliteal artery aneurysms occur in approximately 3%-10% of patients with AAA
- More than 50% of popliteal artery aneurysms occur bilaterally
- Popliteal artery aneurysms may rupture, although rupture is rare
- The most common symptoms at presentation are ischemia due to distal embolism, popliteal artery thrombosis, occlusion, and peroneal nerve compression
- The threshold for repair of asymptomatic aneurysms is controversial (2 cm vs 3 cm)

Questions

1. Which of the following is the most common complication of a popliteal artery aneurysm?
   a. Rupture
   b. Thrombosis or embolism with limb ischemia
   c. Popliteal vein thrombosis
   d. Peroneal nerve palsy

2. Which of the following mechanisms accounts for most AAAs?
   a. Inherited disorder of fibrillin synthesis
   b. Increased concentration of MMPs
   c. Altered shear stress
   d. Infiltration of the vascular wall by lipid-laden macrophages

3. A 72-year-old woman with an AAA has been monitored with yearly abdominal ultrasonography for 5 years. The maximal diameters measured were 3.7 cm at 1 year, 3.7 cm at 2 years, 3.9 cm at 3 years, 4.0 cm at 4 years, and 5.0 cm at 5 years. What do you now recommend?
   a. Abdominal ultrasonography in 6 months
   b. β-Blockers
   c. Doxycycline
   d. Aneurysm repair

4. Which of the following factors is not associated with AAAs?
   a. Male sex
   b. Advancing age
   c. Cigarette smoking
   d. Diagnosis of diabetes mellitus

5. CTA confirmed a 5.0-cm fusiform aneurysm of the descending thoracic aorta in a 74-year-old man. He is asymptomatic. Which of the following management options is most appropriate?
   a. Imaging study (magnetic resonance angiography or CTA) in 6 months to assess the size of the TAA
   b. Administration of doxycycline to decrease the risk of TAA expansion
   c. Endovascular fenestration of the thoracic aorta
   d. Surgical repair of the TAA

Suggested Readings

Ailawadi G, Eliason JL, Upchurch GR Jr. Current concepts in the pathogenesis of abdominal aortic aneurysm. J Vasc Surg. 2003;38:584-8.

American Heart Association. Heart disease and stroke statistics: 2004 update. Dallas (TX): American Heart Association; 2003.

Ashton HA, Buxton MJ, Day NE, et al, Multicentre Aneurysm Screening Study Group. The Multicentre Aneurysm Screening Study (MASS) into the effect of abdominal aortic aneurysm screening on mortality in men: a randomised controlled trial. Lancet. 2002;360:1531-9.

Baxter BT, Pearce WH, Waltke EA, et al. Prolonged administration of doxycycline in patients with small asymptomatic abdominal aortic aneurysms: report of a prospective (Phase II) multicenter study. J Vasc Surg. 2002;36:1-12.

Blankensteijn JD, de Jong SE, Prinssen M, et al, Dutch Randomized Endovascular Aneurysm Management (DREAM) Trial Group. Two-year outcomes after conventional or endovascular repair of abdominal aortic aneurysms. N Engl J Med. 2005;352:2398-405.

Brady AR, Fowkes FG, Greenhalgh RM, et al, UK Small Aneurysm Trial Participants. Risk factors for postoperative death following elective surgical repair of abdominal aortic aneurysm: results from the UK Small Aneurysm Trial. Br J Surg. 2000;87:742-9.

Cole CW, Barber GG, Bouchard AG, et al. Abdominal aortic aneurysm: consequences of a positive family history. Can J Surg. 1989;32:117-20.

Dapunt OE, Galla JD, Sadeghi AM, et al. The natural history of thoracic aortic aneurysms. J Thorac Cardiovasc Surg. 1994;107:1323-32.

Darling RC, Messina CR, Brewster DC, et al. Autopsy study of unoperated abdominal aortic aneurysms: the case for early resection. Circulation. 1977;56 Suppl:II161-4.

Dawson I, Sie R, van Baalen JM, et al. Asymptomatic popliteal aneurysm: elective operation versus conservative follow-up. Br J Surg. 1994;81:1504-7.

Downing R, Grimley RP, Ashton F, et al. Problems in diagnosis of popliteal aneurysms. J R Soc Med. 1985;78:440-4.

Elefteriades JA. Natural history of thoracic aortic aneurysms: indications for surgery, and surgical versus nonsurgical risks. Ann Thorac Surg. 2002;74:S1877-80.

Evans JM, Bowles CA, Bjornsson J, et al. Thoracic aortic aneurysm and rupture in giant cell arteritis: a descriptive study of 41 cases. Arthritis Rheum. 1994;37:1539-47. Erratum in: Arthritis Rheum. 1995;38:290.

EVAR Trial Participants. Endovascular aneurysm repair and outcome in patients unfit for open repair of abdominal aortic aneurysm (EVAR trial 2): randomised controlled trial. Lancet. 2005;365:2187-92.

Isselbacher EM. Thoracic and abdominal aortic aneurysms. Circulation. 2005;111:816-28.

Kerr GS, Hallahan CW, Giordano J, et al. Takayasu arteritis. Ann Intern Med. 1994;120:919-29.

Lederle FA, Johnson GR, Wilson SE, Aneurysm Detection and Management Veterans Affairs Cooperative Study Investigators. Abdominal aortic aneurysm in women. J Vasc Surg. 2001;34:122-6.

Lederle FA, Johnson GR, Wilson SE, et al, Aneurysm Detection and Management (ADAM) Veterans Affairs Cooperative Study Group. Prevalence and associations of abdominal aortic aneurysm detected through screening. Ann Intern Med. 1997;126:441-9.

Lederle FA, Johnson GR, Wilson SE, et al, Aneurysm Detection and Management Veterans Affairs Cooperative Study Investigators. The aneurysm detection and management study screening program: validation cohort and final results. Arch Intern Med. 2000;160:1425-30.

Lederle FA, Johnson GR, Wilson SE, et al, Veterans Affairs Cooperative Study #417 Investigators. Rupture rate of large abdominal aortic aneurysms in patients refusing or unfit for elective repair. JAMA. 2002;287:2968-72.

Lederle FA, Wilson SE, Johnson GR, et al, Aneurysm Detection and Management Veterans Affairs Cooperative Study Group. Immediate repair compared with surveillance of small abdominal aortic aneurysms. N Engl J Med. 2002;346:1437-44.

Panneton JM, Hollier LH. Nondissecting thoracoabdominal aortic aneurysms: Part I. Ann Vasc Surg. 1995;9:503-14.

Prall AK, Longo GM, Mayhan WG, et al. Doxycycline in patients with abdominal aortic aneurysms and in mice: comparison of serum levels and effect on aneurysm growth in mice. J Vasc Surg. 2002;35:923-9.

Prinssen M, Verhoeven EL, Buth J, et al, Dutch Randomized Endovascular Aneurysm Management (DREAM) Trial Group. A randomized trial comparing conventional and endovascular repair of abdominal aortic aneurysms. N Engl J Med. 2004;351:1607-18.

Propranolol Aneurysm Trial Investigators. Propranolol for small abdominal aortic aneurysms: results of a randomized trial. J Vasc Surg. 2002;35:72-9.

Shores J, Berger KR, Murphy EA, et al. Progression of aortic dilatation and the benefit of long-term beta-adrenergic blockade in Marfan's syndrome. N Engl J Med. 1994;330:1335-41.

Singh K, Bonaa KH, Jacobsen BK, et al. Prevalence of and risk factors for abdominal aortic aneurysms in a population-based study: The Tromso Study. Am J Epidemiol. 2001;154:236-44.

Steyerberg EW, Kievit J, de Mol Van Otterloo JC, et al. Perioperative mortality of elective abdominal aortic aneurysm surgery: a clinical prediction rule based on literature and individual patient data. Arch Intern Med. 1995;155:1998-2004.

Szekanecz Z, Shah MR, Harlow LA, et al. Interleukin-8 and tumor necrosis factor-alpha are involved in human aortic endothelial cell migration: the possible role of these cytokines in human aortic aneurysmal blood vessel growth. Pathobiology. 1994;62:134-9.

Tang JL, Morris JK, Wald NJ, et al. Mortality in relation to tar yield of cigarettes: a prospective study of four cohorts. BMJ. 1995;311:1530-3.

The UK Small Aneurysm Trial Participants. Mortality results for randomised controlled trial of early elective surgery or ultrasonographic surveillance for small abdominal aortic aneurysms. Lancet. 1998;352:1649-55.

United Kingdom Small Aneurysm Trial Participants. Long-term outcomes of immediate repair compared with surveillance of small abdominal aortic aneurysms. N Engl J Med. 2002;346:1445-52.

17 Aortic Dissection and Dissection-Like Syndromes

Joshua A. Beckman, MD, MS

Acute aortic syndromes are among the most serious of vascular complications; they require physician suspicion for diagnosis, use of specific medical and surgical therapies, and are fatal if untreated for too long. The disease course of aortic dissection can be dire; the mortality rate is 1% per hour during the first day, 50% by 1 week, and 90% by 3 months. This chapter describes aortic dissection and dissection-like syndromes, including intramural hematoma (IMH), penetrating atherosclerotic ulcer (PAU), and carotid artery dissection.

Aortic Dissection

Epidemiology

Although the estimated incidence of aortic dissection in the United States has decreased over the past 30 years, approximately 2,000 new cases still occur each year. Autopsy studies have suggested an annual incidence of 5 to 10 cases per million, whereas among whites in Minnesota, the rate may be as high as 27 cases per million. Blacks have a higher prevalence of aortic dissection, possibly because of a greater incidence of hypertension. The precise numbers are difficult to determine because up to one-third of patients with an acute aortic dissection die before receiving medical care.

Pathogenesis

An intimal tear is the classic initial event of an aortic dissection. After the intima is exposed to pulsating blood at high pressure, mural separation ensues and is propagated by ventricular systole. The cause of the initial tear is unclear, but the newly recognized syndrome of IMH may provide some insight.

In an IMH, the vasa vasorum ruptures and hemorrhages into the subintimal space, separating the layers of the vessel wall. If the process is confined to the aortic wall, it is considered an IMH. However, if the pressure within the wall is sufficiently high, overt dissection may develop. The relative proportions of aortic dissection and IMH without overt dissection are poorly defined, but in autopsy series of aortic dissection, up to 13% of the decedents had no identifiable tear. A rarer mechanism of aortic dissection is a PAU. Large atherosclerotic ulcers may disrupt the internal elastic lamina of the aorta and cause a local hematoma, aortic pseudoaneurysm, aortic dissection, or aortic rupture.

Classification

Two classification schemes—the DeBakey and Stanford systems—have been used to define aortic dissection. Most physicians use the Stanford system, which categorizes dissections as type A or type B, depending on whether the ascending aorta is involved. Type A dissection involves the ascending aorta, regardless of the location of the aortic tear, whereas type B dissection is limited to the descending aorta. Dissections with retrograde extension to the ascending aorta should be regarded as a dissection that begins in the ascending aorta.

- The Stanford system classifies dissection as type A (involving the ascending aorta) or type B (involving the descending aorta)
- Type A dissections have a very high rate of mortality (1% per hour during the first day) if medical therapy is not effective
- The diagnosis of a type A dissection should prompt urgent surgical consultation and repair

The Stanford system is useful because of its inherent prognostic value and because classification aids in management decisions. Type A dissections have a high mortality rate—up to 1% per hour during the first day if they are not ameliorated considerably with medical therapy. Urgent surgical consultation and repair is therefore indicated for type A dissections. A 6-year series of patients treated with or without surgery showed a mortality rate decrease of more than 50% for the surgically treated group.

In contrast, most patients with type B dissections can be treated medically. The mortality rate in a recent series of type B dissections that were treated medically was approximately 10%. Surgery for type B dissections typically is reserved for patients with evidence of visceral and major organ compromise, limb ischemia, refractory pain, secondary hypertension, or a combination of these symptoms. The risks of mortality and paraplegia are increased for patients who require surgery. Dissection may weaken the wall of the aorta, and therefore patients treated medically are at long-term risk for aneurysm formation. For these patients, aortic size should be monitored regularly, and they should undergo aortic aneurysm repair if they meet the routine repair criteria (discussed in detail in Chapter 16). Risk factors for aortic enlargement include an initial size of 4 cm or larger and a patent false lumen.

- The mortality rate in a recent series of type B dissections treated medically was ≈10%
- Surgery typically is reserved for patients with evidence of visceral and major organ compromise, limb ischemia, and secondary hypertension
- Patients should undergo aortic aneurysm repair if they meet routine repair criteria

Risk Factors

Hypertension is the risk factor most commonly associated with development of aortic dissection. In several large series, hypertension was present in 70% of patients. Aortic dissection also is common in older patients; in the largest cohort of patients with aortic dissection, the mean age was 63 years. Patients with type B dissections generally are older than those with type A dissections. Men are two times more likely than women to have aortic dissection. Other important precipitants of aortic dissection include iatrogenic causes (e.g., catheterization, cardiac surgery), aortic valve disease, and pregnancy.

Although patients with congenital structural abnormalities of the aortic wall or with congenital valve disease (bicuspid aortic valve or unicommissural valves) are a small portion of the population with aortic dissection, they have much higher rates of aortic dissection at younger ages than in age-matched controls. Hereditary connective tissue disorders predispose patients to aortic dissection; the two most common are Marfan syndrome and Ehlers-Danlos syndrome. Marfan syndrome is the most common inherited connective tissue disorder, with an incidence of approximately 1 in 7,000 persons. The disease is attributable to many different fibrillin-1 gene mutations with variable penetrance. Disease manifestations include ectopia lentis, ligamentous redundancy, mitral valve regurgitation, and ascending aortic aneurysm. In the aortic wall, the effects of dedifferentiation of vascular smooth muscle cells, abnormal structural tissue, and increased expression of metalloproteases combine to weaken the aortic wall and increase the likelihood of dissection.

Ehlers-Danlos syndrome is a rare congenital defect of type III collagen production. The most common manifestations include acrogeria, facial features that include a beaked nose and small jaw, thin skin, easy bruising, and vascular rupture. Pathologic examination shows fragmented internal elastic lamina and deposition of glycosaminoglycans in the media of large vessels. In a study of 199 patients with the vascular type of Ehlers-Danlos syndrome (type IV), 80% had a vascular or viscus rupture by age 40 years.

- Hypertension is the risk factor most commonly associated with development of aortic dissection
- Patients with congenital structural abnormalities of the aortic wall or with congenital valve disease have higher rates of aortic dissection at younger ages
- Hereditary connective tissue disorders (Marfan syndrome and Ehlers-Danlos syndrome) predispose patients to aortic dissection

Presentation

Nearly all patients with aortic dissection present with pain or loss of consciousness. Pain occurs in more than 90% of patients with type A and type B dissections. The pain usually is described as sharp or tearing with a sudden onset and may change location. Anterior chest and throat pain is more commonly associated with a type A dissection, whereas pain exclusively in the back signals a type B dissection. The pain of aortic dissection may be confused with that of myocardial infarction or pneumothorax if it is in the chest, or it may be mistaken as pancreatitis or renal colic if it affects the back or abdomen. Patients who present with neurologic symptoms (e.g., stroke or paraplegia) or with throat or neck pain are likely to have arch vessel compromise, extension of the dissection into cerebral vessels, or a combination of the two. Loss of consciousness may result from neurologic involvement or severe hemodynamic embarrassment.

- Pain occurs in more than 90% of patients with type A and type B dissections

Physical findings of aortic dissection may include hypotension or shock, pulse deficits, congestive heart failure, and aortic valvular insufficiency. Each of these findings is associated with an increased risk of mortality. Less common physical findings include superior vena cava syndrome, hematemesis, hemoptysis, and Horner syndrome. Laboratory evaluations, chest radiography, and electrocardiography usually have limited value in the diagnosis of an aortic dissection. No specific blood tests are currently useful for diagnosis. Elevated creatinine levels, which signal new renal failure, are a potent predictor of death and branch vessel involvement.

Methods of Diagnosis

Computed tomography (CT), transesophageal echocardiography (TEE), and magnetic resonance imaging (MRI) provide greater than 90% sensitivity and specificity for the diagnosis of acute aortic dissection. CT and TEE are often preferred in urgent situations because they tend to be readily available. An MRI examination typically requires more time and involves less patient supervision; both are inappropriate for unstable patients. The choice between CT and TEE should be made on the basis of local expertise and availability—the most rapid and most accurate test is the best. In certain settings, one test may be preferred over the other. For a patient with aortic insufficiency or possible cardiac tamponade, TEE provides information about valve function and movement of the heart walls.

Occasionally, despite a strong clinical suspicion, a diagnostic test will not show a dissection. Several possibilities might account for the negative finding. First, TEE cannot image the arch and distal ascending aorta because of the interposed trachea. Second, less common aortic syndromes such as IMH or intimal tear without hematoma may not be detected with this imaging method. If a high index of suspicion exists, a second, complementary modality should be used.

Management

Patients with a diagnosis of aortic dissection or a high clinical suspicion for dissection require rapid initiation of medical therapy, namely pain control and blood pressure reduction. Narcotic analgesia should be instituted to reduce pain. A direct arterial vasodilator to decrease blood pressure and a negative inotropic agent to decrease the force of ventricular contraction are recommended. These medications should be provided intravenously to ensure absorption and facilitate rapid adjustment.

The most commonly recommended vasodilator is intravenous sodium nitroprusside; β-blockers are used most commonly to decrease the force of ventricular contraction. Labetalol combines both properties in a single pharmacologic agent. Calcium-channel antagonists and angiotensin-converting enzyme inhibitors also may be used. For patients with low arterial perfusion pressure, esmolol may be used to rapidly titrate blood pressure and heart rate. Hypotension may be due to compromise of limb perfusion after arterial dissection or development of an aortic dissection flap. If one arm has a higher blood pressure than the other, the medication should be titrated to the higher-pressure limb, especially if a pulse variation between the limbs is noted.

- For patients with an aortic dissection, two therapeutic modalities are recommended
  - Pain control
  - Blood pressure reduction
- Therapy to reduce blood pressure:
  - Intravenous sodium nitroprusside (a direct arterial vasodilator)
  - β-blockers (negative inotropic agents) to decrease the force of ventricular contraction

Presurgical management of patients with pericardial tamponade and type A dissection is poorly defined. In a study of 10 patients with aortic dissection, the mortality rate was high (60%), and pericardiocentesis seemed to worsen outcomes. Most physicians would recommend emergent surgery instead of coronary catheterization. In addition, catheterization does not decrease mortality in these patients.

To minimize the mortality rate, patients with a type A aortic dissection require emergent surgery. Recent series have shown a 50% mortality rate for patients who do not have surgical repair, compared with a 10% to 30% mortality rate for patients who do. The most common causes of death include cardiac tamponade, circulatory failure, aortic rupture, stroke, and visceral ischemia. Older patients and women are less likely to be referred for surgery than younger and male patients. The factors most associated with death include age older than 70 years, abrupt onset of chest pain, hypotension or shock, kidney failure, a pulse deficit, and abnormal electrocardiography findings at presentation. The number of pulse deficits has prognostic value: patients with 2 or more pulse deficits have a 5-day mortality rate of nearly 50%. Although not in common clinical use, endovascular repair techniques are being developed to treat this disease. The most common treatments are surgical repair of the aorta or replacement of the aortic root and aortic valve.

- Patients with a diagnosis of type A aortic dissection require emergent surgery
- The most common causes of death:
  - Cardiac tamponade
  - Circulatory failure

- Aortic rupture
- Stroke
- Visceral ischemia

Medical therapy is the main treatment modality for type B dissections. Patients without evidence of visceral compromise, claudication, progression of the dissection, uncontrolled hypertension, unremitting pain, or Marfan syndrome may be managed medically and have a 30-day mortality rate of about 10%. Limb ischemia, major organ ischemia, or renal failure increases the risk of mortality to 20% by day 2. Some series have reported mortality rates exceeding 70% for renal and mesenteric ischemia. Percutaneous interventions to treat type B dissection are being developed. Abdominal aortic dissections are treated with placement of stents or balloon fenestration of the dissection flap (particularly if the patient is a poor surgical candidate) to restore compromised circulation in a major organ or limb. By maintaining flow through the false lumen, fenestration can increase the long-term risk of aneurysm formation and rupture. Freedom from death or recurrent symptoms is as high as 86% at 14 months for patients undergoing the percutaneous procedure. Endovascular repair also has been used to treat type B dissections, and experience with this procedure is increasing.

Follow-Up

For patients with aortic dissection who receive appropriate treatment, survival rates are approximately 90%, 80%, and 50% at 1, 5, and 10 years, respectively. Death after the index operation typically occurs within 2 years of the event. The most common causes of death are cardiovascular disease or aortic rupture. As many as one-fourth of patients require reoperation within 10 years, most commonly because of aneurysmal expansion of the aorta, which prompts strict radiographic follow-up. Most physicians recommend follow-up with CT or MRI at 3, 6, and 12 months after the index operation and yearly examinations thereafter to monitor aortic expansion. Candidates for aneurysm repair after dissection must meet the same criteria as those having repair of aneurysms without dissection. Initial aortic diameter greater than 4 cm and a patent false lumen are predictive of more rapid expansion and the requirement for repair.

Dissection-Like Syndromes

Intramural Hematoma

IMH is the most common variant of aortic dissection, affecting 5% to 10% of patients with an acute aortic syndrome. Whereas an obvious intimal tear between the lumen and subintimal space occurs in aortic dissection, only intramural hemorrhage with circumferential or longitudinal spread is seen in an IMH. Although definitive proof is lacking, vasa vasorum rupture currently is the accepted mechanism for IMH formation. Increasing pressure in the aortic wall may cause an intimal tear and a classic aortic dissection. Some investigators have posited that invisible microtears are involved in the formation of an IMH.

The presentation of IMH is similar to that of a classic aortic dissection. Abrupt onset of pain is most common, and pain in the chest and back occurs for both. Patients with IMH tend to be older than patients with classic aortic dissection. IMH is more likely to occur in the abdominal aorta, and involvement of the aortic valve is less common. The disease course of an IMH typically becomes obvious soon after diagnosis—showing either regression with hematoma resorption or progression to classic dissection, aneurysm formation, or rupture. Factors that portend a higher risk of morbidity and mortality include involvement of the ascending aorta, aortic diameter exceeding 5 cm, increasing thickness of the hemorrhage on serial radiologic evaluations, and presence of ulceration.

Overall, the mortality rate for IMH is similar to that for classic dissection. As in classic dissection, the IMH location greatly influences prognosis and management. Using the Stanford classification system, a type A IMH is more likely to progress than a type B IMH. One study showed that patients with an IMH had a 30-day mortality rate of 20% and a 5-year mortality rate of 57%. Patients with a type A IMH had an early mortality rate of 8% with surgical therapy and 55% with medical therapy. Patients with a type B IMH who underwent surgery had double the 1-year mortality risk (50%) of those treated medically (23.5%). Risk factors for progression of an IMH (e.g., development of dissection, longitudinal progression of the IMH, or erosion of the aorta) include the presence of a large PAU on the IMH, increasing pleural effusion, a symptomatic PAU, and a type A location. Long-term outcomes are adversely affected by Marfan syndrome, younger age, and lack of β-adrenergic blockade.

The modalities used to diagnose IMH are the same as those used for aortic dissection. Typically, IMH is depicted radiographically as a hemorrhage contained within the vessel wall which does not enter the lumen. After the condition is diagnosed, IMH treatment is similar to that of aortic dissection. Medical therapy that targets blood pressure and ventricular contraction reduction should be instituted. If it is identified during the evaluation of suggestive symptoms, a type A IMH should be repaired surgically and a type B IMH should be managed medically. The management of asymptomatic IMH discovered incidentally is unclear and should be tailored to each patient.

- IMH is the most common aortic dissection variant

- IMH occurs in 5%-10% of patients with an acute aortic syndrome
- The mortality rate for patients with an IMH is similar to that for patients with a classic aortic dissection
- A type A IMH should be repaired surgically, but a type B IMH should be managed medically

Penetrating Atherosclerotic Ulcer

A PAU develops when an inflammatory atherosclerotic plaque penetrates the internal elastic membrane and exposes the media to the lumen. This permits IMH formation, classic aortic dissection, or aortic rupture. A PAU generally occurs in the descending thoracic aorta (the most common site of atherosclerosis) and typically is found in older patients with extensive atherosclerosis. The diagnosis usually is made by CT or MRI, which shows an excrescence beyond the aortic lumen, with mural thickening, displacement of intimal calcium, and sometimes IMH formation. Most physicians recommend surgery for a patient with PAU if the presentation was consistent with an acute event; however, if PAU is discovered incidentally, conservative therapy with radiographic follow-up may be appropriate.

Carotid Artery Dissection

Carotid artery dissection may occur as a result of extension of an aortic dissection or may occur spontaneously in the carotid artery alone. Carotid artery dissections are rare, with an incidence of 2 to 3 cases per 100,000 persons per year in community-based studies and at about half that rate in hospital-based studies. In the Lausanne Stroke Registry of 1,200 consecutive patients, carotid artery dissections were the cause of stroke in 2%. In younger patients, however, carotid dissection caused up to 25% of ischemic strokes. The most common age of presentation is 40 to 50 years, but dissections may occur at any age. The mean age at occurrence in women tends to be 5 to 10 years younger than that in men.

Carotid artery dissection may be idiopathic or the consequence of a known event. Idiopathic events typically are ascribed to a congenital abnormality in the arterial wall, although no specific arteriopathy has been described. Abnormalities most commonly associated include those in Marfan syndrome, Ehlers-Danlos syndrome, polycystic kidney disease, and osteogenesis imperfecta, which characterize about 5% of dissections. However, up to 20% of patients have an unidentified inherited abnormality. Trauma is the most important acquired mechanism of dissection and may originate from a quick blow, motor vehicle accident, heavy vomiting or coughing, or chiropractic manipulation. Other acquired causes include fibromuscular dysplasia, vasculitis, and pregnancy.

Most patients with carotid dissection present with unilateral facial or neck pain and a partial Horner syndrome (miosis, ptosis, but not enophthalmos) from a disruption of the sympathetic nerve fibers that course along the carotid artery. Cerebral or retinal ischemia may develop hours or days later in 50% to 95% of patients. Although few patients have all three manifestations, most have two. Cranial nerve abnormalities are identified in approximately 10% of patients. Approximately 25% "hear" carotid pulsations. A carotid bruit and carotidynia may be noted during the physical examination.

MRI is the modality used most commonly to identify carotid artery dissections, replacing contrast angiography as the diagnostic standard. Some have advocated the use of ultrasonography, reporting that abnormal blood flow is noted in more than 90% of patients; however, a dissection, IMH, or intimal flap is noted in less than one-third of patients.

The treatment of carotid dissection is designed to decrease the rate of thrombosis formation and the possibility of cerebral embolism. Anticoagulation therapy may be used; anticoagulation is typically achieved initially with heparin and then continued with use of warfarin for 3 to 6 months, with a target international normalized ratio of 2.0 to 3.0. Most dissections heal spontaneously. For patients with persistent symptoms, surgical ligation and bypass and percutaneous stenting have been used.

The prognosis of carotid dissection primarily is related to the severity of the initial ischemic event. The mortality rate is less than 5% after a carotid artery dissection, and more than 90% of dissections eventually resolve. Most patients report that head or facial pain resolves within a week. Two-thirds of dissections recanalize, and one-third will decrease in size. Embolic events rarely occur with the development of aneurysms, and the aneurysms do not rupture. After the first 3 months, the risk of recurrence is about 1% per year.

- Mortality due to carotid dissection is less than 5%
- More than 90% of dissections eventually resolve

Questions

1. A 29-year-old pregnant woman presents with severe left facial pain and difficulty seeing with the left eye. She reports upper back pain but no arm weakness or pain. Physical examination shows a left carotid bruit, ptosis, a crescendo-decrescendo murmur at the upper sternal borders, and preserved pulses. What is the most appropriate next step?
   a. Magnetic resonance imaging
   b. Duplex ultrasonography

c. Warfarin anticoagulation therapy
d. Heparin anticoagulation therapy

2. A 69-year-old man presents to the emergency department with severe, sudden-onset back pain. The patient rates the pain as a "5" out of 10 but noted that it was worse before presentation. Physical examination shows a blood pressure of 175/95 mm Hg in the right and left arms, clear lungs, a rapid, regular heart rate without gallop, soft abdomen, and absent pedal pulses on the left side. Electrocardiography shows sinus rhythm and left ventricular hypertrophy. Angiographic imaging is ordered (Figure). Which factor is most associated with poor outcome?

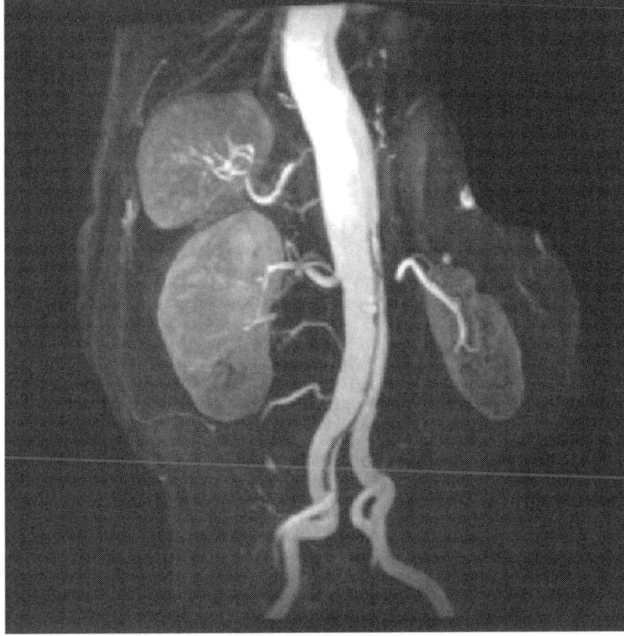

a. Hypertension
b. Left ventricular hypertrophy
c. Persistent back pain
d. Pulse deficit

3. A 69-year-old man presents to the emergency department with severe chest pain that resolves over the course of an hour. His blood pressure is 180/100 mm Hg, but physical examination findings are otherwise unremarkable. Electrocardiography shows T-wave inversions. Chest CT results are shown in the Figure. What is the correct management strategy?
a. Esmolol and nitroprusside infusion, emergent cardiac surgery consultation
b. Oral metoprolol and captopril administration, hospital admission and monitoring, repeated CT in the morning
c. Chewed aspirin, nitroglycerin patch, oral metoprolol, and hospitalization to rule out myocardial infarction

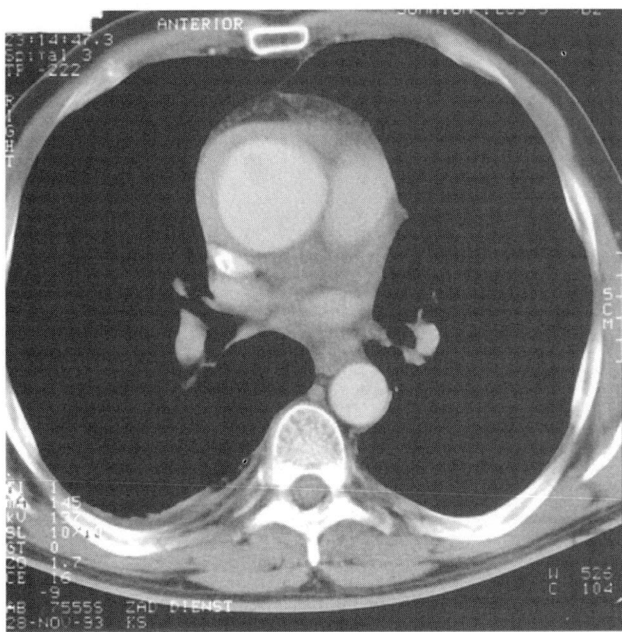

d. Enoxaparin injection, lower extremity venous ultrasonography, inferior vena cava filter placement

4. Which factor is most associated with future aneurysm repair in patients treated for aortic dissection?
a. Hypertension
b. A thrombosed false lumen
c. Aortic diameter of 4.2 cm
d. Dissection extension into the iliac arteries

5. A 63-year-old woman is brought to the emergency department after collapsing at home. Upon arrival, her systolic blood pressure is 70 mm Hg, and she undergoes volume resuscitation. She reports severe chest pain before the collapse and is currently short of breath. Physical examination shows basilar lung crackles, a grade 1/4 diastolic murmur, and absent right radial pulse. Electrocardiography shows ST-segment depressions in the lateral precordial leads. Transthoracic echocardiography shows signs of ascending aortic dissection, pericardial tamponade, and mild aortic valvular insufficiency. What is the most appropriate next step in therapy?
a. Emergent pericardiocentesis
b. Emergent coronary angiography
c. Emergent metoprolol administration
d. Emergent surgical referral

Suggested Readings

Bogousslavsky J, Despland PA, Regli F. Spontaneous carotid dissection with acute stroke. Arch Neurol. 1987;44:137-40.

Cambria RP, Brewster DC, Gertler J, et al. Vascular complications associated with spontaneous aortic dissection. J Vasc Surg. 1988;7:199-209.

Clouse WD, Hallett JW Jr, Schaff HV, et al. Acute aortic dissection: population-based incidence compared with degenerative aortic aneurysm rupture. Mayo Clin Proc. 2004;79:176-80.

Coady MA, Rizzo JA, Hammond GL, et al. Penetrating ulcer of the thoracic aorta: what is it? How do we recognize it? How do we manage it? J Vasc Surg. 1998;27:1006-15.

Doroghazi RM, Slater EE, DeSanctis RW, et al. Long-term survival of patients with treated aortic dissection. J Am Coll Cardiol. 1984;3:1026-34.

Evangelista A, Mukherjee D, Mehta RH, et al, International Registry of Aortic Dissection (IRAD) Investigators. Acute intramural hematoma of the aorta: a mystery in evolution. Circulation. 2005 Mar 1;111:1063-70. Epub 2005 Feb 14.

Gass A, Szabo K, Lanczik O, et al. Magnetic resonance imaging assessment of carotid artery dissection. Cerebrovasc Dis. 2002;13:70-3.

Hagan PG, Nienaber CA, Isselbacher EM, et al. The International Registry of Acute Aortic Dissection (IRAD): new insights into an old disease. JAMA. 2000;283:897-903.

Hirst AE Jr, Johns VJ Jr, Kime SW Jr. Dissecting aneurysm of the aorta: a review of 505 cases. Medicine. 1958;37:217-79.

Januzzi JL, Isselbacher EM, Fattori R, et al, International Registry of Aortic Dissection (IRAD). Characterizing the young patient with aortic dissection: results from the International Registry of Aortic Dissection (IRAD). J Am Coll Cardiol. 2004;43:665-9.

Mehta RH, Suzuki T, Hagan PG, et al, International Registry of Acute Aortic Dissection (IRAD) Investigators. Predicting death in patients with acute type A aortic dissection. Circulation. 2002;105:200-6.

Nienaber CA, Richartz BM, Rehders T, et al. Aortic intramural haematoma: natural history and predictive factors for complications. Heart. 2004;90:372-4.

Pepin M, Schwarze U, Superti-Furga A, et al. Clinical and genetic features of Ehlers-Danlos syndrome type IV, the vascular type. N Engl J Med. 2000;342:673-80. Erratum in: N Engl J Med. 2001;344:392.

Schievink WI. Spontaneous dissection of the carotid and vertebral arteries. N Engl J Med. 2001;344:898-906.

Slonim SM, Nyman U, Semba CP, et al. Aortic dissection: percutaneous management of ischemic complications with endovascular stents and balloon fenestration. J Vasc Surg. 1996;23:241-51.

Stapf C, Elkind MS, Mohr JP. Carotid artery dissection. Annu Rev Med. 2000;51:329-47.

Vilacosta I, Castillo JA, Peral V, et al. Intramural aortic haematoma following intra-aortic balloon counterpulsation: documentation by transoesophageal echocardiography. Eur Heart J. 1995;16:2015-6.

Wheat MW Jr. Acute dissecting aneurysms of the aorta: diagnosis and treatment—1979. Am Heart J. 1980;99:373-87.

Wilson SK, Hutchins GM. Aortic dissecting aneurysms: causative factors in 204 subjects. Arch Pathol Lab Med. 1982;106:175-80.

18 Renal and Mesenteric Artery Disease

Jeffrey W. Olin, DO

Renal Artery Disease

The past decade has seen increased awareness of renovascular disease as a potentially correctable cause of hypertension and renal insufficiency. The association between renal artery stenosis (RAS) and coronary artery disease and congestive heart failure (CHF) has been well studied. Patients with RAS have markedly decreased survival as a result of increased incidence of myocardial infarction and stroke. RAS may present in one of four ways: 1) hypertension; 2) acute or chronic renal failure; 3) CHF, "flash" pulmonary edema, or unstable angina; or 4) incidentally discovered on an imaging test performed for some other reason.

- RAS may present in one of four ways:
  - Hypertension
  - Acute or chronic renal failure
  - CHF, flash pulmonary edema, or unstable angina
  - Discovered incidentally

Incidentally discovered RAS is quite common, but renovascular hypertension occurs in only a minority of all patients with hypertension. RAS is most commonly caused by fibromuscular dysplasia (FMD) or atherosclerosis. The predominant clinical manifestation of FMD is hypertension, which frequently can be cured or substantially improved with percutaneous transluminal angioplasty (PTA). FMD is the primary cause of RAS in young women, whereas atherosclerosis is most often the cause in persons older than 55 years.

Approximately 90% of all renovascular lesions are secondary to atherosclerosis. Atherosclerotic RAS most often occurs at the ostium or the proximal 2 cm of the renal artery. Distal arterial or branch involvement is distinctly uncommon. Most patients with atherosclerotic RAS have one or more of the following features: onset of hypertension before age 30 years or after age 55 years; exacerbation of previously well-controlled hypertension; malignant or resistant hypertension; epigastric bruit (systolic or diastolic); unexplained azotemia; azotemia while receiving angiotensin-converting enzyme (ACE) inhibitors or angiotensin-receptor blockers (ARBs); atrophic kidney or discrepancy in size between the two kidneys; recurrent CHF, flash pulmonary edema, or angina; or atherosclerosis in another vessel (coronary arteries, peripheral arterial disease).

The presence of anatomic RAS does not establish RAS as the cause of the hypertension or renal failure. Primary (essential) hypertension can exist for years before the development of atherosclerotic RAS later in life. Renal revascularization (with PTA, stent placement, or surgery) may result in improved blood pressure control in 50% to 80% of patients, but complete control is unusual in patients with long-standing hypertension. Ischemic nephropathy or flash pulmonary edema almost always occurs in the presence of bilateral renal artery disease or disease with a solitary functioning kidney. Percutaneous or surgical revascularization can lead to improvement or stabilization of renal function and improvement of CHF in carefully selected patients.

- Renal revascularization may result in improved blood pressure control in 50%-80% of patients, but complete control is unusual in patients with long-standing hypertension

Pathogenesis of Hypertension in RAS

A detailed discussion of the pathophysiologic mechanisms of hypertension in renal artery disease is beyond the scope of this chapter. In general, early in the course of the disease, patients with unilateral RAS have a renin-mediated form of hypertension, whereas patients with bilateral RAS or stenosis with only one functioning kidney have a volume-mediated form of hypertension. In patients with volume-mediated hypertension, administration of an ACE inhibitor or ARB does not decrease blood pressure or change renal blood flow. Dietary restriction of sodium or administration of diuretics converts the hypertension to a renin-mediated form and restores sensitivity to ACE inhibitors or ARBs. Functional renal insufficiency may occur when an ACE inhibitor is administered to a patient with bilateral RAS or RAS to a solitary kidney, especially in the volume-contracted state.

- Patients with unilateral RAS have a renin-mediated form of hypertension, whereas patients with bilateral RAS or stenosis to a solitary functioning kidney have a volume-mediated form of hypertension
- In volume-mediated hypertension, administration of ACE inhibitors or ARBs does not decrease blood pressure or change renal blood flow

Pathophysiology of Ischemic Nephropathy

The relationship of ischemic nephropathy to RAS is particularly difficult to fully understand because of several factors. First, no linear relationship exists between the degree of RAS and the degree of renal dysfunction. Second, it is not easy to determine with certainty whether the renal insufficiency is attributable to stenosis of the main renal artery or to parenchymal disease. Third, some patients undergoing renal revascularization have worsening renal function after the procedure. This may be due to atheromatous embolization caused by the procedure or to the natural history of the underlying disease. The development of azotemia while the patient is receiving an ACE inhibitor or ARB indicates the presence of bilateral RAS, RAS to a solitary kidney, or decompensated CHF in the sodium-depleted state.

- There is no linear relationship between the degree of RAS and the degree of renal dysfunction
- It is not easy to determine whether renal insufficiency is due to stenosis of the main renal artery or to parenchymal disease
- Some patients with renal revascularization have worsening renal function after the procedure
- If azotemia develops while the patient is receiving an ACE inhibitor or ARB, it indicates one of the following:
  - Bilateral RAS
  - RAS to a solitary kidney
  - Decompensated CHF in the sodium-depleted state

Two mechanisms exist by which renal functional impairment can occur with the use of antihypertensive agents. The first may involve any antihypertensive agent when a critical perfusion pressure is reached, below which the kidney no longer receives adequate perfusion. This mechanism has been shown with the infusion of sodium nitroprusside in patients with severe bilateral RAS. When the critical perfusion pressure was reached, the urine output, renal blood flow, and glomerular filtration rate decreased and later returned to normal when the blood pressure increased above this critical perfusion pressure. The exact pressure necessary to perfuse a kidney if RAS is present varies with the degree of stenosis and differs among patients.

The second mechanism is confined to patients receiving an ACE inhibitor or ARB and may occur even without a marked change in blood pressure. Patients with high-grade bilateral RAS or RAS to a single functioning kidney may be highly dependent on angiotensin II for glomerular filtration. This is particularly common in patients who receive a combination of ACE inhibitors and diuretics or in patients who follow a sodium-restricted diet. The constrictive effect of angiotensin II on the efferent arteriole allows for the maintenance of normal transglomerular capillary hydraulic pressure, thus allowing continued normal glomerular filtration in the presence of markedly decreased blood flow. When an ACE inhibitor or ARB is administered, the efferent arteriolar tone is no longer maintained and glomerular filtration is therefore decreased. A similar situation occurs in patients with decompensated CHF who are sodium depleted.

Clinical Manifestations of Renal Artery Disease

Prevalence

In a recent population-based study on the prevalence of renovascular disease in a cohort of elderly patients, the 834 participants underwent renal duplex ultrasonography, and 57 (6.8%) were found to have anatomic RAS. The prevalence of RAS was similar in white and black patients (6.9% vs 6.7%).

Several series have determined the prevalence of renovascular disease in patients who have atherosclerotic disease at other sites. In 319 patients reported in six different studies, 44% had bilateral RAS. Other studies have shown that 22% to 59% of patients with peripheral arterial disease have significant RAS. RAS also is common in patients with coronary artery disease. Of 7,758 patients undergoing cardiac catheterization in the Duke University cardiac catheterization laboratory, 3,987 underwent aortography to screen for RAS at the time of catheterization. Of these, 191 (4.8%) had stenosis greater than 75% in the renal artery, and 0.8% had severe bilateral disease. In a series from Mayo Clinic, renal arteries were studied at the time of cardiac catheterization in patients with hypertension. The renal arteries were adequately visualized in 90% and no complications occurred with aortography. RAS was greater than 50% in 19.2% of the patients and was greater than 70% in 7%; bilateral RAS was present in 3.7% of the patients.

- 22%-59% of patients with peripheral arterial disease have significant RAS
- RAS is common in patients with coronary artery disease
- Rates of progression range from 36%-71%

Natural History

Most reports on the natural history of RAS have been retrospective studies, which show the rate of disease progression to range from 36% to 71%. In one series, disease progressed to total occlusion in only 16% of patients over a mean follow-up of 52 months. However, progression to total occlusion occurred more frequently (39%) if initial renal arteriography showed greater than 75% stenosis.

Prospective studies of the anatomic progression of atherosclerotic renovascular disease, using renal duplex ultrasonography, have shown that if the renal arteries were normal, only 8% of patients had disease progression over 36 months. At 3 years, however, 48% of patients had disease progression from less than 60% stenosis to 60% or greater stenosis. In the four renal arteries that progressed to occlusion, all had 60% or greater stenosis at the initial visit. Progression of RAS occurred at an average rate of 7% per year for all categories of baseline disease combined. In one study, 122 patients (204 kidneys) with known RAS were followed up prospectively for a mean of 33 months with duplex ultrasonography. The 2-year cumulative incidence of renal atrophy was 5.5%, 11.7%, and 20.8% in kidneys with a baseline renal artery disease classification of normal, less than 60% stenosis, and 60% or greater stenosis, respectively (P=.009).

Patient survival decreases as the severity of RAS increases; 2-year survival rates are 96% in patients with unilateral RAS, 74% in patients with bilateral RAS, and 47% in patients with stenosis or occlusion to a solitary functioning kidney. In a large study of patients on dialysis, those who progressed to end-stage renal disease secondary to RAS had a median survival of 25 months and a 5-year survival of only 18%.

Fibromuscular Dysplasia

FMD, which accounts for less than 10% of all renal artery disease, is a non-atherosclerotic, non-inflammatory disease that most commonly affects the renal arteries and is the second most common cause of RAS. The most common clinical presentation is hypertension in a young woman. The vessels involved are the renal arteries in 60% to 75% of patients with FMD, extracranial cerebral arteries in 25% to 30%, visceral arteries in less than 10%, and arteries of the extremities in less than 5% of patients. Although atherosclerosis involves the origin and proximal portion of the renal arteries, FMD characteristically involves the distal two-thirds of the artery and can involve the branches.

- FMD accounts for less than 10% of all renal artery disease
- It most commonly affects the renal arteries; the second most common cause of RAS
- FMD characteristically involves the distal two-thirds of the artery and may involve the branches
- Medial fibroplasia is the histologic finding in nearly 80% of all cases of FMD
- Intimal fibroplasia occurs in children and young adults
  - It accounts for approximately 10% of all cases of fibrous lesions

The classification of FMD is important because each type of fibrous dysplasia has distinct histologic and angiographic features, and each type occurs in a different clinical setting (Table 18.1).

Medial fibroplasia is the histologic finding in nearly 80% of all cases of FMD. It tends to occur in women aged 25 to 50 years and often involves both renal arteries. It has a "string of beads" appearance angiographically, with the "bead" diameter larger than the proximal, unaffected artery. Medial fibroplasia responds well to PTA alone.

Intimal fibroplasia occurs in children and young adults and accounts for approximately 10% of all cases of FMD. This lesion is characterized by a circumferential accumulation of collagen inside the internal elastic lamina. Arteriography in intimal fibroplasia shows either a smooth, long area of narrowing or a concentric band-like focal stenosis usually involving the mid portion of the vessel or its branches. Progressive renal artery obstruction and ischemic atrophy of the involved kidney may occur. Although intimal fibroplasia most commonly affects the renal arteries, it may also occur as a generalized disorder, with concomitant involvement of the carotid artery, upper and lower extremities, and mesenteric vessels, and may mimic a necrotizing vasculitis.

Diagnosis of Renovascular Disease

The ideal procedure for imaging of the renovascular system should 1) identify the main renal arteries and accessory vessels; 2) localize the site of stenosis or disease; 3) provide evidence of the hemodynamic significance of the lesion; 4) identify any associated pathology (e.g., abdominal aortic aneurysm, renal mass) that may affect treatment

Table 18.1 Classification of Fibromuscular Dysplasia

Classification	Frequency, %	Pathology	Angiographic appearance
Medial dysplasia			
Medial fibroplasia	75-80	Alternating areas of thinned media and thickened fibromuscular ridges containing collagen; internal elastic membrane may be lost in some areas	"String of beads" appearance—diameter of the "beading" is larger than the diameter of the artery
Perimedial fibroplasia	10-15	Extensive collagen deposition in the outer half of the media	"String of beads" appearance—the "beads" are smaller than the diameter of the artery
Medial hyperplasia	1-2	True smooth muscle cell hyperplasia without fibrosis	Concentric smooth stenosis (similar to intimal disease)
Intimal fibroplasia	<10	Circumferential or eccentric deposition of collagen in the intima; no lipid or inflammatory component; internal elastic lamina fragmented or duplicated	Concentric focal band; long, smooth narrowing
Adventitial (periarterial) fibroplasia	<1	Dense collagen replaces the fibrous tissue of the adventitia and may extend into surrounding tissue	

From Begelman SM, Olin JW. Fibromuscular dysplasia. Curr Opin Rheumatol. 2000;12:41-7. Used with permission.

of the renal artery disease; and 5) detect restenosis after renal artery stent implantation or surgical revascularization.

Angiography

Angiography, once considered the gold standard for arterial imaging, today is rarely required for diagnosing RAS. Usually, one or more of the non-invasive methods can accurately assess the renal arteries. CO_2 and gadolinium are non-nephrotoxic contrast agents that can be particularly useful in patients with renal insufficiency. Although the practice is controversial, some cardiologists perform renal angiography at the time of cardiac catheterization routinely in all patients; others image the renal arteries selectively only in those with clinical clues suggesting the presence of RAS. In one series, renal angiography performed at the time of cardiac catheterization showed only 4.8% of patients to have RAS of more than 75% and only 0.8% to have severe bilateral disease. Similarly, in another prospective evaluation of 297 patients with hypertension, only 19% had RAS greater than 50%, 7% had RAS greater than 70%, and 3.7% had bilateral disease. This study also showed that renal arteries could be evaluated successfully using only 62 mL of contrast agent. Angiography at the time of catheterization is therefore safe, but the yield is low. In addition, evidence suggests that knowing stenosis is present may lead to stenting of the renal artery without definite indication of need.

Duplex Ultrasonography

Duplex ultrasonography combines B-mode imaging with Doppler examination and is an excellent method for detecting RAS. It is the least expensive of the imaging modalities and provides useful information about the degree of stenosis, the kidney size, and other associated disease processes such as aneurysms or obstruction. Duplex scanning also may be helpful for predicting which patients will have improved blood pressure control or renal function after renal artery angioplasty and stenting.

- Duplex ultrasonography is the least expensive imaging modality
- It provides useful information about the degree of stenosis, the kidney size, and other associated disease processes
- Duplex ultrasonography can help predict which patients will have improved blood pressure control or renal function after renal artery angioplasty and stenting

As described in detail in Chapter 7, specific duplex ultrasonographic measurements are used to make the diagnosis of RAS. In the longitudinal view, the peak systolic velocity (PSV) in the aorta is recorded at the level of the renal arteries. The aortic velocity and the highest renal artery PSV are used to calculate the renal-aortic ratio. Because the PSV associated with a significant RAS increases relative to aortic PSV, the renal-aortic ratio can be used to identify severe RAS (Table 18.2). Overall, these duplex ultrasonographic criteria have a sensitivity of 84% to 98% and a specificity of 62% to 99% for diagnosing RAS.

Table 18.2 Duplex Ultrasonographic Criteria for Diagnosis of Renal Artery Stenosis

Stenosis	Duplex criteria
<60%	RAR <3.5
60%-99%	RAR ≥3.5 and PSV >200 cm/s
100% (occlusion)	No flow signal from renal artery Low-amplitude parenchymal signal Small kidney may or may not be present

RAR, renal-aortic ratio; PSV, peak systolic velocity.

Another measure, the renal resistive index (RRI), can be used to provide information about the extent of renal artery disease (see also Chapter 7). The RRI is determined by obtaining a Doppler waveform from the cortical blood vessels of the kidney and measuring PSV and end-diastolic velocity (EDV). The index is calculated with the formula: RRI=(PSV–EDV)/PSV. A retrospective study using Doppler ultrasonography to predict the outcome of therapy in patients with RAS found that, in patients with an RRI higher than 80, 97% had no improvement in blood pressure and 80% had no improvement in renal function. The results suggest that increased RRI is an indication of structural abnormalities in the small blood vessels of the kidney. Such small vessel disease has been seen with longstanding hypertension associated with nephrosclerosis or glomerulosclerosis. However, because several other investigators have refuted this study, the RRI should not be used as the sole criterion to determine the suitability of the patient for renal artery revascularization.

- The RRI is determined by obtaining a Doppler waveform from the cortical blood vessels of the kidney; RRI=(PSV–EDV)/PSV
- The RRI should not be used as the sole criterion to determine suitability for renal artery revascularization

Renal artery duplex ultrasonography is an excellent method for the follow-up of RAS after percutaneous therapy or surgical bypass. Unlike magnetic resonance angiography (discussed below), which can be affected by artifact or scatter produced by the stent, ultrasonographic transmission through the stent is not a problem.

Magnetic Resonance Angiography

Magnetic resonance angiography (MRA) provides excellent imaging of the abdominal vasculature and associated anatomic structures. Contrast-enhanced (with gadolinium) MRA provides superior quality compared with noncontrast studies. MRA has shown a sensitivity of 90% to 100% and a specificity of 76% to 94%. In a meta-analysis of 499 patients who underwent gadolinium-enhanced MRA and catheter angiography (performed less than 3 months apart), the sensitivity and specificity of MRA were 97% and 93%, respectively. MRA accurately identified accessory renal arteries in 82% of patients. However, MRA does not have the same sensitivity and specificity in patients with FMD because the resolution in the smaller blood vessels is not optimal.

- MRA has a demonstrated sensitivity of 90%-100% and a specificity of 76%-94% for diagnosis of RAS

Computed Tomography Angiography

Computed tomography angiography (CTA) is a vascular imaging technique that can be performed rapidly and safely for primary assessment of many vascular diseases. With the advent of multidetector-row CTA, excellent image quality is now possible, with higher resolution than could be obtained previously with single-detector–row technology. Current multidetector-row scanners acquire up to 64 simultaneous interweaving slices.

CTA has several advantages over conventional angiography: 1) volumetric acquisition, which permits visualization of the anatomy from multiple angles and in multiple planes after a single acquisition; 2) improved visualization of soft tissues and other adjacent anatomic structures; 3) less invasiveness and thus fewer complications; and 4) lower cost. CTA also has several advantages over MRA, including wider availability of scanners, higher spatial resolution, absence of flow-related phenomena that may distort MRA images, and the ability to visualize calcification and metallic implants such as endovascular stents or stent grafts. The disadvantages of CTA compared with MRA are exposure to ionizing radiation and the need for potentially nephrotoxic iodinated contrast agents.

The sensitivity of CTA for detecting RAS ranges from 89% to 100% and specificity from 82% to 100%. MRA or duplex ultrasonography may be the preferred imaging modality in patients with impaired renal function.

- CTA has a sensitivity of 89%-100% and a specificity of 82%-100% for assessment of RAS

Captopril Renography

Radionuclide imaging techniques are a non-invasive and safe way to evaluate renal blood flow and excretory function. Addition of an ACE inhibitor such as captopril to isotope renography improves the sensitivity and specificity of the test considerably, especially for patients with unilateral RAS. In most instances of unilateral RAS, the glomerular filtration rate (GFR) of the stenotic kidney decreases by approximately 30% after captopril administration. In contrast, the contralateral normal kidney has increased GFR, urine flow, and salt excretion, despite a decrease in systemic blood pressure.

- Addition of captopril to isotope renography (captopril renography) improves the sensitivity and specificity of the test considerably, especially for patients with unilateral RAS
- In unilateral RAS, the GFR of the stenotic kidney usually decreases by 30% after captopril administration

- In contrast, the normal kidney has increased GFR, urine flow, and salt excretion despite a decrease in systemic blood pressure

Overall, the accuracy of captopril renography for identifying patients with renovascular disease is acceptable, with a sensitivity of 85% to 90% (range, 45%-94%) and specificity of approximately 93% to 98% (range, 81%-100%). Patients with unilateral disease and normal renal function are the best candidates for captopril renography. The presence of significant azotemia or bilateral RAS may adversely affect the accuracy of captopril renography.

Although captopril renography was once the non-invasive diagnostic test of choice for patients with RAS, it is now a secondary screening method because the quality of the images from duplex ultrasonography, CTA, and MRA is superior.

Table 18.3 Indications for PTA With or Without Stent Implantation to Treat Atherosclerotic Renal Artery Stenosis

1) At least 70% stenosis of one or both renal arteries *AND*
   a) An inability to adequately control blood pressure despite a good antihypertensive regimen *OR*
   b) Chronic renal insufficiency not related to another clear-cut cause; disease should be bilateral or comprise stenosis to a solitary functioning kidney
      (The treatment of elevated serum creatinine level in a patient with unilateral disease is controversial, and no clinical trials exist to help guide the clinician.)
2) Dialysis-dependent renal failure in a patient without another definite cause of end-stage renal disease and bilateral disease or severe stenosis to a single kidney
3) Recurrent congestive heart failure or "flash" pulmonary edema not attributable to active ischemia

PTA, percutaneous transluminal angioplasty.

Management of Renal Artery Disease

Medical Therapy

All patients with renal artery disease and hypertension should be treated medically, even if they undergo intervention. A comprehensive risk factor reduction program should be undertaken, because this patient population has markedly increased cardiovascular morbidity and mortality. Many patients have superimposed essential hypertension and require lifelong antihypertensive therapy even after renal artery revascularization. Patients with RAS who are treated solely with medical therapy should be carefully followed up for disease progression, generally with a surveillance program of serial duplex ultrasonographic imaging. Renal function should be evaluated every 3 months.

- Many patients have superimposed essential hypertension and require lifelong antihypertensive therapy even after renal artery revascularization

Percutaneous Transluminal Angioplasty and Stenting

PTA is the treatment of choice for patients with FMD. In contrast, stent implantation is the preferred endovascular therapy for patients with atherosclerosis, especially if the disease involves the ostium or proximal portion of the artery. Since the introduction of stents, surgical revascularization is rarely performed solely for the treatment of renal artery disease.

Despite advances in the technical aspects of PTA and stent implantation, few controlled clinical trials have assessed the effectiveness of renal artery angioplasty and stenting for the control of hypertension or to preserve renal function. Controversy still exists as to the value of renal artery stenting and the appropriate indications for this procedure. The accepted indications for PTA with or without stent implantation for atherosclerotic RAS are shown in Table 18.3.

Because restenosis rates with angioplasty alone are high, endovascular stents offer a significant advantage over angioplasty alone in patients with atherosclerotic disease. The degree of stenosis after stenting approaches zero, and most dissection flaps caused by PTA alone are successfully treated with stents.

For the best results, the lesion should be completely covered, the stent should extend 1 to 2 mm into the aorta in patients with ostial disease, and the stent must be fully expanded. Underdeployment of the stent is a common problem early in an operator's experience. For a less-experienced operator, it may be worthwhile to perform the first several cases with intravascular ultrasonography to be certain the stent is adequately expanded. It is also important to make sure that no postprocedure translesional pressure gradient exists.

In one prospective study, a balloon-expandable stent was placed in 68 patients (74 lesions) with ostial RAS and suboptimal PTA. Patency at 5 years was 84.5% (mean follow-up, 27 months). Restenosis occurred in 8 of 74 arteries (11%), but after reintervention, the secondary 5-year patency rate was 92.4%. Hypertension was cured or improved in 78% of patients. Serum creatinine value did not change significantly after stent implantation.

A meta-analysis of 14 studies (678 patients) compared the technical success, clinical efficacy, and restenosis rates after PTA and stent implantation. Blood pressure was improved in 60% to 80% of patients, and renal function was improved or stabilized in approximately 75% of patients. The restenosis rate among contemporary series was in the range of 11% to 20%.

- PTA is the treatment of choice for patients with FMD
- Renal artery stents:
  - Endovascular stents and angioplasty offer a significant advantage over angioplasty alone in patients with atherosclerotic disease
  - In a meta-analysis of 14 studies (678 patients):
    - Hypertension was improved in 60%-80% of patients
    - Renal function was improved or stabilized in 75% of patients
    - The restenosis rate among contemporary series was 11%-20%

The effect of renal artery stent implantation on preserving renal function was studied in two small series; both used the reciprocal of the serum creatinine value (1/Scr) to determine the rate of deterioration or improvement in renal function. The first study, in which renal artery stents were placed in 32 patients (33 arteries), reported that renal function improved or stabilized in 22 patients (69%). The second study, which included 25 patients with complete follow-up, showed that after stent placement, the slopes of the 1/Scr curves were positive in 18 patients and less negative (than previously) in 7 patients.

Complications of renal artery stent placement include access-related complications such as hematoma, retroperitoneal hemorrhage, pseudoaneurysm, arteriovenous fistula, vessel occlusion, or infection. However, the most serious complications result from atheromatous embolization to the kidneys, bowel, or legs. Stent malposition and rupture of the renal artery are less common complications. The complication rate varies considerably between centers. High-volume centers generally can perform renal artery stenting with minimal morbidity and mortality. Although all studies reported use of an antithrombotic agent during the procedure and most patients were discharged on antiplatelet therapy, the regimens varied.

Embolic protection devices have been used in several series—a wire is placed across the renal artery lesion and a balloon occlusion device or a filter device is deployed in the distal renal artery. This device is designed to capture the atherosclerotic debris caused by angioplasty and stenting, with the goal of preventing atheromatous embolization to the kidneys. In one study using an embolic protection device in 28 patients (32 arteries), the procedure was technically successful in all patients, and visible debris was recovered in all patients. The Cardiovascular Outcomes in Renal Atherosclerotic Lesions (CORAL) randomized multicenter trial, currently recruiting patients with hypertension, aims to compare combined medical therapy and stenting of hemodynamically significant RAS with medical therapy alone. The primary composite cardiovascular and renal end point is cardiovascular or renal death, myocardial infarction, hospitalization for CHF, stroke, doubling of serum creatinine value, and the need for renal replacement. All patients who receive a stent will also receive a distal protection device. Multiple secondary end points will assess quality of life, health policy perspectives, and cost effectiveness. This well-designed trial will provide critically needed information on the utility of renal artery stenting.

Surgical Revascularization

Surgical revascularization now has a much smaller role than it did previously because of the excellent technical results that can be achieved with angioplasty and stent implantation. Many patients can now undergo renal artery stent implantation as an outpatient procedure at a fraction of the cost of surgical revascularization.

Current indications for surgical revascularization include branch disease from FMD that cannot be adequately treated with PTA, recurrent stenosis after stenting (which is extremely rare), or simultaneous aortic surgery (abdominal aortic aneurysm repair or symptomatic aortoiliac disease). In the event of simultaneous aortic surgery, it may be advisable to place a stent in the renal artery first and then proceed with aortic reconstruction. The mortality rate for aortic replacement and renal artery revascularization is higher than for either procedure alone.

Revascularization for Renal Salvage. Patients with bilateral RAS of greater than 70% or severe stenosis to a single functioning kidney are at a markedly increased risk of renal failure. In this patient subgroup, the risk of total occlusion of the renal artery is significant; if occlusion occurs, the outcome is a critical decrease in functioning renal mass with resulting renal failure.

Complete occlusion of the renal artery most often results in irreversible ischemic damage to the involved kidney. However, in some patients with gradual arterial occlusion, the kidney may remain viable because of development of a collateral arterial supply. Clues that can help predict kidney salvage in patients with an occluded renal artery include angiographic demonstration of late filling of the distal renal arterial tree by collateral vessels on the side of total arterial occlusion; a renal size of 8 to 9 cm; functioning of the involved kidney on a renal flow scan; appearance of a nephrogram after a contrast arteriogram; or renal biopsy results showing well-preserved glomeruli and an absence of significant glomerulosclerosis.

Some reports have shown that restoration of renal function in patients with complete occlusion of the renal arteries is feasible with endovascular therapy or surgical revascularization. In a study of 340 patients undergoing surgical renal revascularization between 1987 and 1993, 20 patients were receiving hemodialysis before renal artery repair. Hemodialysis was no longer required in 16 of the 20 patients (80%); two of the 16 resumed dialysis 4 and 6 months after surgery. The long-term survival was better in those who were dialysis independent than in those who required ongoing dialysis therapy. Only two late deaths occurred among the 14 patients not receiving dialysis, versus five late deaths among the six patients who continued to receive dialysis after surgical revascularization (*P*<.01). Another study reported on 304 patients with RAS and serum creatinine levels higher than 2.0 mg/dL who underwent surgical revascularization. With a mean follow-up of 3 years, 83 patients (27.3%) had an improvement in renal function, 160 (52.6%) had no change, and 61 (20.1%) had a worsening of renal function.

The likelihood of renal function improving appears to be dependent on the severity of stenosis in the main renal artery, the rapidity of renal failure development, and the degree of parenchymal damage to the kidney. Several investigators have suggested that parenchymal damage may be the most important determinant of the non-reversibility of renal failure.

Revascularization for Control of CHF or Flash Pulmonary Edema. An emerging indication for renal revascularization is treatment of patients with CHF or flash pulmonary edema. This group of patients most often has significant bilateral RAS or RAS to a solitary functioning kidney and may have no other clear-cut reason (e.g., coronary ischemia) for recurrent CHF.

The mechanism by which RAS causes CHF and pulmonary edema is not well defined. Improvement after stenting may be related in part to the ability to use ACE inhibitors, especially for those with impaired left ventricular function, and the ability to better control volume.

Mesenteric Artery Disease

Acute Mesenteric Ischemia

Acute mesenteric ischemia is a medical emergency. It has many possible causes, including embolization from the heart or proximal vessels and arterial thrombosis. Approximately two-thirds of patients presenting with acute intestinal ischemia are women, with a median age of 70 years. Abdominal pain is universally present, and the pain may be out of proportion to the physical findings. In patients with a delayed presentation, or in those with a high likelihood of non-occlusive mesenteric ischemia, arteriography may be indicated as a diagnostic test. However, for those with an acute presentation and a high likelihood of arterial obstruction or bowel infarction, immediate exploratory surgery is required.

The natural history of acute intestinal ischemia caused by obstruction of intestinal arteries in the absence of treatment is nearly always fatal. Surgical treatment includes laparotomy, revascularization of the ischemic intestine with assessment of intestinal viability after revascularization, and resection of non-viable intestine. A "second look" operation 24 to 48 hours later is generally warranted.

Acute Non-Occlusive Intestinal Ischemia

Intestinal infarction may occur in the absence of fixed arterial obstruction. This usually occurs in persons with severe systemic illness and results in shock and decreased cardiac output. Intestinal infarction often leads to severe prolonged intestinal vasospasm. Drugs such as cocaine, ergotamines, and vasopressors (to treat shock) may also result in severe intestinal vasospasm and infarction.

Non-occlusive mesenteric ischemia is notoriously difficult to diagnose. It should be suspected in patients in shock with abdominal pain and distention. Arteriography is the method of choice for diagnosis. If non-occlusive mesenteric ischemia is confirmed, direct intra-arterial vasodilators should be administered. The presence of continued abdominal symptoms after relief of the vasospasm is a clear indication for laparotomy to search for necrotic bowel.

- Non-occlusive mesenteric ischemia is notoriously difficult to diagnose
- Intestinal infarction may occur in the absence of fixed arterial obstruction
- Arteriography is the method of choice for diagnosis
- If non-occlusive mesenteric ischemia is confirmed, direct intra-arterial vasodilators should be administered to identify necrotic bowel

Chronic Intestinal Ischemia

Chronic intestinal ischemia is usually caused by atherosclerosis; less commonly, it can be caused by giant cell arteritis, Takayasu arteritis, or FMD. Although atherosclerosis of the celiac, superior mesenteric, and inferior mesenteric arteries is common, the clinical manifestations of chronic intestinal ischemia are quite uncommon. It is often thought that severe stenosis or occlusion of two of the three intestinal vessels must be present to induce clinical manifestations, but in some well-documented cases only one vessel was involved, usually the superior mesenteric artery.

The classic presentation is abdominal pain occurring after eating. However, the relationship to food is not always present, perhaps because of unconscious food avoidance. Weight loss invariably occurs owing to reduced caloric intake. A female preponderance has been observed.

Diagnosis of Chronic Intestinal Ischemia

Duplex ultrasonography, CTA, MRA, and catheter-based angiography are all good imaging techniques to demonstrate diseased intestinal vessels. Stenosis or occlusion of the mesenteric vessels is common, although symptomatic intestinal ischemia is rare. No diagnostic tests can establish the diagnosis definitively. The diagnosis relies on the combination of the typical clinical presentation of abdominal pain and weight loss and the presence of other cardiovascular disease, combined with the finding of intestinal arterial obstruction.

- No diagnostic tests can establish the diagnosis of chronic intestinal ischemia definitively
- The diagnosis relies on the combination of the typical clinical presentation:
  - Abdominal pain and weight loss
  - Presence of other cardiovascular disease
  - Presence of intestinal arterial obstruction

Because the atherosclerotic lesions that typically produce intestinal arterial obstruction are usually located at the origin of the celiac, superior mesenteric, and inferior mesenteric arteries, duplex ultrasonography is an effective non-invasive method for diagnosis. Duplex scanning of visceral vessels is technically difficult but can be accomplished in more than 85% of subjects in the elective setting. The test has an overall accuracy of approximately 90% for detection of stenoses greater than 70% or occlusions of the celiac and superior mesenteric arteries, when performed in laboratories experienced in this technique. Both CTA and gadolinium-enhanced MRA are well suited for visualizing the typical atherosclerotic lesions at the origins of the intestinal arteries. All of the non-invasive techniques are less suited for visualizing the more distal intestinal arteries and for diagnosis of some of the more unusual causes of intestinal ischemia. Arteriography remains the gold standard for the diagnosis of chronic intestinal ischemia.

- The atherosclerotic lesions that typically produce intestinal arterial obstruction are usually located at the origin of the celiac, superior mesenteric, and inferior mesenteric arteries
- Duplex scanning has an overall accuracy of ≈90% for detection of >70% diameter stenosis or occlusion of the celiac and superior mesenteric arteries

The natural history of symptomatic chronic intestinal ischemia is only partly known. An unknown percentage of patients have progression to acute intestinal ischemia and the rest have progressive weight loss with ultimate death from starvation. Although it is reasonable to postulate that some of the affected patients must recover spontaneously, no such case has been documented in the literature.

Treatment

Increasingly, reports are showing that percutaneous interventional treatment of intestinal arterial obstructions is possible, with a high technical success rate and few complications in properly selected cases. One study reported on 59 consecutive patients with chronic mesenteric ischemia who underwent stent placement. All patients had clinical follow-up, and 90% had anatomic follow-up with angiography (CTA or conventional) or ultrasonography at least 6 months after the procedure. Success was obtained in 96% (76 of 79 arteries) and symptom relief occurred in 88% (50 patients). With a mean follow-up of 38±15 months (range, 6-112 months), 79% of the patients remained alive and 10 (17%) had recurrence of symptoms. Angiography or ultrasonography at 14±5 months after the procedure showed a restenosis rate of 29%. All patients with recurrent symptoms had angiographic in-stent restenosis and were successfully revascularized percutaneously.

To date, no prospective therapeutic trials have been conducted, and follow-up information is limited. Relief of symptoms and weight gain reliably follow elimination of the arterial obstruction. Several recent reports of concurrent series treated with angioplasty and stenting or surgery indicate that recurrences after percutaneous procedures have been more frequent than after open surgery, but many of the recurrences can be managed by percutaneous interventions. Therefore, it is important for patients to have ultrasonographic surveillance after angioplasty and stenting of the mesenteric arteries. Recurrent symptoms have nearly always indicated recurrent arterial obstruction.

Surgical treatment of chronic intestinal ischemia is accomplished by endarterectomy or bypass grafting, with most surgeons preferring the latter. Long-term patency and relief of symptoms are the rule, with few recurrences. Essentially all symptomatic recurrences are the result of recurrent stenosis or occlusion of visceral arteries or the reconstructions.

Questions

1. An 86-year-old man presented with bilateral 95% stenosis of the renal arteries. His blood pressure was 180/100 mm Hg and serum creatinine value was 1.3 mg/dL. He was started on lisinopril, 40 mg daily. Three weeks later, his blood pressure was 178/98 mm Hg and serum creatinine value was 1.2 mg/dL. What is the most likely reason that his blood pressure and renal function did not change with ACE inhibitor therapy?

a. Bilateral RAS is a volume-mediated form of hypertension, thus the patient did not respond to ACE inhibitors.
b. With such a severe degree of stenosis, the ACE inhibitor is not filtered, thus it has no effect on the kidney.
c. Bilateral RAS is a renin-mediated form of hypertension, thus the patient would require the use of both a diuretic and an ACE inhibitor.
d. The blood pressure is so high that two or more drugs are needed to decrease it to normal levels.

2. A 28-year-old woman presents with blood pressures ranging from 150/92 to 180/104 mm Hg. An epigastric long systolic bruit is detected. Serum creatinine level is 0.7 mg/dL. Angiography of the renal arteries shows that the left renal artery is normal but the right renal artery has a "string of beads" in the mid renal artery, extending for 2 cm into each of two branches off the main renal artery. What is the treatment of choice for this woman?
   a. Start antihypertensive therapy; if the blood pressure is well controlled, no further therapy is needed.
   b. Perform PTA of the right renal artery and the two branches.
   c. Perform stent implantation into the main renal artery and angioplasty in the two branches.
   d. Perform surgical bypass using saphenous vein graft.

3. Renal artery duplex ultrasonography is performed in a 75-year-old woman. Results are shown in the table. Her blood pressure is 170/92 mm Hg and she is receiving hydrochlorothiazide (25 mg/d), lisinopril (40 mg/d), and metoprolol (100 mg/d). The aortic PSV is 55 cm/s.

	Renal artery	
Measurement	**Right**	**Left**
PSV, cm/s	302	190
EDV, cm/s	88	55
Kidney size, cm	10.3	10.5
RRI	0.79	0.69

   How would you interpret these renal artery duplex ultrasonography results?
   a. Renal arteries are normal.
   b. The renal arteries are normal but there is markedly increased resistance within the kidneys.
   c. Results show an 85% stenosis of the right renal artery and a 40% stenosis of the left renal artery.
   d. The left renal artery is narrowed 0%-59%, and the right renal artery shows 60%-99% stenosis.

4. Which of the following is the best indication for renal artery stent implantation?
   a. Increased blood pressure in a 30-year-old woman with perimedial fibroplasia of the left renal artery
   b. A serum creatinine value of 3.5 mg/dL in an 80-year-old man with 95% right RAS and 20% left RAS
   c. A blood pressure of 190/104 mm Hg in a 76-year-old man with 80% bilateral RAS receiving hydrochlorothiazide (25 mg/d), atenolol (100 mg/d), enalapril (10 mg twice daily), and terazosin (10 mg/d)
   d. A blood pressure of 132/80 mm Hg and a serum creatinine value of 1.4 mg/dL in a 65-year-old man taking five drugs for his blood pressure, with 60% right RAS and 40% left RAS

5. A 68-year-old woman was admitted to the medical intensive care unit with septic shock. She was treated with intravenous antibiotics and large doses of pressors. Her systolic blood pressure ranged from 80 to 100 mm Hg. Pressors were discontinued on day 3 because the systolic blood pressures were consistently greater than 100 mm Hg. Later on the third hospital day, severe abdominal pain and marked distention developed. Angiography at that time showed 50% stenosis of the superior mesenteric artery and 60% stenosis of the celiac artery. The inferior mesenteric artery was patent and normal. Irregularities were noted in the intestinal branches, the arcades could not be visualized, and no filling of the intramural vessels was seen. What is the treatment of choice for this patient?
   a. Immediate surgical exploration and resection of ischemic bowel if present
   b. PTA and stent implantation of the celiac and superior mesenteric arteries
   c. Infusion of papaverine into the intestinal vessels
   d. Antibiotics, fluid resuscitation, and expectant waiting

Suggested Readings

Blum U, Krumme B, Flugel P, et al. Treatment of ostial renal-artery stenoses with vascular endoprostheses after unsuccessful balloon angioplasty. N Engl J Med. 1997;336:459-65.

Caps MT, Zierler RE, Polissar NL, et al. Risk of atrophy in kidneys with atherosclerotic renal artery stenosis. Kidney Int. 1998;53:735-42.

Conlon PJ, Little MA, Pieper K, et al. Severity of renal vascular disease predicts mortality in patients undergoing coronary angiography. Kidney Int. 2001;60:1490-7.

Gray BH, Olin JW, Childs MB, et al. Clinical benefit of renal artery angioplasty with stenting for the control of recurrent and refractory congestive heart failure. Vasc Med. 2002;7:275-9.

Hansen KJ, Edwards MS, Craven TE, et al. Prevalence of renovascular disease in the elderly: a population-based study. J Vasc Surg. 2002;36:443-51.

Hansen KJ, Thomason RB, Craven TE, et al. Surgical management of dialysis-dependent ischemic nephropathy. J Vasc Surg. 1995;21:197-209.

Henry M, Klonaris C, Henry I, et al. Protected renal stenting with the PercuSurge GuardWire device: a pilot study. J Endovasc Ther. 2001;8:227-37.

Kasirajan K, O'Hara PJ, Gray BH, et al. Chronic mesenteric ischemia: open surgery versus percutaneous angioplasty and stenting. J Vasc Surg. 2001;33:63-71.

Leertouwer TC, Gussenhoven EJ, Bosch JL, et al. Stent placement for renal arterial stenosis: where do we stand? A meta-analysis. Radiology. 2000;216:78-85.

Mailloux LU, Napolitano B, Bellucci AG, et al. Renal vascular disease causing end-stage renal disease, incidence, clinical correlates, and outcomes: a 20-year clinical experience. Am J Kidney Dis. 1994;24:622-9.

Olin JW, Kaufman JA, Bluemke DA, et al, American Heart Association. Atherosclerotic Vascular Disease Conference: Writing Group IV: imaging. Circulation. 2004;109:2626-33.

Olin JW, Piedmonte MR, Young JR, et al. The utility of duplex ultrasound scanning of the renal arteries for diagnosing significant renal artery stenosis. Ann Intern Med. 1995;122:833-8.

Park WM, Cherry KJ Jr, Chua HK, et al. Current results of open revascularization for chronic mesenteric ischemia: a standard for comparison. J Vasc Surg. 2002;35:853-9.

Pickering TG, Herman L, Devereux RB, et al. Recurrent pulmonary oedema in hypertension due to bilateral renal artery stenosis: treatment by angioplasty or surgical revascularisation. Lancet. 1988;2:551-2.

Radermacher J, Chavan A, Bleck J, et al. Use of Doppler ultrasonography to predict the outcome of therapy for renal-artery stenosis. N Engl J Med. 2001;344:410-7.

Rose R, Bartholomew J, Olin JW. Atheromatous embolization. In: Rutherford RB, editor. Vascular surgery. Vol 1. 6th ed. Philadelphia: Elsevier Saunders; 2005. p. 986-99.

Rundback JH, Sacks D, Kent KC, et al, AHA Councils on Cardiovascular Radiology, High Blood Pressure Research, Kidney in Cardiovascular Disease, Cardio-Thoracic and Vascular Surgery, and Clinical Cardiology, and the Society of Interventional Radiology FDA Device Forum Committee. Guidelines for the reporting of renal artery revascularization in clinical trials. Circulation. 2002;106:1572-85.

Safian RD, Textor SC. Renal-artery stenosis. N Engl J Med. 2001;344:431-42.

Scolari F, Tardanico R, Zani R, et al. Cholesterol crystal embolism: a recognizable cause of renal disease. Am J Kidney Dis. 2000;36:1089-109.

Silva JA, Chan AW, White CJ, et al. Elevated brain natriuretic peptide predicts blood pressure response after stent revascularization in patients with renal artery stenosis. Circulation. 2005 Jan 25;111:328-33. Epub 2005 Jan 17.

Silva JA, White CJ, Collins TJ, et al. Endovascular therapy for chronic mesenteric ischemia. J Am Coll Cardiol. 2006 Mar 7;47:944-50. Epub 2006 Feb 10.

Slovut DP, Olin JW. Fibromuscular dysplasia. N Engl J Med. 2004;350:1862-71.

Tan KT, van Beek EJ, Brown PW, et al. Magnetic resonance angiography for the diagnosis of renal artery stenosis: a meta-analysis. Clin Radiol. 2002;57:617-24.

Textor SC, Wilcox CS. Ischemic nephropathy/azotemic renovascular disease. Semin Nephrol. 2000;20:489-502.

Thomas JH, Blake K, Pierce GE, et al. The clinical course of asymptomatic mesenteric arterial stenosis. J Vasc Surg. 1998;27:840-4.

Watson PS, Hadjipetrou P, Cox SV, et al. Effect of renal artery stenting on renal function and size in patients with atherosclerotic renovascular disease. Circulation. 2000;102:1671-7.

Zierler RE, Bergelin RO, Davidson RC, et al. A prospective study of disease progression in patients with atherosclerotic renal artery stenosis. Am J Hypertens. 1996;9:1055-61.

Zwolak RM, Fillinger MF, Walsh DB, et al. Mesenteric and celiac duplex scanning: a validation study. J Vasc Surg. 1998;27:1078-87.

19 Carotid Artery Disease and Stroke

Michael R. Jaff, DO

Introduction

Stroke is the third leading cause of death in the United States and the second leading cause worldwide (Table 19.1). Over 20% of patients die from acute stroke, and the mortality rate is as high as 50% at 5 years. Stroke is the leading cause of adult disability and is perhaps the atherosclerotic complication most dreaded by patients and their families. More than 750,000 strokes occur annually in the United States, and one-third are due to extracranial carotid atherosclerosis. Although dissection of the internal carotid artery, fibromuscular dysplasia (FMD), arteritis, and trauma may result in cerebrovascular ischemia, atherosclerosis is the most common cause of disease involving the extracranial internal carotid artery.

Table 19.1 Stroke Facts

More than 750,000 strokes occur annually in the United States.
Approximately 30% of all strokes are attributable to extracranial atherosclerotic carotid artery disease.
Stroke is the third leading cause of death in the United States.
Stroke is the most common cause of disability for adults in the United States.

Extracranial Carotid Artery Stenosis and Stroke Risk

The risk of stroke increases as the severity of carotid stenosis increases. The stroke rate for patients with carotid stenosis of 75% or less is 1.3% per year, whereas the rate is 10.5% per year if stenosis is greater than 75%. In the North American Symptomatic Carotid Endarterectomy Trial (NASCET), symptomatic patients with 70% to 99% carotid stenosis had a 26% risk of ipsilateral stroke and a 28% risk of any stroke over 2 years of follow-up. However, the risk of subsequent stroke may differ on the basis of the initial cerebrovascular symptom. A retinal transient ischemic attack (TIA) such as amaurosis fugax was associated with an annual stroke rate of 2%. During more than 7 years of follow-up, the cumulative rate of cerebral infarction was 14% for patients with amaurosis fugax and 27% for patients with hemispheric TIA as the initial cerebrovascular symptom. The NASCET study showed a 2-year risk of fatal and non-fatal stroke of 17% after transient monocular blindness and 42% after hemispheric TIA.

- The risk of stroke increases as the severity of the carotid stenosis increases
- In the NASCET study, the cumulative rate of cerebral infarction was 14% for patients with amaurosis fugax and 27% for patients with hemispheric TIA as the initial cerebrovascular symptom

Regardless of the anatomic location, carotid plaque increases the risk of stroke. The pathogenesis of stroke in extracranial carotid stenosis is a function of decreased vessel diameter, superimposed thrombosis, and embolization of thrombotic material. This has been shown by transcranial Doppler ultrasonography in patients with transient monocular blindness. Certain alterations in plaque morphology may lead to clinical symptoms; as in the coronary circulation with acute coronary syndromes, plaque rupture has been postulated to result in acute stroke. In contrast to the pathophysiology of acute coronary syndromes, only a minority of symptoms of atherosclerotic carotid artery stenoses are caused by thrombotic occlusion or hemodynamic impairment; most symptoms are a result of emboli (plaque rupture, ulceration).

Progression of Carotid Stenosis

The rate of disease progression for established extracranial carotid artery stenosis is approximately 20% to 40%. In one prospective natural history study of 232 patients with mild or moderate carotid stenosis (<50% and 50%-79%, respectively), carotid duplex ultrasonography (CDUS) was performed annually for a mean of 7 years. Disease progressed in 23% of the patients, half of whom had progression to severe stenosis (80%-99%) or occlusion. Risk of progression to severe stenosis or occlusion was higher for patients with stenosis initially categorized as 50% to 79% than for those with stenosis less than 50%.

More recently, in a study of 425 asymptomatic patients with 50% to 79% carotid stenosis, progression of stenosis was observed in 17% of 282 arteries that were evaluated by at least 2 serial CDUS examinations (mean follow-up, 38 months). The incidence of ipsilateral stroke, however, was low despite the rate of disease progression (0.85% at 1 year, 3.6% at 3 years, 5.4% at 5 years). Nonetheless, all natural history studies have shown that more severe stenoses are associated with increased risks of disease progression and subsequent stroke. Of 242 asymptomatic patients with different degrees of carotid stenosis, 35 patients (14%) had a stroke or TIA. However, patients with 80% to 99% carotid stenosis had an annual neurologic event rate of 20.6%.

Internal carotid artery occlusion is an unpredictable clinical dilemma. In a retrospective review of 167 patients with carotid occlusion who presented with no symptoms (27%), stroke (43%), or TIA (17%), 30 patients (18%) had a stroke during follow-up (mean, 39 months), 67% (20) of which were ipsilateral to the occlusion. Consistent with other reports, heart disease was the cause of death in 22 of the 54 patients (41%) who died during follow-up. The contralateral stroke event rate was 33%; the 5-year stroke-free rate for patients with stenoses of 50% to 99% was slightly lower than that for patients with stenoses less than 50% (77% vs 94%; *P*=.08).

Plaque ulceration clearly increases the risk of subsequent stroke. As in the coronary arterial bed, the pathophysiology of plaque rupture, foam cell infiltration, and thinning of the fibrous cap occurs more often in patients with symptomatic (rather than asymptomatic) carotid stenosis. During 2 years of follow-up of medically treated patients in the NASCET study, plaque ulceration increased the risk of ipsilateral stroke from 26.3% to 73.2% as the degree of stenosis progressed from 75% to 99%. For patients without plaque ulceration, the 2-year stroke risk was 21.3%, regardless of the degree of stenosis.

History and Physical Examination

Perhaps the most important aspect of the evaluation of patients with extracranial carotid artery disease is determining both the symptomatic status of the patient and the degree of stenosis. Treatment options and their outcomes vary greatly depending on whether the carotid artery stenosis is symptomatic.

Symptoms suggestive of cerebral ischemia are categorized by the location and amount of the brain affected and by the duration and reversibility of the symptoms. For example, transient retinal ischemia (amaurosis fugax) is described as a "dark shade" or loss of vision in one visual field that typically resolves within minutes. Symptoms such as aphasia and contralateral hemiparesis or hemiparesthesia may originate from the dominant hemisphere. Non-dominant hemispheric ischemia results in a patient's lack of awareness of symptoms (anosognosia). Posterior circulation ischemia (vertebrobasilar insufficiency) causes symptoms of dysarthria, diplopia, vertigo, syncope, transient confusion, or a combination of the these symptoms. A reversible ischemic neurologic deficit is a similar phenomenon with symptoms lasting up to 24 hours. A stroke (cerebrovascular accident) is a more permanent manifestation of cerebral ischemia, with symptoms lasting more than 24 hours.

Palpation of the carotid artery upstroke gives non-specific physical findings. A diminished carotid upstroke might suggest cardiac valvular pathology or a global decrease in left ventricular systolic function. In fact, occlusion of the internal carotid artery often is accompanied by a normal carotid upstroke because the internal carotid artery is located cephalad to the angle of the mandible. However, the finding of a cervical bruit has clinically significant implications.

Carotid Bruits and the Risk of Cardiovascular Disease

Cervical bruits may have several causes (Table 19.2). Estimates of the prevalence of asymptomatic carotid bruits in adults range from 1% to 2.3% for patients aged 45 to 54

Table 19.2 Causes of Cervical Bruits

	Bruit		
Cause	Systolic only	Diastolic only	Systolic and diastolic
Carotid atherosclerosis	✓	✓	✓
Thyrotoxicosis	✓	✓	✓
Transmitted cardiac murmur			
Aortic stenosis	✓		
Aortic insufficiency		✓	
Arteriovenous fistula			✓
Venous hum	✓		✓

years and 8.2% for patients 75 years or older. However, in a selected series of patients scheduled to undergo vascular surgical procedures, the incidence of cervical bruits ranged from 6% to 16% (mean prevalence, 10%). The risk of a carotid bruit developing in patients aged 65 years or older is approximately 1% per year, nearly twice the rate in patients aged 45 to 54 years.

The implications of an asymptomatic carotid bruit are vast. The incidence of subsequent stroke for a patient with an asymptomatic carotid bruit ranges from 1.5% annually to 2.1% in 3 years, as shown by the European Carotid Surgery Trial. In this study, the 3-year risk of stroke for 127 patients with severe carotid stenosis (70%-99%) was 5.7%.

This association of asymptomatic carotid bruits with subsequent stroke may not be as strong in the elderly population. In a study of 241 nursing home residents (mean age, 86 years), 12% had asymptomatic carotid bruits. Incidence varied with age—8% for patients aged 75 to 84 years, 10% for those aged 85 to 94 years, and 13% for patients aged 95 years or older. However, the 3-year incidence of stroke was the same for patients with a bruit (10%) and without a bruit (9%). Of interest, the bruit was undetectable during follow-up in 60% of the surviving residents, with no occurrences of stroke or cerebrovascular events.

The presence of a carotid bruit does not adequately predict the severity of carotid stenosis. In a substudy of the NASCET, 1,268 patients with recent transient cerebral ischemia or non-disabling stroke were examined for the presence of a carotid bruit. Of these patients, 58% had a bruit localized to the ipsilateral carotid artery, 31% had a carotid bruit involving the contralateral vessel, and 24% had bilateral carotid bruits. The sensitivity and specificity of a focal bruit to predict high-grade ipsilateral carotid stenosis was 63% and 61%, respectively. The absence of a bruit lowered the pretest probability of a 70% to 99% carotid stenosis from 52% to 40%.

In addition to the risk of subsequent cerebrovascular events in patients with asymptomatic carotid bruits, the incidence of coronary artery disease and coronary mortality in this patient group is much higher than that of the general population. One landmark study of 506 patients with extracranial carotid artery disease and symptomatic or asymptomatic bruits showed that approximately 35% had severe coronary artery disease that required revascularization or that had progressed to an inoperable status.

The prevalence of severe coronary artery disease in patients with symptomatic and asymptomatic carotid artery disease translates into increased mortality rates. In a study of 444 men with asymptomatic carotid artery stenosis (mean follow-up, 4 years), the mortality rate was 37%. Of these deaths, 61% were due to coronary artery disease. Multivariate analysis showed that diabetes mellitus, abnormal electrocardiography findings, and the presence of intermittent claudication were associated with increased mortality risk (2 or 3 risk factors showed annual mortality rates of 11.3% and 13%, respectively).

- The presence of a carotid bruit does not predict the severity of carotid stenosis
- Incidence of coronary artery disease and coronary mortality in patients with carotid disease is much higher than that in the general population
- A study of 506 patients with extracranial carotid artery disease and symptomatic or asymptomatic bruits showed that 35% had severe coronary artery disease that required revascularization or that had progressed to an inoperable status

Differential Diagnosis of Cerebral Ischemia, Stroke, and Carotid Artery Disease

There are many causes of stroke other than carotid artery disease (Table 19.3). The most common cause is an embolic event, most often from a cardiac source. If a cardiac cause is suspected, electrocardiography and echocardiography can be used to identify non-valvular atrial fibrillation, rheumatic mitral valve disease, and cardiac chamber thrombi (prior myocardial infarction). A common source of cerebral emboli is aortic arch atherosclerosis, which is identified with transesophageal echocardiography. Paradoxic emboli must be thoroughly investigated with transesophageal echocardiography, especially now that new percutaneous methods for closure of occult patent foramen ovale make this procedure less risky and invasive than surgery. Other uncommon causes of stroke include intracranial tumors, intracerebral hemorrhage (rupture of an aneurysm), central nervous system vasculitis, and intracranial arteriovenous malformations.

Although carotid artery atherosclerosis is the most common cause of extracranial carotid artery stenosis and stroke, other causes must be considered. Lacunar infarcts,

Table 19.3 Causes of Cerebrovascular Ischemia or Infarction

Thrombosis due to atherosclerosis
Embolization
Hemorrhage
Rupture of intracranial aneurysm or arteriovenous malformation
Intracranial infection (i.e., meningitis)
Cerebrovascular arteritis
Cerebral venous thromboembolism
Hypercoagulability
Carotid artery dissection
Moyamoya disease
Fibromuscular dysplasia of the internal carotid artery
Complicated migraine
Lacunar infarcts

embolization, intracranial hemorrhage, and rupture of intracranial aneurysms or arteriovenous malformations are, in descending order of frequency, important pathologic entities. Some (e.g., traumatic injury to the carotid artery) are simple to identify on the basis of medical history, physical examination, and imaging studies. Other causes are challenging to identify because they may be associated with a multitude of symptoms, including acephalgic complex migraine and atypical manifestations of epilepsy. FMD of the internal carotid artery and spontaneous carotid artery dissection are two vascular conditions that may mimic cerebral ischemia caused by carotid artery atherosclerosis; these conditions must be understood by the vascular medicine specialist.

FMD of the Carotid Artery

FMD is classified on the basis of the arterial layer involved—intima, media, or adventitia. Although many physicians consider FMD to affect only the renal arteries, the internal carotid artery also is commonly involved. FMD typically affects women in their 40s. Medial fibroplasia is the most common form of FMD and is characterized angiographically as a "string of beads," in which the "beads" are larger in diameter than the normal artery. FMD usually affects the mid and distal segments of the artery. Patients may present with a myriad of symptoms such as headache, pulsatile tinnitus, and vague symptoms that do not commonly reflect true cerebral ischemia. In addition, if a cervical bruit is identified during a routine physical examination, CDUS may be used to evaluate it, which may show turbulence with an increase in peak systolic velocities in the mid and distal internal carotid artery.

The natural disease course of medial fibroplasia of the internal carotid artery is relatively benign. Some suggest reassurance and no therapy for incidentally discovered carotid FMD. For patients with symptoms that may be attributable to carotid FMD, antiplatelet therapy with aspirin is recommended. No data are available for other antiplatelet agents (ticlopidine, clopidogrel, long-acting dipyridamole, and aspirin). For symptomatic lesions that do not respond to antiplatelet therapy, percutaneous therapy (carotid artery angioplasty) usually is preferred over surgical graduated intraluminal dilatation, despite the lack of comparative trials. Physicians must recall that an association between carotid FMD and intracranial aneurysms is often noted.

Carotid Artery Dissection

Spontaneous dissection of the carotid or vertebral arteries accounts for only 2% of all strokes, but it is the second most common cause of stroke in younger patients. Spontaneous carotid dissection tends to occur at age 40 to 50 years. Although patients may present after a catastrophic event, they typically have pain on one side of the head that is accompanied by partial Horner syndrome (ptosis, miosis, and anhidrosis). After this "warning" presentation, many patients (50%-95%) will present with cerebral or retinal ischemia. Carotid dissection flaps typically begin distal to the carotid bulb.

In the appropriate clinical scenario, diagnostic tests are recommended. The initial diagnostic algorithm begins with duplex ultrasonography, which can identify the dissection flap, true and false lumens, and differential flow patterns in the two channels. However, if the dissection is small or begins cephalad to the angle of the mandible, the dissection may not be detected. Magnetic resonance angiography (MRA) and, more recently, multidetector computed tomography angiography (CTA) are replacing traditional angiography as the imaging methods of choice for detecting carotid artery dissection.

The conventional treatment of carotid dissection is medical, with anticoagulation therapy (heparin and warfarin) or antiplatelet therapy. A meta-analysis did not prove the superiority of one regimen over the other. However, most physicians tend to offer anticoagulation therapy initially. If symptoms resolve, antiplatelet therapy replaces anticoagulation therapy after 3 to 6 months; antiplatelet therapy is used for a longer course (potentially lifelong). Revascularization with surgery or endovascular therapy currently is reserved for patients with persistent or recurrent symptoms of ischemia despite adequate anticoagulation.

- Spontaneous dissection of the carotid arteries is the second most common cause of stroke in younger patients
- Conventional treatment of carotid dissection includes anticoagulation therapy (heparin and warfarin) or antiplatelet therapy

Risk Factors for Stroke and Carotid Artery Disease

Control of several modifiable risk factors, in particular hypertension, diabetes mellitus, dyslipidemia, and tobacco use, is integral to stroke prevention. For example, patients with diabetes mellitus have twice the risk of stroke and carotid artery disease than patients without diabetes mellitus. Similarly, smokers have increased risk for all stroke subtypes; the relative risk is 2.58 when compared with patients who have never smoked. Low levels of high-density lipoprotein cholesterol and a high ratio of total to high-density lipoprotein cholesterol are risk factors for carotid atherosclerosis, although hypercholesterolemia is not a strong independent risk factor for stroke.

As many as 60% of all strokes are attributable to hypertension, and the incidence and mortality rates increase with blood pressures above 110/75 mm Hg. An estimated two-thirds of stroke risk in the general population is attributable to hypertension. Clinical trials of antihypertensive therapy have shown that even a modest decrease in blood pressure decreases the incidence of stroke. Many prospective trials suggest a linear relationship between blood pressure and stroke risk, but other (largely cohort) studies have suggested a J-shaped phenomenon that shows increased stroke rates at the very high and very low blood pressure levels. An evaluation of 7 meta-analyses of randomized trials suggests that the relationship is linear with a 31% risk reduction with every 10-mm Hg decrease in systolic blood pressure.

Atherosclerosis of the extracranial carotid arteries is a leading cause of stroke. Hypertension promotes the development of atherosclerosis at the bifurcation of the common carotid artery into the internal and external carotid arteries. Carotid atherosclerosis generally is most severe within 2 cm of the common carotid artery bifurcation and often involves the posterior wall of the vessel.

In a series of 3,602 patients, the presence of hypertension predicted the severity of carotid atherosclerosis, as evaluated by high-resolution B-mode ultrasonographic assessment of intimal-medial thickness, carotid plaque score, and maximal percentage of stenosis. The presence of hypertension may be as important as plaque morphology and severity for prediction of neurologic events. A prospective study of serial carotid ultrasonography showed that hypertension, plaque echolucency, and lesion progression predicted patient symptoms.

Patients with diabetes mellitus are twice as likely to have a stroke. Tobacco use is a well-documented risk factor for cerebrovascular ischemia. Use of oral contraceptives and active tobacco use together form an important combination of risk factors that may result in hypercoagulability.

Carotid atherosclerosis risk increases as the number of risk factors for stroke (e.g., hypertension, diabetes mellitus, tobacco use, and dyslipidemia) increases. One study of almost 4,000 patients showed that the incidence of mild carotid stenosis (25%-49%) increased from 2.4% in patients without risk factors to 18.6% in patients with three risk factors. Similarly, the incidence of severe (≥50%) carotid stenoses increased from 0.6% for patients with no stroke risk factors to 5% for patients with three risk factors.

- Approximately 60% of all strokes are attributable to hypertension
- Even a modest decrease in blood pressure decreases the incidence of stroke (a 10-mm Hg decrease in systolic blood pressure is associated with a 31% risk reduction)
- Carotid atherosclerosis risk increases as the number of stroke risk factors (hypertension, diabetes mellitus, tobacco use, and dyslipidemia) increases

Diagnostic Tests for Carotid Artery Disease

Intra-arterial digital subtraction angiography is the diagnostic standard for identifying carotid artery stenosis and measuring its severity. Although serious complications are associated with cerebral arteriography, in skilled centers, these risks approach 1% morbidity and 0.1% mortality. However, this test is an impractical means of establishing the presence of carotid artery stenosis because it is invasive and cost prohibitive.

If the patient has ischemic symptoms, computed tomography (CT) of the brain should be performed initially; CT may show hemorrhagic infarction, subarachnoid hemorrhage, tumor, intracranial aneurysm, and arteriovenous malformation. Magnetic resonance imaging of the brain is a more sensitive indicator of small and hyperacute infarcts and necrosis caused by the ischemia. For patients with a cervical bruit or at high risk of carotid stenosis, CDUS, MRA, and CTA are reliable and non-invasive tests.

- CDUS, MRA, and CTA are the preferred non-invasive diagnostic tests for carotid artery disease

Carotid Duplex Ultrasonography

CDUS uses B-mode and Doppler ultrasonography to detect focal increases in systolic and end-diastolic velocities, which may be used to indicate moderate and severe extracranial carotid artery stenosis. State-of-the-art centers use a combination of gray-scale, color-flow, Doppler, and, in certain circumstances, "power Doppler" techniques to perform a complete CDUS examination. The gray-scale image provides information about the location of the major extracranial carotid arteries (common carotid, internal carotid, external carotid, and vertebral arteries). It also assesses plaque composition (heterogeneous [fibrous] plaque and homogeneous [fatty] plaque) and plaque ulceration. The color-flow image facilitates rapid localization of the arterial stenosis, but the Doppler evaluation most reliably defines the presence and severity of carotid artery stenosis. However, inaccurate determinations of the severity of stenosis may result from improper CDUS procedure. CDUS is the ideal modality for evaluating the adequacy of revascularization over time. Some centers use transcranial Doppler in conjunction with CDUS to determine collateral pathways in the intracranial circulation. In addition, cerebral vasospasm is well visualized with this technique.

Magnetic Resonance Angiography

MRA uses the energy generated by controlled proton shifts in an electromagnetic field to produce a three-dimensional image of the carotid artery bifurcation, which can be used to detect carotid artery stenoses. High-quality MRA requires administration of a contrast agent, commonly gadolinium, via a peripheral venous catheter. Accuracy of MRA is less operator-dependent than Doppler ultrasonography. However, interpretation of the source images and image postprocessing are important. Reformatted images do not determine stenosis severity accurately. In fact, without gadolinium, the two-dimensional time-of-flight images overestimate stenoses (moderate stenoses appear severe, severe stenoses appear occluded). In addition, patients who are severely ill, morbidly obese, or claustrophobic, or who have an implanted cardiovert-er-defibrillator or pacemaker should not undergo MRA evaluation.

CDUS and MRA have similar reported sensitivities (83%-86%) and specificities (89%-94%). A meta-analysis of these imaging modalities showed that they have the same capacity to detect complete carotid artery occlusion and stenosis greater than 70%. Current algorithms commonly use the results of two imaging modalities to determine the anatomic options for carotid revascularization.

Multidetector CTA

More recently, multidetector CTA has been used to identify patients with carotid artery stenosis. Early experience with first-generation devices showed a sensitivity of 85% to detect stenosis of 70% to 99%, with a specificity of 93%. Calcification at the area of significant stenosis impairs image interpretation. In addition, CTA is not practical for serial surveillance of a carotid stenosis because the test requires considerable external beam radiation and administration of an iodinated contrast medium.

Invasive Arteriography

Angiography is considered the gold standard for assessing cerebrovascular arteries. Given the progressive improvement in non-invasive imaging techniques, cerebrovascular arteriography is infrequently required as a diagnostic test. However, if two non-invasive tests performed by expert laboratories have discordant findings, angiography is indicated. The major drawback of invasive angiography is the risk of adverse events associated with the procedure. In the Asymptomatic Carotid Atherosclerosis Study (ACAS) trial, a 1.2% risk of stroke was attributable to angiography.

Treatment of Carotid Artery Disease With or Without Cerebral Ischemia

Medical Treatment of Carotid Artery Disease: Stroke Prevention

Aggressive risk-factor intervention is the cornerstone of any treatment for carotid artery disease. Treatment of hypertension, even for patients with mildly elevated blood pressure, decreases the risk of stroke. In a meta-analysis of hypertension treatment trials, an average decrease in blood pressure of only 5.8 mm Hg resulted in a 43% decrease in the incidence of stroke. A recent meta-analysis of seven randomized, secondary-prevention trials of antihypertensive therapy for patients with previous stroke or TIA confirmed that the prevention of vascular events was associated with the magnitude of blood pressure reduction.

Data assessing the benefit of antihypertensive therapy in patients with carotid stenosis are limited, partially because of concerns about blood pressure reduction in patients with severe carotid stenosis. One meta-analysis evaluated patients from two major randomized carotid endarterectomy trials and one major randomized trial of antiplatelet therapy. Among medically treated patients with symptomatic carotid atherosclerosis, elevated blood pressure was associated with increased stroke risk. In patients with bilateral carotid stenoses of 70% or greater, however, those with lower systolic blood pressure had more events. Although the results were interesting, the study was observational and had only a small number of absolute events. Because of these limitations, it is not possible to make definitive recommendations to avoid lowering blood pressure in patients with bilateral carotid atherosclerosis. If blood pressure is lowered, it should be done so cautiously. The antihypertensive agent of choice for patients with carotid atherosclerosis should not differ from published guidelines.

Antiplatelet therapy, specifically aspirin (81-325 mg/d), results in a 25% relative risk reduction compared with placebo. The CAPRIE (Clopidogrel vs Aspirin in Patients at Risk of Ischaemic Events) trial did not show a decrease in stroke risk with clopidogrel when compared with aspirin alone. Long-acting dipyridamole added to aspirin for secondary stroke prevention has some benefit. Combination antiplatelet therapy with aspirin and clopidogrel, which is effective for patients with acute coronary syndromes, recently was shown to offer no decrease in the rate of neurologic events and had a significant increase in serious hemorrhagic events when compared with aspirin alone. No data support the use of anticoagulation therapy with warfarin to decrease the risk of stroke in patients who do not have atrial fibrillation or another indication for systemic anticoagulation.

Large studies of lipid-lowering therapy, predominantly with statins (HMG-CoA reductase inhibitors), have shown significant rates of stroke reduction. Patients with atherosclerotic carotid artery disease should receive lipid-lowering therapy to achieve National Cholesterol Education Program guideline levels.

- Antiplatelet therapy with aspirin (81-325 mg/d) results in a relative risk reduction when compared with placebo
- The CAPRIE trial showed no reduction in stroke risk with clopidogrel when compared with aspirin alone
- Combination antiplatelet therapy with aspirin and clopidogrel shows no decrease in neurologic event rates but shows a significant increase in serious hemorrhagic events when compared with aspirin-only therapy
- No data support the use of warfarin to decrease the risk of stroke in patients without atrial fibrillation or other conditions requiring systemic anticoagulation
- Lipid-lowering therapy, predominantly with statins, decreases stroke rate

Surgical Therapy

Carotid endarterectomy (CEA) is well established as the surgical procedure of choice for treatment of extracranial carotid artery disease. The preferred method of performing CEA is debated; major points of contention include patching the vessel versus primary closure, use of shunting during the procedure, standard endarterectomy versus eversion endarterectomy, and use of regional versus general anesthesia. The procedure is safe and effective when performed by a highly skilled and experienced surgeon. Most professional medical organizations agree that the perioperative morbidity and mortality rates for CEA are 3% for asymptomatic patients, 6% for symptomatic patients, and 10% for patients with a restenotic CEA site.

The NASCET and the European Carotid Surgery Trial showed that CEA was superior to medical therapy for the prevention of stroke in symptomatic patients with high-grade carotid stenosis (70%-99%), despite a 6% incidence of perioperative stroke and death. When compared with the best medical therapy, CEA also showed clinically significant benefits in symptomatic patients with moderate-severity stenosis (50%-69%).

For patients with asymptomatic carotid stenosis of 60% to 99% and acceptable perioperative risk status, evidence suggests that CEA is more effective than medical therapy for prevention of stroke. This was first shown in the ACAS trial, in which the 5-year absolute risk reduction was slightly greater than 1% per year. The prospective multicenter Asymptomatic Carotid Surgery Trial reported outcomes in 3,120 patients who were randomly assigned to receive medical therapy or CEA. In this series, the risk of perioperative stroke and death was 3.1%. The 5-year risk of stroke was decreased from 11% for medically treated patients to 3.8% for those undergoing CEA (P<.001).

One study examined mortality rates for all Medicare patients (N=113,300) who underwent CEA during the same period in which the randomized CEA trials were conducted. This study reported a 30-day mortality rate threefold greater than that reported in the randomized prospective trials. This raises a question about whether the rates of perioperative stroke and death shown in prospective randomized multicenter trials can be achieved in community-based settings.

- For symptomatic patients with high-grade carotid stenosis (70%-90%), CEA is superior to medical therapy for prevention of stroke
- For asymptomatic patients with 60%-99% carotid stenosis, CEA is more effective than medical therapy for stroke prevention

Percutaneous Therapy

Carotid artery stent (CAS) placement recently has become an acceptable alternative for selected patients at increased risk of serious complications during CEA. The procedure used in one large-scale multicenter prospective trial (comparing CAS placement with CEA in high-risk patients) and in many industry-sponsored prospective multicenter single-arm registries involves a self-expanding metallic alloy stent and a distal embolic protection device (EPD). EPDs capture the debris potentially released during stent placement and prevent embolization of particulate matter to the brain. Carotid stenting currently is recommended as an alternative to CEA for patients with anatomic or medical comorbid conditions that place them at high surgical risk (Table 19.4).

The Carotid and Vertebral Artery Transluminal Angioplasty Study (CAVATAS) was a prospective trial of 504 patients randomly assigned to undergo CEA (n=253) or carotid angioplasty (n=251, only 26% of whom received a stent). Using an end point of disabling stroke or death by 30 days, no difference was measured between the angioplasty (10%) and surgical groups (9.9%).

The first large prospective multicenter trial to compare CEA to CAS with EPD in high-risk patients was the SAPPHIRE (Stenting and Angioplasty with Protection in Patients at High Risk for Endarterectomy) study. Patients were randomly assigned to receive a CAS with distal protection (n=159) or to undergo CEA (n=151). Other patients who were too high risk for CEA and had CAS placement (n=406) or who were not candidates for CAS and underwent CEA (n=7) were followed up in a prospective

Table 19.4 Comorbid Conditions of Patients With High Surgical Risk

Anatomic condition
High cervical lesion that would require jaw disarticulation for CEA
Ostial common carotid artery lesion that would require median sternotomy
Contralateral internal carotid artery occlusion
Prior neck irradiation
Restenosis of prior CEA site
Contralateral laryngeal nerve palsy
Tracheal stoma
Medical condition
Class III or IV congestive heart failure
Left ventricular ejection fraction <30%
Unstable angina pectoris
Recent myocardial infarction
Severe chronic obstructive pulmonary disease
Need for coronary artery bypass graft surgery

CEA, carotid endarterectomy.

single-arm registry. In the randomized group, the primary (combined) end point was the 30-day incidence of stroke, death, and myocardial infarction and was designed to assess non-inferiority of CAS to CEA. The incidence rate was lower for the CAS group (4.8%) than for the CEA group (9.6%), but the difference was not statistically significant (P=.14). For registry patients, the 30-day incidence was 7.8% for those who received a CAS and 14.7% for those who underwent CEA. The surgical group also had an excess of cranial nerve injuries (5.3%), versus no such injuries in the stent group. The 1-year combined end point was 11.9% for the CAS group and 19.9% for the CEA group (P<.05).

The Carotid Revascularization Using Endarterectomy or Stenting Systems phase 1 study enrolled 397 patients who either were symptomatic and had greater than 50% carotid artery stenosis (n=128) or were asymptomatic and had greater than 75% stenosis (n=269). Treatment was solely at the discretion of the investigator; 254 patients were treated with endarterectomy, and 143 underwent CAS placement using a distal EPD. No difference in combined death and stroke rates was observed between the two groups at 1 year (CEA, 13.6%; CAS, 10.0%).

The Carotid Revascularization with Endarterectomy versus Stent Trial, sponsored by the National Institutes of Health, currently is enrolling patients, and the results of several prospective single-arm registries are being released. Controversy persists among investigators and clinicians about the safety and efficacy of CAS with EPD in non–high-risk asymptomatic patients with moderate or severe carotid artery stenosis. The industry-sponsored ACT 1 Trial (Carotid Stenting vs Surgery of Severe Carotid Artery Disease and Stroke Prevention in Asymptomatic Patients) has begun enrollment, and several other trials are in the planning stages. These studies may provide data on the large population of asymptomatic patients with carotid artery stenosis.

Questions

1. Which test is most likely to determine the cause of left-sided hemiplegia in a 63-year-old right-handed man?
   a. Erythrocyte sedimentation rate
   b. Transcranial Doppler ultrasonography
   c. Brain CT
   d. Transesophageal echocardiography
   e. Hemoglobin A_{1c}

2. What is the most important clue from the history or physical examination for determining the need for and method of revascularization of a carotid artery?
   a. The finding of a cervical bruit
   b. The absence of a temporal artery pulse
   c. Evidence of tendinous xanthomas on the olecranon bursa
   d. Classic description of repeated episodes of aphasia for the previous 24 hours
   e. The number of pack-years that the patient smoked cigarettes

3. Which of the following diagnostic algorithms is most correct?
   a. Cervical bruit→Digital subtraction arteriography
   b. Cervical bruit→CDUS→Digital subtraction arteriography
   c. Symptoms of cerebral ischemia→Diffusion-weighted magnetic resonance imaging
   d. Symptoms of cerebral ischemia→Two-dimensional time-of-flight MRA
   e. Cervical bruit→MRA→Multidetector CTA→Digital subtraction arteriography

4. A 61-year-old woman has a left systolic and diastolic cervical bruit. Which of the following would most likely explain this physical examination finding?
   a. An 80%-99% ipsilateral internal carotid artery stenosis with a patent contralateral internal carotid artery
   b. Mitral stenosis
   c. Left ventricular ejection fraction of 20%
   d. An ipsilateral jugular vein thrombosis
   e. An 80%-99% ipsilateral internal carotid artery stenosis with a contralateral "string sign"

5. Which treatment strategy is optimal for a 77-year-old man with a 90% right internal carotid artery stenosis, transient left-arm hemiplegia, and a contralateral left internal carotid artery occlusion?
   a. Antihypertensive therapy, aspirin, and statins
   b. Antihypertensive therapy, aspirin, clopidogrel, and statins
   c. Antihypertensive therapy, aspirin, clopidogrel, statins, and CAS

d. Antihypertensive therapy, aspirin, clopidogrel, statins, and CEA
e. Antihypertensive therapy, aspirin, statins, and CEA after 6 weeks of observation

Suggested Readings

Bock RW, Gray-Weale AC, Mock PA, et al. The natural history of asymptomatic carotid artery disease. J Vasc Surg. 1993;17:160-9.

CAPRIE Steering Committee. A randomised, blinded, trial of clopidogrel versus aspirin in patients at risk of ischaemic events (CAPRIE). Lancet. 1996;348:1329-39.

CaRESS Steering Committee. Carotid Revascularization Using Endarterectomy or Stenting Systems (CaRESS) phase 1 clinical trial: 1-year results. J Vasc Surg. 2005;42:213-9.

CAVATAS Investigators. Endovascular versus surgical treatment in patients with carotid stenosis in the Carotid and Vertebral Artery Transluminal Angioplasty Study (CAVATAS): a randomised trial. Lancet. 2001;357:1729-37.

Executive Committee for the Asymptomatic Carotid Atherosclerosis Study. Endarterectomy for asymptomatic carotid artery stenosis. JAMA. 1995;273:1421-8.

Grundy SM, Cleeman JI, Merz CN, et al, National Heart, Lung, and Blood Institute, American College of Cardiology Foundation, American Heart Association. Implications of recent clinical trials for the National Cholesterol Education Program Adult Treatment Panel III guidelines. Circulation. 2004;110:227-39. Erratum in: Circulation. 2004;110:763.

Halliday A, Mansfield A, Marro J, et al, MRC Asymptomatic Carotid Surgery Trial (ACST) Collaborative Group. Prevention of disabling and fatal strokes by successful carotid endarterectomy in patients without recent neurological symptoms: randomised controlled trial. Lancet. 2004;363:1491-502. Erratum in: Lancet. 2004;364:416.

Hertzer NR, Young JR, Beven EG, et al. Coronary angiography in 506 patients with extracranial cerebrovascular disease. Arch Intern Med. 1985;145:849-52.

McGovern PG, Burke GL, Sprafka JM, et al, The Minnesota Heart Survey. Trends in mortality, morbidity, and risk factor levels for stroke from 1960 through 1990. JAMA. 1992;268:753-9.

North American Symptomatic Carotid Endarterectomy Trial Collaborators. Beneficial effect of carotid endarterectomy in symptomatic patients with high-grade carotid stenosis. N Engl J Med. 1991;325:445-53.

Sauve JS, Thorpe KE, Sackett DL, et al, The North American Symptomatic Carotid Endarterectomy Trial. Can bruits distinguish high-grade from moderate symptomatic carotid stenosis? Ann Intern Med. 1994;120:633-7.

Wennberg DE, Lucas FL, Birkmeyer JD, et al. Variation in carotid endarterectomy mortality in the Medicare population: trial hospitals, volume, and patient characteristics. JAMA. 1998;279:1278-81.

Yadav JS, Wholey MH, Kuntz RE, et al, Stenting and Angioplasty With Protection in Patients at High Risk for Endarterectomy Investigators. Protected carotid-artery stenting versus endarterectomy in high-risk patients. N Engl J Med. 2004;351:1493-501.

20 Patient Selection and Diagnosis for Endovascular Procedures

Christopher J. White, MD

Introduction

The concept of non-surgical revascularization was introduced by Charles Dotter and was further advanced with the development of balloon dilation catheters by Andreas Gruntzig. Endovascular intervention (EI) has evolved over the past 25 years in a stepwise fashion. Early EI procedures used bulky equipment, required large access catheters, and were limited to balloon dilation. Procedures were initially offered only to patients who were not surgical candidates. As the catheters evolved and developed lower profiles, they were used in more anatomic locations, including the upper and lower extremities, renal and mesenteric circulations, and the supraclavicular arteries.

Durability, or prolonged vascular patency, has traditionally been better with surgical procedures, but recently stents have been shown to be better in many vascular distributions. The use of stents has shifted the balance in treatment away from conventional surgical therapies and toward endovascular therapy. There is currently a better understanding of differences in restenosis rates by anatomic region, which also affects treatment selection. For example, the superficial femoral artery, the renal artery, and the internal carotid artery all have nominal diameters of approximately 6 mm, yet the restenosis rates for these three vascular beds, with the same stents placed, are markedly different. Clearly, the intimal hyperplastic response differs among vascular beds and should be factored into the patient's treatment plan.

- The superficial femoral, renal, and internal carotid arteries all have nominal diameters of approximately 6 mm, but the restenosis rates for all three vascular beds, with the same stents placed, are markedly different

Currently, EI is considered a safe and effective means of restoring blood flow in selected patients, and if a patient is a candidate for either open or percutaneous surgery, EI is considered the therapy of choice.

General Evaluation

For all patients being considered for possible peripheral revascularization, the history should be directed at their chief concern; patients also should undergo a general medical evaluation with attention directed to the status of the entire cardiovascular, pulmonary, and renal systems. Atherosclerosis is a systemic disease; therefore, risk factor assessment, screening tests for cardiovascular diseases, and optimization of medical therapy are required.

A cardiovascular history establishes the presence of atherosclerotic risk factors, including the presence of other common manifestations of atherosclerosis such as cerebrovascular, renal, cardiac, and lower extremity symptoms. A complete physical examination should include all pulses, listening for bruits over the carotids, palpation of the abdominal aorta and common femoral arteries, examination of the legs and feet, and auscultation of the heart and lungs.

General laboratory data required before planning an EI include electrocardiography, serum electrolytes, fasting blood sugar, renal function studies, complete blood count, coagulation status (international normalized ratio, prothrombin time, activated partial thromboplastin time), and stool Hemoccult. If the patient has active lung disease, chest radiography and pulmonary function testing are appropriate.

Standard premedication before planned EI includes aspirin therapy (81-325 mg daily). The use of additional antiplatelet agents (clopidogrel or ticlopidine) is optional; however, they are frequently used for carotid and cerebrovascular interventions. No objective evidence has shown that the use of these more expensive therapies improves procedural success or decreases complications, as has been shown for coronary artery intervention.

- Proper planning for EI requires appropriate history, physical examination, and general laboratory data
- Standard premedication before EI includes aspirin therapy (81-325 mg/d)
- Additional antiplatelet agents (clopidogrel or ticlopidine) are optional; these therapies are not proven to increase procedural success or decrease complications

Selection Criteria

Patient Selection

Patient selection for EI depends on both anatomic and functional criteria. In general, the selection of patients for surgical revascularization and EI are similar, although a lower threshold for symptom limitations is often accepted for EI of lower extremity lesions. Elderly patients and those with severe medical comorbid conditions (cardiopulmonary disease, diabetes mellitus, renal insufficiency) are preferentially treated with EI versus open surgery.

Conventional open surgery remains the treatment of choice for patients at low to moderate surgical risk who may require carotid endarterectomy. Unless such patients are enrolled in a clinical trial, they should not be offered carotid stenting as an alternative to carotid endarterectomy. In no other vascular bed is open surgery clearly the treatment of choice, although conventional surgery is an attractive option in many circumstances. For example, in patients with limb-threatening ischemia or acute limb ischemia who are not suitable candidates for EI, open surgery is the treatment of choice.

There is debate in the literature regarding the efficacy of EI for patients with long (≥10 cm) occlusions or diffuse stenotic disease. Some of these patients may be better served by open surgery than EI, but attempted EI rarely, if ever, compromises the success of a later approach with open surgery. For this reason, in experienced centers, conventional surgery is reserved for patients who are not candidates for EI or in whom attempted EI has failed.

Clinical equipoise—collective professional uncertainty regarding treatment—seems to exist between open surgery and endovascular therapy for abdominal aortic aneurysm repair. Decisions regarding individual patient therapy should be based on the treating physician's experience, the patient's preference, the patient's comorbid conditions, and the suitability of the lesion for endograft repair.

- Conventional open surgery remains the treatment of choice for patients at low to moderate surgical risk who require carotid endarterectomy
- The efficacy of EI for long (≥10 cm) occlusions or diffuse stenotic disease is debated
- In experienced centers, conventional surgery is reserved for patients who are not candidates for EI or in whom attempted EI has failed
- Clinical equipoise exists between open surgery and endovascular therapy for abdominal aortic aneurysm repair

Anatomic Criteria

Several anatomic criteria are important for choosing between EI and open surgery for a given patient. These include the ability to gain vascular access to the target lesion, a reasonable likelihood of crossing the lesion with a guidewire, and the expectation that an angioplasty catheter or device can be advanced to the lesion to successfully recanalize it. A favorable procedural result is more likely in stenoses than occlusions, in larger-diameter than smaller-diameter vessels, in discrete rather than longer (≥3 cm) lesions, and in patients with milder rather than more severe symptoms. Anatomic criteria also include the objective assessment of lesion severity. Severity may be assessed with invasive angiography or non-invasively with magnetic resonance angiography (MRA), computed tomography angiography (CTA), or duplex imaging.

The availability of endovascular stents (balloon and self-expandable) has significantly extended the anatomic subset of patients who can be considered as candidates for percutaneous revascularization, particularly for those with longer lesions and occlusions. The limiting factor for non-surgical revascularization of the aortoiliac vessels is the ability to pass a guidewire across the lesion. Regardless of the balloon dilation result, the option of stent placement offers a reliable and reproducible method to recanalize these vessels.

Anatomic criteria for aortic arch vessel and supraclavicular procedures must take into account the tortuosity, calcification, and embolic potential of the aortic arch and arch vessels. A severely unwound aortic arch or tortuous arch vessels may present a high risk for complications with an endovascular approach and can be approached more safely with conventional surgery.

- Anatomic criteria to be considered for aortic arch vessel and supraclavicular procedures must include the tortuosity, calcification, and embolic potential of the aortic arch and arch vessels

When considering renal or mesenteric artery revascularization, the status of the abdominal aorta must be taken into account. A very diseased, shaggy, abdominal aorta may dictate specific endovascular approaches, such as the "no-touch" technique. A history of atheroembolization should be considered a contraindication to renal intervention. Finally, if the vessels arise from the aorta with an acute downward orientation, an upper extremity approach (axillary, brachial, or radial) is indicated.

In-Stent Restenosis

An interesting phenomenon is the differential rate of in-stent restenosis related to intimal hyperplasia in different vascular beds. At best, the rate of restenosis for superficial femoral artery lesions is between 30% and 50%, for renal artery lesions is 10% to 15%, and for carotid artery lesions is less than 5%. It is generally assumed that in-stent restenosis merits at least one attempt at repeat percutaneous therapy before referral for surgical therapy. However, restenosis in the superficial femoral artery is much more likely to be resistant to percutaneous therapies and more likely to benefit from surgical bypass.

Vascular Access

The initial consideration for an EI is the choice of vascular access site. The target lesion dictates the most desirable arterial access site. For example, for carotid lesions, retrograde common femoral access is preferred, because gaining catheter access to the aortic arch vessels is generally easier from below them. For mesenteric lesions, brachial access is often chosen to take advantage of the cephalic orientation of these vessels arising from the abdominal aorta. Other considerations include the presence of occlusive disease or a dialysis fistula, which may limit the choice of access sites.

Contraindications

Relative anatomic contraindications to EI include lesions likely to generate atheroemboli and lesions that are undilatable because of calcification. Relative clinical contraindications include any instances in which the risks of the procedure outweigh the potential benefits.

Functional Criteria

The functional significance of peripheral vascular stenosis is reflected by the associated symptoms. Functional criteria may be objective or subjective. Examples of objective assessments of ischemia include the ankle-brachial index, duplex velocity measurements, and translesional pressure gradients. Walking distance on a treadmill is another way to objectively assess the functional limitation due to a lower extremity vascular stenosis. Subjective assessments include abdominal discomfort after meals, leg cramping with walking, or resting leg pain at night.

When selecting patients for revascularization therapy, it is appropriate in many cases to require that the patient had previous failure of conservative therapy (exercise, pharmacologic intervention, risk factor modification) before subjecting the patient to the risks of either surgery or EI.

- It is appropriate to require previous failure of conservative therapy before considering revascularization therapy for a patient
- Before being considered for percutaneous or surgical revascularization therapy, symptomatic patients with anatomically suitable lower extremity lesions should have either:
  - Failure of a reasonable attempt at medical therapy for lifestyle-limiting claudication
  - Demonstrated critical limb ischemia

Patients with symptomatic lower extremity lesions that are anatomically suitable should have prior failure of a reasonable attempt at medical therapy for lifestyle-limiting claudication or demonstration of critical limb ischemia before being considered candidates for percutaneous or surgical revascularization therapy. If a patient presents for percutaneous intervention with limb-threatening ischemia (gangrene, non-healing ulcer, or rest pain), multilevel disease is likely to be present. Simply improving "inflow" without addressing more distal flow-limiting lesions may not solve the problem. However, for patients with moderate to severe symptomatic carotid artery stenoses, a trial of medical therapy before revascularization is not appropriate. Based on level I clinical trial evidence, these patients should be revascularized.

- Multilevel disease is likely to be present in a patient with limb-threatening ischemia; simply improving "inflow" by percutaneous intervention without addressing distal flow-limiting lesions may not solve the problem

Asymptomatic patients usually are not considered candidates for revascularization because the potential benefit does not justify the known procedural risks, but asymptomatic patients may be considered for revascularization in specific instances. The first such indication is moderate to severe carotid artery stenosis (≥60%) in an asymptomatic patient; level I evidence supports revascularization of these patients. If the carotid stenosis is 80% or greater and the patient is at increased risk for carotid artery endarterectomy, randomized trial evidence suggests that carotid stent placement with an embolic protection device is indicated. Based on the natural history of carotid artery lesions, revascularization of the asymptomatic carotid stenosis, in experienced hands, is the correct procedure.

Another circumstance in which an asymptomatic stenosis or occlusion would be considered for intervention is if a patient with an asymptomatic iliac lesion requires common femoral artery access for a cardiac procedure. In this case, it is appropriate to treat the iliac stenosis. Similarly, if placement of an intra-aortic counterpulsation balloon is necessary, it is appropriate to perform femoral or iliac angioplasty to gain access. Finally, in a patient with a femoral or brachial access complication, it would be appropriate to dilate an asymptomatic stenosis to allow catheter access to treat the access site complication.

When selecting patients for EIs, it is important to understand any additional condition they have that could affect the procedure. This might include diabetes mellitus, renal insufficiency, a history of contrast reactions, and adverse anticoagulation status. Appropriate planning and patient preparation are required in these circumstances.

Diagnostic Assessment

When assessing patients with peripheral vascular disease for revascularization, supportive data in the form of diagnostic testing are desirable to confirm a clinical diagnosis. Typically, non-invasive testing is preferred over invasive testing. Choices include physiologic testing, such as Doppler ultrasonography (duplex) and ankle-brachial index, and anatomic assessment with imaging studies, including ultrasonography, MRA, and CTA.

Non-Invasive Testing

Testing should be directed by clinical information, attempting to confirm a clinical hypothesis based on history or physical examination data. With the exception of well-established screening programs in high-risk populations (e.g., carotid duplex ultrasonography in coronary bypass patients), indiscriminate non-invasive testing is discouraged. No single non-invasive test is best overall. The selection of the test is based on the preference of the treating physician, patient concerns (e.g., claustrophobia for MRA, renal function for CTA, obesity for renal ultrasonography), technician skill level, and cost. Generally, confirmatory non-invasive testing is not encouraged. If clinical suspicion is high and the non-invasive test is either indeterminate or contradictory, invasive testing is required to answer the question.

Invasive Testing

Invasive testing includes physiologic or functional testing. Physiologic testing includes the hemodynamic measurement of translesional pressure gradients and the determination of fractional flow reserve. Occasionally, a borderline resting gradient is augmented with a vasodilator to amplify the severity of the vascular disease. Invasive imaging can be done with intravascular ultrasonography or angiography. Typically, invasive testing is reserved for patients who meet the minimum criteria for revascularization. In other words, if a patient with claudication has been characterized by non-invasive testing and is well compensated with pharmacologic therapy and a walking program, invasive angiography is not required because there is no indication for revascularization.

Questions

1. A patient with poorly controlled hypertension on three medications undergoes screening renal Doppler ultrasonography, which gives inconclusive results. What would be your next step?
- **a.** Invasive angiography
- **b.** Non-invasive CTA
- **c.** Non-invasive MRA
- **d.** Radionuclide renal scanning with an angiotensin-converting enzyme inhibitor

2. A patient with a systolic blood pressure gradient of 50 mm Hg between arms (right>left) is undergoing diagnostic angiography to determine the presence of coronary artery disease. Which of the following would most likely necessitate additional angiography of the brachiocephalic vessels?
- **a.** Left arm claudication when weight lifting
- **b.** Planned coronary artery bypass grafting
- **c.** Retrograde left vertebral flow on duplex ultrasonography
- **d.** Abnormal results of Allen test on the left arm

3. A patient presents on two medications for recurrent uncontrolled hypertension and with ultrasonographic evidence of left renal in-stent restenosis. The original stent placement procedure had been complicated by a small shower of "atheroemboli" to both feet, which resolved over several weeks without tissue loss. What would be your recommendation now?
- **a.** Angiography and possible re-intervention from the arm
- **b.** MRA/CTA to confirm in-stent restenosis

c. Add additional medications to control blood pressure
d. Refer for left renal bypass

4. A 67-year-old man recently had a transient ischemic attack secondary to a 75% narrowing of the right internal carotid artery. Angiography shows an unfavorable type 3 (unwound, calcified, tortuous) aortic arch. He expresses a strong preference for avoiding open surgical therapy. What would be your recommendation?
   a. Carotid stent with emboli protection with a direct carotid puncture
   b. Medical therapy with aspirin and dipyridamole
   c. Attempt carotid stent placement with femoral access
   d. Recommend surgical revascularization

5. A 55-year-old board certified vascular surgeon has an MRA showing a severe (>80%) discrete right internal carotid artery stenosis. He is asymptomatic, and the stenosis was found after a carotid bruit was heard during an insurance-required physical examination. He understands his treatment options, he is willing to pay for any unreimbursed expenses, and he came to you for a carotid stent. What would you do?
   a. Offer him a stent since he is well informed about the risks and benefits
   b. Recommend he have carotid endarterectomy
   c. Offer him aspirin and clopidogrel medical therapy
   d. Ask him to return in 3 months for follow-up duplex ultrasonography

Suggested Readings

Barnett HJ, Taylor DW, Eliasziw M, et al, North American Symptomatic Carotid Endarterectomy Trial Collaborators. Benefit of carotid endarterectomy in patients with symptomatic moderate or severe stenosis. N Engl J Med. 1998;339:1415-25.

Dotter CT, Judkins MP. Transluminal treatment of arteriosclerotic obstruction: description of a new technic and a preliminary report of its application. Circulation. 1964;30:654-70.

Executive Committee for the Asymptomatic Carotid Atherosclerosis Study. Endarterectomy for asymptomatic carotid artery stenosis. JAMA. 1995;273:1421-8.

Gruntzig A, Hopff H. Percutaneous recanalization after chronic arterial occlusion with a new dilator-catheter (modification of the Dotter technique) [German]. (Translated by A Gruntzig.) Dtsch Med Wochenschr. 1974;99:2502-11.

Halliday A, Mansfield A, Marro J, et al, MRC Asymptomatic Carotid Surgery Trial (ACST) Collaborative Group. Prevention of disabling and fatal strokes by successful carotid endarterectomy in patients without recent neurological symptoms: randomised controlled trial. Lancet. 2004;363:1491-502. Erratum in: Lancet. 2004;364:416.

Johnston KW. Balloon angioplasty: predictive factors for long-term success. Semin Vasc Surg. 1989;2:117-22.

North American Symptomatic Carotid Endarterectomy Trial Collaborators. Beneficial effect of carotid endarterectomy in symptomatic patients with high-grade carotid stenosis. N Engl J Med. 1991;325:445-53.

Wilson SE, Sheppard B. Results of percutaneous transluminal angioplasty for peripheral vascular occlusive disease. Ann Vasc Surg. 1990;4:94-7.

Yadav JS, Wholey MH, Kuntz RE, et al, Stenting and Angioplasty With Protection in Patients at High Risk for Endarterectomy Investigators. Protected carotid-artery stenting versus endarterectomy in high-risk patients. N Engl J Med. 2004;351:1493-501.

21 Endovascular Techniques I: Catheters and Diagnostic Angiography

Mark C. Bates, MD, FACC

History

The term "catheter" originated from the Greek word *"kath-eter,"* meaning "to send down." Claude Bernard (a well-known French physiologist) was credited in the mid 1800s as being the first to use the term "catheter" to describe a tube used in an animal model to measure cardiac pressures. However, the use of tubular structures to access the bladder or blood vessels predated Bernard's work by thousands of years. *Sushruta Samhita*, an Indian surgical text from 1000 BC, reported the insertion of wood tubes smeared with liquid butter into the bladder for removal of urine and management of strictures or installation of medication. Archeologists in Egypt have discovered evidence to suggest that doctors circa 400 BC used hollow reeds and brass pipes as means to study heart valve function in cadavers.

The first successful documented medical use of an intravascular catheter in humans was in 1667, when a tube was placed in a vessel and used to perform the first documented blood transfusion. In the 1800s a Parisian master metal cutter and instrument designer, Joseph-Frederic-Benoit Charriere, developed the French scale for measuring catheter size. French size (F) is synonymous with Charriere size (CH) and equals one-third millimeter.

- 1 F = 1 CH = 0.33 mm—used to describe the outer diameter (O.D.) of a catheter and the inner diameter (I.D.) of a sheath

In 1929, Werner Forssmann, after studying the writings of Bernard, advanced a rubber ureteral catheter into the right side of his own heart, performing the first documented heart catheterization in a living human. He was ostracized initially by the medical community for his unorthodox approach but was ultimately awarded the Nobel Prize. Sven Seldinger developed the first percutaneous technique for inserting catheters into blood vessels in 1953. In the following years, significant advances in catheter technology and imaging have shaped the field of modern angiology.

The centuries of pioneering work that have gone into catheter development are beyond the scope of this chapter, but it is important to understand this history and the foundation of knowledge that led to the clinical success we now enjoy.

Catheter Characteristics

Terms and Definitions

– I.D., inner diameter of a catheter—usually measured in inches for a guide catheter and in French size for a sheath.
– O.D., outer diameter of a catheter—usually measured in French size. Diagnostic catheters and guides are described by O.D. and sheaths are described by I.D.
– Flexibility—an indication of the bending stiffness of the material. The flexural modulus is a coefficient of elasticity, which represents the ratio of stress to strain as a material is deformed under dynamic load.
– Kink resistance—refers to the ability of a tube to withstand bending and coiling without deforming or kinking (a fold in the wall). Kinking weakens the structural strength of the tube and can also block or slow the transference of media through the tube. Kink resistance is, to a large extent, a function of wall thickness and shore hardness.
– Lubricity (coefficient of friction)—measures the frictional properties or tackiness of a material. A low coefficient of friction is usually desired in medical applications to minimize bodily trauma and tissue irritation.

– Shore hardness—the relative resistance of a material's surface to indentation by an indenter of specified dimensions under specified load. Shore hardness refers to the general stiffness of a material. The hardnesses are measured according to the Durometer and Rockwell scales.
– Tensile strength—a measure of the force required to stretch a plastic and the percentage of stretching the plastic can withstand before breaking. Ultimate tensile strength is the maximum stress a material withstands at the point of rupture. Good tensile strength allows for design of thinner wall thicknesses, which result in smaller diameters. High tensile strength also aids in ease of catheter insertion. Related to this is "ultimate elongation," which is the total elongation by percentage of a sample at the point of rupture.
– Torque—a measure of force related to the rotational stability of the tube. If rotated at one end, a tube with a high degree of torque will rotate at nearly the same ratio at the other (untouched) end. A high degree of torque can be desirable in invasive applications. Braiding of tubes is a method used to increase torque.
– Biocompatibility—the suitability of materials for biomedical applications. Tests used to screen for suitable plastic materials include implants in research animals, injection of resin extracts into animals to detect toxic responses, and tissue culture on resins and resin extracts using mammalian and human cells. Other tests include hemolysis testing, intracutaneous injection of rabbits, systemic toxicity in mice, cell growth inhibition of aqueous extracts, and total and extractable heavy metals and buffering capability.
– Thrombogenicity—the tendency of an agent to cause blood clot formation around the invasive area. This is an adverse phenomenon that can lead to further complications. In plastics applications, a smooth surface is desirable to avoid activation of the clotting mechanism. Hydrophilic surfaces are known to prevent absorption of protein and cells and therefore prevent the blood clotting immune response. The more hydrophilic the plastic, the less foreign the material is to the body.

Contemporary Catheter Design and Materials

Catheter Materials

Early catheters were made from the naturally occurring materials rubber and latex. Biocompatibility issues and the lack of coaxial support (column strength) in rubber and latex led to the use of inert thermoelastic polymers in the 1950s. One of the most popular catheter materials used today is nylon, a polyamide resin, which has a very high melting point and is inert. Other plastics such as polyurethane, polyvinyl chloride, polyethylene, and silicone rubber are also used, depending on the catheter performance characteristics desired.

Catheter Construction

Understanding how a catheter is constructed helps in understanding its characteristics and how it will behave in the body. A key advance in catheter design came from Robert Stevens in the early 1960s—incorporating a metal braid into a catheter polymer. This greatly improved torque response and selective catheter performance. Today, many diagnostic catheters have a flat or fine wire braid and are labeled "braided." The use of a braided catheter may be preferred in tortuous anatomy or if substantial columnar catheter support is needed. Braiding also increases kink resistance, shore hardness, and tensile strength. Although guide catheters have multiple layers, most diagnostic catheters are made of a single polymer with or without a braid.

- The use of a braided catheter may be preferred for tortuous anatomy or if significant columnar catheter support is needed

The outer layer of the catheter determines lubricity, biocompatibility, and thrombogenicity. For example, catheters coated with hydrophilic fluoropolymers reduce resistance and improve tracking as the catheter is navigated through tortuous or diseased vessels.

Non-Selective Angiography

Non-selective angiography is performed by placing a catheter with multiple side holes, a "flush catheter" (Fig. 21.1), into the parent vessel; it usually requires the use of a power injector to obtain diagnostic information regarding the vessel and branches. Non-selective power injection angiography should never be performed with an end-

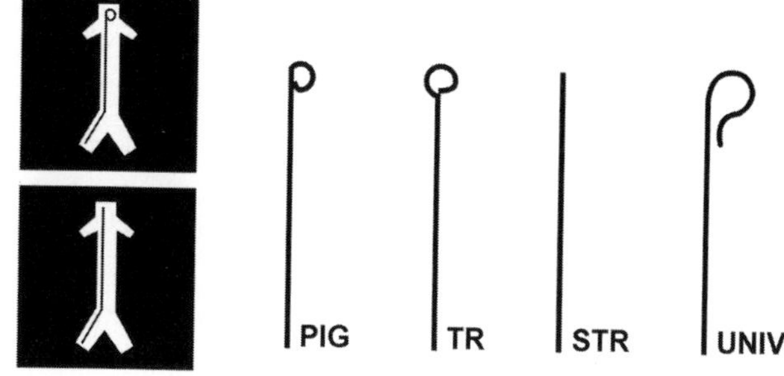

Fig. 21.1 Examples of non-selective "flush" catheters. PIG, pigtail; STR, straight; TR, tennis racket; UNIV, universal.

hole catheter because of the inherent risk of inadvertent injection into a small side branch or atheromatous plaque. Meticulous catheter flushing, beginning with blood withdrawal, is important before any forward injection of saline or contrast material.

Each catheter has a threshold for maximum contrast injection volume over time. The injection flow rate threshold can be estimated by understanding Poiseuille's law:

$$\text{Volume flow rate } (\bar{F}) = \frac{\text{pressure decrease along the tube}}{\text{resistance to flow}}$$

$$\text{Resistance to flow (R)} = 8\eta L/\pi r^4$$

$$\bar{F}=(P_1-P_2)\pi r^4/8\eta L$$

Where: P_1=pressure at entry point; P_2=pressure at exit point; r=radius of tube; η=viscosity of fluid; and L=length of tube.

Catheter length and internal radius are important variables in this equation. Side holes in the catheter reduce the effective catheter length, whereas tapering the tip decreases the effective internal diameter. Changing catheter lumen radius has a greater effect on resistance than does changing length because it is a fourth-order variant. For example, if a 5F pigtail catheter with a 0.038-in wire lumen is 65 cm long, the maximal flow rate for a power injection is 33 mL/s. The same catheter with a length of 110 cm has a maximum flow rate of 26 mL/s. If the maximal flow rate is exceeded, the pressure in the system increases. Most power injectors are set to abort injection when a predetermined pressure is exceeded. If the predetermined safe acceptable injection flow rate is exceeded, most diagnostic catheters will rupture (at 1,050-1,200 pounds per square inch). Fortunately, the injector tubing or connecters frequently yield before the catheter does, but it is the operator's responsibility to make sure catheter tolerances are never exceeded.

- Maximal flow tolerance of a catheter is determined by catheter I.D., length, presence or absence of distal taper or side holes, and viscosity of material being injected
- An end-hole catheter should not be used for non-selective power injection

Abdominal Angiography

Static abdominal angiography is typically used to evaluate the abdominal aorta and visceral branches. If the diagnostic objective is to exclude aorto-ostial renal artery stenosis, a slight left anterior oblique (LAO) view can provide the best definition of both renal ostia. Many advocate using a tennis racket or universal catheter to allow preferential filling of the renal arteries, decrease dilution, and decrease the overlying artifact that is frequently seen from the cephalad spray of the pigtail catheter into the superior mesenteric or celiac system. Occasionally, cranial angulation is needed to see the renal ostia in patients with infrarenal abdominal aortic aneurysmal disease because of the frequently anterior trajectory of the proximal neck.

The pigtail catheter is typically stationed at the level of L1 with the image intensifier in the lateral projection to evaluate the origin of the celiac and mesenteric system. One of the most feared complications of abdominal angiography is inadvertent power injection into the thoracic artery and the artery of Adamkiewicz, which results in permanent paralysis. This serious complication can be avoided by appropriate positioning of the catheter below T12 and being certain that the flush catheter is freely moving in the aorta before injection of contrast material.

Aortic Arch Angiography

The origin of the great vessels is usually best visualized in the LAO projection. The optimum image window can be defined by simply shifting the image intensifier in the LAO direction until the foreshortening of the pigtail catheter on fluoroscopy is completely eliminated, which suggests that the image intensifier is perpendicular to the arch profile. With rare exception, selective angiography of the great vessels should not be performed without first performing non-selective imaging of the aortic arch so that definition of complex atherosclerotic disease and anatomic variations of the arch are clearly delineated before navigating a catheter into the target vessel.

Image angulation that may assist in defining ostial disease includes LAO for the great vessels, aortic arch, and renal arteries (for most patients); lateral view to steep right anterior oblique (RAO) for mesenteric vessels; contralateral oblique for the internal iliac ostium; and ipsilateral oblique for the common femoral bifurcation. It is the responsibility of the angiographer to understand the potential satellite non-vascular issues when interpreting the results of non-selective angiography. Disease entities such as renal cell carcinoma on nephrography, or the silhouette of an abdominal aneurysm with mural thrombus in the abdominal aorta, must not be missed.

Basic Knowledge for Non-Selective Angiography

- Meticulous catheter flushing is important before any forward injection of saline or contrast
- The pigtail catheter must be freely moving within the aorta before any power injection to avoid inadvertent injection into a small side branch and to minimize the risk of atheroembolization

- The pressure tolerance and volume injection thresholds of each catheter should never be exceeded during a power injection
- Image angulation that may assist in defining ostial disease in non-selective angiography:
  - Great vessels/aortic arch: LAO
  - Renal arteries: LAO for most patients
  - Mesenteric vessels: lateral view to steep RAO
  - Internal iliac ostium: contralateral oblique
  - Common femoral bifurcation: ipsilateral oblique
- The angiographer must understand the potential satellite non-vascular issues when interpreting the results of non-selective angiography

Selective Angiography

For the purpose of this discussion, selective angiography is defined as the direct injection of contrast material in a preformed catheter positioned under fluoroscopic guidance into a target vessel. Several principles are fundamental to selective angiography.

– First, a selective catheter should never be advanced forward without being led by a guidewire.

– Second, hemodynamic assessment at the tip of the catheter should be performed before any forward injection of contrast or saline to avoid inadvertent injection of clot from the catheter tip, barotrauma to the vessel wall, atheroembolism, or vessel dissection.

– Third, gentle movement of the catheter is important to allow torque to be transmitted to the distal tip. Torque response is determined by catheter polymer characteristics and the presence or absence of a braid.

– Fourth, polymer-based hydrophilic catheters markedly improve tracking and can be essential for access of a contralateral limb in a patient with a steep aortoiliac bifurcation or distal aortoiliac tortuosity.

In regions of the vascular tree with substantial vessel overlap or eclipsed by a metal prosthesis, a clear understanding of the anatomy in a 3-dimensional plane is important to profile the vessels correctly and to obtain definitive diagnostic information. The anatomy can vary significantly from patient to patient, so there is no definitive menu of views. Suggested views for specific vessel families are noted throughout this chapter with the caveat that individual anatomic variation can be considerable.

Carotid and Vertebral Angiography

In the absence of azotemia, carotid and vertebral angiography should be preceded by aortic arch angiography. The selective catheter of choice for carotid angiography depends on the characteristics of the aortic arch. Various pre-shaped catheters are available for carotid angiography and, for the purpose of discussion, these are separated into three categories: passive (Fig. 21.2), intermediate (Fig. 21.3), and active (Fig. 21.4). Treatment of patients with complex aortic arch anatomy can be challenging, and they are more likely to require the use of active catheters. For example, elderly patients with long-standing hypertension can have a so-called "unwound" aorta (type III arch), which can be difficult to access with a simple angled catheter. Also, patients with the normal anatomic variant of the left carotid artery originating from the innominate artery ("bovine arch"), which occurs in 7% of patients, may require more active diagnostic catheters. The origin of the

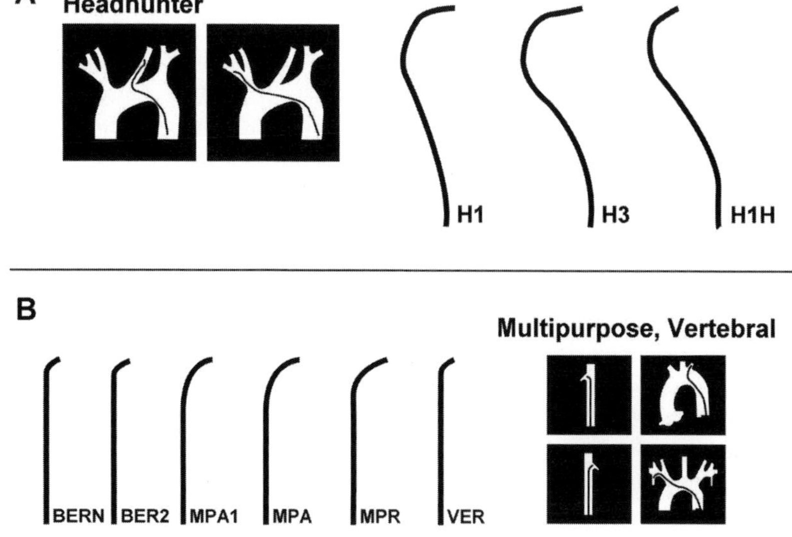

Fig. 21.2 Examples of passive catheters. *A*, Passive carotid access (headhunter) catheters. The headhunter catheters (H1, H3, H1H) naturally reflect into the great vessels and are used as workhorse systems for access in patients with a type I arch and without bovine right carotid anatomy. *B*, Passive (multipurpose, vertebral) catheters. The Bernstein catheter (BERN, BER 2) is similar to the vertebral (VER); both catheters have shorter tips than the multipurpose (MPA, MPA1, MPR). The Bernstein hydrophilic catheter and the glidewire are a good combination for simple arch access.

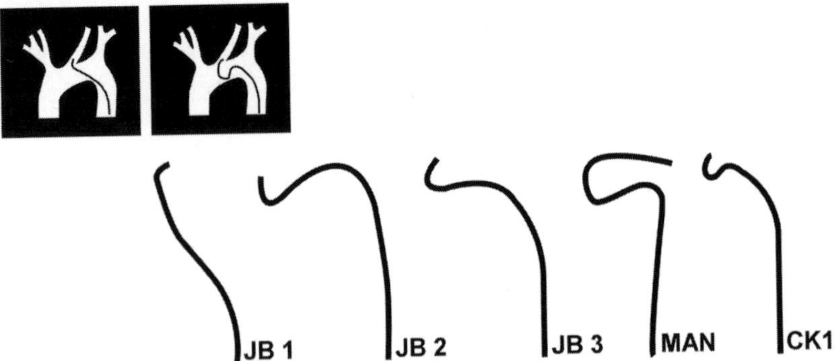

Fig. 21.3 Examples of intermediate catheters include the Bentson (JB 1, JB 2, JB 3; Cordis Corp, Miami Lakes, Florida), Mani (MAN; Cordis Corp), and CK1 catheters, as well as the Vitek (Cook Inc, Bloomington, Indiana; not pictured). They require less manipulation in the aorta than the "active" catheters (see Fig. 21.4) and can be used for access in type II and III arches.

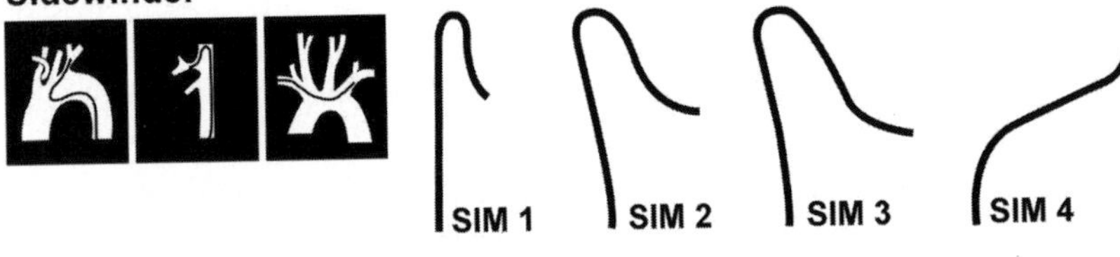

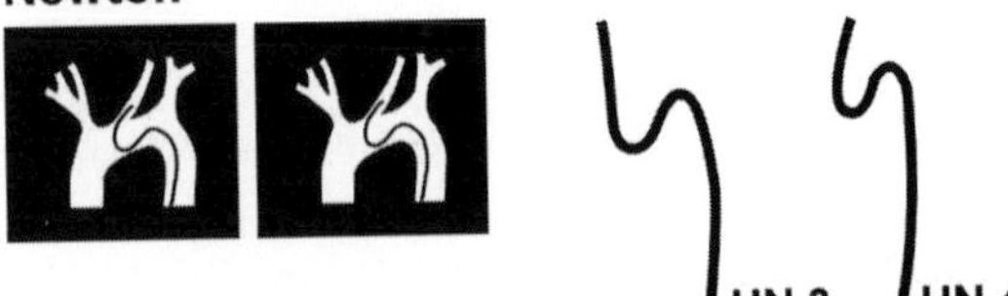

Fig. 21.4 Examples of active catheters include the sidewinder and Newton (Merit Medical, South Jordan, Utah) curves. These catheters are more active and may require maneuvers to get into the preformed shape. Of the several models of the Simmons sidewinder (SIM 1, SIM 2, SIM 3, SIM 4), the SIM 2 may be needed for complex type III arch cases and is shaped in the left subclavian artery. The Newton (HN 3, HN 4) is much easier to shape in the aorta and can facilitate access in type II or III arches.

left vertebral artery from the aortic arch is less common (0.5%) but is also considered a normal anatomic variant.

The Simmons sidewinder is considered an "active catheter" because it must be shaped in the ascending aorta; this process can be a source of atheroemboli or embolic complication. The best-accepted technique for shaping the Simmons sidewinder catheter is performed in the LAO view. The catheter is advanced over a wire into the aortic arch. The wire is removed and the catheter is flushed. The catheter is retracted and the tip positioned so the left subclavian artery can be imaged. A wire is then advanced into the left subclavian artery using fluoroscopic guidance. The sidewinder catheter is advanced over the wire until the secondary curve is approaching the subclavian origin. The wire is then retracted into the secondary curve and the catheter is advanced and rotated, allowing it to prolapse into the ascending aorta until the tip is freely moving. The catheter can then be rotated into the great vessel of interest and retracted into the target carotid or vertebral artery.

With any catheter manipulation, particularly in the region of the extracranial cerebrovascular system, it is important to use meticulous fluoroscopic guidance. Always lead with a wire and follow with the hemodynamic principles of checking for damping of pressure before any injection.

The type of diagnostic catheter used for carotid angiography is a matter of operator preference. Most cases can be done with an angled glide catheter or another "passive" glide system. Views that are suggested for evaluating the extracranial carotid artery and great vessels include ipsilateral oblique or true lateral for the internal carotid artery and external carotid artery ostium; LAO for the origins of the left common carotid, left subclavian, and innominate arteries; and RAO for the origins of the right common carotid, right and left vertebral, left internal mammary, and right subclavian arteries.

Suggested Views for Extracranial Carotid Arteries and Great Vessels

- Internal carotid artery: ipsilateral oblique or true lateral

- External carotid artery ostium: ipsilateral oblique or true lateral
- Origin of left common carotid artery: LAO
- Origin of right common carotid artery: RAO
- Origin of right vertebral artery: RAO
- Origin of left vertebral artery: RAO
- Origin of left internal mammary artery: RAO
- Origin of left subclavian artery: LAO
- Origin of innominate artery: LAO
- Origin of right subclavian artery: RAO

Upper Extremity Angiography

Navigation of a selective catheter into the left upper extremity is performed in the LAO projection and then shifted to the anterior-posterior (AP) projection as the catheter is advanced over a wire. If selecting the right subclavian artery, it is sometimes helpful to use the RAO view to define the subclavian origin while the catheter is advanced into the right upper extremity.

The upper extremity vessels distal to the axillary arteries are more sensitive to catheter manipulation and spasm. Vasodilator therapy should be administered before power injection in the distal upper extremity in a patient with pronounced pericatheter spasm. Papaverine (30-60 mg) is used to release spasm in the digital arteries in patients with vasoreactive conditions.

In patients with suspected thoracic outlet syndrome, stationing the catheter in the axillary artery and monitoring pressure during abduction and provocative maneuvers may be beneficial. If a significant gradient is generated during provocative maneuvers, the catheter is retracted proximal to the subclavian axillary transition, and angiographic confirmation of vessel encroachment during these maneuvers confirms the diagnosis.

Visceral Angiography

Multiple catheter shape options are available for imaging the visceral vessels, as detailed in Fig. 21.5. The celiac and superior mesenteric arteries are most easily engaged in the lateral view, but selective angiography typically also requires an AP imaging profile to view branch vessels. Administration of glucagon (0.5-1 unit) 1 minute before superior mesenteric angiography decreases the bowel gas artifact and improves image quality. Continued imaging through the levophase during mesenteric angiography with a long slow contrast injection is important for definition of the mesenteric venous system if mesenteric vein thrombosis is a consideration. The distal superior mesenteric artery distribution should be examined for microaneurysms or angiographic stigmata of vasculitis.

Renal Angiography

A popular myth is that the right renal artery projects posteriorly and thus is best seen in the RAO view. Typically, however, the right renal artery arises slightly anteriorly and is best seen in the AP to LAO projection. It is important during selective renal angiography to meticulously evaluate the renal parenchyma to exclude non-vascular pathology, including, but not limited to, hydronephrosis and renal cell carcinoma. If fibromuscular dysplasia is suspected, multiple oblique views may be required to further define the anatomy. Quantitative measurement of any renal artery aneurysm and presence or absence of concentric calcium deposition is important in defining the natural history of fibromuscular dysplasia and must be part of the strategy for defining the needed views of obliquity.

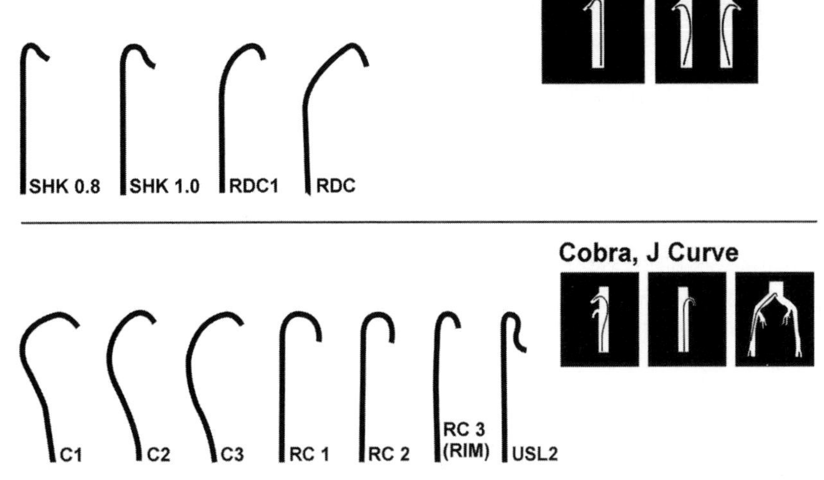

Fig. 21.5 Visceral catheter shapes. The shepherd hook (SHK 0.8, SHK 1.0), renal double curve (RDC, RDC1), cobra (C1, C2, C3; based on length of the secondary curve), RC 1, RC 2, RIM, and universal (USL2) catheters can be used for visceral angiography and contralateral access. The Judkins right coronary catheter (JR4, not shown) is also used for imaging of renal arteries.

Contralateral Lower Extremity Access

Most contralateral leg access can be simply achieved by wire access via a pigtail, internal mammary artery, RIM, J-cath, Omni-sos, or other universal flush catheter. Baseline angiography of the aortic bifurcation is performed, and the catheter is retracted into the distal aorta so the tip is facing the contralateral iliac artery. The best view to define the aorta is typically AP, but occasionally an oblique view is needed because the aorta can be rotated, particularly in elderly women. The wire is then advanced into the contralateral external iliac artery and the catheter advanced over the wire into the target second- or third-order station for angiography.

Access to the contralateral lower extremity is particularly challenging in patients with a high aortoiliac bifurcation, abdominal ectasia or aneurysmal change, previous aortobifemoral surgery, or distal native aortic tortuosity. In these cases, it may be best to start with a more supportive catheter like the Omni-sos or universal. The catheter is retracted into the bifurcation over a regular hydrophilic angled wire (glidewire). The hydrophilic wire tip is then turned to address the lateral iliac wall and advanced into the contralateral external iliac artery. Often the wire must be advanced deep into the contralateral superficial femoral or profunda femoris artery to provide "anchor" support to advance the universal flush catheter forward. If the universal flush catheter will not advance, an angled braided hydrophilic catheter (glide catheter) can be used, and this combination allows access to the contralateral limb in most cases. Occasionally, a Simmons sidewinder or more aggressive curve is needed, but this should be considered only in unusual cases in which brachial access or ipsilateral approach is not advised.

Questions

1. A 64-year-old, right-handed carpenter presents with right arm claudication and becomes dizzy when using a hammer. He has a normal right carotid pulse and decreased right arm blood pressure compared with the left. Duplex ultrasonography shows right vertebral flow reversal. What is most likely to be the best view to image the lesion?
- **a.** Left anterior oblique
- **b.** Straight AP
- **c.** Right anterior oblique
- **d.** True lateral
- **e.** AP cranial

2. What is the O.D. of a 6F diagnostic catheter?
- **a.** 6 CH
- **b.** 1.98 mm
- **c.** 0.78 in
- **d.** All of the above

3. To shape a Simmons sidewinder catheter for selective imaging of the great vessels in a patient with a type III aortic arch, what should the operator do?
- **a.** Gently advance the catheter into the aortic arch with the tip in the left coronary cusp until the preformed shape is assumed within the arch proper.
- **b.** Place the tip of the catheter in the left carotid artery and, after test injections of contrast, advance the catheter into the left common carotid artery until it assumes its preformed shaped in the ascending aorta.
- **c.** Advance the catheter into the aortic arch and, after meticulous flushing, navigate a hydrophobic wire or other soft-tip wire into the left subclavian artery over which the catheter is advanced until the secondary curve addresses the subclavian ostium. At this point, the wire is retracted into the secondary curve and the catheter advanced and rotated until it forms its preformed shape in the ascending aorta.
- **d.** Move the catheter into the thoracic aorta until the tip engages a thoracic branch, then advance until the catheter assumes its preformed shape. Advance the catheter over the arch and then retract it into the targeted great vessel.
- **e.** All of the above can be used.

4. During non-selective abdominal angiography, the power injector suddenly stops injection when the preset pressure threshold of 900 pounds per square inch (psi) is exceeded. What should the operator do?
- **a.** Increase the threshold to 1,200 psi and proceed with injection
- **b.** Withdraw blood from the catheter and flush
- **c.** Make certain the flush catheter is moving freely within the aorta
- **d.** Evaluate all connections and tubing for kinks or obstruction
- **e.** b, c, and d

5. During carotid angiography with an end-hole hydrophilic catheter, attempts to withdraw blood and flush the catheter are unsuccessful because of suspected occlusion of the catheter or kink in the catheter. What should the operator do?
- **a.** Remove the catheter over a wire
- **b.** Remove the catheter and flush outside the body
- **c.** Proceed with power injection
- **d.** Inject a small amount of heparinized saline forward to clear the catheter

6. A patient enters the hospital with a suspected congenital arteriovenous malformation between the renal artery and renal vein. For non-selective angiography of the abdominal aorta, the need is anticipated for a high volume of contrast material. A 6F, 0.035-in wire–compatible, 100-cm length pigtail catheter is selected. During attempts to inject 60 mL of contrast over 2 seconds, the power injector tubing splits and contrast is sprayed throughout the room. How may this situation have been avoided?

- **a.** Utilization of a 65-cm pigtail catheter from the same family
- **b.** A better understanding by the operator regarding the maximal flow rate for the catheter selected
- **c.** The appropriate setting of a pressure limit on the power injector below the threshold for the injector tubing or catheter selected
- **d.** Use of a high-flow pigtail catheter that is 100 cm in length but has a larger internal diameter
- **e.** Dilution of the contrast material
- **f.** All of the above

7. During abdominal angiography, the patient has severe back pain followed by hypotension and loss of motor and sensory function below the waist. This complication:

- **a.** Could have been avoided by stationing the catheter below T12.
- **b.** Could have been avoided by making certain that the catheter was free moving in the aorta before injection.
- **c.** May be improved by venting of the spinal fluid, but this is based on anecdotal experience.
- **d.** Is likely to result in long-term paralysis.
- **e.** All of the above.

8. Baseline aortic arch angiography in a patient before selective left carotid angiography shows that the left carotid artery originates from the brachiocephalic trunk approximately 1 cm distal to the brachiocephalic ostium. This finding:

- **a.** Is a normal anatomic variant
- **b.** Occurs in as many as 7% of patients
- **c.** May require the utilization of a more "active" catheter like the Simmons sidewinder, Vitek, or Newton catheter for selective angiography
- **d.** All of the above

9. A patient enters the hospital with severe right foot pain and absent right pedal pulses. The patient has documented severe osteoarthritis that required bilateral hip and knee replacements. Traditional angiography with bilateral lower extremity runoff shows luminal irregularity and calcification but no focal area of significant stenosis. What would be the next best diagnostic test?

- **a.** Erythrocyte sedimentation rate and additional serologic testing for vasculitis
- **b.** Cardiac work-up for possible embolic source
- **c.** Steep oblique image intensifier angulation or cross table views of the ipsilateral popliteal and tibioperoneal system before moving the patient off the table
- **d.** Venous studies of the right lower extremity

Suggested Readings

Baum S, Pentecost MJ, editors. Abrams' angiography: interventional radiology. 2nd ed. Philadelphia: Lippincott Williams & Wilkins; 2006.

Osborn AG. Diagnostic cerebral angiography. 2nd ed. Philadelphia: Lippincott Williams & Wilkins; 1999.

Singh H, Cardella JF, Cole PE, et al, Society of Interventional Radiology Standards of Practice Committee. Quality improvement guidelines for diagnostic arteriography. J Vasc Interv Radiol. 2003;14:S283-8.

Spies JB, Bakal CW, Burke DR, et al, Standards of Practice Committee of the Society of Cardiovascular and Interventional Radiology. Standards for interventional radiology. J Vasc Interv Radiol. 1991;2:59-65.

Uflacker R, editor. Atlas of vascular anatomy: an angiographic approach. Baltimore: Williams & Wilkins; 1997.

22 Endovascular Techniques II: Wires, Balloons, and Stents

Ian R. McPhail, MD

Wires

Angiography wires come in all shapes, sizes, intricacies, and capabilities. Variables include diameter, length, tip shape, visibility, hydrophilic coating, tip and shaft stiffness, docking, and torque properties. Major classification is often by size, grouping 0.035/0.038-in and 0.014/0.018-in diameter wires. Access wires for the femoral approach and for diagnostic angiography of large and medium-sized vessels are usually 0.035 inches in diameter, with J-shaped or soft floppy tips that are unlikely to inadvertently enter an unwanted branch vessel or initiate a dissection during access or catheter exchange. Their usual construction is a core wire with an outer spiral wrap, allowing the tip to be straightened for insertion by applying tension to the wrap over the core with one hand.

These wires have little directional control and rely on large, open vessels for passage or shaped catheter manipulation for steering. They have soft to medium shaft stiffness and are often used as the working wire for interventions on larger vessels. Wires with similar tips but much stiffer shafts (such as 0.035-in wires) are useful in obtaining access through heavily scarred groins in which a dilator might kink a standard wire, for straightening tortuous iliac segments and endografting the aorta, and for work in the great vessels. Shaped or shapeable tips, on a shaft responsive to torque (especially with a hydrophilic coating), are invaluable in accessing branch vessels and crossing stenoses. Hydrophilic wires are essential in tortuous vessels, recanalization work, and crossing the aortic bifurcation from a contralateral approach. However, hydrophilic wires are more difficult to handle (slippery when wet and sticky when dry), potentially more traumatic, and should not be used as routine access or working wires.

Small-diameter wires, as used in the coronary arteries, have become increasingly popular for peripheral access and interventions. For example, the micropuncture set uses a small needle with a 0.018-in wire to obtain access. The dilator system is introduced and the 3F/0.018-in inner dilator is removed from within the 4F/0.035-in outer dilator, allowing for the insertion of a standard 0.035-in access wire. This is an extremely useful system for entering arm vessels and the internal jugular vein, especially under ultrasonographic guidance. The sharp, fine needle is also good for cutting through scar tissue and for entering the small femoral arteries of some young women and children. Catheter exchanges, positioning, and primary branch access are usually performed with 0.035-in wires. However, 0.014/0.018-in systems are superb tools for intervention on smaller vessels and have been adopted by most operators. The 0.014-in wires dominate coronary work. These wires generally have a shapeable tip that is visible under fluoroscopy. They are less traumatic than thicker wires and are conveniently paired with low-profile balloons and stents that easily cross tight lesions. A hydrophilic coating may be applied to all or just the tip of the wire. Tip length and shaft properties vary. Rapid exchange balloons (described below) and stents are commonly paired with these smaller wires.

Several specific recommendations can be made for using wires. 1) Choose the wire diameter, length, tip configuration, coating, and handling properties specifically for the task at hand. 2) If the wire does not advance easily, do not just force it. 3) Do not use a hydrophilic-coated wire through a needle; the coating might shear off. 4) If a wire with a spiral wrap gets caught on something (e.g., the apex of an inferior vena cava filter or the tip of a needle), do not pull on it or the wrap will unravel. Instead, advance the wire, preferably with catheter support. 5) Either the soft or stiff end of a wire can be partially advanced through a catheter to change the shape of the distal end of the catheter (e.g., open it up). 6) Choose hydrophilic wires (vs non-hydrophilic "working wires") for tortuous vessels and for crossing difficult lesions.

Wire Do's and Don'ts

- Do select the correct wire (diameter, length, tip, stiffness, torque control, visibility) for the job
- If the wire doesn't go in easily, don't just push
- Don't use a hydrophilic-coated wire through a needle; the coating might shear off
- If a wire with a spiral wrap gets caught on something, don't pull or the wrap will unravel. Instead, advance the wire, preferably with catheter support
- Either the soft or stiff end of a wire can be partially advanced through a catheter to change the shape of the distal end of the catheter
- Choose hydrophilic wires for tortuosity and crossing difficult lesions vs non-hydrophilic "working wires"

Balloons

This discussion will focus on high-pressure, non-elastic angioplasty balloons (as opposed to low-pressure, elastomeric balloons used for vessel occlusion, embolectomy, or fixation). Current angioplasty balloons are available in many diameters and lengths. Made with a thin wall of materials such as polyethylene terephthalate or nylon, they tend to maintain their shape and size under high inflation pressure (typically 8-20 atm and sometimes as high as 30 atm). Of these 2 materials, polyethylene terephthalate is stronger and the balloon can have a thinner wall and lower profile; nylon is weaker but softer and deflates more easily, facilitating removal. Of note, inflating a balloon with undiluted high-viscosity contrast fluid may make it difficult to deflate and remove.

Per Laplace's law, wall stress increases with balloon radius for a given pressure. Therefore, larger balloons tend to have lower burst pressures; this can be overcome with various reinforcing materials. The following equation defines the stress on a typical angioplasty balloon:

Radial (hoop) stress = (pressure × radius)/(2 × thickness)

Because radial stress is greater than longitudinal, balloons usually tear along their long axis rather than circumferentially. A longitudinal tear may be less likely to catch on a lesion or stent than a circumferential tear and less likely to perforate a vessel than would a high-pressure jet from a pinhole-type balloon rupture.

Balloon length should be based on the length and shape of the target lesion. One that is too long can traumatize adjacent "normal" endothelium; this also applies to the "shoulders" of the balloon. A balloon that is too short may "squirt" out of position during inflation.

Aside from being able to position a balloon of the desired size across the lesion and inflate it to adequate pressure, the most important property in practice is the issue of balloon compliance. Compliance refers to the relationship between changes in volume and pressure. A compliant balloon increases in diameter as pressure increases. A non-compliant balloon reaches its predetermined nominal maximum diameter and enlarges very little as inflation pressure increases. This property of non-compliant balloons concentrates force on the resistant part of a stenosis without assuming a "dog bone" configuration and overdilating the adjacent vessel. Balloon compliance is also important when expanding a stent. A compliant balloon will continue to expand beyond its stated diameter as pressure is increased, which allows the operator to size the balloon conservatively (i.e., undersize slightly for safety) and then expand the balloon further, if desired, by increasing the pressure.

Balloons may be mounted on shafts to accept either smaller (0.014/0.018-in) or larger (0.035/0.038-in) wire diameters—generally for use in smaller and larger vessels, respectively. Imaging through the sheath or guide catheter with the balloon in situ is easier with the smaller systems, and they can cross very tight lesions through tortuous access.

The balloon may be mounted on a shaft that takes the wire through the full length of the shaft ("over-the-wire" systems) or one that takes the wire only through its distal end, with the wire exiting out the side of the shaft a short distance back from the balloon ("rapid exchange"). The advantages of an over-the-wire system are that wire exchange can be performed with the balloon in situ and that contrast material can be injected through the shaft lumen where the wire passes. However, a long wire is required, which can be cumbersome. Rapid exchange systems use a shorter wire and facilitate faster balloon placement and exchange, usually with less wire movement.

Cryoplasty balloons produce a cold thermal injury to the vessel by inflating with liquid nitrous oxide that turns to gas. These balloons have recently received considerable attention in the media, but their superiority remains unproven. Cutting balloons have blades that are brought into contact with the vessel wall during inflation and are useful in resistant lesions.

Balloon Do's and Don'ts

- Do not use undiluted high-viscosity contrast material in a balloon or it may be difficult to deflate
- Choose balloon length carefully. One that is too long can traumatize adjacent "normal" endothelium; this also applies to the "shoulders" of the balloon. A balloon that is too short may "squirt" out of position during inflation

- If the balloon bursts before successful dilation, a larger balloon is even more likely to burst (due to Laplace's law)
- Laplace's law for a cylinder: Tension = Pressure × Radius
- Compliant balloons enlarge with increasing pressure; non-compliant balloons concentrate force on the stenosis rather than assuming a "dog bone" shape
- Over-the-wire balloons allow wire exchange and distal contrast injection through the balloon catheter shaft; rapid exchange balloons facilitate shorter wires

Stents

Vascular stents are metal frameworks that support the lumen from within. Much of what is known about stents has been learned in the coronary circulation. In 1994, the results of 2 clinical trials, from the Benestent Study and Stent Restenosis Study (STRESS), established stents as superior to balloon angioplasty alone in preventing restenosis in the coronary circulation. The US Food and Drug Administration (FDA) approved the first balloon-expandable coronary stent that same year, and use of this type of stent has skyrocketed since, including broad application in the peripheral vasculature. Stents work well to prevent acute recoil after angioplasty, maximize lumen diameter, and "tack down" dissection flaps. However, although stents support the lumen, they also increase the risk of subacute thrombosis and incite intimal hyperplasia. The thrombosis problem can be largely overcome with antiplatelet therapy and high-pressure balloon inflation.

Drug-eluting stents and newer stent designs have lower restenosis rates. However, neither the use of clopidogrel nor the use of drug-eluting stents has been proven effective in the peripheral circulation. Furthermore, surprisingly few good, prospective, randomized trials have published data supporting the benefit of stents in the periphery; these stents are often used "off label" (e.g., bronchial- or biliary-approved stents used in the vasculature) in clinical practice. Current stents may be broadly classified as balloon-expandable or self-expanding.

Balloon-Expandable Stents

Balloon-expandable stents rely on inflation of an angioplasty balloon to expand the stent from its collapsed configuration and push it into contact with the vessel wall. Most contemporary stents are factory-mounted on the balloon. They have become much easier to use since the early days of the stiff but strong unmounted Palmaz-Schatz stent. Computer-guided laser cutting of alloy tubes has facilitated the manufacture of complex new stent designs with vastly improved handling properties. Many interdependent variables determine stent design, including size, configuration, and material composition. Longitudinally oriented struts seem favorable for patency, but transverse elements are needed for flexibility. Lower profile (thinner in the radial direction) struts also seem to be associated with less restenosis and allow a smaller delivery system. Large interstices (i.e., a low mesh density) mean that smaller struts are indenting the vessel wall and providing less surface coverage. The small struts put higher local pressure on the wall and incite more intimal hyperplasia. Thus, radial strength, wall coverage, and delivery system size are some of the competing elements in stent design.

Other interconnected variables include foreshortening, expandability, and flexibility. The less a stent foreshortens when it is deployed, the easier it is to achieve precise placement. Expandability allows for a smaller size in the collapsed state and some play in the final diameter. Although balloon-expandable stents are not nearly as flexible as self-expanding stents, some degree of flexion is still required of balloon-expandable stents to facilitate passage through tortuous access vessels. The alloys used vary in strength, vessel response, and visibility under fluoroscopy. Earlier stents were stainless steel, with newer designs favoring cobalt-chromium alloys. The most biocompatible material has yet to be determined. Magnesium-based and other absorbable stents are under investigation.

Self-Expanding Stents

As the name implies, self-expanding stents are released from their constraining delivery mechanism and expand within the vessel until the stent reaches its predetermined maximum diameter or is constrained by the vessel wall. Basic configurations include spiral and mesh. They are much more flexible than balloon-expandable stents and will recoil if a compressive force is applied. They are also available in larger sizes. These properties are invaluable in applications such as use in the superficial femoral and carotid territories where the vessels are subject to bending or movement.

The archetypal self-expanding stent is the Wallstent. It is well known to most practitioners. The stent is made of a low-iron-content (safe for use with magnetic resonance imaging [MRI]) biomedical superalloy braided into a mesh cylinder. It is elongated when constrained in the delivery system and shortens considerably as it is deployed distally to proximally, back along the delivery catheter. Therefore, the tip can be accurately positioned during the initial phase of deployment, but it is very difficult to know where the back end of the stent will end up. It is flexible and not prone to kinking, but difficulties with accurate placement have led to more widespread use of nitinol self-expanding stents.

Nitinol (a "shape memory alloy") derives its name from nickel-titanium/Naval Ordnance Laboratory, referring to the components of the alloy and the site of its discovery in 1961. Nitinol stents are appealing because they revert to their original shape when warmed to body temperature. This allows both a compact delivery system and an outward radial force in the vessel after placement. The stents are MRI safe, flexible, and foreshorten little. Accurate placement is much easier than with the Wallstent, although they are difficult to see under fluoroscopy and usually have marker dots at both ends. Despite their flexibility, nitinol stents have been prone to fracture in the superficial femoral artery, which is associated with decreased patency.

Coil stents consist of a continuous coil of wire. Early coronary versions included the GRII and the Wiktor stents, which had poor patency. The IntraCoil is FDA approved for the femoropopliteal arterial segment. The main advantage is flexibility; this stent has been used across joint lines. However, limited surface area is in contact with the vessel wall, which may result in higher restenosis rates. One technical peculiarity of the IntraCoil is that it should not be oversized. It is recommended that the stent diameter match the vessel lumen diameter, rather than oversizing slightly as is the norm with other types of stents. An oversized coil stent will result in a tilted coil configuration.

Another special type of self-expanding stent is the Gianturco Z. Approved for use in the airways, it comes in large diameters and is useful for vascular applications such as the vena cava. Very large interstices allow placement across large branches while preserving patency.

Other Types of Stents

Covered Stents

"Covered stents" and "stent grafts" are terms loosely used to describe metal stents that are either covered or lined with fabric (usually polytetrafluoroethylene). Examples include the lined Viabahn, which is FDA approved for the superficial femoral artery, and the covered Wallgraft, which is approved for tracheobronchial use. The addition of fabric means a larger delivery system is involved. Benefits include the ability to treat aneurysms and perforations while maintaining lumen patency. Superior patency over traditional stents in atheromatous disease has not been proven, and covered stents may fail by abrupt thrombosis.

Drug-Eluting Stents

The most recent and dramatic advance in stent design is the drug-eluting stent. These stents provide local release of a drug to prevent restenosis. Agents used include the anti-proliferative drugs sirolimus and paclitaxel. FDA approved for coronary use since 2003, they have become popular, with substantially lower restenosis rates than bare metal stents. However, they are expensive, and patients must remain on clopidogrel for 6 months after placement to prevent thrombosis. Early studies have been done in the periphery including the renal, superficial femoral artery, and tibial territories, with mixed results.

Non-Invasive Imaging After Stent Placement

Non-invasive imaging is complicated by stent placement. Most contemporary stents are not ferromagnetic and are therefore MRI safe. (Web sites such as www.mrisafety.com are useful online references for various intravascular devices. If in doubt, check with the manufacturer.) Some stents can be imaged with MRI. Others leave a black void on the scan, which can be misinterpreted as an occlusion. Ultrasonography can assess flow through stents. Considerable artifact can be produced by stents when imaged by computed tomography, but this seems to be less of an issue with newer scanners and larger vessels.

- Balloon-expandable stents are more rigid and precise
- Self-expanding stents are more flexible and available in larger sizes
- Flexible stents should be used in vessels prone to movement
- Covered stents are generally used for aneurysms and perforations (iatrogenic or traumatic)

Questions

1. All of the following are advantages of self-expanding stents over balloon-expandable stents except:
a. Greater flexibility
b. Longer available stent lengths
c. Superior overall long-term patency
d. Recoil in response to external compression

2. The compliant balloon you are using breaks when attempting to treat a tight non-calcified lesion. The balloon size seems slightly oversized compared with the adjacent vessel diameter, but the central portion of the lesion never expanded beyond 50% before the balloon broke. Your next step should be:
a. A larger non-compliant balloon
b. A balloon-expandable stent
c. A self-expanding stent
d. A non-compliant balloon of the same size

3. All of the following are true of balloon-expandable stents except:
   a. Precise placement is easier than with self-expanding stents
   b. Gold coatings favor patency
   c. Horizontal struts favor flexibility
   d. They are less flexible than self-expanding stents

4. A flow-limiting dissection results after you dilate an external iliac artery stenosis from a contralateral approach through a sheath over the aortic bifurcation. Your first choice should be:
   a. Puncture the affected side and place a self-expanding stent
   b. Place a self-expanding stent through the indwelling sheath
   c. Place a balloon-expandable stent through the indwelling sheath
   d. Puncture the affected side and place a balloon-expandable stent

5. An external iliac artery angioplasty is complicated by vessel rupture with brisk bleeding and a sudden decrease in blood pressure. After reinflating the balloon to control bleeding, your next step should be:
   a. Deflate the balloon after 10 minutes to see if the bleeding stops, and perform no further intervention if the bleeding has stopped
   b. Refer for emergent open surgical repair
   c. Prepare to place a covered stent
   d. Coil embolize the external iliac artery with plans for subsequent femoral-femoral crossover bypass graft

Suggested Readings

Fischman DL, Leon MB, Baim DS, et al, Stent Restenosis Study Investigators. A randomized comparison of coronary-stent placement and balloon angioplasty in the treatment of coronary artery disease. N Engl J Med. 1994;331:496-501.

Palmaz JC. Intravascular stents in the last and the next 10 years. J Endovasc Ther. 2004;11 Suppl 2:II200-6.

Palmaz JC, Bailey S, Marton D, et al. Influence of stent design and material composition on procedure outcome. J Vasc Surg. 2002;36:1031-9.

Serruys PW, de Jaegere P, Kiemeneij F, et al, Benestent Study Group. A comparison of balloon-expandable-stent implantation with balloon angioplasty in patients with coronary artery disease. N Engl J Med. 1994;331:489-95.

Serruys PW, Kutryk MJ, Ong AT. Coronary-artery stents. N Engl J Med. 2006;354:483-95.

23 Aortoiliac Intervention

Christopher J. White, MD

Introduction

Patients with aortoiliac occlusive disease may present with a full range of symptoms, from mild claudication to limb-threatening ischemia. The severity of symptoms is multifactorial and depends on the severity of the occlusive lesion, the presence of collateral vessels, and the presence of multilevel vascular disease. In the case of isolated terminal aorta stenoses, both legs generally are equally affected, although disparities in collateral circulation may render one limb more ischemic than the other.

The initial assessment of a patient with suspected aortoiliac occlusive disease should include a physical examination for signs of peripheral ischemia, distal embolization, and the status of the peripheral pulses. Both rest and exercise ankle-brachial index (ABI) should be measured. A mild impairment in the resting ABI may be markedly exaggerated with exercise. Segmental ABIs with pulse-volume recordings can indicate the presence or absence of multilevel occlusive disease. Another helpful test in the preprocedural assessment of these patients is the duplex examination (Doppler and ultrasonography). The duplex scan provides information regarding the presence or absence of abdominal aortic aneurysmal disease and indicates the severity of occlusive lesions. If the presence of aneurysmal disease is not certain, abdominal computed tomography or magnetic resonance imaging may be performed.

Aortoiliac Angiography

Vascular access for aortoiliac angiography may be obtained from the upper extremity (radial, brachial, or axillary approach) or via a femoral (ipsilateral or contralateral) artery. Using a standard Seldinger technique, arterial access is obtained, and a 4F to 6F vascular sheath is inserted. Heparin administration is optional. A pigtail catheter or other angiographic catheter is advanced to the level of the renal arteries over a guidewire. Diagnostic aortography is used to demonstrate inflow and outflow of the target lesion, and runoff angiography is performed to visualize the lower extremity circulation. A "working view" of the lesion is obtained to serve as a "road map." Bony landmarks or an external radiopaque ruler is helpful to guide intervention. When performing diagnostic aortography, it is important to image the renal arteries and any collateral circulation in the pelvis. Occasionally, it is necessary to obtain additional selective or angulated views of the terminal aorta and common iliac arteries to define the extent of the stenosis.

Abdominal Aorta Intervention

Distal abdominal aortic disease conventionally has been treated with endarterectomy or bypass grafting. Frequently, distal aortic occlusive disease accompanies occlusive disease of the common or external iliac arteries. The potential advantages of a percutaneous technique compared with aortoiliac reconstruction are substantial in that general anesthesia and abdominal incision are not required, and percutaneous therapy is associated with a shorter hospital stay and lower morbidity. Although axillofemoral extra-anatomic bypass offers a lower-risk surgical alternative for patients with terminal aorta occlusive disease and severe comorbid conditions, it has the disadvantages of a lower patency rate than direct surgical bypass of the lesions and requires that surgical intervention of a normal vessel be performed to achieve inflow.

- Axillofemoral extra-anatomic bypass is a lower-risk surgical alternative for patients with terminal aorta occlusive disease and severe comorbid conditions
- Disadvantages are lower patency rate than direct surgical bypass of the lesion and requirement for surgical intervention of a normal vessel to achieve inflow

Since 1980, balloon angioplasty has been used successfully in the terminal aorta. An extension of this strategy has been the use of endovascular stents in the treatment of infrarenal aortic stenoses. Although balloon dilation of these lesions has been reported to be effective, the placement of stents offers a more definitive treatment with a larger acute gain in luminal diameter, scaffolding of the lumen to prevent embolization of debris, and enhanced long-term patency compared with balloon angioplasty alone. Excellent results at late follow-up (mean, 48 months) were reported in 24 patients treated with infrarenal aortic stents, with no in-stent restenosis.

- Balloon dilation of infrarenal lesions is reportedly effective, but stent placement is a more definitive treatment
- Advantages of stents:
  - The acute gain in luminal diameter is larger
  - Scaffolding of the lumen helps prevent embolization of debris
  - Long-term patency is enhanced

Stents are an attractive therapeutic option for the management of large artery occlusive disease to maintain or improve the arterial luminal patency after balloon angioplasty. The efficacy of stents versus balloon angioplasty for aortic stenoses has not been demonstrated in randomized trials.

Iliac Artery Intervention

Iliac artery intervention is an important skill for the cardiovascular interventionalist to master, not only to improve blood flow to the lower extremities, but also to preserve vascular access for what may be lifesaving cardiovascular therapies such as coronary intervention, insertion of an intra-aortic counterpulsation balloon, or treatment of vascular access complications. Indications for iliac intervention to relieve symptomatic lower extremity ischemia include 1) lifestyle-limiting or progressive claudication, 2) ischemic pain at rest, 3) non-healing ischemic ulcerations, and 4) gangrene. A major principle of angiographic imaging is to demonstrate the angiographic anatomy of the inflow and outflow vessels before performing intervention.

- Indications for iliac intervention to relieve symptomatic lower extremity ischemia include:
  - Lifestyle-limiting or progressive claudication
  - Ischemic pain at rest
  - Non-healing ischemic ulcerations
  - Gangrene

Subsets of patients and lesions ideally suited to balloon angioplasty have been proposed (Table 23.1); contraindications are listed in Table 23.2. Clinical success is more likely 1) with stenoses than with occlusions, 2) with aortoiliac disease than with femoropopliteal or tibioperoneal disease, and 3) in patients with claudication than in those requiring limb salvage (Table 23.3). The primary success rate of angioplasty for selected iliac artery stenoses is more than 90%, with 5-year patency rates between 80% and 85%; iliac occlusions, however, have a lower procedural success rate (33%-85%). The clinical benefit of percutaneous transluminal angioplasty (PTA) versus medical therapy in iliac lesions has been demonstrated in a randomized trial with end points that included relief of symptoms, improvement in walking distance, and continued patency of the affected artery.

Table 23.1 Ideal Iliac Artery Lesions for PTA

Stenotic lesion
Non-calcified lesion
Discrete (≤3 cm) lesion
Patent runoff vessels (≥2)
Non-diabetic patient

PTA, percutaneous transluminal angioplasty.

Table 23.2 Relative Contraindications for Iliac Artery PTA

Occlusion
Long lesion (≥5 cm)
Aortoiliac aneurysm
Atheroembolic disease
Extensive bilateral aortoiliac disease

PTA, percutaneous transluminal angioplasty.

Table 23.3 Patency After Iliac PTA by Clinical and Lesion Variables

	Patency, %		
Variables	**1-year**	**3-year**	**5-year**
ST/CL/GR	81	70	63
ST/LS/GR	65	48	38
OC/CL/PR	61	43	33
OC/LS/PR	56	17	10

CL, claudication; GR, good runoff; LS, limb-threatening ischemia; OC, occlusion; PR, poor runoff; PTA, percutaneous transluminal angioplasty; ST, stenosis.

- PTA has shown clinical benefit (relief of symptoms, improvement of walking distance, and patency of the affected artery) versus medical therapy in iliac lesions
- The primary success rate of PTA for selected iliac artery stenoses is >90%, with 5-year patency rates of 80%-85%
- Iliac occlusions have a lower procedural success rate (33%-85%)

The long-term patency of iliac vessels treated with balloon angioplasty is influenced by both clinical and anatomic variables. Restenosis rates tend to be lower in non-diabetic male patients with claudication and in those with discrete non-occlusive stenoses with good distal runoff (Table 23.3). Conversely, restenosis is more likely to occur in diabetic female patients with rest pain and in diffuse and lengthy occlusive lesions with poor distal runoff.

Traditional surgical therapy for iliac obstructive lesions includes aortoiliac and aortofemoral bypass, which are reported to have 74% to 95% 5-year patency, comparable to balloon angioplasty. In a series of 105 consecutive patients undergoing aortofemoral bypass, of which 58% were treated for claudication, the operative mortality was 5.7%, the early graft failure rate was 5.7%, and the 2-year patency was 92.8%.

- Traditional surgical therapy for iliac obstructive lesions includes aortoiliac and aortofemoral bypass
  - Reported 74%-95% patency
  - Comparable to angioplasty
- Endovascular stents have improved the success rate for PTA of the iliac arteries

Balloon angioplasty of selected lesions compares favorably with surgical therapy. A randomized trial comparing PTA with bypass surgery for 157 iliac lesions found no significant difference between PTA and surgery for death, amputations, or loss of patency at 3 years. At 3-year follow-up, ABI was not significantly different between the surgery group and the PTA group (Table 23.4). In another randomized controlled trial of surgery versus angioplasty in 102 patients with severe claudication and limb-threatening ischemia, the hemodynamic effect was no different at 1 year for revascularization by angioplasty or surgery. Therefore, on the basis of these clinical trials, the current recommendation is for percutaneous therapy before surgical therapy if a patient is a candidate for either procedure.

Table 23.4 ABI in Patients Treated With PTA or Surgery for Iliac Lesions*

	ABI†		
Treatment	**Baseline**	**Post-treatment**	**3-year F/U**
PTA	0.50±.01	0.78±.04	0.80±.07
Surgery	0.50±.02	0.82±.03	0.78±.05

ABI, ankle-brachial index; F/U, follow-up; PTA, percutaneous transluminal angioplasty.
*Differences not significant.
†Mean±SD.

Endovascular stents have improved the success rates for PTA of the iliac arteries. Because of the large diameter of the iliac vessels, the risk of thrombosis or restenosis after iliac placement of metallic stents is quite low. It is debated whether primary or provisional stent placement is the "best" strategy for iliac lesions. Data supporting primary iliac stent placement come from a meta-analysis of more than 2,000 patients from eight reported angioplasty (PTA) series and six stent series. The patients who received iliac stents had a statistically higher procedural success rate and a 43% decrease in late (4-year) failures compared with those treated with balloon angioplasty alone.

In a relatively small randomized trial comparing provisional stenting (stent placement for unsatisfactory balloon angioplasty results) with primary stenting in iliac arteries, pressure gradients across the lesions after primary stent placement (5.8±4.7 mm Hg) were significantly lower than after PTA alone (8.9±6.8 mm Hg) but not after provisional stenting (5.9±3.6 mm Hg). The primary technical success rate, defined as a postprocedural gradient less than 10 mm Hg, was not different between primary (81%) and provisional stenting (89%). The use of provisional stenting avoided stent placement in 63% of the lesions and still achieved an acute hemodynamic result equivalent to that with primary stenting. Longer-term follow-up is necessary to evaluate the feasibility and safety of this approach and the effects of provisional stenting on late patency.

Primary iliac placement of balloon-expandable stents has been evaluated in a multicenter trial in 486 patients followed up for as long as 4 years (mean±SD, 13.3±11 months). Using life table analysis, clinical benefit was seen in 91% of the patients at 1 year, 84% at 2 years, and 69% at 43 months of follow-up. The angiographic patency rate of the iliac stents was 92%. Complications were predominantly related to the arterial access site. Thrombosis of the stent occurred in five patients. A preliminary report from a European randomized trial of primary iliac balloon-expandable stent placement versus balloon angioplasty showed a 4-year patency rate of 92% for the stent group versus 74% for the balloon angioplasty group (Table 23.5).

One observational study compared the non-randomized results of iliac stenting versus surgery in patients with TransAtlantic Inter-Society Consensus (TASC) type B and C lesions (Table 23.6). The study showed no difference in rates of limb salvage and patient survival at 5 years, but vessel patency was decreased in limbs with poor runoff with stents compared with surgery. Endovascular procedures are used to treat most lesions (TASC type A, B, and C not involving the common femoral artery), with open

Table 23.5 Randomized Trial of Iliac PTA Versus Stent Placement

	Procedure	
Result	**Stent (*n*=123)**	**PTA (*n*=124)**
Technical success, %	98.4	91.9
Hemodynamic success, %	97.6	91.9
Clinical success, %	97.6	89.5
Complications, %	4.1	6.5
Patency (4-year), %	91.6	74.3

PTA, percutaneous transluminal angioplasty.

Table 23.6 Morphologic Stratification of Iliac Lesions

TASC A lesions
Single stenosis of CIA or EIA (unilateral or bilateral) <3 cm in length
TASC B lesions
Single stenosis of iliac artery, not involving CFA, of 3-10 cm in length
Two stenoses of CIA or EIA, not involving CFA, <5 cm
Unilateral CIA occlusion
TASC C lesions
Bilateral stenoses of CIA and/or EIA, not involving CFA, of 5-10 cm in length
Unilateral EIA occlusion not involving CFA
Unilateral EIA stenosis extending into CFA
Bilateral CIA occlusion
TASC D lesions
Extensive stenoses of entire CIA, EIA, and CFA of >10 cm
Unilateral occlusion of CIA and EIA
Bilateral EIA occlusions
Iliac stenosis adjacent to AAA or iliac aneurysm

AAA, abdominal aortic aneurysm; CFA, common femoral artery; CIA, common iliac artery; EIA, external iliac artery; TASC, TransAtlantic Inter-Society Consensus.

surgery reserved for more complex anatomic problems (TASC type C involving the common femoral artery and type D) or endovascular failures.

Iliac stent placement also may be used as an adjunct to surgical bypass procedures. In a 14-year study of 70 consecutive patients, clinical results have been encouraging for use of iliac angioplasty with or without stent placement to preserve inflow for femoro-femoral bypass. Seven years after surgery, patients requiring treatment of the inflow iliac artery with angioplasty or stent placement had good results, similar to those without iliac artery disease. These results suggest that percutaneous intervention can provide adequate long-term inflow for femoro-femoral bypass as an alternative to aortofemoral bypass in patients at increased risk for major surgery.

It has been debated whether stent architecture or composition (e.g., nitinol vs stainless steel) has an effect on restenosis rates. The recently completed CRISP-US (Cordis Randomized Iliac Stent Project–United States) trial showed no difference in outcomes between nitinol and stainless steel iliac artery stents at 1 year.

- The CRISP-US trial failed to show any differences between nitinol and stainless steel iliac artery stents at 1 year

Balloon-expandable stents offer greater radial force in heavily calcified, bulky iliac lesions and allow greater precision for placement, which is particularly useful in ostial lesions. Self-expanding stents are longitudinally flexible and can be delivered more easily from the contralateral femoral access site. The self-expanding stents also allow for normal vessel tapering and are particularly suited to longer lesions in which the proximal vessel can be several millimeters larger than the distal vessel.

- Balloon-expandable stents offer:
  - Greater radial force in heavily calcified, bulky iliac lesions
  - Greater precision for placement, particularly useful in ostial lesions

Conclusion

Percutaneous therapy for aortoiliac disease has substantially changed the standard of care by which patients are currently treated. It is unusual in hospitals with qualified interventionalists for a patient to undergo aortofemoral bypass surgery for aortoiliac occlusive disease if a percutaneous approach is feasible.

Questions

1. The severity of lower extremity ischemic symptoms depends on all of the following except:
   a. Multilevel lesions
   b. Presence of collateral circulation
   c. Severity of the occlusive lesion
   d. Blood pressure control

2. A patient reporting lower extremity claudication with walking one block is referred for consideration of iliac intervention. On examination, femoral pulses are normal. What screening test can you perform to assess the severity of the iliac stenosis?
   a. Ankle-brachial index
   b. Ankle-brachial index at rest and exercise
   c. Magnetic resonance angiography
   d. Computed tomography angiography

3. Which of the following statements is true?

- **a.** Axillofemoral bypass has lower operative risk and equivalent patency to aortofemoral bypass graft surgery.
- **b.** Balloon angioplasty for aortoiliac stenoses yields patency results equal to surgery after 3 years.
- **c.** Primary stenting is associated with lower postprocedural pressure gradients than provisional stenting.
- **d.** Stainless steel self-expanding stents yield superior long-term patency to nitinol self-expanding stents.

4. Which of the following would not be considered a favorable lesion criterion for percutaneous iliac intervention?
   - **a.** Focal calcification
   - **b.** Short, discrete occlusion
   - **c.** Two or more patent runoff vessels
   - **d.** Lesion length of 2 cm

5. Which of the following is the strongest contraindication to iliac intervention?
   - **a.** Spontaneous atheroembolization to the feet
   - **b.** Bilateral internal iliac (hypogastric) occlusions
   - **c.** History of a hypercoagulable state (protein S deficiency)
   - **d.** An occlusion >10 cm long

Suggested Readings

Ameli FM, Stein M, Provan JL, et al. Predictors of surgical outcome in patients undergoing aortobifemoral bypass reconstruction. J Cardiovasc Surg (Torino). 1990;31:333-9.

Bosch JL, Hunink MG. Meta-analysis of the results of percutaneous transluminal angioplasty and stent placement for aortoiliac occlusive disease. Radiology. 1997;204:87-96. Erratum in: Radiology. 1997;205:584.

Dormandy JA, Rutherford RB, TASC Working Group. Management of peripheral arterial disease (PAD). TransAtlantic Inter-Society Consensus (TASC). J Vasc Surg. 2000;31:S1-S296.

Holm J, Arfvidsson B, Jivegard L, et al. Chronic lower limb ischaemia: a prospective randomised controlled study comparing the 1-year results of vascular surgery and percutaneous transluminal angioplasty (PTA). Eur J Vasc Surg. 1991;5:517-22.

Martinez R, Rodriguez-Lopez J, Diethrich EB. Stenting for abdominal aortic occlusive disease: long-term results. Tex Heart Inst J. 1997;24:15-22.

Richter G, Noeldge G, Roeren T. First long-term results of a randomized multicenter trial: iliac balloon-expandable stent placement versus regular percutaneous transluminal angioplasty. In: Liermann DD. Stents: state of the art and future developments. Morin Heights (Canada): Polyscience Publications; 1995. p. 30-5.

Samal AK, White CJ. Percutaneous management of access site complications. Catheter Cardiovasc Interv. 2002;57:12-23.

Sullivan TM, Childs MB, Bacharach JM, et al. Percutaneous transluminal angioplasty and primary stenting of the iliac arteries in 288 patients. J Vasc Surg. 1997;25:829-38.

Tetteroo E, Haaring C, van der Graaf Y, et al, Dutch Iliac Stent Trial Study Group. Intraarterial pressure gradients after randomized angioplasty or stenting of iliac artery lesions. Cardiovasc Intervent Radiol. 1996;19:411-7.

Whyman MR, Fowkes FG, Kerracher EM, et al. Randomised controlled trial of percutaneous transluminal angioplasty for intermittent claudication. Eur J Vasc Endovasc Surg. 1996;12:167-72.

Wilson SE, Wolf GL, Cross AP. Percutaneous transluminal angioplasty versus operation for peripheral arteriosclerosis: report of a prospective randomized trial in a selected group of patients. J Vasc Surg. 1989;9:1-9.

24 Diseases of the Aorta

Jon S. Matsumura, MD
Timothy M. Sullivan, MD

Aortic Dissection

Dissection of the aorta is characterized by separation of the layers of the aortic wall. Classically, this is thought to occur when there is an intimal-medial tear of varying depth leading to entry of blood into the "false lumen." Another theory is that primary intramural bleeding ruptures into the aortic lumen. In either case, the dissection extends as blood flow forces the tear along the aortic wall.

This process can affect any branch of the aorta from the coronary orifices to the iliac arteries. Dissection of branch arteries can often cause ischemia of the recipient organ if the dissection flap obstructs flow. The dissection can also lead to arterial malperfusion, through so-called "dynamic" mechanisms. Specifically, differential outflow resistance and pressure between the true and false lumens can lead to collapse of the true lumen; this compromises blood flow when the flap drapes over and covers the orifices of branches fed off the true lumen. The dissection can also extend retrograde toward the aortic valve, causing acute aortic insufficiency and left ventricular failure.

Finally, the dissection can perforate through the entire aortic wall and rupture, leading to intrapericardial, mediastinal, pleural, retroperitoneal, or intraperitoneal hemorrhage. The false lumen can also dilate and, often over a more prolonged time course, lead to aneurysm of the aorta or dissected branch vessels. These aneurysms can cause symptoms from mass effects (commonly compressing the left mainstem bronchus, left recurrent laryngeal nerve, or esophagus), thrombosis, embolization, and vessel rupture.

- Dissection of branch arteries often causes ischemia of the affected organ when the dissection flap obstructs flow. The dissection can also lead to arterial malperfusion through so-called "dynamic" mechanisms

Dissection is frequently encountered in practice; most reports suggest that the incidence is higher in males. Population-based studies show that mortality from thoracic aortic dissection is less than that for ruptured abdominal aortic aneurysms, but acute dissection is a more common aortic emergency than ruptured aneurysm. Thoracic aortic dissection has been reported in teenagers, but the incidence increases markedly after age 50 years (median age, 69 years in men, 76 years in women). Dissection involves the ascending aorta in roughly two-thirds of patients and, in the other one-third, is limited to the descending thoracic and thoracoabdominal aorta.

Clinical presentation typically is excruciating, sudden, tearing pain that originates in the interscapular area and radiates to the low back and abdomen. Such pain in a middle-aged patient with hypertension should raise the index of suspicion for dissection. Location of pain may correlate with dissection (i.e., substernal chest pain and ascending aortic involvement) but not reliably so; up to 10% of patients with acute dissection have no chest or back pain. Dissection can be associated with discrepant upper extremity blood pressure and with acute ischemia of the lower extremities, spinal cord, kidneys, and intestines.

Occasionally, the pulse examination varies with time because the dissection extends distally and the true lumen dynamically collapses. Electrocardiography often shows left ventricular hypertrophy due to hypertension and may show acute ischemic changes if the coronary arteries are involved. Chest radiography may demonstrate cardiomegaly, widened mediastinum with loss of the aortic knob, deviation of the trachea to the right, downward displacement of the left mainstem bronchus, or left pleural effusion. Dissection is definitively diagnosed and accurately staged by transesophageal echocardiography, computed tomography (CT), or magnetic resonance imaging. Unfortunately, aortic dissection is also known as a "masquerader," and diagnosis can be missed until autopsy. Chronic dissections are typically asymptomatic unless complicated by aneurysmal enlargement.

- 10% of patients with acute dissection have no chest or back pain
- Transesophageal echocardiography, CT, or magnetic resonance imaging can be used for definitive diagnosis and accurate staging of dissection

Aortic dissection is arbitrarily defined as acute when identified less than 14 days from onset; otherwise, it is considered chronic. Dissections are classified, on the basis of the extent of aorta involved, by two common schemes. DeBakey, in 1965, identified three types of dissection: type I involves the ascending aorta and a variable portion of the thoracic or thoracoabdominal aorta; type II is limited to the ascending aorta; and type III involves the descending thoracic aorta without (IIIa) or with (IIIb) extension into the abdominal aorta. In 1970, Daily proposed the Stanford classification; dissections involving the ascending aorta were classified as type A, and those without ascending aortic involvement, type B.

The natural history of acute type A and B dissections in untreated patients is markedly different. The risk of early death from dissections involving the ascending aorta (DeBakey types I and II, Stanford type A) is substantially higher than for lesions isolated to the descending aorta (DeBakey type III, Stanford type B). Life-threatening complications in dissections that involve the ascending aorta include intrapericardial rupture, acute aortic valvular insufficiency, and coronary occlusion. Because of these differences in natural history, the treatment of acute type A and B dissections is also different. Hence, staging of acute dissection is an essential early priority because type A dissections usually require urgent surgical treatment.

Most agree that the immediate treatment of uncomplicated type B dissections is medical, including strict blood pressure control, negative inotropic management, and close clinical and radiographic surveillance in an intensive care setting. Blood pressure control may paradoxically improve malperfusion if it results in less dynamic collapse of the true lumen. Indications for urgent intervention or operation in patients with acute type B dissection include intractable pain, uncontrollable hypertension, bleeding (typically left hemothorax), or peripheral vascular complications, such as ischemia of the gut, kidney, spinal cord, or lower extremity. Surgical repair can involve extra-anatomic bypass, fenestration, or aortic replacement. Recently, endovascular alternatives (including balloon fenestration and aortic stent graft repair) have become more established, especially given the morbidity associated with direct surgical repair in this high-risk group of patients. Patients with chronic type B dissection are at risk of late aneurysm formation and should be followed up with CT or magnetic resonance imaging. Surgical or endovascular repair is typically indicated for thoracic aortic diameters greater than 6 cm.

- Staging of acute dissection is an essential early priority because type A dissections usually require urgent surgical repair
- Indications for intervention in type B dissection include intractable pain, uncontrollable hypertension, bleeding, or peripheral vascular complications

Aortic Aneurysm

Abdominal Aorta

Abdominal aortic aneurysms (AAAs) are the most common "true" aneurysms (aneurysms affecting all three layers of the arterial wall) encountered in clinical practice. An aneurysm is defined as a dilatation of an artery to 1.5 to 2 times the diameter of the normal adjacent artery. Small aneurysms are rarely symptomatic; smaller aortic and peripheral aneurysms may present with embolism or thrombosis, but rupture is the primary threat for larger aortic aneurysms. A ruptured AAA carries a mortality rate greater than 75% and is the 13th leading cause of death in adults in the United States. AAAs are associated with aneurysms of the thoracic aorta, visceral aorta, and iliac and popliteal arteries. Risk factors for AAA include male sex, increasing age, hypertension, cigarette smoking/chronic obstructive pulmonary disease, and family history of AAA.

Most studies suggest that the maximum aneurysm diameter increases at a rate of approximately 10% per year; thus, small aneurysms typically grow at a slower rate than larger ones. Some aneurysms, however, grow more rapidly or in a "staccato" pattern, making close surveillance imperative. As the aortic wall dilates, the aneurysm sac fills with laminated thrombus; laminated thrombus does not protect the wall from rupture (despite its apparent thickness) and may be associated with increased aneurysm growth rates. Unless the patient has symptomatic arterial thromboembolism, radiographic detection of AAA thrombus does not deserve additional therapy such as anticoagulation. Although most aortic aneurysms are asymptomatic unless they rupture (with resultant severe abdominal and back pain and shock), some aneurysms present with subacute pain. Less than 10% of AAAs are the inflammatory variant, which may present with chronic back pain, low-grade fever, elevated erythrocyte sedimentation rate, and hydronephrosis due to retroperitoneal fibrosis.

- Risk factors for AAA include male sex, increasing age, hypertension, cigarette smoking or chronic obstructive pulmonary disease, and family history
- Unless a patient has symptomatic arterial thromboembolism, radiographic detection of AAA thrombus does not warrant additional therapy such as anticoagulation

AAAs are frequently identified incidentally in an imaging study obtained for another reason. They can be difficult to palpate on physical examination, especially in obese patients. As of 2007, AAA screening is a coverable benefit under Medicare in the United States for 65-year-old men and women with family history of AAA and men who ever smoked. B-mode ultrasonography is the initial diagnostic test of choice to screen for and follow small AAAs. CT is typically performed if the AAA is being considered for repair or if ultrasonography results are indeterminate, as in obese patients or if the AAA extends proximally near the renal arteries or distally into the iliac arteries. Catheter angiography, because it images only the arterial flow lumen, can severely underestimate the diameter of an aortic aneurysm because the dilated arterial segment may have preserved lumen size owing to sac thrombus.

- As of 2007, AAA screening is a Medicare-covered benefit for 65-year-old men and women with family history of AAA and men who ever smoked

On the basis of current evidence (studies primarily of men), a general rule is that asymptomatic AAAs smaller than 5.5 cm in diameter should be followed up with radiographic surveillance every 3 to 12 months, and larger AAAs should be repaired. However, therapeutic plans may require individualization based on the patient's risks of aneurysm rupture, surveillance compliance, risks of intervention, and life expectancy.

- In general, asymptomatic AAAs <5.5 cm diameter should be followed up with radiographic surveillance every 3-12 months; larger AAAs should be repaired

Table 24.1 Estimated Risk of Rupture for Abdominal Aortic Aneurysms

Aneurysm diameter, cm	Annual risk of rupture, %
≤4	~0
>4-5	0.5-5
>5-6	3-15
>6-7	10-20
>7-8	20-40
>8	30-50

Several factors have been associated with the risk of aneurysm rupture, including aneurysm size (Table 24.1), female sex, family history of AAA, uncontrolled hypertension, cigarette smoking, and chronic obstructive pulmonary disease (Table 24.2). Size is the most important independent risk factor for rupture; the risk of rupture appears to increase substantially as the aneurysm increases in size from 5 to 6 cm. Those less than 4 cm in diameter have an extremely low risk of rupture, whereas those greater than 6 cm have an annual rupture risk of more than 10% to 20%. Some studies have suggested that women have an increased risk of rupture of even small aneurysms and that the risk of rupture of a 5-cm aneurysm in a female is roughly equivalent to that of a 6-cm aneurysm in a male. Saccular aneurysms may be at greater risk of rupture than fusiform, cylindrical aneurysms. A rate of aneurysm expansion greater than 1 cm per year, although not a conclusive risk factor for rupture independent of diameter, is also considered an indication for repair in many centers.

- Aneurysm size is the most important independent risk factor for rupture
- Women may have an increased risk of aneurysm rupture

Risk associated with intervention varies on the basis of patient, hospital, and surgeon factors. Most centers report operative mortality between 0% and 8% stratified by patient risks (average, 4%) after elective, open AAA

Table 24.2 Risk Assessment for AAA Rupture

	Risk		
Variable	Low	Average	High
Aneurysm diameter, cm	≤5	>5-6	>6
Smoking or COPD	None, mild	Moderate	Severe, taking corticosteroids
Hypertension	None	Controlled	Poorly controlled
Aneurysm shape	Fusiform	Saccular	Very eccentric
Wall stress	Low (35 N/cm^2)	Medium (40 N/cm^2)	High (45 N/cm^2)
Sex	...	Male	Female

AAA, abdominal aortic aneurysm; COPD, chronic obstructive pulmonary disease.

Table 24.3 Operative Mortality Risk for Elective Open Surgical Repair of AAAs

	Mortality risk		
Variable	**Low (0%-3%)**	**Moderate (>3%-7%)**	**High (>7%)**
Age, y	<70	70-80	>80
Cardiac disease	No overt disease	Stable CAD, EF >35%	Significant CAD, EF <25%
Other comorbid conditions	None	Mild COPD	Severe COPD Oxygen dependence FEV_1 <1 L/s Creatinine >3 mg/dL Liver disease
Anatomy	Normal	Adverse	Adverse

AAAs, abdominal aortic aneurysms; CAD, coronary artery disease; COPD, chronic obstructive pulmonary disease; EF, ejection fraction; FEV_1, forced expiratory volume in 1 second.

repair (Table 24.3). Risk factors for operative mortality include advanced age and cardiac (congestive heart failure, ischemic heart disease), renal, and pulmonary diseases. Female sex also appears to be an independent risk factor for perioperative death. Analysis of the patient allows for categorization into low (0%-3%), moderate (>3%-7%), or high (>7%-10%) risk subsets, on the basis of age, medical comorbidities, and anatomic factors associated with operative repair. Larger hospital volume, larger surgeon volume, and vascular surgery certification have been associated with improved outcomes. Decision making should include consideration of the risks of elective repair (Table 24.4).

Endovascular repair has become an increasingly popular option for the repair of AAAs. This procedure is less invasive and allows for exclusion of the aneurysm sac with a stent graft placed via femoral artery access. Endovascular aortic aneurysm repair (EVAR) has a shorter procedure time, decreased blood loss, fewer complications, less perioperative mortality, and more rapid and complete recovery compared with open surgical repair. Strict anatomic requirements are necessary to provide for adequate fixation of the stent graft to the adjacent infrarenal aorta and the iliac arteries (Table 24.5). Treatment of aneurysms outside these guidelines increases the risk of adverse outcomes, including conversion to open repair and AAA rupture.

Table 24.5 Anatomic Criteria for Endovascular Repair of AAA With Aortic Stent Grafts

Proximal neck	Common iliac arteries	External iliac arteries
Minimum length, 15 mm Maximum diameter, 28 mm Angulation, <60°	Maximum diameter, variable	>7 mm Diameter (for access from a femoral approach)

AAA, abdominal aortic aneurysm.

Disadvantages of EVAR include late complications such as stent graft migration, device failure, and endoleak. Various types of endoleak have been described (Table 24.6). "Endotension" is used to describe excluded aneurysms, which remain pressurized and may continue to enlarge without identifiable endoleak. Strategies for managing patients after EVAR are anecdotal and vary among experts. A common strategy is based on the type of endoleak. Type I and III endoleaks are regarded as having higher potential for rupture and should be repaired when possible. Patients with type II endoleaks (the most common type) and stable or shrinking aneurysms may be followed up. Type II leaks

Table 24.4 Current Recommendations for Elective AAA Repair

- For average-risk patients, a threshold of 5.5 cm diameter is appropriate for elective repair of AAA. Rapid expansion of the aneurysm (>1 cm/y) and patient preference (for 4.5-5.5 cm diameters) could prompt earlier repair.
- Endovascular repair of smaller-diameter AAAs is currently not justified.
- For women, elective repair of 4.5- or 5-cm AAAs may be appropriate.
- Endovascular repair is a comparable alternative to open surgery and is best indicated in patients with appropriate anatomy. The use of endovascular repair in patients with unfavorable anatomy increases the likelihood of rupture and conversion to open repair.

AAA, abdominal aortic aneurysm.

Table 24.6 Classification of Endoleaks After Endovascular AAA Repair

Classification	Type of leak
Type I	At attachment site
Type II	Branch flow leak (inferior mesenteric, lumbar, accessory renal arteries)
Type III	Graft failure or component disconnection
Type IV	Graft porosity
Type V	Endotension (continued aneurysm expansion without detectable endoleak)

AAA, abdominal aortic aneurysm.

associated with aneurysm enlargement may benefit from retreatment. Often, type II leaks can be embolized with coils or glue to obliterate the endoleak nidus.

Because of uncertainty about the durability of EVAR, patients must be followed up indefinitely (typically with CT) to evaluate for endoleak, device migration, material fatigue, and aneurysm expansion. Although open surgical repair remains the gold standard for most patients with AAA, randomized clinical trials have shown EVAR to have less perioperative mortality and morbidity and shorter recovery time; however, it is associated with more late complications. These studies with early device designs found equivalent survival with EVAR or surgery in later follow-up. Randomized trials using currently approved devices are ongoing.

- In randomized clinical trials, endovascular repair of AAA is an alternative to surgery with less perioperative mortality and morbidity, shorter recovery time, and more late complications. Survival in later follow-up with early device designs was equivalent to that with surgery

Isolated Iliac Artery Aneurysms

Iliac artery aneurysms as isolated entities (i.e., without associated AAA) are rare. Because of their location, they can be difficult to identify on physical examination. The common iliac artery is most frequently involved, followed by the internal iliac artery; external iliac aneurysms are extremely rare. There is a male predominance, and half are bilateral. The natural history of iliac aneurysms, unlike that of AAAs, is not well defined. Most series suggest that they should be repaired at a maximum diameter of between 3 and 4 cm, although a higher threshold may be appropriate because of the increased morbidity of open repair of isolated iliac aneurysms.

Iliac aneurysms may be treatable with an endovascular technique, providing a good proximal "neck" is present. A distal "landing zone" can typically be provided by the external iliac artery if the ipsilateral internal iliac can be sacrificed by coil embolization. The effective occlusion of an iliac artery was once thought to require the contralateral iliac artery to be patent to reduce the risk of pelvic ischemia or buttock claudication. However, some groups have found bilateral hypogastric sacrifice to be relatively safe if not associated with microembolization or hypotension. If a proximal neck does not exist in the ipsilateral common iliac artery, treatment of the entire aortoiliac segment could be required.

Thoracic Aorta

Aneurysms of the thoracic aorta are, like abdominal aneurysms, potentially lethal. Aneurysm size substantially affects the risk of rupture and mortality. For aneurysms of the descending thoracic aorta, a 6-cm diameter seems to be the cutoff point, above which the risk of complications increases markedly, and corresponds to a yearly risk of dissection or rupture of at least 7% and a mortality rate of 12%. Although elective surgical repair of thoracic aortic aneurysms is associated with considerable perioperative risk, long-term survival is excellent. Because surgical treatment of thoracic and thoracoabdominal aortic aneurysms can be associated with severe morbidity and mortality (including paraplegia, depending on the extent of the aneurysm), elective repair of descending aortic aneurysms is typically recommended at a 6- to 6.5-cm diameter. For the ascending aorta, elective repair is recommended at a diameter of 5 to 5.5 cm. If significant aortic valve disease is present, repair at a smaller size might be indicated. Endovascular repair of selected thoracic aortic aneurysms is an appealing alternative to open surgical repair. One thoracic endoprosthesis device, a nitinol-supported expanded polytetrafluoroethylene tube graft (Table 24.7, Fig. 24.1), is currently approved by the US Food and Drug Administration for thoracic EVAR, but others are in clinical trial.

Table 24.7 Results of Endovascular Repair of Thoracic Aortic Aneurysms

Complications within 30 d	Incidence*	
Any major	45 (32)	
Bleeding complications, all	12 (9)	
Any endoleak	5 (4)	
Pulmonary	14 (10)	
Cardiac	4 (3)	
Vascular trauma/thrombosis	20 (14)	
Stroke	5 (4)	
Paraplegia/paraparesis	4 (3)	
Death	2 (1.5)	
	Incidence*	
Late events	**1 year**	**2 year**
Migration, proximal	0/97 (0)	3/68 (4)
Migration, components	1/84 (1)	4/61 (7)
Endoleak	7/97 (7)	6/68 (9)
Size decrease ≥5 mm	23/83 (28)	24/64 (38)
Size increase ≥5 mm	6/83 (7)	11/64 (17)
Endovascular revision	1	1
Conversion to open surgery	1 (1)	0
Ruptures	0	0
Aneurysm-related death	2 (1.5)	0

*Values are no. of patients (%).

From Makaroun MS, Dillavou ED, Kee ST, et al, GORE TAG Investigators. Endovascular treatment of thoracic aortic aneurysms: results of the phase II multicenter trial of the GORE TAG thoracic endoprosthesis. J Vasc Surg. 2005;41:1-9. Used with permission.

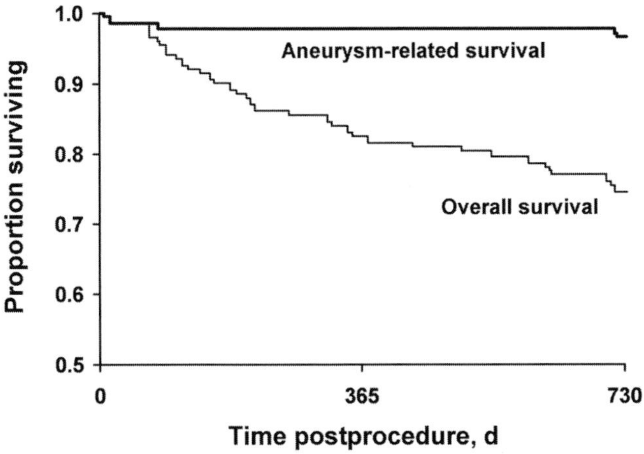

Fig. 24.1 Survival after endovascular repair of thoracic aortic aneurysms with a thoracic endoprosthesis device. (From Makaroun MS, Dillavou ED, Kee ST, et al, GORE TAG Investigators. Endovascular treatment of thoracic aortic aneurysms: results of the phase II multicenter trial of the GORE TAG thoracic endoprosthesis. J Vasc Surg. 2005;41:1-9. Used with permission.)

- Elective repair of descending aortic aneurysms is typically recommended at a 6- to 6.5-cm diameter
- For the ascending aorta, elective repair is recommended at a diameter of 5 to 5.5 cm

Questions

1. What is the most important factor when evaluating a patient for endovascular aortic aneurysm repair?
   a. Iliac artery length
   b. Maximum aneurysm diameter
   c. Proximal aortic neck length and diameter
   d. Hypogastric artery patency

2. A type II endoleak is due to:
   a. A tear in the graft fabric
   b. Perigraft flow at the aortic neck
   c. Porosity of the graft fabric
   d. Retrograde flow from a patent branch vessel

3. Which statement regarding aortic dissection is correct?
   a. Ruptured aneurysms are more common emergencies than acute aortic dissections.
   b. Thoracic aortic dissection is more common in persons younger than 50 years.
   c. Dissection involves the ascending aorta in two-thirds of patients and is limited to the descending or abdominal aorta in one-third of patients.
   d. Half of all patients with acute aortic dissection have no pain associated with it.

4. Which type of endoleak is often managed without intervention but with continued monitoring?
   a. Type I endoleak
   b. Type II endoleak with stable aneurysm sac size
   c. Type II endoleak with enlarging aneurysm sac
   d. Type III endoleak

5. Which statement regarding AAA is correct?
   a. The presence of laminated thrombus in the AAA is an indication for anticoagulation.
   b. Most AAAs are asymptomatic until they rupture.
   c. A man with a 5-cm AAA has a 10%-20% per year risk of death from AAA rupture.
   d. Women with AAAs have a decreased risk of rupture relative to men.

6. Randomized trials comparing aortic endografts with open aneurysm repair:
   a. Demonstrate decreased 30-day mortality
   b. Involve patients with lower rates of heart disease, diabetes mellitus, and hypertension in the endovascular group
   c. Lack randomization and proper controls
   d. Demonstrate higher short-term morbidity in the endovascular group

7. Postoperative endograft surveillance involves:
   a. Lifelong CT at periodic intervals
   b. Physical examination alone
   c. Baseline abdominal radiographs and CT at 3-month intervals for 1 year
   d. Yearly CT for 2 years

Suggested Readings

Brewster DC, Cronenwett JL, Hallett JW Jr, et al, Joint Council of the American Association for Vascular Surgery and Society for Vascular Surgery. Guidelines for the treatment of abdominal aortic aneurysms: report of a subcommittee of the Joint Council of the American Association for Vascular Surgery and Society for Vascular Surgery. J Vasc Surg. 2003;37:1106-17.

Coady MA, Rizzo JA, Hammond GL, et al. Surgical intervention criteria for thoracic aortic aneurysms: a study of growth rates and complications. Ann Thorac Surg. 1999;67:1922-6.

Daily PO, Trueblood HW, Stinson EB, et al. Management of acute aortic dissections. Ann Thorac Surg. 1970;10:237-47.

Davies RR, Goldstein LJ, Coady MA, et al. Yearly rupture or dissection rates for thoracic aortic aneurysms: simple prediction based on size. Ann Thorac Surg. 2002;73:17-27.

DeBakey ME, Henly WS, Cooley DA, et al. Surgical management of dissecting aneurysms of the aorta. J Thorac Cardiovasc Surg. 1965;49:130-49.

Dillavou ED, Muluk S, Makaroun MS. Is neck dilatation after endovascular aneurysm repair graft dependent? Results of 4 US

Phase II trials. Vasc Endovascular Surg. 2005;39:47-54.
Hiatt MD, Rubin GD. Surveillance for endoleaks: how to detect all of them. Semin Vasc Surg. 2004;17:268-78.
Kasirajan V, Hertzer NR, Beven EG, et al. Management of isolated common iliac artery aneurysms. Cardiovasc Surg. 1998;6:171-7.
Lederle FA, Wilson SE, Johnson GR, et al, Aneurysm Detection and Management Veterans Affairs Cooperative Study Group. Immediate repair compared with surveillance of small abdominal aortic aneurysms. N Engl J Med. 2002;346:1437-44.
Makaroun MS, Dillavou ED, Kee ST, et al, GORE TAG Investigators. Endovascular treatment of thoracic aortic aneurysms: results of the phase II multicenter trial of the GORE TAG thoracic endoprosthesis. J Vasc Surg. 2005;41:1-9.
Miller DC. Acute dissection of the descending thoracic aorta. Thorac Surg Clin. 1992;2:347-78.
Stavropoulos SW, Baum RA. Catheter-based treatments of endoleaks. Semin Vasc Surg. 2004;17:279-83.
Tonnessen BH, Sternbergh WC III, Money SR. Late problems at the proximal aortic neck: migration and dilation. Semin Vasc Surg. 2004;17:288-93.
Towne JB. Endovascular treatment of abdominal aortic aneurysms. Am J Surg. 2005;189:140-9.
The UK Small Aneurysm Trial Participants. Mortality results for randomised controlled trial of early elective surgery or ultrasonographic surveillance for small abdominal aortic aneurysms. Lancet. 1998;352:1649-55.

25 Carotid Angioplasty and Stenting

Timothy M. Sullivan, MD, FACS, FACC

Introduction

Cerebrovascular accident, or stroke, is the third leading cause of death in the United States, surpassed only by heart disease and malignancy. Stroke accounts for 10% to 12% of all deaths in industrialized countries. Almost one in four men and one in five women aged 45 years can expect to have a stroke if they live to age 85 years. In a population of one million, 1,600 people will have a stroke each year. Only 55% of these will survive 6 months, and a third of the survivors will have significant problems caring for themselves. As our population ages, the total number of people affected by stroke will continue to increase unless historic stroke rates decrease in the future.

The etiology of stroke is multifactorial. Ischemic stroke accounts for about 80% of all first-ever strokes, whereas intracerebral hemorrhage and subarachnoid hemorrhage are responsible for 10% and 5%, respectively. Most ischemic strokes are linked to complications of atheromatous plaques. The most frequent site of such an atheroma is the carotid bifurcation. Although the prevention of stroke in the general population has largely focused on the control of hypertension, a substantial number of strokes are preventable by the identification and treatment of carotid disease, especially as the population ages.

- Cerebrovascular accident, or stroke, is the third leading cause of death in the United States, surpassed only by heart disease and malignancy
- Ischemic stroke accounts for about 80% of all first-ever strokes
- Intracerebral hemorrhage and subarachnoid hemorrhage are responsible for 10% and 5%, respectively
- Most ischemic strokes are linked to complications of atheromatous plaques

Surgical endarterectomy of high-grade carotid lesions, both symptomatic and asymptomatic, has been identified as the treatment of choice for stroke prophylaxis in most patients when compared with "best medical therapy" (risk factor reduction and antiplatelet agents), as shown by the NASCET (North American Symptomatic Carotid Endarterectomy Trial) and ACAS (Asymptomatic Carotid Atherosclerosis Study) trials. In the NASCET study, the risk of endarterectomy-related disabling stroke or death was 1.9% with a 3.9% risk of minor stroke (5.8% risk of stroke and death overall). In the ACAS trial, the surgical risk of major stroke or death was 0.6%, excluding the 1.2% risk of stroke caused by diagnostic arteriography (overall risk of stroke and death, 2.3%). Carotid endarterectomy (CEA) is being performed in increasing numbers of patients and now represents the most frequent surgical procedure performed by vascular surgeons.

Despite the proven efficacy of CEA in the prevention of ischemic stroke, great interest has been generated in carotid angioplasty and stenting (CAS) as an alternative to surgical therapy. The use of angioplasty and stenting techniques in the coronary and peripheral circulation stimulated investigation into the application of this technology to the carotid circulation, especially in patients who are poor surgical candidates. Therefore, as CAS evolved as an alternative therapy to CEA, several studies attempted to define a group of patients who might be better served with non-surgical interventional therapy.

In one study of 2,228 consecutive CEA procedures in 2,046 patients from 1989 to 1995, the stroke and mortality rates for CEA as an isolated procedure were exemplary—1.8% and 0.5%, respectively, for a combined rate of 2.3%. In addition, no statistical difference was found in stroke and mortality rates among asymptomatic patients, patients presenting with hemispheric transient ischemic attack (TIA), or those undergoing surgery for stroke with minimal residua. Patients having combined CEA and coronary artery bypass grafting had higher rates of perioperative stroke (4.3%) and death (5.3%) than patients having isolated CEA. Carotid reoperations were also associated with higher rates of stroke (4.6%) and death (2.0%). These data suggest that CEA can be performed safely in large groups of unselected patients, but they also may give some insight into categories of patients who are at increased risk of adverse events with operative intervention.

- Patients having combined CEA and coronary artery bypass grafting had higher rates of perioperative stroke and death than patients having isolated CEA
- Carotid reoperations are also associated with higher rates of stroke and death

A follow-up study attempted to retrospectively identify a subgroup of patients who were at increased procedural risk with CEA and therefore may be better served by CAS. A total of 3,061 CEA procedures were examined from a prospective database over a 10-year period. A high-risk cohort was identified, which included patients with severe coronary artery disease (requiring angioplasty or bypass surgery within the 6 months before CEA), severe chronic obstructive pulmonary disease, or renal insufficiency (serum creatinine >3.0 mg/dL) or history of congestive heart failure. The rate of the composite end point of stroke, death, or myocardial infarction (MI) was 3.8% for the entire group (stroke 2.1%, MI 1.2%, death 1.1%). This composite end point occurred in 44 of the 594 patients considered high risk (7.4%), significantly more frequently than in those in the low-risk category (71 of 2,467 [2.9%]; $P<.001$).

Other authors have questioned whether any patient is truly at "high risk" for CEA; conflicting data exist regarding the extent to which factors such as very distal lesions, reoperations, cervical radiation, and contralateral carotid occlusion increase surgical risk. Subsequent trials have therefore focused on medically compromised, high-risk patients as those who may benefit from an alternative procedure such as CAS. This chapter will examine the indications, techniques, and results of this novel therapy.

Indications

The basic indications for CAS do not differ from those for standard surgical CEA:

1) Asymptomatic lesions that fall within the "80% to 99%" stenosed range on duplex ultrasonography, which correlates with angiographic stenosis of at least 60%. Most clinical trials of CAS in asymptomatic patients require angiographic stenosis of at least 80% for study inclusion.
2) Symptomatic patients (hemispheric TIA, amaurosis fugax, or stroke with minimal residua) with at least 70% angiographic stenosis. Patients with symptomatic, ulcerated stenoses greater than 50% may benefit from endarterectomy; this has not yet been extrapolated to carotid intervention.

Possible indications for CAS in "high-risk" patients are shown in Table 25.1, and relative contraindications to the procedure are listed in Table 25.2.

Table 25.1 Indications for CAS in "High-Risk" Patients

Severe cardiac disease
- Requiring coronary PTA or CABG
- History of congestive heart failure

Severe chronic obstructive pulmonary disease
- Requiring home oxygen
- FEV_1 <20% of predicted

Severe chronic renal insufficiency
- Serum creatinine >3.0 mg/dL
- Currently on dialysis

Prior carotid endarterectomy (restenosis)
- Contralateral vocal cord paralysis

Surgically inaccessible lesions
- At or above the 2nd cervical vertebra
- Inferior to the clavicle

Radiation-induced carotid stenosis

Prior ipsilateral radical neck dissection

CABG, coronary artery bypass grafting; CAS, carotid angioplasty and stenting; FEV_1, forced expiratory volume in 1 second; PTA, percutaneous transluminal angioplasty.

Table 25.2 Contraindications to CAS

Inability to obtain femoral artery access
Unfavorable aortic arch anatomy
Severe tortuosity of the common or internal carotid arteries
Severely calcified or undilatable stenoses
Lesions containing fresh thrombus
Large amount of laminated thrombus at the site of patch angioplasty (prior CEA) on duplex ultrasonography
Extensive stenoses (>2 cm)
Critical (>99%) stenoses
Lesions adjacent to carotid artery aneurysms
Preload-dependent states; severe aortic valvular stenosis
Contrast-related issues
  Chronic renal insufficiency
  Previous life-threatening contrast reaction

CAS, carotid angioplasty and stenting; CEA, carotid endarterectomy.

Results of CAS

Short-Term Results

The short-term results of CAS are largely dependent on the presence or absence of cerebral embolization. With the relatively recent addition of cerebral protection to the procedure, associated stroke risk seems to have decreased. Admittedly, however, improvements in devices and technology have created a "moving target," making evaluation of results difficult at best.

The SAPPHIRE (Stenting and Angioplasty with Protection in Patients at High Risk for Endarterectomy) trial of CAS in high-risk patients is the only industry-sponsored, US Food and Drug Administration (FDA)-approved trial to date that was randomized: patients were randomly assigned to undergo CAS (*n*=159) or CEA (*n*=151). A separate registry was compiled of patients believed to be too high risk for surgery who underwent CAS (*n*=406) or patients who were not suitable candidates for CAS and underwent CEA (*n*=7).

The study sought to evaluate the combined end point of major adverse events including stroke, death, and MI, and was designed to test non-inferiority of CAS compared with CEA. Most of the patients were asymptomatic; only 30.2% of the CAS group and 28.5% of the CEA group were symptomatic. At 30 days, the risk of stroke in the two groups was almost identical (CAS, 3.1%; CEA, 3.3%; *P*>.99). One patient in the CAS group (0.6%) and three patients in the CEA group (2.0%) died within 30 days (*P*=.36). Significantly more patients in the CEA group had periprocedural MI (6.6%) than did patients in the CAS group (4.4%) (*P*<.05). Of note, most of the MIs were non–Q-wave, identified on routine postprocedural laboratory studies, including three of seven in the CAS group and eight of ten in the CEA group. The composite end point did not reach statistical significance (CAS, 4.4%; CEA, 9.9%; *P*=.08).

At 1 year, the end points that reached statistical significance included major ipsilateral stroke (CAS, 0%; CEA, 3.3%; *P*=.03) and MI (CAS, 2.5%; CEA, 7.9%; *P*=.04). The results in the stent registry group (*n*=413) included 20 strokes (4.8%), 9 deaths (2.2%), and 7 periprocedural MIs (1.7%) at 30 days. These results will likely be used to support FDA approval of the stent and filter protection device used in this important study.

The ARCHeR (ACCULINK for Revascularization of Carotids in High-Risk Patients) trial represents another industry-sponsored study of a stent and a filter embolic protection device. The ARCHeR trial differs from SAPPHIRE in that it is a registry of high-risk patients rather than a randomized trial and is a series of three multicenter, nonrandomized, prospective studies that ultimately enrolled 581 high-risk patients from 48 centers. Angiographic stenosis of at least 50% for symptomatic patients and 80% for asymptomatic patients was required for inclusion. For the first portion of the study, stents were placed without embolic protection (159 patients), which was added in the two subsequent groups (422 patients). The primary end points were death, stroke, or MI within 30 days, and ipsilateral stroke from 31 to 365 days. At 30 days, the risk of the composite end point was 8.3%, and the risk of stroke or death was 6.9%; most strokes were minor. The risk of major or fatal stroke was 1.5%. The risk of ipsilateral stroke at 1 year was 1.3%, yielding a risk of the primary composite end point of 9.6% at 1 year.

Stent Implantation, Restenosis, and Duplex Follow-Up

Restenosis has proved to be a substantial clinical problem after endovascular therapy in several vascular beds, including the coronary and renal arteries. Before the routine use of stents in conjunction with percutaneous transluminal angioplasty (PTA), one study followed up 12 patients with symptomatic carotid stenosis treated with PTA alone. The immediate result of angioplasty was a decrease in the mean percent stenosis from 82% to 51%. Six of the 12 patients showed further improvement in lumen diameter of greater than 14% at 1 year—from a mean of 47% stenosis immediately after PTA to 28% at follow-up angiography. Obviously, substantial arterial remodeling occurs after carotid PTA.

In a prospective study of 108 patients undergoing CAS, restenosis of greater than 50% occurred in 15 patients (14%). Elevated levels of C-reactive protein 48 hours after intervention, indicative of a systemic inflammatory response, correlated strongly with restenosis at 6 months (*P*=.01). Both residual stenosis of 10% to 30% and restenosis after prior stent implantation were independent predictors of restenosis in this study. In another series of 222 patients having successful carotid artery stenting, several factors were predictive of restenosis. By univariate analysis, female sex and age older than 75 years were statistically predictive of restenosis; by multivariate analysis, older age, female sex, implantation of multiple stents, and higher postprocedural percent stenosis were associated with an increased risk of restenosis.

Another study identified loss of proximal stent apposition as a risk factor for restenosis. In addition, most restenoses were found on routine follow-up and were asymptomatic, a finding that has been confirmed by others. These studies suggest that several patient- and procedure-related factors are associated with restenosis after CAS. Although the reported incidence of restenosis is variable, ranging from 1.8% to 75%, most studies report restenosis rates between 5% and 10% at 12 to 24 months.

- Most stent restenoses are found on routine follow-up and are asymptomatic

Because of the nature of CAS (the plaque is not removed, simply displaced), the duplex criteria for restenosis used to follow patients up after CEA may not apply. In one study of 170 stented carotid arteries, prospective duplex criteria for the presence of stenosis included peak systolic velocity greater than 125 cm/s, internal:common carotid artery velocity ratio greater than 3, and intrastent doubling of velocity. Although very few stents showed significant restenosis, duplex ultrasonography was able to accurately identify restenosis, which correlated with angiographic findings at 1 year.

On the basis of these data, baseline duplex ultrasonography after CAS, which can be correlated with completion angiography and followed over time, is imperative. This policy will lead to fewer false-positive duplex studies. From the data presented, several recommendations regarding follow-up in patients having CAS can be made:

1) Duplex ultrasonographic follow-up of stented carotid arteries is an important tool to identify patients with restenosis. Early restenosis is typically secondary to myointimal hyperplasia.
2) Because follow-up duplex ultrasonography studies may be difficult to interpret on the basis of traditional velocity criteria, a baseline study is imperative; this must be correlated with the degree of residual stenosis at the completion of the CAS procedure. Subsequent studies should be performed at 3, 6, and 12 months, and at 6- to 12-month intervals thereafter.

Current evidence suggests that a peak systolic velocity of 150 cm/s or less in the internal carotid artery correlates with a normal vessel (0%-19% stenosis). Elevation of the peak systolic velocity and the internal:common carotid artery velocity ratio (>80% increase) may be even more important criteria in determining significant restenosis after CAS. Identification of high-grade restenosis typically warrants further evaluation with contrast angiography. Most patients having recurrent stenosis complicating CAS can be safely treated with repeat angioplasty.

- Duplex ultrasonographic follow-up of stented carotid arteries is an important tool to identify patients with restenosis
- Early restenosis is typically secondary to myointimal hyperplasia
- A baseline study must be correlated with the degree of residual stenosis at the completion of the CAS procedure
- Subsequent studies should be performed at 3, 6, and 12 months, and at 6- to 12-month intervals thereafter
- Most patients having recurrent stenosis complicating CAS can be safely treated with repeat angioplasty

Technical Aspects of CAS

Anatomy

The anatomy of the cerebral circulation, from the aortic arch to the capillary level, is important to the planning of CAS. Several anatomic considerations are particularly germane to the procedure. The configuration of the aortic arch is perhaps the first anatomic challenge to consider. With advancing age, the apex of the arch tends to become displaced distally. This change in arch configuration makes selective catheterization of the brachiocephalic vessels more challenging and influences the choice of catheter. The operator should become familiar with various selective catheters, including those which enable deep cannulation of the common carotid artery; this facilitates ultimate passage of a guidewire for delivery of a sheath. As the level of the object vessel's origin increases in distance from the dome of the arch, the degree of difficulty in obtaining guidewire and sheath access increases. Cannulation of a left common carotid artery arising from a common brachiocephalic trunk (bovine arch) may be particularly difficult; a bovine arch should be identified on preprocedural contrast aortography or magnetic resonance aortography. A complete study of all structures is essential, including the aortic arch and origins of the brachiocephalic trunks.

The presence of tandem lesions along the course of the cerebral circulation is likewise an important consideration in treatment planning. Proximal common carotid artery lesions may require intervention before internal carotid artery revascularization, in order to provide safe access to the internal carotid artery. Tortuosity of the internal carotid is also relevant; although most internal carotid arteries are relatively straight, extreme tortuosity may preclude safe passage of a guidewire or protection device and may exclude patients from safe intervention. The anatomy and configuration of the external carotid artery is typically not an important consideration in carotid intervention, even if this vessel is iatrogenically stenosed or covered with a bare stent.

Finally, collateral circulation (or lack thereof) through the circle of Willis is an important consideration that may profoundly influence procedural strategy. The status of the contralateral internal carotid artery, the vertebrobasilar system, and the intracranial collaterals may affect the type of embolic protection to be used. Anatomic variations in the circle of Willis are the rule rather than the exception. A "complete" circle is present in less than half of all cases. Common variations include a hypoplastic

(10%) or absent A1 segment and a plexiform (10%-33%) or duplicated (18%) anterior communicating artery. Anomalies of the posterior portion of the circle of Willis occur in half of all cases, including a hypoplastic (33%) or absent posterior communicating artery. Careful attention should be paid, on preprocedural angiography or intracranial magnetic resonance angiography, to the anterior and posterior communicating arteries. Patients with limited collateral circulation may have reversible neurologic symptoms with inflation of a protection balloon or during angioplasty of the target lesion. They may also be at higher risk for permanent neurologic deficits, because their limited collateral blood supply is less likely to compensate for any iatrogenic arterial occlusions complicating the procedure.

- A "complete" circle of Willis is present in less than half of all persons

Cerebral Protection During CAS

Stroke remains the most devastating complication of procedures (both surgical and interventional) directed at the extracranial carotid artery. Although stroke can have several causes, most are due to cerebral embolization of atheromatous debris or thrombus. CEA can be performed without mobilization and dissection of the carotid bulb, but the same cannot be said for CAS, in which the lesion must be crossed with a guidewire, balloon, and stent. This requirement has led to the development of devices to prevent atheromatous embolization during critical portions of the procedure. Most would predict that unprotected angioplasty and stenting of high-grade, ulcerated carotid lesions would produce stroke rates of at least 25%, but even with relatively crude equipment and a lack of cerebral protection, early series of CAS produced stroke rates far below this level.

Even if cerebral emboli do not produce major stroke, they may cause substantial cognitive impairment. In a prospective study of 100 patients monitored with transcranial Doppler during carotid intervention, microemboli were detected during 92% of procedures. Although most emboli were characteristic of air (and not associated with adverse clinical events), more than 10 particulate emboli correlated with significant deterioration in postoperative cognitive function. In a study of the embolic potential of carotid plaques during experimental angioplasty, an average of 133 emboli per angioplasty were measured; lesion severity correlated significantly with increased maximum size of embolic particles (P=.01). Patients receiving statin therapy for more than 4 weeks preoperatively had significantly fewer emboli of smaller size (P=.02).

In a clinical study of the use of a distal balloon occlusion system during CAS, the median number of particles, their maximum diameter, and their maximum area were significantly higher in patients who had periprocedural neurologic complications. Three phases of the procedure are associated with an increased risk of embolization: predilatation, stent deployment, and post dilatation.

Devices for Cerebral Embolic Protection

Three types of embolic protection—distal balloon occlusion, distal filter protection, and reversal of internal carotid flow—are currently available for use in the carotid artery; use of the methods is either a part of FDA-approved clinical trials or "off label" with devices approved for non-carotid use. The first research group to use an angioplasty technique involving temporary occlusion of the internal carotid artery during manipulation of ulcerated plaques subsequently reported on a triple-coaxial catheter system allowing angioplasty with cerebral protection in 13 patients. Cholesterol crystals of 600 to 1,200 microns were aspirated at the time of intervention.

One device approved for aorto-coronary saphenous vein graft intervention, used in the MAVErIC (Evaluation of the Medtronic AVE Self-Expanding Carotid Stent System with Distal Protection in the Treatment of Carotid Stenosis) trial of carotid intervention, has been used off label extensively during carotid intervention. Advantages of this device include its low profile, ease of crossing the target lesion, procedural simplicity, and its ability to aspirate large particulate debris after intervention. Disadvantages include potential incomplete occlusion of the internal carotid artery in patients with particularly large arteries (the device can be inflated to 3-6 mm in diameter) and inability to aspirate exceptionally large particles into the suction catheter after intervention. In addition, as flow is diverted into the external carotid artery, emboli may travel by this route and into the ipsilateral middle cerebral artery via periorbital and ophthalmic artery collaterals.

A small percentage of patients with an incomplete circle of Willis and an "isolated" cerebral hemisphere may be intolerant of even temporary internal carotid occlusion. The same device was evaluated in 75 CAS procedures; four patients (5%) had development of transient neurologic symptoms during balloon occlusion which resolved with deflation and restoration of internal carotid flow. Embolic material was aspirated from the internal carotid artery in all patients; no patients had major or minor stroke within 30 days.

A great deal of interest has been generated in filter protection devices in an attempt to trap large particulate debris while maintaining flow in the internal carotid; this not only provides continued cerebral perfusion during intervention, but also allows angiography of the target vessel during various phases of the procedure. The pore size of all currently available filters is greater than 100 microns;

thus, they allow passage of smaller particles that may not cause clinically significant neurologic events but may cause silent neuronal injury. These filters may also be difficult to pass across particularly severe stenoses because of their larger profile when compared with balloon occlusion devices. Filters that are not completely apposed to the vessel wall may allow emboli to pass around the device and into the distal cerebral circulation.

- The pore size of all currently available cerebral embolic protection filters is greater than 100 microns

Another device induces reversal of flow in the internal carotid artery by occluding the common and external carotid arteries via balloon occlusion of the external carotid and creation of a temporary arteriovenous shunt between the internal carotid artery and the femoral vein. This device, although potentially more cumbersome than other protection devices, may produce "complete" protection by preventing any emboli from traveling to the intracranial circulation.

In a study of 1,202 CAS procedures from 1994 to 2002, 33% of patients had a cerebral protection device used during their procedures. The overall stroke rate was 4.4%; the risk of stroke reached its maximum during the period of September 1996 to September 1997 (9.1%) and reached its nadir during the final year of the study (0.6%). Improvements in technique, equipment, pharmacotherapy, and the use of neuroprotection seem to have contributed substantially to the improved results.

Protection devices are not without potential problems and complications including abrupt vessel closure secondary to iatrogenic dissection, inability to retrieve the device, transient loss of consciousness, and tremors and fasciculations secondary to device-induced cerebral ischemia. Nevertheless, it seems reasonable, on the basis of the available evidence, to consider using embolic cerebral protection devices in most CAS procedures.

Pharmacologic Adjuncts for the Prevention of Intraprocedural Stroke

The pharmacologic prevention of thromboembolic events during CAS is modeled after the literature regarding prevention of these events during percutaneous coronary interventions. Intravenous heparin should be administered to maintain an activated clotting time of at least 250 to 300 seconds. Antiplatelet therapy consists of aspirin and clopidogrel orally before the procedure and for 1 month after. Antiplatelet therapy with glycoprotein IIB/IIIA antagonists has been shown to decrease thromboembolic complications during percutaneous coronary procedures. Although there has been some interest in applying these agents to patients undergoing CAS, early data suggest that they offer no significant benefit and may increase the risk of intracerebral hemorrhage.

Complications After CAS

Embolic stroke is the most common serious complication reported with CAS; its incidence may be affected by the use of cerebral protection devices. Advanced age and the presence of long or multiple lesions have been implicated as independent predictors of stroke. As with most procedures, a significant learning curve must be overcome by the physician. Other complications have also been cited, including prolonged bradycardia and hypotension, deformation of balloon-expandable stents, stent thrombosis, and Horner syndrome. Cerebral hyperperfusion with associated seizures and intracranial hemorrhage have also been reported.

Future Directions

Based on the preliminary results of clinical trials of CAS in high-risk patients, the results of this procedure appear equivalent to those for CEA in this subgroup. The addition of cerebral protection, along with improvements in stents and better patient selection will likely add to its safety. The next logical question to be asked is whether low-risk patients can be safely treated with CAS. The Carotid Revascularization Endarterectomy versus Stent Trial (CREST) will attempt to provide a definitive answer. This important study contrasts the relative efficacy of CEA and CAS in preventing the primary outcomes of stroke, MI, or death at 30 days, and ipsilateral stroke at 4 years of follow-up. The primary criteria for eligibility are carotid stenosis of at least 50% and hemispheric TIA or non-disabling stroke. It is anticipated that 2,500 patients will be enrolled and randomly assigned. The outcome is not anticipated for several years, but randomization is the only way to definitively study this issue.

CAS is an evolving technique that shows considerable promise in the treatment of patients with carotid occlusive disease. CEA, however, remains the treatment of choice for most patients with bifurcation disease, both symptomatic and asymptomatic. At present, certain high-risk subsets of patients, especially those with cardiopulmonary disease and those with surgically unfavorable lesions, benefit from endovascular therapy.

- In high-risk patients, the results of CAS appear equivalent to those for CEA
- CEA remains the treatment of choice for most patients with bifurcation disease, both symptomatic and asymptomatic

Questions

1. The risk of stroke and death after CEA in the NASCET trial of surgery versus best medical therapy in symptomatic patients was:
   a. <1%
   b. 4.3%
   c. 5.8%
   d. 9.5%

2. In the ACAS trial, the risk of stroke and death after CEA in asymptomatic patients was:
   a. <1%
   b. 2.3%
   c. 3.5%
   d. 5.8%

3. The 30-day risk of stroke, death, and MI in the ARCHeR trial of carotid stenting in high surgical risk patients was:
   a. 2.3%
   b. 5.8%
   c. 6.9%
   d. 8.3%

4. CAS has been advocated for use in patients believed to be at high risk with surgical CEA. The SAPPHIRE study randomly assigned high-risk patients to CAS or CEA based on several specific criteria that included all of the following *except*:
   a. Age >65 years
   b. Lesions below the clavicle
   c. Restenosis after CEA
   d. Severe cardiac disease
   e. Severe renal disease

5. The incidence of restenosis after carotid angioplasty is typically reported as between 5% and 10% at 18 to 24 months after intervention. Of the following, which has *not* been associated with an increased risk of restenosis after CAS?
   a. Elevated levels of C-reactive protein after CAS
   b. Common carotid artery diameter >7 mm
   c. Incomplete stent apposition
   d. Female sex
   e. Residual stenosis after CAS

Suggested Readings

Bicknell CD, Cowling MG, Clark MW, et al. Carotid angioplasty in a pulsatile flow model: factors affecting embolic potential. Eur J Vasc Endovasc Surg. 2003;26:22-31.

Bonita R. Epidemiology of stroke. Lancet. 1992;339:342-4.

Chakhtoura EY, Hobson RW II, Goldstein J, et al. In-stent restenosis after carotid angioplasty-stenting: incidence and management. J Vasc Surg. 2001;33:220-5.

Christiaans MH, Ernst JM, Suttorp MJ, et al, Antonius Carotid Endarterectomy, Angioplasty, and Stenting Study Group. Restenosis after carotid angioplasty and stenting: a follow-up study with duplex ultrasonography. Eur J Vasc Endovasc Surg. 2003;26:141-4.

Crawley F, Clifton A, Markus H, et al. Delayed improvement in carotid artery diameter after carotid angioplasty. Stroke. 1997;28:574-9.

Criado FJ, Lingelbach JM, Ledesma DF, et al. Carotid artery stenting in a vascular surgery practice. J Vasc Surg. 2002;35:430-4.

Executive Committee for the Asymptomatic Carotid Atherosclerosis Study. Endarterectomy for asymptomatic carotid artery stenosis. JAMA. 1995;273:1421-8.

Gaunt ME, Martin PJ, Smith JL, et al. Clinical relevance of intraoperative embolization detected by transcranial Doppler ultrasonography during carotid endarterectomy: a prospective study of 100 patients. Br J Surg. 1994;81:1435-9.

Gray WA, Hopkins LN, Yadav S, et al, ARCHeR Trial Collaborators. Protected carotid stenting in high-surgical-risk patients: the ARCHeR results. J Vasc Surg. 2006;44:258-68.

Hertzer NR, O'Hara PJ, Mascha EJ, et al. Early outcome assessment for 2228 consecutive carotid endarterectomy procedures: the Cleveland Clinic experience from 1989 to 1995. J Vasc Surg. 1997;26:1-10.

Khan MA, Liu MW, Chio FL, et al. Predictors of restenosis after successful carotid artery stenting. Am J Cardiol. 2003;92:895-7.

Lal BK, Hobson RW II, Goldstein J, et al. In-stent recurrent stenosis after carotid artery stenting: life table analysis and clinical relevance. J Vasc Surg. 2003;38:1162-8.

Mozes G, Sullivan TM, Torres-Russotto DR, et al. Carotid endarterectomy in SAPPHIRE-eligible high-risk patients: implications for selecting patients for carotid angioplasty and stenting. J Vasc Surg. 2004;39:958-65.

New G, Roubin GS, Iyer SS, et al. Outcomes from carotid artery stenting in over 1,000 cases from a single group of operators [abstract]. J Am Coll Cardiol. 2003;41 Suppl A:79A.

North American Symptomatic Carotid Endarterectomy Trial Collaborators. Beneficial effect of carotid endarterectomy in symptomatic patients with high-grade carotid stenosis. N Engl J Med. 1991;325:445-53.

Ohki T, Parodi J, Veith FJ, et al. Efficacy of a proximal occlusion catheter with reversal of flow in the prevention of embolic events during carotid artery stenting: an experimental analysis. J Vasc Surg. 2001;33:504-9.

Ouriel K, Hertzer NR, Beven EG, et al. Preprocedural risk stratification: identifying an appropriate population for carotid stenting. J Vasc Surg. 2001;33:728-32.

Schillinger M, Exner M, Mlekusch W, et al. Acute-phase response after stent implantation in the carotid artery: association with 6-month in-stent restenosis. Radiology. 2003 May;227:516-21. Epub 2003 Mar 20.

Theron J, Raymond J, Casasco A, et al. Percutaneous angioplasty of atherosclerotic and postsurgical stenosis of carotid arteries. AJNR Am J Neuroradiol. 1987;8:495-500.

Tübler T, Schlüter M, Dirsch O, et al. Balloon-protected carotid artery stenting: relationship of periprocedural neurological complications with the size of particulate debris. Circulation. 2001;104:2791-6.

Whitlow PL, Lylyk P, Londero H, et al. Carotid artery stenting protected with an emboli containment system. Stroke. 2002;33:1308-14.

Yadav JS, Roubin GS, Iyer S, et al. Elective stenting of the extracranial carotid arteries. Circulation. 1997;95:376-81.

Yadav JS, Wholey MH, Kuntz RE, et al, Stenting and Angioplasty With Protection in Patients at High Risk for Endarterectomy Investigators. Protected carotid-artery stenting versus endarterectomy in high-risk patients. N Engl J Med. 2004;351:1493-501.

26 Endovascular Treatment of Renal and Mesenteric Arterial Stenosis

Haraldur Bjarnason, MD

Renal Artery Occlusive Disease

Epidemiology

Renal artery stenosis is associated with hypertension, renal insufficiency, or a combination of both conditions, and is often silent and asymptomatic. Renal artery disease can be primary (affecting the main renal arteries) or secondary to systemic disease such as diabetes mellitus (affecting the parenchyma vessels). This chapter will focus on disease affecting the main renal arteries.

Hypertension has been estimated to affect approximately 50 million persons in the United States and approximately 1 billion worldwide. Atherosclerotic renal artery disease is estimated to be a causative factor in 1% to 3% of patients with arterial hypertension and in 20% to 25% of patients who respond inadequately to medical therapy. The condition is also thought to be the cause of renal failure in 5% to 15% of adult patients who eventually require dialysis. Kidneys supplied by renal arteries with atherosclerotic occlusion or stenoses have a high incidence of atrophy over a relatively short period of observation.

Renal artery occlusive disease is associated with coronary, cerebrovascular, and peripheral arterial disease. The prevalence of significant (>50% luminal diameter narrowing) renal artery stenosis was 6.3% for unilateral lesions and 1.3% for bilateral disease in a group of patients undergoing coronary angiography. New or progressive renal artery stenosis was noted in 11.1% of patients after an average follow-up of 2.6 years. These findings agree with data from other studies. Postmortem cadaver studies have shown a 4.3% to 24% incidence of renal artery stenosis, and studies of patients older than 40 years showed renal artery stenosis in 10.4% (2.9% bilateral) of patients with history of stroke and in 12% (3.4% bilateral) of patients with history of myocardial infarction.

Fibromuscular dysplasia is also a causative factor for renal artery hypertension, responsible for less than 10% of cases of renal artery stenosis. Fibromuscular dysplasia mainly affects young women at an age of 15 to 50 years but is not uncommonly observed in older patients. Even though fibromuscular dysplasia is most common in the renal arteries (60%-70% of patients with known fibromuscular dysplasia), it is also found in the carotid arteries, vertebral arteries, and other visceral and peripheral arteries. If the renal arteries are involved, the disease is bilateral in 35% of the cases.

- Renal artery stenosis can cause hypertension and renal functional impairment, or a combination of both
- Renal artery stenosis is the cause of 1%-3% of all cases of hypertension and 20%-25% of difficult-to-treat hypertension
- In 5%-15% of patients who eventually require dialysis, renal artery stenosis is the main causative factor
- Fibromuscular dysplasia of the renal arteries causes <10% of renal artery stenoses

Etiology

The most common causes of renal artery stenosis are atherosclerosis and fibromuscular dysplasia, but many other conditions also can cause renal artery stenosis, some of which are listed in Table 26.1. Only atherosclerosis and fibromuscular dysplasia are of general practicality; the others are infrequently encountered in clinical practice.

Atherosclerotic renal artery stenosis is responsible for approximately 90% of all renal artery stenoses. It typically affects the ostium and the proximal one-third of the renal artery, but in advanced cases the disease can affect the entire main renal artery and even extend into the renal artery branches (Fig. 26.1).

Table 26.1 Causes of Renal Artery Stenosis

Cause	Affected segment	Incidence, %
Atherosclerosis	Ostium and proximal 1/3 of artery	90
Fibromuscular dysplasia	Mid and distal 1/3 of artery	10
Takayasu arteritis	Ostium and proximal part of artery	<1
Neurofibromatosis, type 1	All	<1
Radiation	All	<1
Renal artery entrapment by diaphragmatic crus	Entire artery	<1
Moyamoya	Proximal 1/3 more frequent	<1
Trauma	All	<1

A

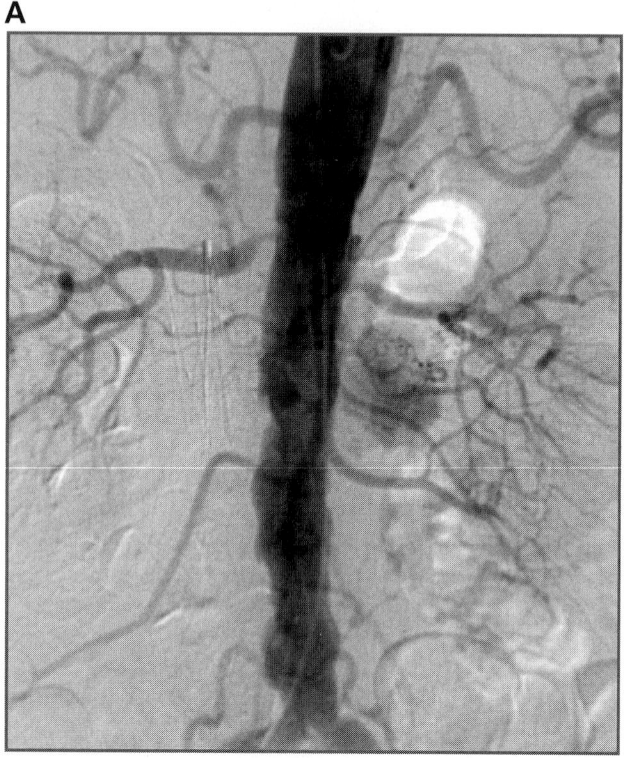

B

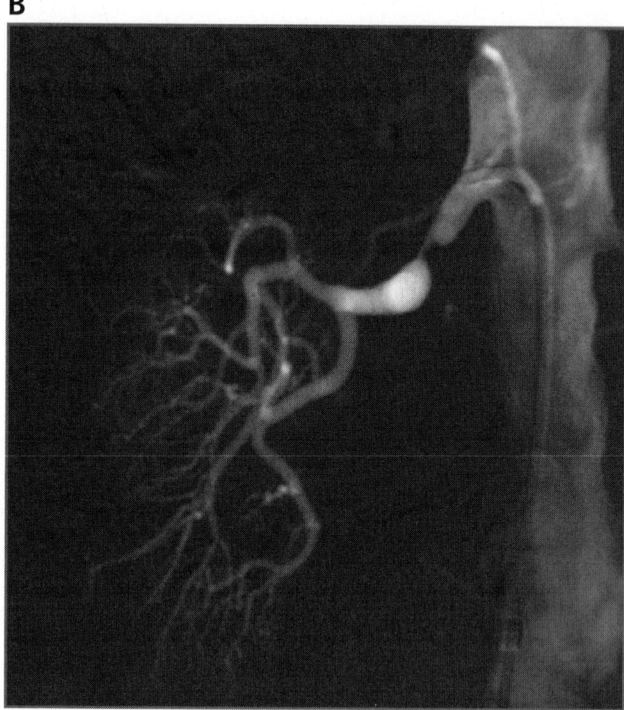

Fig. 26.1 Angiographic images of renal artery stenosis. *A*, Typical bilateral renal artery stenosis confined to the ostia of both renal arteries. Note the irregularity of the aortic lumen caused by atherosclerosis. The ostial lesions are part of the aortic atherosclerotic plaque. *B*, Unusual atherosclerotic stenosis of the body of the right renal artery.

Fibromuscular dysplasia causes about 10% of cases of renal artery stenosis and can be roughly divided into several main categories based on the affected layers of the vessel wall.

1) Medial fibroplasia represents the most common type; it affects the media but not the intima, internal elastic lamina, or adventitia. It is characterized by the so-called "string of beads," which are relatively short saccular dilated areas separated by bands or webs of fibrotic tissue causing relative stenosis of the vessel. The combination of stenotic webs and turbulence in ectatic areas may cause a hemodynamically significant stenosis within the vessel (Fig. 26.2).
2) Perimedial fibroplasia, which affects the arterial wall at the junction of the media and adventitia, is characterized by longer stenotic segments caused by a collar of elastic tissue. This results in elongated narrowing and less prominent beading.
3) Intimal fibroplasia constitutes less than 10% of all fibroplasias and commonly presents as a concentric, long, smooth stenosis that can resemble Takayasu arteritis or temporal (giant cell) arteritis, usually seen in larger arteries. This can also appear as a redundant artery.
4) Adventitial (periarterial) hyperplasia presents as long segments of tubular smooth narrowing.

Fibromuscular dysplasia most commonly affects the mid to distal portion of the main renal artery. The branch vessels are also commonly affected, but the ostium and the proximal one-third of the vessel are rarely involved.

A

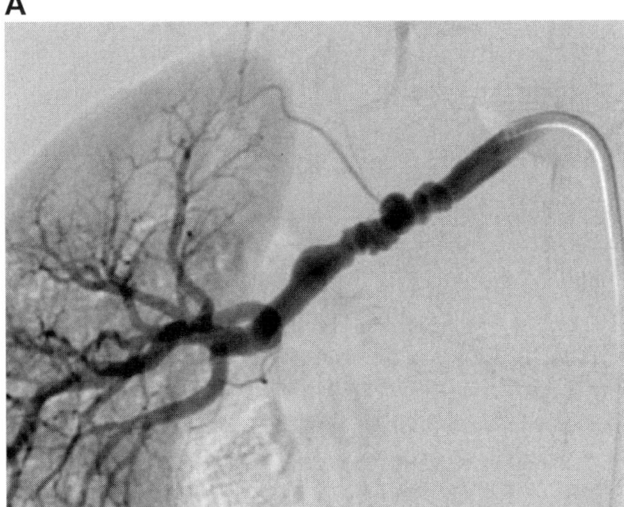

B

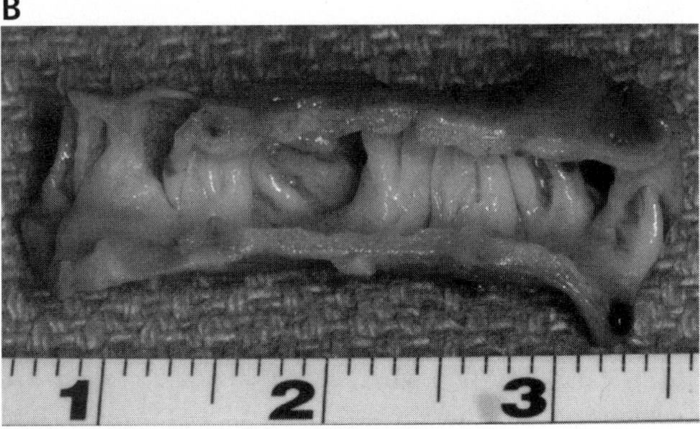

Fig. 26.2 Medial fibromuscular dysplasia. *A*, Typical angiographic findings of medial fibromuscular dysplasia in the right main renal artery. Note the alternating web-like stenosis and almost aneurysmal areas between. *B*, Surgical specimen from a renal artery with medial fibromuscular dysplasia, with findings similar to those seen by angiography.

Aneurysms and dissection are not uncommon complications of fibromuscular dysplasia. Aneurysms can rupture, causing severe life-threatening bleeding. Such aneurysms are usually treated surgically or can sometimes be embolized using endovascular techniques. Spontaneous dissections are also well-recognized complications of fibromuscular dysplasia. Dissections may cause decreased flow through the involved vascular bed or occlusion. The dissection flap tends to continue into more peripheral branch vessels, leading to branch vessel occlusion with infarcts or severe renal ischemia in smaller or larger portions of the kidney. Both of these complications are associated with renovascular hypertension.

- 90% of renal artery stenoses are caused by atherosclerosis and the remaining 10% by fibromuscular dysplasia
- Atherosclerotic stenoses are usually confined to the ostium and proximal one-third of the main renal artery
- Fibromuscular dysplasia usually affects the mid to distal portion of the vessel and often includes the branch vessels
- Both fibromuscular dysplasia and atherosclerotic disease of the renal arteries are progressive conditions
- The so-called "string of beads" is typical of medial fibromuscular dysplasia, the most common type
- Renal atrophy is seen in kidneys affected with fibromuscular dysplastic and atherosclerotic renal artery stenosis

Natural History

Atherosclerotic and fibromuscular renal artery stenoses are both progressive conditions. Using angiography, investigators have shown that the severity of fibromuscular dysplasia progresses in 37% of the cases, on the basis of increasing numbers of aneurysms, worsening obstructions, and new lesions.

The complicated "string of beads" appearance of medial fibroplasia makes it difficult to estimate disease progression by angiography. Cortical thickness has been shown to decrease over time in kidneys with unilateral fibromuscular dysplasia and hypertension. This same trend was not seen in patients with essential hypertension. However, renal failure is rare in patients with fibromuscular dysplasia. In a study of healthy kidney donors undergoing preoperative angiography, the incidence of fibromuscular dysplasia was 3.8%, and 26.6% of those who did not donate had subsequent development of hypertension over the following 7.5 years.

Atherosclerotic renal artery stenosis is also progressive; 51% of patients with atherosclerotic disease of the renal artery will have substantial progression over 5 years. A follow-up study using duplex scanning evaluated 295 kidneys over 33 months. Baseline study results included 56 normal renal arteries, 96 with less than 60% stenosis, and 143 with 60% stenosis or more. Overall progression of the stenosis occurred in 91 patients (31%). Progression was common (49%) in the most severely stenotic group, compared with 28% in the moderate stenosis group; renal artery stenosis developed in 18% of the initially normal renal arteries during the study period. Nine occlusions occurred, two in the group with less than 60% stenosis (2.1%) and seven (4.9%) in the group with at least 60% stenosis.

In a separate paper from the same group of investigators, renal artery obstruction caused renal atrophy over 2-year follow-up in 20.8% of patients with at least 60% stenosis and in 11.7% of those with less than 60% stenosis. In patients with no stenosis, renal size decreased in 5.5% of the population. Similar findings have been reported in other studies, demonstrating progression of the renal artery stenosis, with less than 50% stenosis seen in only 11.1% of patients over 2.6 years.

Endovascular Treatment

Endovascular treatment of renal artery stenosis involves either percutaneous transluminal angioplasty or a combination of angioplasty and stent placement. Stents are almost exclusively placed in the renal arteries by using an angioplasty balloon (balloon-expandable rather than self-expanding stents).

Atherosclerosis and fibromuscular dysplasia respond very differently to angioplasty and will therefore be discussed separately. Stents are now used almost exclusively for atherosclerotic renal artery stenoses, whereas stent placement is infrequently indicated in the treatment of fibromuscular dysplasia.

Historically, surgery was the accepted standard of therapy for renal artery fibromuscular dysplasia, but it has now been replaced by angioplasty. Many small, retrospective studies with short follow-up have been published on the outcomes of angioplasty for renal artery fibromuscular dysplasia, but longitudinal studies reporting long-term outcomes are rare. The reported technical success rates for angioplasty vary from 83% to 100%, with reported cure rates of 22% to 59%. Improvement is commonly seen in 21% to 79% of treated patients; 2% to 26% will have no improvement in blood pressure after angioplasty for fibromuscular dysplasia. Complications are infrequent, occurring in up to 14%; most are minor and related to vascular access.

A recently published report of 59 patients treated with angioplasty for fibromuscular dysplasia (the longest reported follow-up was 7 years) showed a 24% cure rate and a 39% improvement in hypertension. Seven patients had compromised renal function before angioplasty; five still had normal renal function 7 years after angioplasty, and in two patients renal function was unchanged from before angioplasty.

Complications of angioplasty are relatively few, and the procedure has become safer with improved equipment. Renal artery rupture and dissections appear to be less common now than in the early days of angioplasty, perhaps related to improved balloons and guidewires, better patient selection, and improved periprocedural care. The success of angioplasty for fibromuscular dysplasia appears to be inversely related to the duration of hypertension before angioplasty and to age greater than 50 years. The outcome appears to be worse with a concomitant history of atherosclerotic coronary or carotid artery disease.

Compared with the relatively good outcomes after angioplasty for fibromuscular dysplasia, balloon angioplasty alone has not been as successful in treating atherosclerotic renal artery stenosis. This is most likely because of the high degree of elastic recoil in atherosclerotic arteries compared with that encountered in fibromuscular webs. The restenosis rate after angioplasty alone varies widely but has been reported to be from 10% to 46%. Angioplasty (without stent placement) has a higher technical success rate when applied to atherosclerotic lesions in the mid portion of the main renal artery (72%-82%) than in ostial lesions (success rate ≈60%).

Stents are now almost uniformly used for all ostial lesions and almost all atherosclerotic renal artery stenoses (Fig. 26.3). One current report quotes a technical success rate for stents of 94% to 100% and a restenosis rate of 11% to 23%, with an improvement in blood pressure control in 50% to 80% and stabilization of renal function in 60% to 70%.

A

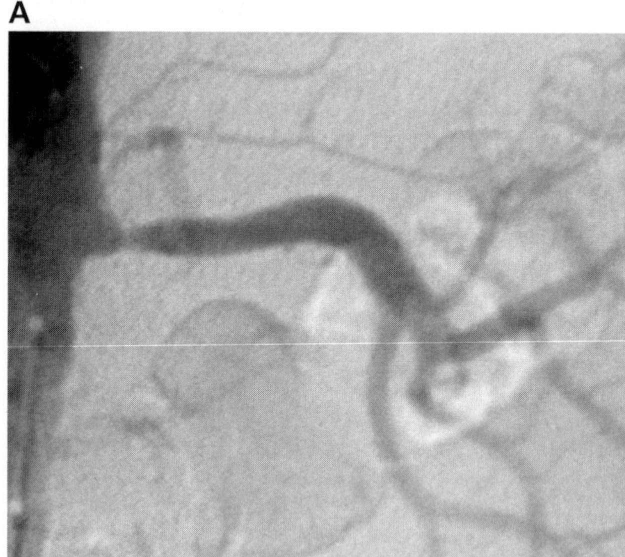

B

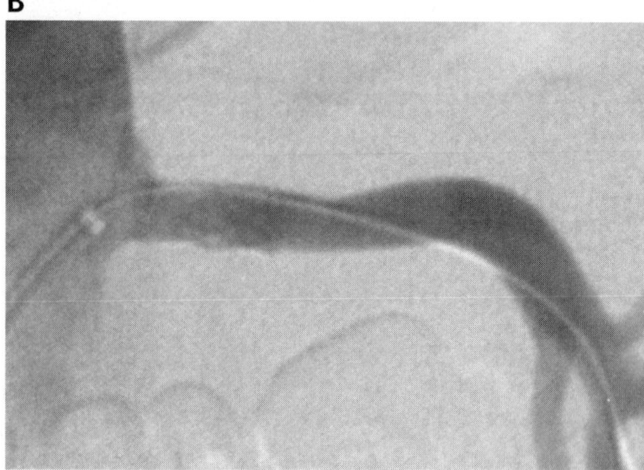

Fig. 26.3 Preprocedural and postprocedural images of angioplasty and stent placement for renal artery stenosis. *A*, Angiographic image demonstrates a short stenosis of the left renal artery close to or at the ostium. The severity of the stenosis is approximately 70% based on vessel diameter. *B*, After placement of a balloon-expandable stent, the lumen has been restored. The stent should extend slightly (1-2 mm) into the aortic lumen for an ostial stenosis.

Renal function at the time of stent placement strongly predicts patency and expected survival after intervention. In patients with normal renal function, 3-year survival is 94%, 74% if serum creatinine is between 1.5 and 2.0 mg/dL, and 52% if serum creatinine is greater than 2.0 mg/dL.

- The cure rate with angioplasty for renal artery fibromuscular dysplasia is approximately 25%, and some improvement can be expected in approximately 40%
- Stent placement is now the preferred treatment for most patients with atherosclerotic renal artery disease
- The technical success rate for renal artery stent placement for atherosclerotic stenosis is >90%
- The restenosis rate is 15%-20% after renal artery angioplasty and stenting; improvement in blood pressure control can be expected in >50% and stabilization or improvement in >60%

Imaging the Renal Arteries

Conventional angiography is still considered the best anatomic study for evaluating patients with renal artery stenosis. Duplex ultrasonography can be very helpful and should be the first imaging study in patients suspected of having renal artery stenosis. The quality of renal ultrasonography depends on the operator and on other variables such as body habitus, but even so, the sensitivity of duplex scanning has been reported to be 98%, with 98% specificity and high positive and negative predictive values.

In many practices, computed tomography angiography (CTA) is now replacing conventional angiography as the anatomic test of choice for evaluating renal arteries. The images are comparable to those of conventional angiography, vessels can be evaluated in three dimensions, and CTA offers options for clarifying anatomy which may be better than with conventional angiography. Exposure of the patient to radiation from renal CTA is comparable to that from catheter angiography.

Magnetic resonance angiography (MRA) is also a good test to evaluate the anatomy of the renal arteries. It has lower resolution than CTA or conventional angiography but is excellent for patients with impaired renal function because the contrast agent (gadolinium) is relatively non-nephrotoxic.

Mesenteric Arterial Occlusive Disease

This discussion will focus on atherosclerotic lesions, which are responsible for more than 90% of all cases of chronic mesenteric ischemia. It is crucial to understand the basic vascular supply to the bowel. The supply from the stomach to the distal rectum is provided by 3 major vessels: the celiac artery, the superior mesenteric artery, and the inferior mesenteric artery. A rich collateral vascular bed exists between these three vessels. Asymptomatic stenosis of one or more of the three arteries is not uncommon; one angiographic study showed more than 50% stenosis of either the celiac or superior mesenteric artery in 27% of asymptomatic patients. The usual symptom of chronic mesenteric ischemia is abdominal pain, which typically starts 30 minutes after food intake (postprandial pain) and may last for up to 3 hours. Patients exhibit "food fear" with resultant weight loss.

Epidemiology

Chronic mesenteric ischemia is rare, with an incidence of only 2 to 4 patients per 100,000, and affects mostly elderly women. Acute mesenteric ischemia accounts for approximately 0.1% of all hospital admissions. Estimates suggest that only 20% to 50% of these patients have underlying mesenteric artery stenosis. Most patients with atherosclerotic mesenteric artery stenosis have classic symptoms of chronic mesenteric ischemia before acute occlusion develops. This allows for corrective intervention—either surgical or endovascular—on the mesenteric vessels, thus averting an acute event.

- Chronic mesenteric ischemia is more common in elderly women
- The incidence of chronic mesenteric ischemia is low (2-4 per 100,000 patients)

Etiology

The cause of chronic mesenteric ischemia in most cases (>90%) is atherosclerosis, but many other causes have been associated with the condition (Table 26.2). Approximately half of patients with chronic mesenteric ischemia also have significant coronary artery disease and peripheral vascular disease.

- Atherosclerotic changes in the central mesenteric arteries are the most common causes of chronic mesenteric ischemia
- A large proportion of patients with chronic mesenteric ischemia have coronary or carotid artery disease

Natural History

Even less is known about the natural history of chronic mesenteric ischemia than about that of renal artery stenotic disease. The disease is progressive, and some patients with mesenteric artery stenosis eventually have symptoms of chronic mesenteric ischemia. In a 1998 study

Table 26.2 Causes of Chronic Mesenteric Arterial Occlusion

Cause	Affected segment	Incidence, %
Atherosclerosis	Ostium and first portion	90
Median arcuate ligament compression syndrome	Ostium celiac >> superior mesenteric artery	<5
Fibromuscular dysplasia	Main artery	<5
Takayasu arteritis	Ostium and proximal part of artery	<1
Giant cell arteritis (temporal arteritis)	Main artery	<1
Radiation	All	<1
Thromboangiitis obliterans	All	<1
Mesenteric vein thrombosis	Venous	<1

of 60 patients with severe angiographic mesenteric stenosis, four (7%) had development of mesenteric ischemia, one of whom presented with acute mesenteric ischemia and subsequently died. These four patients belonged to a cohort of 15 (27%) that had three-vessel disease (superior mesenteric, celiac, and inferior mesenteric artery). None of the other patients had symptoms of mesenteric ischemia during the study period.

The mortality rate for patients with asymptomatic mesenteric arterial stenosis is high. Over a mean follow-up of 2.6 years, 40% of the patients in one study (29 of 72, 12 with less severe disease) died from other causes and only one from acute mesenteric ischemia. Although highly controversial, the practice of prophylactic intervention in asymptomatic patients with significant three-vessel mesenteric artery stenosis is recommended by the authors of this study. They also suggest that patients with asymptomatic one- or two-vessel disease be followed up closely.

- Patients with silent mesenteric arterial stenosis of two or more arteries should be followed up on a regular basis; there are currently no data to support intervention in asymptomatic patients
- Patients with mesenteric artery stenosis have a high mortality rate from other causes

Endovascular Treatment

Surgical management has traditionally been the treatment of choice for chronic mesenteric ischemia, but endovascular therapy (angioplasty alone or with stent placement) has become commonplace in the management of these patients. The outcomes are highly variable, with frequent complications (19%-54%) and significant mortality (0%-17%) after surgical repair. Surgical options include endarterectomy and bypass using synthetic or autologous conduits.

Most atherosclerotic lesions occur in the ostium or the first two to three centimeters of the vessel but can extend into the more distal aspects in some patients (Fig. 26.4). Initial technical success after endovascular repair is typically greater for ostial lesions (95%) than for more distal lesions. Most reports indicate technical success rates between 88% and 100%, with long-term symptom relief in the range of 61% to 91%. The restenosis rate is relatively low, with primary patency rates of 60% to 85% and secondary patency rates up to 100%. Recurrence rates are higher for celiac intervention, possibly because of the cruciate ligament, which may compress a stent in the celiac artery. Angioplasty and stent placement are not advocated for the treatment of celiac artery stenosis caused by compression by the median ligaments.

A recent paper on stenting the superior mesenteric and/or celiac artery in 14 patients reported technical success in 17 of 18 treated arteries (94%). No perioperative deaths or major morbidity was reported; mean hospital stay was 2 days. The mean length of follow-up was 13 months, during which restenosis developed in 8 patients (57%), with a mean of 9 months from the initial procedure to the time of reintervention. Seven patients were treated with repeat angioplasty or placement of an additional stent. Subsequent fatal acute mesenteric ischemia developed in one of the patients.

A recent abstract from Mayo Clinic reported outcomes of surgical and endovascular treatment for chronic mesenteric ischemia in 229 consecutive patients. Surgical revascularization was performed in 146 patients (265 vessels) and endovascular revascularization with either angioplasty alone or angioplasty and stent placement was performed in 83 patients (105 vessels). Surgical revascularization resulted in higher early morbidity and longer hospitalization but no greater mortality than in the endovascular group. Incidences of recurrent symptoms and restenosis were significantly higher, and reintervention was needed more commonly, in the endovascular group than in the surgically treated group. The recommendation was that surgical revascularization should be offered to "good risk" patients, whereas endovascular revascularization should be reserved for patients who were at high surgical risk.

- Surgical bypass is the preferred therapy for most patients with low surgical risk and chronic mesenteric ischemia

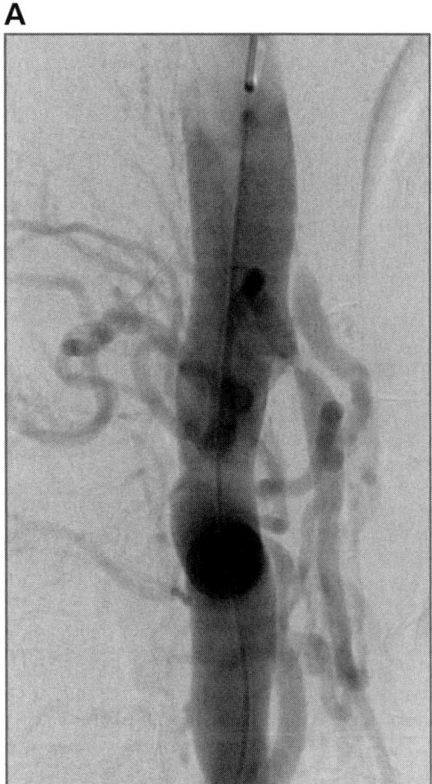

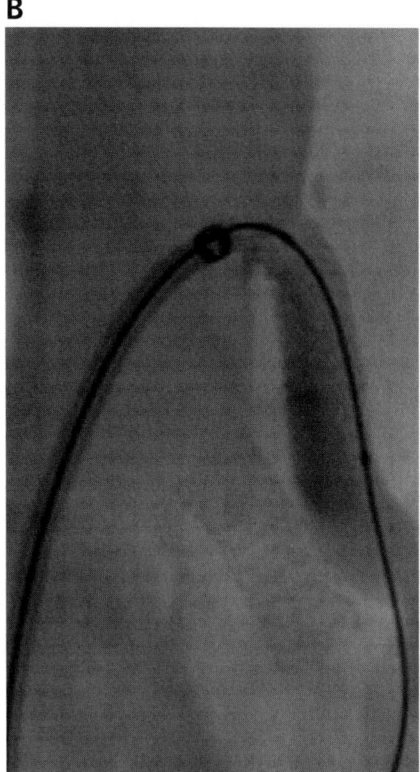

Fig. 26.4 Preprocedural and postprocedural images of angioplasty and stent placement for mesenteric artery stenosis. *A*, Lateral aortography showing tight stenosis of the celiac axis origin and the superior mesenteric artery origin caused by atherosclerosis. (The head is toward the top of the image.) *B*, After placement of balloon-expandable stents across both ostial stenoses, a good lumen was restored with subsequent good clinical response.

- Clinical success for mesenteric artery angioplasty and stenting is in the range of 60%-90%

Imaging the Mesenteric Arteries

Angiography is still regarded as the gold standard for arterial imaging of the mesenteric arteries. Over the past 5 to 10 years, considerable progress has been made in both CTA (with introduction of multislice scanners) and MRA. Ultrasonography with Doppler should still be the first imaging study for suspected chronic mesenteric arterial disease. Color Doppler can identify narrow areas of the vessels, but Doppler peak-velocity measurements give an accurate indication of the severity of the vascular disease.

For mesenteric arterial disease, a peak systolic velocity of more than 275 cm/s, either in the celiac or superior mesenteric artery, predicts a 70% stenosis with a sensitivity of 92% and a specificity of 96%. Like renal duplex ultrasonography, this technique is dependent on operator experience and patient body habitus.

In recent years, CTA has become an excellent tool for anatomic evaluation of the mesenteric circulation. This is largely due to the multislice CT scanners that can cover the entire body in less than 10 seconds and obtain sub-millimeter resolution. MRA is also a good study for anatomic evaluation but does not have the resolution of CTA or conventional angiography and may therefore be somewhat less predictable.

Questions

1. Which statement regarding fibromuscular dysplasia is true?
   a. It is more common in men.
   b. The renal arteries are the only affected visceral arteries.
   c. It can be seen in the iliac arteries.
   d. Fibromuscular dysplasia usually resolves by age 20 years.

2. Which of the following can cause renal artery stenosis?
   a. Neurofibromatosis
   b. Radiation
   c. Trauma
   d. Takayasu arteritis
   e. All of the above

3. Which statement is true?
   a. Aneurysms are common complications of fibromuscular dysplasia.
   b. Atherosclerosis constitutes approximately 10% of all renal artery stenoses, and fibromuscular dysplasia, 90%.
   c. Atherosclerotic stenoses are most common in the main body of the main renal artery rather than at the ostium.

d. "String of beads" is a phrase often used for angiographic changes seen with neurofibromatosis.

4. Which statement is true regarding endovascular treatment of renal artery stenosis?
   a. For renal artery stenosis caused by atherosclerosis, angioplasty alone is usually sufficient treatment.
   b. After angioplasty for renal artery stenosis caused by fibromuscular dysplasia, hypertensive cure can be expected in more than 95% of cases.
   c. Atherosclerotic stenosis of the renal artery ostium is now almost uniformly treated with stent placement.
   d. Three-year survival cannot be predicted by preprocedural creatinine value in patients undergoing renal artery intervention.

5. Regarding chronic mesenteric ischemia, which statement is true?
   a. The majority of patients with chronic mesenteric ischemia are women.
   b. An important artery for chronic mesenteric ischemia is the inferior epigastric artery.
   c. Coronary disease is rare in patients with chronic mesenteric ischemia.
   d. Almost no collateral circulation exists between the major mesenteric arteries.

6. Which is *not* true of chronic mesenteric ischemia and its management?
   a. Most mesenteric artery stenoses are central or ostial.
   b. Stent placement is not indicated for median arcuate ligament compression syndrome.
   c. Clinical success can be expected in 60%-90% of patients treated with angioplasty and stenting for chronic mesenteric artery ischemia.
   d. Patients with chronic mesenteric ischemia rarely die from other causes.

Suggested Readings

Alhadad A, Mattiasson I, Ivancev K, et al. Revascularisation of renal artery stenosis caused by fibromuscular dysplasia: effects on blood pressure during 7-year follow-up are influenced by duration of hypertension and branch artery stenosis. J Hum Hypertens. 2005;19:761-7.

Brown DJ, Schermerhorn ML, Powell RJ, et al. Mesenteric stenting for chronic mesenteric ischemia. J Vasc Surg. 2005;42:268-74.

Caps MT, Perissinotto C, Zierler RE, et al. Prospective study of atherosclerotic disease progression in the renal artery. Circulation. 1998;98:2866-72.

Caps MT, Zierler RE, Polissar NL, et al. Risk of atrophy in kidneys with atherosclerotic renal artery stenosis. Kidney Int. 1998;53:735-42.

Chobanian AV, Bakris GL, Black HR, et al, National Heart, Lung, and Blood Institute Joint National Committee on Prevention, Detection, Evaluation, and Treatment of High Blood Pressure; National High Blood Pressure Education Program Coordinating Committee. The Seventh Report of the Joint National Committee on Prevention, Detection, Evaluation, and Treatment of High Blood Pressure: the JNC 7 report. JAMA. 2003 May 21;289:2560-72. Epub 2003 May 14. Erratum in: JAMA. 2003;290:197.

Cleveland TJ, Nawaz S, Gaines PA. Mesenteric arterial ischaemia: diagnosis and therapeutic options. Vasc Med. 2002;7:311-21.

Mounier-Vehier C, Lions C, Jaboureck O, et al. Parenchymal consequences of fibromuscular dysplasia renal artery stenosis. Am J Kidney Dis. 2002;40:1138-45.

Razavi M, Chung HH. Endovascular management of chronic mesenteric ischemia. Tech Vasc Interv Radiol. 2004;7:155-9.

Safian RD, Textor SC. Renal-artery stenosis. N Engl J Med. 2001;344:431-42.

Salifu MO, Haria DM, Badero O, et al. Challenges in the diagnosis and management of renal artery stenosis. Curr Hypertens Rep. 2005;7:219-27.

Sharafuddin MJ, Olson CH, Sun S, et al. Endovascular treatment of celiac and mesenteric arteries stenoses: applications and results. J Vasc Surg. 2003;38:692-8.

Slovut DP, Olin JW. Fibromuscular dysplasia. N Engl J Med. 2004;350:1862-71.

Tan KT, van Beek EJ, Brown PW, et al. Magnetic resonance angiography for the diagnosis of renal artery stenosis: a meta-analysis. Clin Radiol. 2002;57:617-24.

Thomas JH, Blake K, Pierce GE, et al. The clinical course of asymptomatic mesenteric arterial stenosis. J Vasc Surg. 1998;27:840-4.

van de Ven PJ, Kaatee R, Beutler JJ, et al. Arterial stenting and balloon angioplasty in ostial atherosclerotic renovascular disease: a randomised trial. Lancet. 1999;353:282-6.

van Jaarsveld BC, Krijnen P, Pieterman H, et al, Dutch Renal Artery Stenosis Intervention Cooperative Study Group. The effect of balloon angioplasty on hypertension in atherosclerotic renal-artery stenosis. N Engl J Med. 2000;342:1007-14.

Watson PS, Hadjipetrou P, Cox SV, et al. Effect of renal artery stenting on renal function and size in patients with atherosclerotic renovascular disease. Circulation. 2000;102:1671-7.

Zalunardo N, Tuttle KR. Atherosclerotic renal artery stenosis: current status and future directions. Curr Opin Nephrol Hypertens. 2004;13:613-21.

27 Endovascular Therapy for Brachiocephalic Vessels

David P. Slovut, MD, PhD, FACC
J. Michael Bacharach, MD, MPH, FACC

Subclavian and Innominate Artery Intervention

Anatomy

The aortic arch typically gives rise to three great vessels: the brachiocephalic trunk, which bifurcates into the right subclavian artery and right common carotid artery; the left common carotid artery; and the left subclavian artery. In 20% to 30% of the population, the brachiocephalic trunk and left common carotid artery share a common origin. In 7% of persons, the left common carotid artery arises as a branch off the innominate artery, a variant known as a bovine arch. Arch anomalies include left arch with aberrant right subclavian artery (0.4%-2.0% incidence), right arch with aberrant left subclavian artery (the most common type of right arch and a frequent cause of symptomatic vascular ring), and right arch with mirror-image branching (associated with cyanotic congenital heart defects).

- In 20%-30% of cases, the brachiocephalic trunk and left common carotid artery share a common origin
- Upper extremity occlusive disease accounts for only 5%-6% of all cases of limb ischemia, much less frequent than lower extremity ischemia

Etiology of Occlusive Disease

Upper extremity occlusive disease occurs much less frequently than disease of the lower extremity, accounting for only 5% to 6% of all cases of limb ischemia. Several types of subclavian artery occlusive disease (with different causes) are amenable to percutaneous revascularization, including that due to atherosclerotic disease, Takayasu arteritis, fibromuscular dysplasia, giant cell arteritis, and radiation-induced arteriopathy.

Atherosclerosis is the most common cause of large vessel stenosis. Occasionally, small vessel obstruction occurs as ulcerated plaques from the large vessel stenoses shower emboli to the digits, producing painful focal discoloration of the fingertips, splinter hemorrhages, or livedo reticularis. Atherosclerosis affects the left subclavian artery three to five times more often than the right. Most lesions are proximal to the origin of the vertebral artery, whereas 10% involve the artery both proximal and distal to the vertebral artery and 10% are found distal to the origin of the vertebral artery.

Takayasu arteritis (also known as aortic arch arteritis and "pulseless disease") is a chronic, idiopathic vasculitis involving the aorta, great vessels, and coronary and pulmonary arteries. It occurs predominantly in women, with higher prevalence rates reported in Asian and South American countries. Fibromuscular dysplasia is a non-atherosclerotic, non-inflammatory vascular disease that most commonly affects the renal and internal carotid arteries. In the upper extremities, fibromuscular dysplasia is identified most frequently in the subclavian arteries but has been described in the brachial and axillary arteries. Giant cell arteritis, also referred to as temporal arteritis, predominates in women older than 60 years. The disease produces a spectrum of symptoms including headache, vision loss, and intermittent jaw and tongue claudication. Giant cell arteritis involves the subclavian, axillary, or brachial arteries in 15% of cases.

Other causes of upper extremity ischemia include drugs (e.g., cocaine, ergotamine, methamphetamine), collagen vascular disease, iatrogenic injury, and thoracic outlet syndrome (TOS), which may present as a neurologic syndrome diagnosed by electromyography. In less than 5% of cases, TOS results from a vascular abnormality caused by compression of the subclavian artery or vein. Patients are often young and may report arm ache and fatigue, particularly when raising the arm above the head. Patients with proximal thrombosis or distal embolization may present with Raynaud syndrome, ulceration of the digits, or gangrene. Non-invasive testing with thoracic outlet maneuvers can provoke symptoms or signs of arterial compression. TOS is not amenable to percutaneous revascularization; cervical or first rib resection is required to relieve the compression.

- In less than 5% of cases, TOS results from a vascular abnormality caused by compression of the subclavian artery or vein
- TOS is not amenable to percutaneous revascularization; cervical or first rib resection is required to relieve the compression

Indications for Intervention

Patients with upper extremity ischemia may report symptoms such as arm or hand claudication, arm paresthesias, or rest pain. Lower limb ischemia is sometimes seen in patients who have undergone extra-anatomic bypass such as axillofemoral bypass grafting. Inflow disease is an uncommon but important cause of late graft failure. Up to 25% of patients who undergo axillofemoral bypass grafting have significant atherosclerotic disease in the inflow arteries. In vertebral-subclavian steal syndrome, upper extremity exertion leads to retrograde vertebral flow and neurologic symptoms including vertigo, syncope, ataxia, diplopia, motor deficits, and intermittent arm claudication. In coronary-subclavian steal syndrome, blood is diverted from the coronary circulation to the arm via the internal mammary artery graft during arm exercise. Symptoms include angina or infarction. The syndrome can be diagnosed by an image-based stress test (nuclear, echocardiographic, or magnetic resonance imaging [MRI]) after arm exercise.

- In vertebral-subclavian steal syndrome, upper extremity exertion leads to retrograde vertebral flow and neurologic symptoms including vertigo, syncope, ataxia, diplopia, motor deficits, and intermittent arm claudication
- In coronary-subclavian steal syndrome, blood is diverted from the coronary circulation to the arm via the internal mammary artery graft during arm exercise

Subclavian artery stenosis is associated with a favorable natural history. Many patients with high-grade stenosis and mild upper extremity claudication become asymptomatic as collaterals develop. In asymptomatic patients, subclavian intervention may be performed before coronary artery bypass grafting using the internal mammary artery or extra-anatomic bypass grafting, or to preserve inflow to the internal mammary artery in patients who may undergo bypass in the future. In patients with other brachiocephalic lesions, especially concomitant carotid artery disease, it may be reasonable to revascularize the subclavian artery. To date, no prospective, multicenter, randomized trials of subclavian artery intervention have been performed. Retrospective case series have demonstrated reasonable durability, with patency rates of 75% to 85% at 35- to 60-month follow-up.

Patient Assessment and Treatment

Subclavian artery stenosis is considered significant if the pressure difference between arms is more than 20 mm Hg. Segmental arm pressures and Doppler waveforms can be measured above the elbow, below the elbow, and above the wrist while insonating the radial artery at the wrist. Abnormal waveforms and decreased pressures at the above-elbow cuff site indicate subclavian or axillary artery occlusive disease. Digital plethysmography may show a peaked waveform in vasospasm and a damped waveform in occlusive disease. Elevated velocities in the stenotic segment and a peak velocity ratio of more than 5.5 by duplex ultrasonography are consistent with greater than 75% diameter stenosis.

Several specific ultrasonographic findings are seen in steal syndrome: reversal of vertebral flow throughout the cardiac cycle, bidirectional vertebral flow (forward in systole, retrograde in diastole), and normal flow with the patient at rest. In the latter two situations, inducing arm hyperemia by inflating a blood pressure cuff to suprasystolic pressure for 5 minutes may unmask steal phenomenon. With cuff deflation, patients with steal have flow reversal or biphasic vertebral flow. Computed tomography angiography (CTA), magnetic resonance angiography (MRA), or invasive angiography of the aortic arch and great vessels can be used to determine the extent of brachiocephalic artery involvement and aid in planning revascularization. During invasive angiography, the left anterior oblique view is useful for delineating the left subclavian artery, whereas the right anterior oblique view with caudal angulation permits visualization of the innominate bifurcation.

Before the advent of percutaneous transluminal angioplasty, surgical revascularization was the primary therapeutic modality for patients with symptomatic subclavian artery occlusive disease. Commonly used extrathoracic methods for subclavian artery revascularization include carotid-subclavian, carotid-axillary, or axillo-axillary bypass using polytetrafluoroethylene or polyethylene terephthalate grafts and subclavian-carotid transposition. Surgical repair produces excellent long-term patency (>90%) with low morbidity and mortality.

For catheter-based therapy, arterial access is obtained via the femoral artery in most cases. The brachial approach or combined femoral and brachial approach can be useful in treating patients with total subclavian artery occlusion. After access is achieved, heparin should be administered until the activated clotting time is greater than 250 seconds; alternatively, bivalirudin can be used. Although it has not been reported specifically for subclavian intervention, bivalirudin has been associated with a low rate of ischemic events and bleeding in patients undergoing renal, iliac, and femoral artery intervention.

The stenotic lesion is crossed with a 0.035-in guidewire. If the brachial approach is used, the guidewire can be advanced into the abdominal aorta, snared, and exteriorized via a groin sheath, a maneuver that permits the use of a smaller brachial artery sheath. A 7F guiding sheath is positioned across the stenosis. Lesions may be treated with balloon angioplasty alone or stenting, although long-term patency is greater with stenting (Fig. 27.1). If possible, the stent should be positioned to avoid covering the vertebral artery. Balloon-expandable stents are preferable for use with ostial lesions, whereas self-expanding nitinol stents are favored for tortuous vessels and lesions distal to the vertebral artery where stent compression is possible. Vasospasm is treated with intra-arterial nitroglycerin (200 μg) or papaverine (10-40 mg). Antiplatelet therapy should consist of aspirin, 325 mg orally per day indefinitely, and clopidogrel, 300 mg loading dose followed by 75 mg orally for 4 weeks after stenting.

- Subclavian artery stenosis is considered significant if a pressure gradient >20 mm Hg is found between brachial artery measurements

A

B

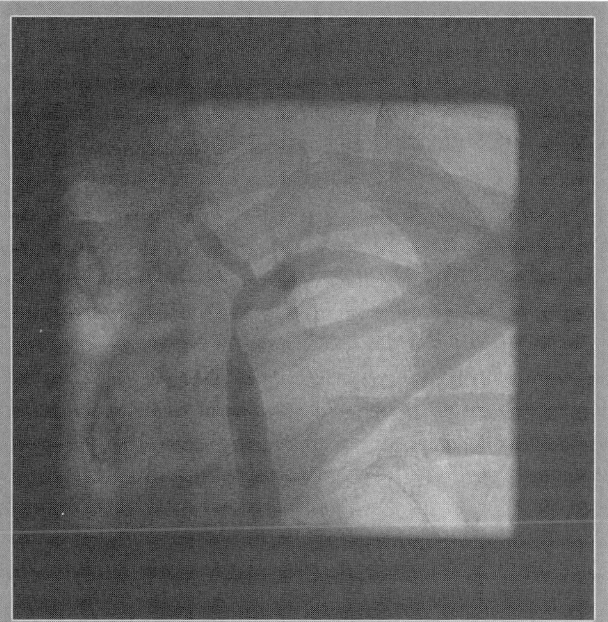

C

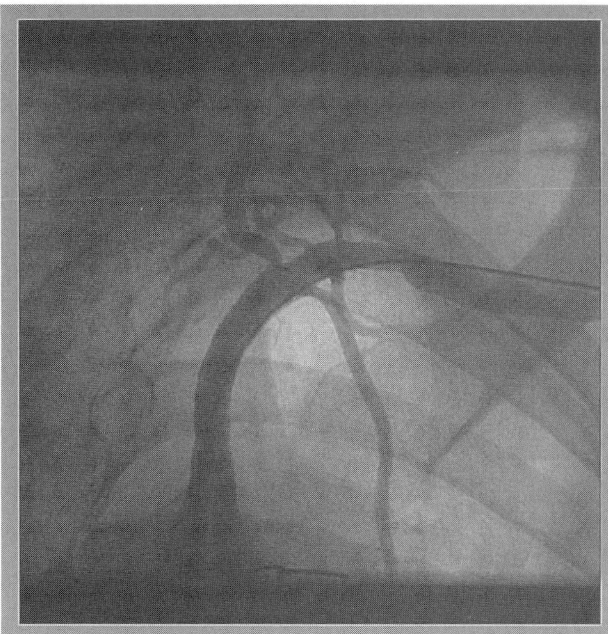

Fig. 27.1 Angiographic images of balloon angioplasty and stenting of upper extremity arteries. *A*, Composite image shows contrast injection via the left main coronary artery with dye traveling retrograde up the internal mammary artery graft to fill the distal left subclavian artery. *B*, Selective injection of the left subclavian artery shows critical stenosis. The vertebral artery, but not the internal mammary artery, is seen in this injection. *C*, After balloon angioplasty, wide luminal patency is re-established. The internal mammary artery graft now fills antegrade.

- Retrograde vertebral artery flow persists briefly after dilating subclavian artery lesions, which protects the posterior circulation from emboli; consequently, use of embolic protection devices is not warranted
- Technical success rates for treating stenotic lesions are >90%, whereas the rate for total occlusions is 50%-60% in most series; the rate for major adverse events (e.g., stroke and death) is 2%

Distal embolic complications are infrequent. Retrograde vertebral artery flow can persist briefly after dilating subclavian artery lesions, which may protect the posterior circulation from emboli. Consequently, use of embolic protection devices is usually not warranted. In general, the vertebral artery remains patent if it originates from a non-stenotic segment of the subclavian artery. If associated vertebral artery stenosis is present, or if the subclavian lesion encroaches on the vertebral artery, the artery should be protected with a guidewire during subclavian artery dilatation. If the vertebral artery is compromised, simultaneous inflation using kissing technique may be performed. Treatment of ostial right subclavian stenoses merits placement of a safety wire in the common carotid artery. For restenotic lesions, balloon angioplasty, cutting balloon angioplasty, or repeat stenting may be performed.

Technical success rates for treating stenotic lesions are greater than 90%, and the rate for total occlusions is 50% to 60% in most series. Major adverse events (e.g., stroke and death) occur in less than 2%. Minor complications include transient ischemic attack, distal embolization to the arm or hand, reperfusion edema with or without compartment syndrome, and access-related brachial artery thrombosis. Long-term results are excellent, with primary patency rates higher than 90% at 1 year and secondary patency rates of 80% to 90% at 5 years.

In Takayasu arteritis, medical therapy consists of corticosteroids and antiplatelet agents. Revascularization is indicated for severe cerebral or upper extremity ischemia. Ideally, revascularization is performed during the quiescent phase of the disease. In patients with active disease (e.g., fever, musculoskeletal pain, or elevated erythrocyte sedimentation rate), prednisone (1 mg/kg per day) should be administered before intervention and continued for 6 months. Methotrexate (7.5 mg/wk) may be added in patients who are unresponsive to prednisone. Compared with patients with atherosclerosis, those with Takayasu arteritis are younger, more likely to be female, and present with upper extremity claudication rather than gangrene. In contrast to atherosclerotic disease, Takayasu arteritis produces diffuse transmural fibrotic arterial lesions that typically require higher inflation pressures to dilate. Although long-term symptomatic relief is excellent, restenosis occurs in 26% of patients. Disease activity should be controlled strictly with immunosuppressive therapy. In patients with giant cell arteritis, case reports suggest excellent immediate and long-term outcome with upper extremity balloon angioplasty.

Innominate Artery Occlusive Disease

Innominate artery occlusive disease is seen infrequently. When present, it is often accompanied by carotid or subclavian artery stenosis. In contrast to carotid artery occlusive disease, the natural history of innominate artery occlusive disease is poorly understood. Patients may present with an asymptomatic blood pressure disparity between arms, or with upper extremity claudication, cerebrovascular steal, transient ischemic attack, or stroke. Transthoracic surgical repair consists of aorto-innominate bypass or aortocarotid bypass with reimplantation of the subclavian artery. Innominate endarterectomy and cervical reconstruction are used less commonly. Transthoracic operation is preferred in patients with embolic disease who require exclusion of the embolic source and revascularization of the distal innominate artery. Graft patency is excellent. The combined stroke and death rate is up to 16%. Overall patient survival after transthoracic reconstruction is 73% at 5 years and 52% at 10 years. Percutaneous revascularization with balloon angioplasty alone or stenting provides excellent medium-term patency (>90%) with low morbidity and mortality.

Aneurysmal Disease

Aneurysms of the subclavian and axillary arteries are seen in atherosclerotic disease, trauma, vasculitides, and TOS. Covered stents have been used for more than a decade to treat abdominal aortic aneurysms and have been used successfully to exclude subclavian artery aneurysms.

Trauma, whether blunt or penetrating, can produce a spectrum of injuries ranging from intimal tear to pseudoaneurysm to complete transection. Traditionally, most vascular injuries to the head and neck warrant surgical repair.

An aneurysm is seen in 60% of patients with an aberrant subclavian artery (Kommerell diverticulum). The abnormality may be discovered incidentally or during investigation for symptoms such as cough and progressive dysphagia for solids (dysphagia lusoria). Surgical treatment is indicated because of the risk of rupture.

Vertebral and Basilar Artery Intervention

Anatomy

The blood supply to the medulla, pons, and mid brain is derived from the vertebrobasilar system. The vertebral artery is divided into four segments: V1 (extraosseous, extending from its origin to the transverse foramen of C_6), V2 (foraminal, extending from the transverse foramen of C_6 to C_1), V3 (extraspinal, extending from the exit of the transverse foramen of C_1 to the foramen magnum), and V4 (intradural, extending from the foramen magnum to the basilar artery) (Fig. 27.2). The left vertebral artery is dominant in 75% of the population and arises directly from the aorta in 1% to 5%; pronounced tortuosity of the V1 segment is observed in 40%. The basilar artery arises from the confluence of the vertebral arteries. The posterior inferior cerebellar artery (PICA) typically originates from the intradural segment of the vertebral artery but can arise from the extracranial vertebral artery 5% to 18% of the time. In 0.2% of cases, the vertebral artery has an anomalous ending at the PICA. In rare cases, the PICA is absent and the ipsilateral anterior inferior cerebellar artery supplies the territory.

- The blood supply to the medulla, pons, and mid brain is derived from the vertebrobasilar system
- Symptoms of posterior circulation ischemia include diplopia, blurred vision, vertigo, gait disturbance, episodic perioral numbness, or drop attacks

Extracranial Vertebral Artery Occlusive Disease

In general, vertebrobasilar territory ischemia results from luminal compromise of both vertebral arteries or their inflow vessels (i.e., synchronous innominate and left subclavian artery lesions). Mechanisms of vertebrobasilar ischemia include embolization from the aorta or heart, thrombotic cerebral ischemia from ulcerated plaque, and low-flow states, in which symptoms develop when blood flow is inadequate to support neuronal function. Potential causes of low-flow states include atherosclerosis of the vertebral arteries or small intracranial branches, steal syndromes, vasculitides, fibromuscular dysplasia, and vertebral artery impingement. Symptoms of posterior circulation ischemia include diplopia, blurred vision, vertigo, gait disturbance, episodic perioral numbness, or drop attacks. Stereotypical movements such as extend-

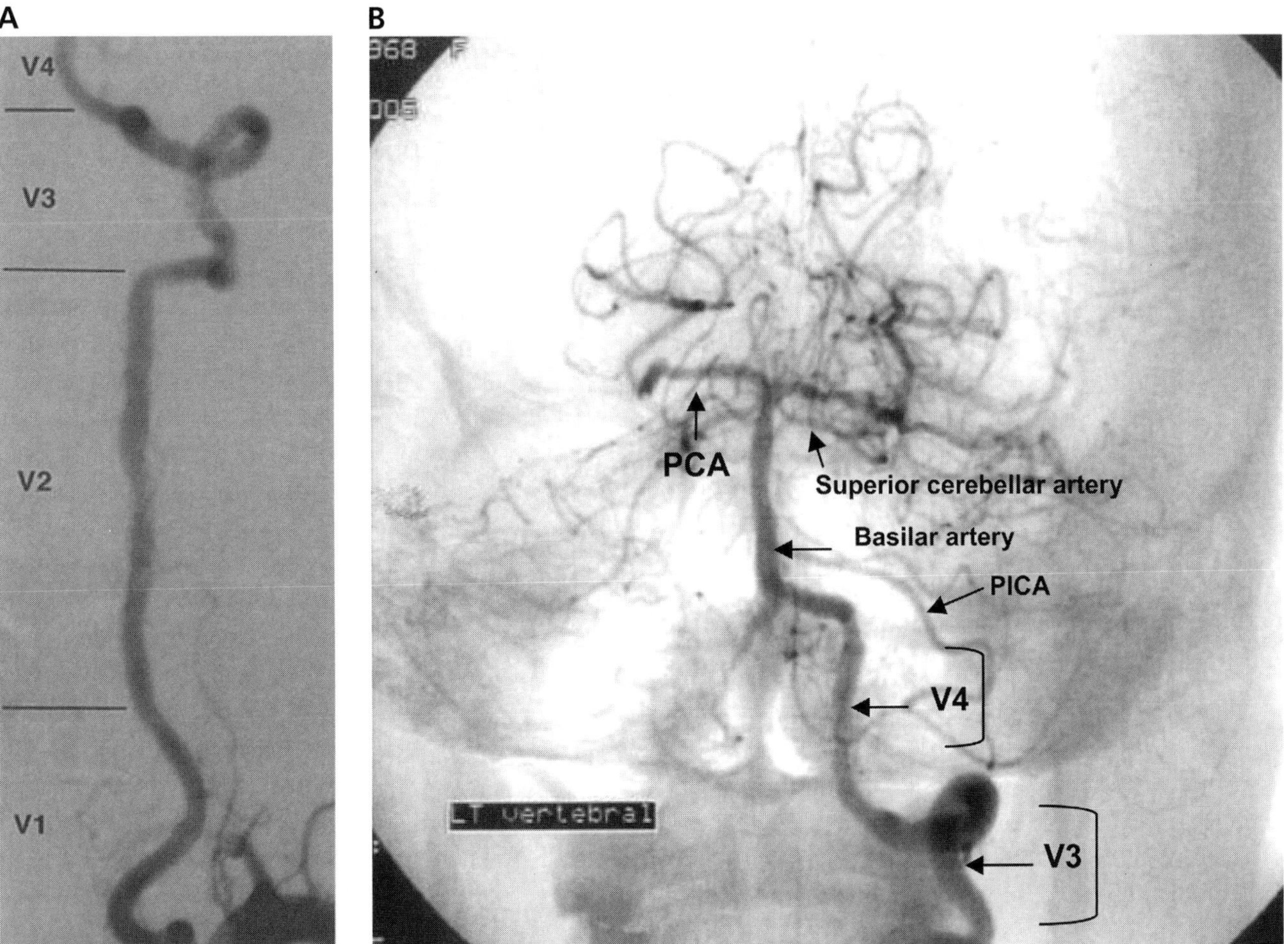

Fig. 27.2 Angiographic images showing the segments of the vertebral artery. *A*, The extracranial vertebral artery segments, V1-V4. *B*, The intracranial vertebral artery segments. PCA, posterior cerebral artery; PICA, posterior inferior cerebellar artery.

ing the neck or turning the head in a particular direction may provoke symptoms. Non-specific symptoms include headache, nausea, vomiting, and tinnitus. Initial therapy consists of platelet inhibitors or anticoagulation. Revascularization is indicated if symptoms persist despite medical management.

Doppler examination of the vertebral arteries in vertebrobasilar ischemia shows reversal of flow or bidirectional flow. MRA, CTA, or invasive 4-vessel cerebral angiography using digital subtraction provides more definitive imaging when revascularization is being contemplated. An anteroposterior view with 20° cranial angulation typically provides good visualization of the entire extracranial vertebral artery. Multiple orthogonal views, including anteroposterior and lateral views, should be obtained to fully evaluate the high cervical and intracranial vertebrobasilar circulation.

Surgical treatment of the vertebral artery can be technically challenging. Approaches to surgical revascularization include vertebral to common carotid artery transposition, vertebral endarterectomy, vertebral vein patch angioplasty with or without suture plication of the artery, and bypass from the subclavian artery to the vertebral artery. Complications—including Horner syndrome, lymphocele, recurrent laryngeal nerve palsy, immediate thrombosis, and chylothorax—after proximal vertebral artery reconstruction occur in up to 15% of cases. In some series, the rate of vertebral artery thrombosis approaches 9%.

Catheter-based intervention has gained favor for treatment of symptomatic vertebral artery lesions. Before the procedure, patients should receive aspirin, 325 mg orally, and a loading dose of clopidogrel (300 mg orally followed by 75 mg orally once daily for 4 weeks). Femoral artery access is favored, although the brachial approach may be used. Heparin, 50 to 70 U/kg, is administered to achieve an activated clotting time greater than 250 seconds. A 6F Judkins right, headhunter, vertebral artery, or internal mammary artery catheter is used to engage the subclavian artery. A 6F or 7F guiding catheter is advanced to the stenosis over a 0.035-in wire. A buddy wire may be positioned in the distal subclavian artery to provide additional stability for the guiding catheter. The lesion is traversed with a 0.014-in steerable guidewire. Predilation is performed with a balloon that is undersized compared with the reference vessel diameter. For ostial lesions, low-profile balloon-expandable coronary stents are preferred. The proximal portion of the stent is positioned with 1 or 2 cells protruding into the subclavian artery to prevent prolapse of subclavian artery plaque into the vertebral artery. For distal vertebral artery lesions, balloon-expandable or self-expanding stents may be used. Additional dilatation of the stent can be required to produce complete stent expansion. Oversizing the postdilation balloon is inadvisable because of the risk of perforation, dissection, or extrusion of plaque through the stent struts.

Distal embolic protection devices have been used rarely in the vertebral artery. Compared with the internal carotid artery, the vertebral artery is smaller and more tortuous, which can make finding an adequate landing zone for the embolic protection device problematic. Placement of an embolic protection device should be considered if the vertebral artery diameter is larger than 3.5 mm, if the distal landing zone is relatively free of tortuosity, and if the target lesion is ulcerated. Minimal sedation is given during the procedure to facilitate neurologic monitoring. Neurologic status should be assessed after each major procedural step (e.g., placement of the guiding catheter, balloon dilation, and stent deployment). Only anecdotal data exist regarding the use of glycoprotein IIb/IIIa inhibitors in vertebral artery intervention.

Procedural success is achieved in more than 90% of vertebral artery interventions; most patients improve or become asymptomatic. Long-term angiographic follow-up shows moderate to severe in-stent restenosis in up to 43% of cases, but most patients with restenosis remain asymptomatic. Drug-eluting stents have not been tested or approved for use in the vertebral artery. Close follow-up including duplex ultrasonography is warranted to monitor these patients. Repeat intervention is performed for symptom recurrence.

- Placement of an embolic protection device should be considered if the vertebral artery diameter is larger than 3.5 mm, if the distal landing zone is relatively free of tortuosity, and if the target lesion is ulcerated
- Procedural success is achieved in more than 90% of vertebral artery interventions; most patients improve or become asymptomatic

Vertebral Artery Dissection

The source of a vertebral artery dissection is usually an intimal tear, which allows pressurized blood to enter the artery wall and form an intramural hematoma. Subintimal dissection usually leads to stenosis of the arterial lumen; subadventitial dissection can produce aneurysmal dilatation of the artery. Dissection may occur spontaneously after blunt trauma or chiropractic manipulation, which can stretch the vertebral artery over the lateral mass of the second cervical vertebra. Spontaneous dissection is seen more commonly in fibromuscular disease, Marfan syndrome, Ehlers-Danlos type IV syndrome, and cystic medial necrosis. Patients may report sudden pain in the back of the neck or head. Physical examination may indicate signs of posterior circulation ischemia.

Approximately 90% of vertebral artery dissections are found at the level of the first and second cervical vertebrae. In the other cases, the dissection occurs just before the artery enters the intervertebral foramen. Dissections can be diagnosed using gadolinium-enhanced MRA, CTA, or conventional angiography. Angiographic features of dissection include tapering, stenosis, abrupt vessel occlusion, intimal flaps, or luminal filling defects. Intramural hematoma can spiral along the length of the dissected segment and appear as a crescent shape adjacent to the vessel lumen. Most vertebral artery dissections heal spontaneously. Anticoagulation therapy with intravenous heparin followed by 3 to 6 months of oral warfarin is recommended to decrease the potential for secondary thromboembolic complications. Long-term outcomes are excellent. Surgery or catheter-based intervention is reserved for continued symptoms despite maximum anticoagulation therapy or the presence of an aneurysm causing recurrent thromboembolism or threatened rupture.

- Most vertebral artery dissections heal spontaneously
- Anticoagulation with intravenous heparin followed by 3-6 months of oral warfarin is recommended to decrease the potential for secondary thromboembolic complications

Vertebral Artery Trauma

Blunt and penetrating trauma may produce a spectrum of arterial injuries ranging from dissection to pseudoaneurysm formation to arterial transection. Some of these lesions are amenable to percutaneous treatment. For example, embolization of vertebral artery pseudoaneurysms can be performed by coaxial placement of a microcatheter in the pseudoaneurysm and injection of gelfoam pledgets or polyvinyl alcohol.

Intracranial Vertebral Artery Occlusive Disease

Intracranial stenosis accounts for 8% to 10% of the estimated 600,000 ischemic strokes each year. Symptomatic intracranial vertebral or basilar artery stenosis is associated with significant morbidity and mortality. In one series of 102 medically treated patients, 14% had recurrent stroke and 21% died during a mean follow-up of 15 months. The high mortality rate was attributed to severe neurologic deficits with brainstem stroke and to associated complications such as pneumonia, systemic infection, and respiratory failure. Stroke-free survival was 76% at 12 months and 48% at 5 years.

Retrospective studies in patients with symptomatic intracranial artery stenosis have suggested that warfarin is more effective than aspirin in preventing stroke. This conclusion, however, was not supported by the prospective, randomized WASID study (Warfarin versus Aspirin for Symptomatic Intracranial Disease), which compared aspirin (650 mg orally twice per day) with warfarin (international normalized ratio [INR] target, 2-3) in 569 patients with symptomatic intracranial artery stenosis. Over a mean follow-up of 1.8 years, study medications were discontinued in 28.4% of patients receiving warfarin and 16.4% of patients receiving aspirin (P<.001). The INR was subtherapeutic 22.7% of the time and supratherapeutic 14.1% of the time. The primary end point (ischemic stroke, brain hemorrhage, or death from vascular causes other than stroke) was reached in 22.1% of patients in the aspirin group and 21.8% of patients in the warfarin group (P=.83). Secondary end points (ischemic stroke in any vascular territory, ischemic stroke in the territory of the stenotic intracranial artery, and a composite of ischemic stroke, death from vascular causes other than stroke, and nonfatal myocardial infarction) were similar between groups. Conversely, the mortality rate (4.3% aspirin vs 9.7% warfarin; P=.02) and major hemorrhage rate (3.2% aspirin vs 8.3% warfarin; P=.01) were higher in the warfarin group. The WASID study suggests that aspirin is the preferred therapy for patients with symptomatic intracranial artery stenosis.

The prognosis is poor for patients with symptomatic intracranial atherosclerosis in whom antiplatelet therapy fails. The median time to recurrent transient ischemic attack, stroke, or death is 36 days; 53% of patients with a recurrent event had a stroke or died. Interest is growing in using endovascular methods in patients with symptomatic intracranial stenosis. The SSYLVIA study (Stenting of Symptomatic Atherosclerotic Lesions in the Vertebral or Intracranial Arteries) was a prospective, non-randomized, multicenter trial that evaluated the safety of a balloon-expandable stent for the cerebral vasculature. The trial included 23 lesions in the intracranial vertebral, basilar, or posterior cerebral artery. Stent placement was successful in 95% of cases and procedural success achieved in 88.5%. Three ischemic strokes were observed within 30 days of stenting. At 6-month follow-up, restenosis was seen in 25% of pre-posterior inferior cerebellar vertebral arteries and 32% of intracranial lesions. The majority of patients (61%) with restenosis were asymptomatic.

- The WASID study suggests that aspirin is the preferred therapy for patients with symptomatic intracranial artery stenosis
- The prognosis is poor for patients with symptomatic intracranial atherosclerosis in whom antiplatelet therapy fails

In another series (21 lesions, 18 patients), intervention was performed for patients in whom medical therapy failed and who were considered high risk for imminent stroke. The technical success rate was high, as was the complication rate. Disabling ischemic stroke was seen in 11%, intracranial hemorrhage in 17%, and major extracranial hemorrhage in 22% of patients. The use of systemic anticoagulation that is mandatory during endovascular intervention predisposes patients to intracranial hemorrhage; adjunctive use of glycoprotein IIb/IIIa inhibitors further increases the risk. Diffusion-weighted MRI may provide a means of identifying patients at the greatest risk of hemorrhagic conversion.

To date, prospective, randomized trials comparing medical therapy and intervention in the posterior circulation have not been performed. Although intracranial vertebral angioplasty is technically feasible, complications from the procedure can be life threatening.

Basilar Artery Occlusion

Basilar artery occlusion accounts for 20% of ischemic strokes. The onset of symptoms can be gradual or sudden; the most devastating manifestation is the locked-in syndrome. Mortality rates exceed 85% if the basilar artery is not recanalized. Intra-arterial thrombolysis has been used to treat basilar artery occlusion. In one series of 40 patients, thrombolysis with urokinase was initiated within 5.5 hours of symptom onset. At 3 months, outcome was favorable in 35% and poor in 23%, and 17 patients (42%) died. Favorable clinical outcome was associated with minimal neurologic impairment before treatment and when recanalization was achieved.

- Basilar artery occlusion accounts for 20% of ischemic strokes

Administration of intra-arterial thrombolytic agents requires a dedicated neurointerventional service and can be performed only at major referral centers. Even with a dedicated service, unacceptable delays can occur between symptom onset and treatment. Intravenous therapy was examined as an alternative to intra-arterial administration in a series of 50 consecutive patients with angiographically verified basilar artery occlusion and a clinical syndrome consistent with posterior circulation compromise in a previously independently functioning person. Major causes of occlusion included vertebrobasilar thromboembolism (44%), cardioembolic phenomenon (32%), and vertebral artery dissection (14%). Treatment delays of up to 12 hours were allowed for sudden loss of consciousness and quadriparesis and up to 48 hours for gradually progressive symptoms such as ophthalmoplegia, dysarthria, and bilateral weakness. Exclusion criteria included signs of intracranial bleeding on CT or absence of brainstem reflexes. Alteplase 0.9 mg/kg was infused with a 10% bolus over 1 hour. The overall recanalization rate was 52%, favorable neurologic outcome, 24%, and 3-month survival rate, 60%. Unconsciousness as a presenting symptom did not preclude a good outcome.

Additional strategies for treating basilar artery occlusion include mechanical thromboaspiration and fragmentation, mechanical recanalization with catheter thrombectomy, angioplasty, and stenting, as well as intra-arterial thrombolysis with stent placement. Potential complications include intracranial hemorrhage, thromboembolic occlusion, brainstem infarct owing to damage of small perforating arteries, major extracranial vascular complication, and death.

Questions

1. A 65-year-old woman presents with left arm and leg weakness lasting 12 hours. MRA 2 weeks earlier showed high-grade stenosis (*arrow*) of the innominate artery (Figure [I, inferior; L, left, R, right, S, superior]). Upon presentation to the emergency department, CT of the head shows no evidence of hemorrhage. What is the optimal treatment strategy?
   - **a.** Immediate catheter-directed thrombolysis
   - **b.** Immediate angioplasty with provisional stent placement

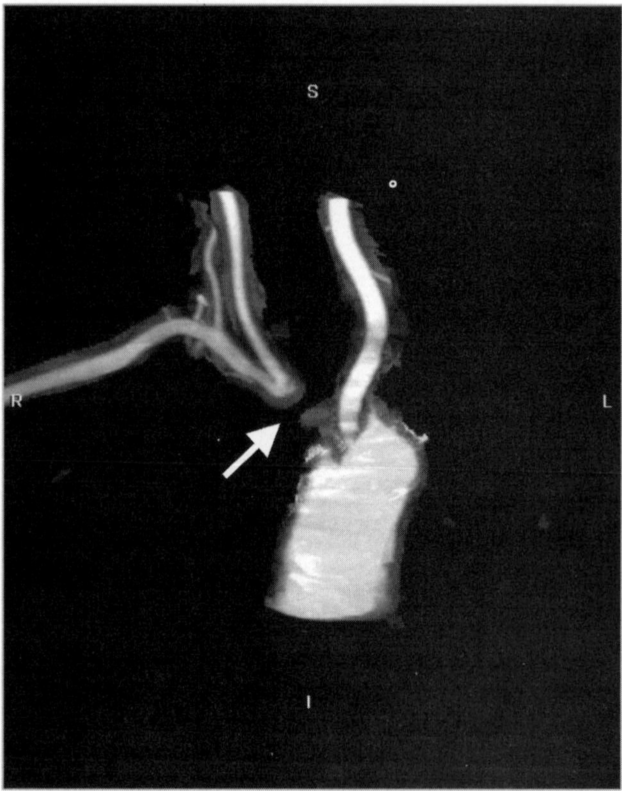

Figure for Question 1.

c. Aorta-to-carotid bypass in 5-7 days
d. Innominate artery atherectomy in 5-7 days

2. During placement of a thoracic endoprosthesis for a descending thoracic aneurysm, the physician inadvertently covers the left subclavian artery with the graft. What is the most likely sequelae for the patient?
   a. No symptoms
   b. Vertigo and diplopia
   c. Intermittent arm claudication
   d. Left arm paralysis

3. What is the most common arch abnormality associated with symptoms?
   a. Left arch with aberrant right subclavian artery
   b. Right arch with aberrant left subclavian artery
   c. Right arch with mirror-image branching
   d. Double arch with both arches patent

4. Based on results of a recent randomized trial, which of the following constitutes optimal therapy for patients with symptomatic intracranial artery stenosis?
   a. Aspirin, 650 mg orally twice daily
   b. Clopidogrel, 75 mg orally once daily
   c. Warfarin with an INR target of 2-3
   d. Ticlopidine, 250 mg orally once daily

5. A 43-year-old man presents with diplopia and near syncope after a motor vehicle crash. MRI of the head was negative. CT was performed (Figure). What is the optimal management strategy at this point?
   a. Anticoagulation with heparin followed by 6 months of warfarin
   b. Percutaneous transluminal angioplasty of the vertebral artery
   c. Administration of intra-arterial thrombolysis
   d. Bypass from the subclavian to the vertebral artery

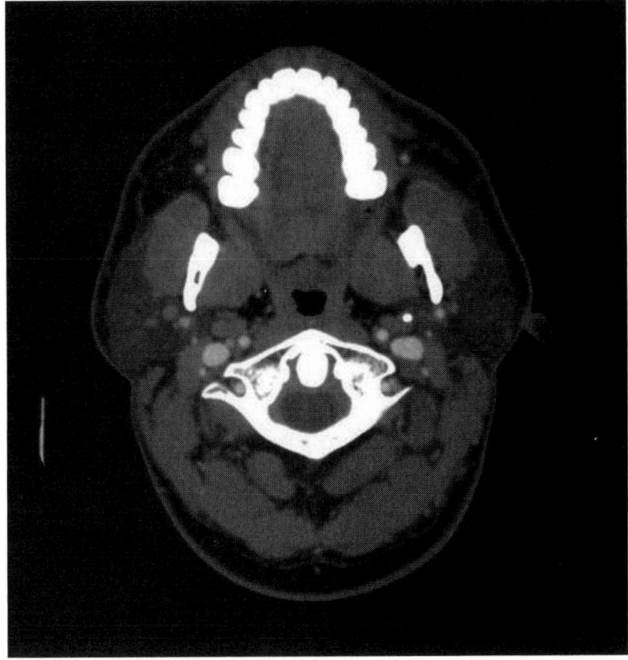

Figure for Question 5. (Courtesy of S. Ramee, MD, Ochsner Clinic.)

Suggested Readings

Allie DE, Hall P, Shammas NW, et al. The Angiomax Peripheral Procedure Registry of Vascular Events Trial (APPROVE): in-hospital and 30-day results. J Invasive Cardiol. 2004;16:651-6.

Arnold M, Nedeltchev K, Schroth G, et al. Clinical and radiological predictors of recanalisation and outcome of 40 patients with acute basilar artery occlusion treated with intra-arterial thrombolysis. J Neurol Neurosurg Psychiatry. 2004;75:857-62.

Bates MC, Broce M, Lavigne PS, et al. Subclavian artery stenting: factors influencing long-term outcome. Catheter Cardiovasc Interv. 2004;61:5-11.

Chimowitz MI, Lynn MJ, Howlett-Smith H, et al, Warfarin-Aspirin Symptomatic Intracranial Disease Trial Investigators. Comparison of warfarin and aspirin for symptomatic intracranial arterial stenosis. N Engl J Med. 2005;352:1305-16.

De Vries JP, Jager LC, Van den Berg JC, et al. Durability of percutaneous transluminal angioplasty for obstructive lesions of proximal subclavian artery: long-term results. J Vasc Surg. 2005;41:19-23.

Gupta R, Schumacher HC, Mangla S, et al. Urgent endovascular revascularization for symptomatic intracranial atherosclerotic stenosis. Neurology. 2003;61:1729-35.

Hatano T, Tsukahara T, Ogino E, et al. Stenting for vertebrobasilar artery stenosis. Acta Neurochir Suppl. 2005;94:137-41.

Henry M, Amor M, Henry I, et al. Percutaneous transluminal angioplasty of the subclavian arteries. J Endovasc Surg. 1999;6:33-41.

Hoffman GS, Weyand CM, editors. Inflammatory diseases of blood vessels. New York: Marcel Dekker; 2002.

Ligush J Jr, Criado E, Keagy BA. Innominate artery occlusive disease: management with central reconstructive techniques. Surgery. 1997;121:556-62.

Lindsberg PJ, Soinne L, Tatlisumak T, et al. Long-term outcome after intravenous thrombolysis of basilar artery occlusion. JAMA. 2004;292:1862-6.

Min PK, Park S, Jung JH, et al. Endovascular therapy combined with immunosuppressive treatment for occlusive arterial disease in patients with Takayasu's arteritis. J Endovasc Ther. 2005;12:28-34.

Osborn AG. Diagnostic cerebral angiography. 2nd ed. Philadelphia: Lippincott Williams & Wilkins; 1999.

Qureshi AI, Ziai WC, Yahia AM, et al. Stroke-free survival and its determinants in patients with symptomatic vertebrobasilar stenosis: a multicenter study. Neurosurgery. 2003;52:1033-9.

Schievink WI. Spontaneous dissection of the carotid and vertebral arteries. N Engl J Med. 2001;344:898-906.

SSYLVIA Study Investigators. Stenting of Symptomatic Atherosclerotic Lesions in the Vertebral or Intracranial Arteries (SSYLVIA): study results. Stroke. 2004 Jun;35:1388-92. Epub 2004 Apr 22.

Sullivan TM, Gray BH, Bacharach JM, et al. Angioplasty and primary stenting of the subclavian, innominate, and common carotid arteries in 83 patients. J Vasc Surg. 1998;28:1059-65.

Thijs VN, Albers GW. Symptomatic intracranial atherosclerosis: outcome of patients who fail antithrombotic therapy. Neurology. 2000;55:490-7.

Weber W, Mayer TE, Henkes H, et al. Efficacy of stent angioplasty for symptomatic stenoses of the proximal vertebral artery. Eur J Radiol. 2005 Nov;56:240-7. Epub 2005 Jun 14.

Wehman JC, Hanel RA, Guidot CA, et al. Atherosclerotic occlusive extracranial vertebral artery disease: indications for intervention, endovascular techniques, short-term and long-term results. J Interv Cardiol. 2004;17:219-32.

28 Endovascular Treatment of Lower Extremity Occlusive Arterial Disease

Daniel G. Clair, MD

Etiology of Peripheral Arterial Disease

Peripheral arterial disease (PAD) of the lower extremities most commonly results from atherosclerosis causing progressive narrowing of the arteries in the lower extremities. Atherosclerosis is a systemic disease that is the leading cause of death in Western countries. It involves the deposition of lipids, connective tissue, inflammatory cells, and other debris within the media of the vessel wall. Although the formation of lesions in the vasculature involves several causative factors, the relationship between inflammation and serum lipid deposition within the arterial wall is important. Understanding this link and determining means to limit the inflammatory process will likely be significant in decreasing the progression of disease.

Prevalence and Significance of PAD

The risk of PAD increases substantially with age; current estimates for its prevalence in the United States in persons older than 40 years range from 3.5% to 5%, as determined by an ankle-brachial index less than 0.9. Only a portion of these persons, however, will actually have clinical sequelae of PAD. This prevalence continues to increase with age and in those older than 70 years is between 14% and 15%. Currently, about 5 million adults are affected by PAD; this number can be expected to increase to 7 million by 2020.

Of interest, male sex does not appear to be associated with an increased incidence of PAD, and in some age categories the incidence may be higher in women than men. Numerous studies have assessed risk factors and their relationships to PAD occurrence (Table 28.1). Although it is important to understand the significance of this disease in terms of the number of persons affected, it is also imperative to appreciate its clinical significance and the association of PAD with other cardiovascular and cerebrovascular diseases.

Table 28.1 Risk Factors Associated With Peripheral Arterial Disease

Risk factor	Odds ratio
African American	2.83
Smoking	4.46
Hypertension	1.75
Hypercholesterolemia	1.68
Diabetes mellitus	2.71
Renal dysfunction	2.00
Coronary artery disease	2.54
Cerebrovascular disease	2.42
Congestive heart failure	1.20
Any cardiovascular disease	2.69
Advanced age	2.9
Elevated fibrinogen	1.4
Elevated body mass index	1.2

- The incidence of PAD increases with age; 14%-15% of persons older than 70 years will be affected by PAD
- Most patients present without symptoms

Natural History

Only one-third of those with PAD are symptomatic. If symptoms are present, the most common is intermittent claudication, which seems to be more common in men than women—40% of men and only 13% of women with objectively measured disease report this symptom. Of those with claudication, only a small number will eventually have severe limb-threatening complications. Over a 10-year period, 30% of patients with claudication will have rest pain and only 23% will have an ischemic ulcer. In addition, a patient with claudication will, over time, lose an average of 9 meters of walking distance per year. This progression is clearly worse in persons who smoke. For those affected with PAD who have disease progression to critical limb ischemia, the risk of primary amputation ranges from 10% to 40%. For patients in whom revascularization cannot be attempted—because of anatomic unsuitability or medical comorbidities—the likelihood of amputation is 40% over the ensuing 6 months. In these patients with PAD, the risk of infrainguinal disease progression is much lower than the risk of associated coronary artery disease. PAD is an excellent marker for the presence of coronary artery disease.

Symptomatic coronary artery disease can be identified clinically in up to 40% of patients with PAD; the addition of stress testing or cardiac catheterization can reveal its presence in 60% and 90% of patients, respectively. In addition to the markedly elevated incidence of coronary artery disease, patients with PAD also have an increased incidence of cerebrovascular disease. The association of PAD with atherosclerosis in other vascular beds has led to increased mortality in this patient group, which can be as high as six times the mortality in age-matched controls. Patients with PAD have been documented, in some studies, to have 5-year mortality rates of 30% to 50%. It is imperative that clinicians caring for patients with PAD look for atherosclerosis in other vascular territories.

- Approximately one-third of persons with PAD have symptoms, the most common being intermittent claudication
- PAD is an important marker for coronary artery disease, which is associated with significantly increased mortality in PAD patients

Clinical Presentation

Most people with PAD are asymptomatic; they may have had only a diminished pulse noted on physical examination. Patients with a decreased pulse should be assessed for atherosclerotic risk factors. If present, modification of these risk factors may retard disease progression and is a critical aspect of caring for this complex group of patients.

The most common presenting clinical symptom of PAD is intermittent claudication (a Latin derivative meaning "to limp"), a reproducible tightness or cramping of the lower extremity with exertion. Claudication is usually relieved by rest and is readily reproducible at a defined walking distance. The pain can occur in various muscle groups of the lower extremity and may involve the buttock, thigh, calf, foot, or toes. The location of the muscle group affected can be a marker for the location of the culprit atherosclerotic lesion. However, it is only possible to be certain that the level of obstruction is above the affected area of the leg. For example, calf claudication could be due to aortoiliac, femoral, or popliteal disease, and it would be unusual for disease of the femoral artery to cause buttock claudication.

A smaller group of patients presents with limb-threatening or critical limb ischemia due to PAD. These patients have rest pain, ischemic ulceration, or gangrene. Rest pain usually occurs at night and is most common in the toes or distal forefoot. The patient usually describes either rubbing the foot or getting up to walk to relieve the pain. Pain relief usually results from the addition of gravitational pressure to the arterial pressure perfusing the affected extremity and to a decrease in venous return during dependency. In severe situations, the patient may present with pronounced swelling in the foot from extended dependency. This can create confusion as to whether venous disease or arterial disease is present. Careful history and physical examination, along with objective testing, can distinguish between the different causes of the pain. More severe ischemia of the limb can lead to ischemic ulceration, often precipitated by minor trauma.

Patients with the most significant degree of ischemia present with ischemic ulceration and gangrene. These ulcers are usually located in the distal foot. Patients often have considerable pain associated with the ulcer and most have associated pain at rest. Pain can be absent, however, especially in patients with diabetes mellitus with peripheral neuropathy. On examination, the physical findings are consistent with severe ischemia and absence of palpable pulses in the foot. Many of these patients also may have had prior claudication, although claudication does not necessarily precede the development of an ischemic ulcer.

- In only a minority of patients, intermittent claudication progresses to critical limb ischemia, defined as rest pain or ischemic ulceration

To objectively compare different patients with PAD, several classifications for the extent of limb ischemia have been devised. The two most common stratification schemes are the Fontaine (Table 28.2) and the Rutherford classifications (Table 28.3). The relationship of extent of disease to clinical presentation is helpful when comparing therapies

Table 28.2 Fontaine Classification of Chronic Limb Ischemia

Stage	Presentation
I	Asymptomatic
IIa	Mild claudication
IIb	Moderate to severe claudication
III	Rest pain
IV	Ulcer or gangrene

Table 28.3 Rutherford Classification of Peripheral Ischemia

Grade	Category	Presentation
0	0	Asymptomatic
I	1	Mild claudication
	2	Moderate claudication
	3	Severe claudication
II	4	Ischemic rest pain
	5	Minor tissue loss
III	6	Major tissue loss

and evaluating outcomes of various forms of therapy. By objectively comparing groups of patients with similar clinical presentations, these classifications allow the results of a given therapy to be assessed in patients with similar disease extent and presentation.

Evaluation of the Lower Extremity Arterial System

To assess the lower extremity arteries, it is necessary to understand the arterial anatomy of the lower extremity. The clinician must know the named branches of the lower extremity arterial system and the areas of the limb they supply. In addition, the examiner must understand the anatomic position of these vessels to reliably ascertain their presence by palpation or Doppler insonation. Of these arteries, those that can be directly assessed by physical examination include the common femoral, popliteal, dorsalis pedis, and posterior tibial. Occasionally, a collateral branch of the peroneal artery can also be palpated just anterior to the lateral malleolus. Pulse quality is usually recorded as 2 for normal, 1 for present but diminished, and 0 for absence of pulse. Pulse examination and the scoring classification should be prominently noted in the patient's medical record.

Non-invasive tests of the lower extremity circulation (ankle-brachial index, pulse volume recording, transcutaneous oximetry) can determine the extent and often the location of the obstruction. The findings of these tests, along with non-invasive evaluation of the arterial system using either magnetic resonance angiography or computed tomography angiography, can direct planned therapy. The use of non-invasive testing is discussed in other chapters.

To standardize evaluation of the extent of disease in the lower extremity vessels, a working group was created to devise a classification scheme that is based on anatomic extent, morphologic assessment, and location of lesions within the vascular system. This group, comprising experts from the United States and Europe, developed the TransAtlantic Inter-Society Consensus (TASC) classification strategy and made recommendations regarding appropriate therapy for different lesions. The recommendations vary by the location and extent of the lesion. Briefly, this stratification allows the classification of lesions as A, B, C, or D, based on morphologic criteria, and is location specific for the vasculature of the lower extremity below the inguinal ligament (Table 28.4). Data regarding interventional and surgical therapeutic outcomes for lesions of the femoropopliteal segment indicate that interventional therapy has clear benefit over surgical therapy for type A lesions and that surgical therapy is the treatment of choice for type D lesions. For type B and C lesions, more information is necessary to make definitive therapeutic recommendations.

Therapeutic Options

The treatment of peripheral vascular disease can vary from medical therapy (including exercise therapy) to open surgical reconstruction of the lower extremity arteries. Various factors can influence the choice regarding whether to

Table 28.4 TASC Classification of Lesions of the Lower Extremity Vessels

TASC lesion type	Location: Femoropopliteal segment	Location: Infrapopliteal segment
A	Single stenosis <3 cm of CFA or SFA	Single stenosis <1 cm in tibial or peroneal vessel
B	Single stenosis of 3-10 cm, not involving distal popliteal artery	Multiple focal stenoses <1 cm in tibial or peroneal vessel
	Heavily calcified stenosis up to 3 cm	One or two focal stenoses, each <1 cm at tibial trifurcation
	Multiple lesions, each <3 cm (stenosis or occlusion)	Short tibial or peroneal stenosis in conjunction with femoropopliteal PTA
	Single or multiple lesions in the absence of continuous tibial runoff to improve inflow for distal surgical bypass	
C	Single stenosis or occlusion >5 cm	Stenosis of 1-4 cm
	Multiple stenoses or occlusions, each 3-5 cm with or without heavy calcification	Occlusions of 1-2 cm in the tibial or peroneal vessels
		Extensive stenoses of the tibial trifurcation
D	Complete CFA or SFA occlusion or complete popliteal and proximal trifurcation occlusions	Tibial or peroneal occlusions >2 cm
		Diffusely diseased tibial or peroneal vessels

CFA, common femoral artery; PTA, percutaneous transluminal angioplasty; SFA, superficial femoral artery; TASC, TransAtlantic Inter-Society Consensus.

proceed with invasive therapy for this condition, including patient age, severity of claudication, location and extent of disease, presence and severity of critical limb ischemia, medical comorbid conditions, and the risk-benefit ratio of the proposed procedure.

Interventional Therapies

Angioplasty

Several options exist for interventional therapy of arterial lesions of the lower extremity (Table 28.5). By far the most commonly used modality is angioplasty, for which two different methods can be used. The first involves advancing a guidewire intraluminally through a stenosis or an occlusion and inflating a balloon catheter within the vessel lumen. More recently, subintimal angioplasty has been used increasingly for occlusive lesions in the lower extremities. This method has increased the acute technical success rate of traversing occlusive lesions to 80% to 90%. Although outcomes for long segments treated with this technique are similar to those with standard angioplasty, the ability to achieve treatment success represents a significant advance. Success rates for femoropopliteal angioplasty vary depending on several factors. Factors associated with less favorable outcomes include poor runoff, diabetes mellitus, renal failure, increasing lesion length and complexity, popliteal (vs femoral) artery, critical limb ischemia (vs claudication), and occlusion (vs stenosis).

Angioplasty patency rates for femoropopliteal lesions in patients with claudication at 1, 3, and 5 years are 75%, 60%, and 55% for stenotic lesions and 65%, 50%, and 40% for occlusions. With limb ischemia, expected results at the same time points are 60%, 45%, and 40% for severe, short-distance claudication and 50%, 30%, and 25% for patients with critical limb ischemia. For favorable lesions in patients with claudication, angioplasty can be an ideal therapy, but it can be less than optimal for complex lesions affecting those with diabetes mellitus, renal insufficiency, and limb-threatening ischemia. Recently, however, data from a randomized trial in patients suitable for interventional or surgical therapy support an "either-or" approach. In this trial comparing angioplasty with surgery for critical limb ischemia, similar amputation-free survival rates were seen for the two therapies, with a lower cost in the short term for angioplasty. This study also clearly documented the significant mortality risk in these patients, with a 40% to 50% 5-year mortality rate.

Table 28.5 Options for Interventional Treatment of Lower Extremity Arterial Disease

Treatment	12-mo patency, %	Notes
Angioplasty		
With claudication	50-75	TASC A and B lesions
With critical limb ischemia	40-60	TASC A and B lesions
Cryoplasty	70	Lesions <8 cm and minimal calcification
Cutting balloon angioplasty	No data	
Laser	60-80	Assisted angioplasty
Mechanical atherectomy	80	30% Assisted angioplasty
Stent	60-80	TASC A and B lesions
Drug-eluting stent	80-100	Decreases to 60% at 2 years
Covered stent	60-80	TASC A and B lesions
Brachytherapy	60-80	Difficult application

TASC, TransAtlantic Inter-Society Consensus.

- Multiple factors can affect therapeutic intervention for PAD: medical comorbidities (specifically diabetes and renal failure), extent of PAD, and the nature and extent of the proposed revascularization
- The most commonly performed interventional procedure for lower extremity arterial disease is angioplasty, with expected 12-month patency rates of 50%-75% in TASC A and B lesions

Cryoplasty

Cryoplasty is a technique that combines the pressure of angioplasty with cold energy by delivering nitrous oxide to inflate a non-compliant balloon. Catheters are available in various lengths and diameters. This technology has been evaluated in a registry of 102 patients with occlusive disease of the femoropopliteal segment. In these lesions, varying from TASC types A through C (15% as occlusions; average lesion length, 4.7 cm), the 9-month primary patency rate by duplex ultrasonography was 70%. However, clinical patency was 82% because only 16 patients required reintervention during the follow-up period. Only 8.8% of lesions required stenting for either dissection or significant residual stenosis. There are no data on the use of this device in the treatment of infrapopliteal lesions.

Cutting Balloon Angioplasty

In cutting balloon angioplasty, the balloon contains three or four sharp microtomes fixed longitudinally about the outer surface of a non-compliant balloon. Radial expansion of the balloon results in longitudinal incisions in the plaque, thereby relieving hoop stress in the arterial wall. These devices are available in diameters from 2 to 8 mm and lengths of 10 to 20 mm. Data are not available on the use of this device in the femoropopliteal segment but are available from a single-institution study of its use in the infrapopliteal segment. In 73 patients with 93 vessels treated, the technical success rate was 80% and improved to 100% when adjunctive stenting was included. Limb salvage in this group was 89.5%, but data for luminal patency were not available. These balloons have also been used to treat vein graft stenoses in the lower extremities. In some situations they allow improved early results in recalcitrant lesions when compared with angioplasty alone. Information about their use in the femoral and popliteal arteries is not yet available.

Laser

Laser technology has been used to recanalize arteries for several years. Lasers currently in use deliver lower energy than those previously used, which limits the degree of tissue penetration. The device often requires the addition of angioplasty to achieve adequate luminal caliber. In a randomized trial comparing laser-assisted angioplasty with angioplasty alone in patients with complex femoropopliteal occlusive disease, the initial technical success rates were similar in the two groups (85% laser vs 91% angioplasty), with the same primary patency rate (49%) in the two groups. A smaller proportion of the patients with laser-assisted angioplasty required stenting (42%) than did those with angioplasty alone (59%; *P*=.02).

Lasers also have been used in the infrapopliteal arteries. In the LACI 2 (Laser Angioplasty for Critical Limb Ischemia) trial, 145 patients who were poor surgical candidates (with 155 critically ischemic limbs) were treated. The average vessel length treated was 16.2 cm. Limb salvage at 1 year was 93%, and reintervention was required in only 15% of limbs. This compares favorably with reported results for angioplasty of the infrapopliteal vessels.

Mechanical Atherectomy

The recent introduction of a new debulking device, a mechanical atherectomy catheter, has made another technique available to the endovascular specialist. The device removes plaque with a rotating blade and captures the plaque in a catheter housing that requires intermittent emptying. It has been assessed in a voluntary registry of device users in patients with femoropopliteal occlusive disease, which involved the treatment of 1,047 lesions in 505 patients with a mean superficial femoral artery (SFA) lesion length of 7.7 cm. Only 25% of patients required adjunctive therapy and 5% required stenting. The rate of freedom from target lumen revascularization was 80% at 12 months. No data regarding vessel patency were given from this registry. Randomized data are needed to adequately assess outcomes in comparison to angioplasty in the femoropopliteal segment.

The results of mechanical atherectomy in the infrapopliteal segment are not as well defined, but a small study reporting results for 27 lesions in 17 patients gives some insight. In this study, the primary technical success rate was 93%, with 30% of lesions requiring adjunctive therapy. No mid- or long-term data are available for treatment of this segment, making it impossible to compare this technique with angioplasty alone.

- Laser-assisted angioplasty and mechanical atherectomy have been shown to decrease the incidence of stenting requirements in treating lower extremity arterial disease

Stenting

Stent placement in the femoropopliteal arteries has been used for several years; results appear to be improving with the introduction of flexible nitinol stents. These devices, however, have also been increasingly scrutinized because of stent fracture (which may also be related to recurrent stenosis). Currently, most devices used in the femoropopliteal segment are of the self-expanding and flexible type because results with balloon-expandable stents were disappointing.

Although stents have been increasingly used in the femoropopliteal segment, no convincing data exist to show that primary stenting dramatically improves outcome. However, stenting can improve outcomes after suboptimal balloon angioplasty. In two recent reports that assessed outcomes in femoropopliteal segment stenting, 12-month patency for stented lesions was 50% to 60%. In an assessment designed to evaluate drug-eluting stents in the femoropopliteal segment, the patency rate at 6 months was 100% in the non–drug-eluting stent arm for 8-cm SFA lesions. Further evaluation of the results with nitinol stents for occlusive disease is warranted.

Drug-Eluting Stents

Data are now available from two randomized trials assessing outcomes for drug-eluting stents in the SFA. In the SIROCCO I and II trials (Sirolimus-Eluting versus Bare Nitinol Stent for Obstructive Superficial Femoral Artery Disease), as the name implies, patients were randomly assigned to sirolimus-eluting or non–drug-eluting, nitinol self-expanding stents. The first of these trials showed early decrease in intimal hyperplasia with the sirolimus-eluting stents; however, problems with stent fracture were significant and the data have not been formally published. Early results were encouraging (restenosis rates: 0% for drug-eluting vs 23.5% for nitinol stents), but later results failed to show long-term benefit. These results—substantial restenosis rates and stent fractures—led to changes in stent design and drug delivery method. In the second trial (SIROCCO II), 6-month data showed a significant decrease in restenosis in the drug-eluting stent group (0% vs 7.7%). The effects have not been sustained in the long term, however, with 18-month data showing a lack of improved patency in the drug-eluting stents (restenosis rate: 20.7% for drug-eluting stents vs 17.9% for non–drug-eluting stents). Currently, a randomized trial is evaluating the use of paclitaxel-eluting stents in the SFA.

Few studies have evaluated the method of drug elution or the dose of anti-restenotic agent best suited to treating the SFA. Given that vessel volumes and wall thicknesses are very different from those in the coronary arteries, it is unlikely that dosing in the same manner will result in similar outcomes. Work must continue to identify the best drug, dosing, and elution method to treat this arterial segment with drug-eluting stents. Until this is better clarified, these devices will remain available only as part of investigational studies.

Covered Stents

Several studies have reported the use of covered stents in the infrainguinal vessels, and each has assessed the results of covered stent therapy for lesions within the SFA. Early results showed high technical success rates (>95%), but the 12-month primary patency rates were comparable to those seen with angioplasty alone for favorable lesions (60%-80%). These devices can prove helpful for treating dissection and eccentric plaque and for significant residual stenosis after primary angioplasty, but the future role of this technology remains unclear.

Brachytherapy

Brachytherapy has been used in conjunction with angioplasty and stenting below the inguinal ligament, but difficulties in dosing continue to make its use problematic. In one study, restenosis rates were decreased by gamma radiation dosed at the time of angioplasty and were similarly decreased in the group treated with external beam irradiation after intervention and stenting. However, decreased restenosis rates have not been seen uniformly with radiation after intervention. In the Vienna-5 trial, the results were not as promising in patients undergoing stent placement in conjunction with radiotherapy. Nevertheless, more studies have documented the efficacy of radiation in limiting restenosis than have shown no benefit. The extent of this benefit, however, remains unclear. Results are awaited from the PARIS (Peripheral Artery Radiation Investigational Study) II trial, a randomized prospective study comparing angioplasty alone with angioplasty in conjunction with intraluminal radiation.

In the setting of acute interventions, the application of this technology has not been easy, and the extended time necessary to perform this therapy is problematic. Its applicability is currently limited because of the difficulty in delivering the radiation dose to the vessel wall.

- Radiotherapy and drug-eluting stents have the potential to improve long-term outcomes of infrainguinal intervention; however, difficulties with application of these technologies have limited their widespread use

Summary

Endovascular treatment of lesions below the inguinal ligament is compromised by the high incidence of recurrent narrowing, secondary to intimal hyperplasia. Several factors are associated with this phenomenon, including lesion length, lesion morphology, and associated medical comorbidities. As the age of patients with this problem continues to increase, so does the number of their associated comorbid conditions. In addition, many patients are not ideal surgical candidates because of inadequate autologous conduit or limited target vessels. These patients are candidates for interventional therapy, with the understanding that recurrence rates will be high. For patients with low surgical risk, the vascular therapist must decide whether intervention or surgery offers the best initial treatment; classification of the lesion according to TASC criteria may be of benefit. Patients with TASC A and B lesions can likely be offered interventional therapy initially, whereas those with TASC D lesions must understand that with endovascular therapy the risk of recurrence is high. When other issues that affect outcome (runoff status, presence of diabetes mellitus or renal disease) are factored into the decision, the choice may be to forego interventional therapy and opt for surgery.

- Despite extensive research into interventional modalities for treatment of lower extremity atherosclerotic disease, all treatments are associated with some degree of recurrence and an inability to achieve long-term patency

Adjunctive therapies remain appropriate in specific settings, as outlined above. Although indications exist for these adjunctive therapies, no method has been clearly proven to radically alter outcomes when compared with angioplasty alone in this area of the peripheral vasculature. It is hoped that in the near future advances in the technologies of these adjunctive therapies will improve the outcomes of intervention in this region to allow their more widespread application with lower risk of recurrence.

Questions

1. All of the following are associated with an increased risk of PAD except:
   a. Coronary artery disease
   b. Diabetes mellitus
   c. Male sex
   d. Hypertension
   e. Cerebrovascular disease

2. Most patients with PAD present with:
   a. Claudication
   b. Rest pain
   c. Ischemic ulcer
   d. Gangrene
   e. None of the above

3. Which of the following is *not* associated with an increased risk of failure of a lower extremity intervention?
   a. Renal failure
   b. Diabetes mellitus
   c. Coronary artery disease
   d. Critical limb ischemia
   e. Calcification

4. What is the most frequently used technique for treating PAD in the lower extremities?
   a. Angioplasty
   b. Cryoplasty
   c. Atherectomy
   d. Laser
   e. Drug-eluting stents

5. Which classification was developed to create a uniform standard for assessing PAD lesion morphology?
   a. Rutherford classification
   b. Fontaine classification
   c. TASC classification
   d. Rutherford-Becker score
   e. Rooke ratio

Suggested Readings

Ansel GM, Sample NS, Botti CF Jr III, et al. Cutting balloon angioplasty of the popliteal and infrapopliteal vessels for symptomatic limb ischemia. Catheter Cardiovasc Interv. 2004;61:1-4.

Bolia A, Miles KA, Brennan J, et al. Percutaneous transluminal angioplasty of occlusions of the femoral and popliteal arteries by subintimal dissection. Cardiovasc Intervent Radiol. 1990;13:357-63.

Bray PJ, Robson WJ, Bray AE. Percutaneous treatment of long superficial femoral artery occlusive disease: efficacy of the Hemobahn stent-graft. J Endovasc Ther. 2003;10:619-28.

Centers for Disease Control and Prevention (CDC). Lower extremity disease among persons aged > or = 40 years with and without diabetes: United States, 1999-2002. MMWR Morb Mortal Wkly Rep. 2005;54:1158-60.

Charo IF, Ransohoff RM. The many roles of chemokines and chemokine receptors in inflammation. N Engl J Med. 2006;354:610-21.

Diehm N, Shang A, Silvestro A, et al. Association of cardiovascular risk factors with pattern of lower limb atherosclerosis in 2659 patients undergoing angioplasty. Eur J Vasc Endovasc Surg. 2006 Jan;31:59-63. Epub 2005 Nov 2.

Dillavou E, Kahn MB. Peripheral vascular disease: diagnosing and treating the 3 most common peripheral vasculopathies. Geriatrics. 2003;58:37-42.

Dormandy JA, Rutherford RB, TASC Working Group (TransAtlantic Inter-Society Consensus). Management of peripheral arterial disease (PAD). J Vasc Surg. 2000;31:S1-S296.

Duda SH, Bosiers M, Pusich B, et al. Endovascular treatment of peripheral artery disease with expanded PTFE-covered nitinol stents: interim analysis from a prospective controlled study. Cardiovasc Interv Radiol. 2002 Sep-Oct;25:413-8. Epub 2002 Jun 4.

Gray BH, Laird JR, Ansel GM, et al. Complex endovascular treatment for critical limb ischemia in poor surgical candidates: a pilot study. J Endovasc Ther. 2002;9:599-604.

Hartung O, Otero A, Dubuc M, et al. Efficacy of Hemobahn in the treatment of superficial femoral artery lesions in patients with acute or critical ischemia: a comparative study with claudicants. Eur J Vasc Endovasc Surg. 2005;30:300-6.

Howell MA, Colgan MP, Seeger RW, et al. Relationship of severity of lower limb peripheral vascular disease to mortality and morbidity: a six-year follow-up study. J Vasc Surg. 1989;9:691-6.

Krueger K, Zaehringer M, Bendel M, et al. De novo femoropopliteal stenoses: endovascular gamma irradiation following angioplasty: angiographic and clinical follow-up in a prospective randomized controlled trial. Radiology. 2004 May;231:546-54. Epub 2004 Apr 2.

Laird J, Jaff MR, Biamino G, et al. Cryoplasty for the treatment of femoropopliteal arterial disease: results of a prospective, multicenter registry. J Vasc Interv Radiol. 2005;16:1067-73.

Morgan JH III, Wall CE Jr, Christie DB, et al. The results of superficial femoral, popliteal, and tibial artery stenting for peripheral vascular occlusive disease. Am Surg. 2005;71:905-9.

Novo S, Coppola G, Milio G. Critical limb ischemia: definition and natural history. Curr Drug Targets Cardiovasc Haematol Disord. 2004;4:219-25.

O'Hare AM, Katz R, Shlipak MG, et al. Mortality and cardiovascular risk across the ankle-arm index spectrum: results from the Cardiovascular Health Study. Circulation. 2006;113:388-93.

Pokrajac B, Potter R, Wolfram RM, et al. Endovascular brachytherapy prevents restenosis after femoropopliteal angioplasty: results of the Vienna-3 randomised multicenter study. Radiother Oncol. 2005;74:3-9.

Zabakis P, Kardamakis DM, Siablis D, et al. External beam radiation therapy reduces the rate of re-stenosis in patients treated with femoral stenting: results of a randomised study. Radiother Oncol. 2005;74:11-6.

Zeller T, Frank U, Burgelin K, et al. Initial clinical experience with percutaneous atherectomy in the infragenicular arteries. J Endovasc Ther. 2003;10:987-93.

29 Thrombolytic Therapy for Arterial and Venous Occlusive Disease

J. Michael Bacharach, MD, MPH, FACC
David P. Slovut, MD, PhD, FACC

Introduction

For decades, surgical thrombectomy and bypass grafting have been mainstay therapy for acute limb-threatening ischemia. Historically, surgical treatment has been associated with in-hospital mortality rates of 15% to 25% and amputation rates of more than 25%. Percutaneous catheter-directed thrombolysis has emerged as an alternative to surgery for restoring arterial patency. In the 30 years since McNicol and colleagues first performed directed local delivery of streptokinase, substantial progress has been made in the clinical application of thrombolytic therapy for peripheral arterial occlusive disease. Various infusion techniques and catheters have been developed. It is now known that lysis occurs most effectively when the infusion catheter is seated within the thrombus and thrombolytic drug is delivered directly into the clot, which improves the likelihood of clot lysis within a shorter period of time. With intra-arterial infusion of tissue plasminogen activator (tPA), effective clot lysis has been achieved in as few as 4 to 8 hours. Faster and more efficacious clot lysis can be achieved by combining thrombolysis with catheter-directed mechanical and rheolytic thrombectomy. Today, catheter-directed thrombolytic therapy offers a well-established method for treating peripheral arterial and venous occlusions.

Catheter-Directed Intra-Arterial Thrombolysis

Patient Selection

Common indications for intra-arterial thrombolysis include:

1) Acute thrombosis with a threatened but viable extremity (successful thrombolysis permits time for definitive surgical or endovascular revascularization without irreparable ischemic limb damage);
2) Embolic or thrombotic occlusion of native arteries, saphenous vein grafts, or prosthetic grafts;
3) Thrombotic or embolic complications after angiography or endovascular intervention;
4) Acute thrombosis of a popliteal aneurysm (thrombolysis may significantly increase the chance of successful limb salvage); and
5) Patients with wound complications or comorbid conditions that make surgical revascularization technically unfeasible or excessively risky.

Determining the degree of ischemia is important when selecting patients to undergo thrombolysis and predicting long-term outcomes. Thrombolytic therapy should not be used for patients with an immediately threatened limb. Evidence of substantial sensory or motor impairment suggests that irreversible damage is imminent. These patients should undergo immediate surgical revascularization. Patients with lesser degrees of ischemia are generally candidates for thrombolysis (Table 29.1). Because of bleeding risk, thrombolysis may be contraindicated in some patients. Relative contraindications are considered in relation to available alternatives and the experience of the treating physician.

Patients with a low probability of a successful outcome after catheter-directed thrombolysis should undergo surgery as first-line therapy. Common indications for operative thromboembolectomy include acute embolic occlusion of large arteries; severely ischemic limb in which the viability is imminently threatened; acute postoperative bypass graft occlusion or thrombosis, because patients are at substantial risk of hemorrhage (most postoperative graft failure is associated with technical error); and modest ischemia with symptoms of claudication

Table 29.1 Recommendations for Thrombolytic Therapy for Acute Limb Ischemia

Class I: evidence for and/or general agreement that the treatment is beneficial, useful, and effective

- Catheter-based thrombolysis is an effective and beneficial therapy and is indicated for patients with acute limb ischemia (Rutherford categories I and IIa) of less than 14 days' duration. (Level of evidence: A)

Class IIa: weight of evidence/opinion is in favor of usefulness/efficacy

- Mechanical thrombectomy devices can be used as adjunctive therapy for acute limb ischemia due to peripheral arterial occlusion. (Level of evidence: B)

Class IIb: usefulness/efficacy is less well established by evidence/opinion

- Catheter-based thrombolysis or thrombectomy may be considered for patients with acute limb ischemia (Rutherford category IIb) of more than 14 days' duration. (Level of evidence: B)

From ACC/AHA guidelines for the management of patients with peripheral arterial disease (lower extremity, renal, mesenteric, and abdominal aortic): a collaborative report from the American Associations for Vascular Surgery/Society for Vascular Surgery, Society for Cardiovascular Angiography and Interventions, Society for Vascular Medicine and Biology, Society of Interventional Radiology, and the ACC/AHA Task Force on Practice Guidelines (Writing Committee to Develop Guidelines for the Management of Patients With Peripheral Arterial Disease): summary of recommendations. J Vasc Interv Radiol. 2006;17:1383-98. Used with permission.

(the risk-benefit ratio does not favor catheter-directed thrombolysis).

- Thrombolytic therapy should not be used in patients with an immediately threatened limb; these patients should undergo immediate surgical revascularization
- Patients with a low probability of a successful outcome after catheter-directed thrombolysis should undergo surgery as first-line therapy

Choice of Thrombolytic Agent

All thrombolytic agents currently in use are plasminogen activators. These agents do not directly degrade fibrinogen to fibrin but act as proteolytic enzymes that convert plasminogen to plasmin. Plasmin is the active molecule that cleaves fibrin polymer to cause the dissolution of thrombus.

Urokinase (UK) was the predominant agent used for peripheral thrombolysis in the 80s and 90s. Because of its efficacy, predictability, lack of immunogenicity, and decreased bleeding complications compared with streptokinase, UK administration became the standard of care for catheter-directed thrombolysis in the United States. However, UK was removed from the US market in late 1998 because of concerns about the safety of its production. The agent was reintroduced in 2002 and remains available but is not actively promoted.

Other thrombolytic agents available in the United States include recombinant tPA (rtPA), the third-generation thrombolytic agent reteplase, and tenecteplase. Reteplase is a recombinantly derived mutant version of tPA that was initially developed and approved for bolus infusion treatment of acute myocardial infarction. Compared with rtPA, reteplase has a longer half-life (13-15 minutes), higher fibrin specificity, and lower fibrin affinity, which may improve the ability of the agent to penetrate clot and decrease hemorrhagic complications. Tenecteplase is modified rtPA with a longer half-life and greater fibrin specificity, which decreases fibrinogenolysis. The tPAs, particularly rtPA, have been used widely for thrombolysis in peripheral arterial and venous occlusive disease.

Several comparative studies and pooled analyses have been performed to determine which fibrinolytic agent provides the optimal combination of efficacy and safety. UK and tPA offer improved thrombolysis and fewer complications than streptokinase. In three retrospective studies comparing UK with streptokinase, clot lysis occurred in 80% of patients receiving UK and in 52% of patients receiving streptokinase. Studies using tPA at a dosage of 0.05 to 0.1 $mg \cdot kg^{-1} \cdot h^{-1}$ have shown lysis in 93% to 100% of patients. Intra-arterial infusion of reteplase at 0.5 U/h was associated with 96% technical success, a low rate of hemorrhagic complications, and no intracerebral bleeding.

Although several groups have proposed various guidelines for thrombolytic administration, no consensus yet exists regarding optimal dosing or delivery mode for these agents. A Cochrane Database review of arterial thrombolysis evaluated six randomized trials to assess optimal methods for infusing fibrinolytic drugs in patients with peripheral arterial ischemia. Substantial heterogeneity and disparate outcome measures among studies did not allow for meaningful statistical comparison of variables such as vessel patency, time to thrombolysis, and angiographic success. Instead, clinically relevant variables such as limb salvage, amputation, major amputation, death, major hemorrhage, and cerebrovascular accident were examined. The review concluded that high-dose and "accelerated" regimens decreased the duration of thrombolysis but were more labor intensive and had slightly more bleeding complications than did low-dose regimens. Intravenous systemic lysis should not be used for treatment of peripheral arterial ischemia. The use of glycoprotein IIb/IIIa antagonists remains unproven in peripheral vascular thrombolysis.

Patency

Early patency rates for intra-arterial thrombolysis of native arteries vary from 56% to 100%. For bypass grafts, immediate success rates range from 60% to 80%. Factors that predict successful thrombolysis include the ability to pass a guidewire into or through the clot, shorter duration of occlusion, location of the occlusion (proximal vs distal), and presence of patent distal vessels by angiography or audible Doppler signals.

Short-term patency decreases as the degree of ischemia worsens. In one study, patients with single-segmental occlusions and non-threatening ischemia had a 30-day patency rate after thrombolysis of 100%. In patients with more severe ischemia and tandem lesions in contiguous segments, 30-day patency was 84%; this decreased to only 63% in the patient group with the worst ischemia. Long-term patency decreases further with greater degrees of ischemia. In another study, patients with the most severe ischemia, as evidenced by tissue loss, had a 5-year postlysis patency of 51%, compared with 95% patency in patients with only mild claudication.

The extent to which anatomic location of the occlusion influences patency is not entirely known. A study comparing iliac and femoropopliteal lesions reported 6-month patency rates of 92% and 48%, respectively. Patency rates were greater for suprainguinal grafts than for infrainguinal bypass grafts (70% vs 26%). Other studies, however, have failed to demonstrate a statistical difference when comparing cumulative patency between suprainguinal and infrainguinal bypass grafts.

The duration of occlusion appears to affect the initial success of lysis and short-term patency but has little effect on long-term patency. The 2-week patency rate was 58% for thrombotic occlusions of less than 6 months' duration and 36% for occlusions lasting longer than 6 months. Cumulative patency of successfully opened lesions was not influenced by duration of occlusion.

The most important determinant of long-term patency for both native arteries and bypass grafts is whether the underlying stenotic lesion that precipitated the thrombotic event has been identified and corrected (Fig. 29.1). One study demonstrated this convincingly in a group of patients treated for femoropopliteal occlusions. In patients who had an untreated residual stenosis in the reopened arterial segment, 6-month patency was only 48%, compared with 77% in patients without residual stenoses. The influence of persistent hemodynamically significant lesions on bypass graft patency was even more pronounced. The 6-month patency rate for infrainguinal grafts without persistent stenosis was 80%, versus only 7% for grafts with persistent lesions. Another study reported a 1-year patency rate of 86% in bypass grafts that had correctable lesions, compared with 37% in lysed grafts with lesions that could not be corrected.

Another important factor influencing long-term bypass graft patency is graft material. Higher patency rates have been shown for vein grafts than for prosthetic grafts. The

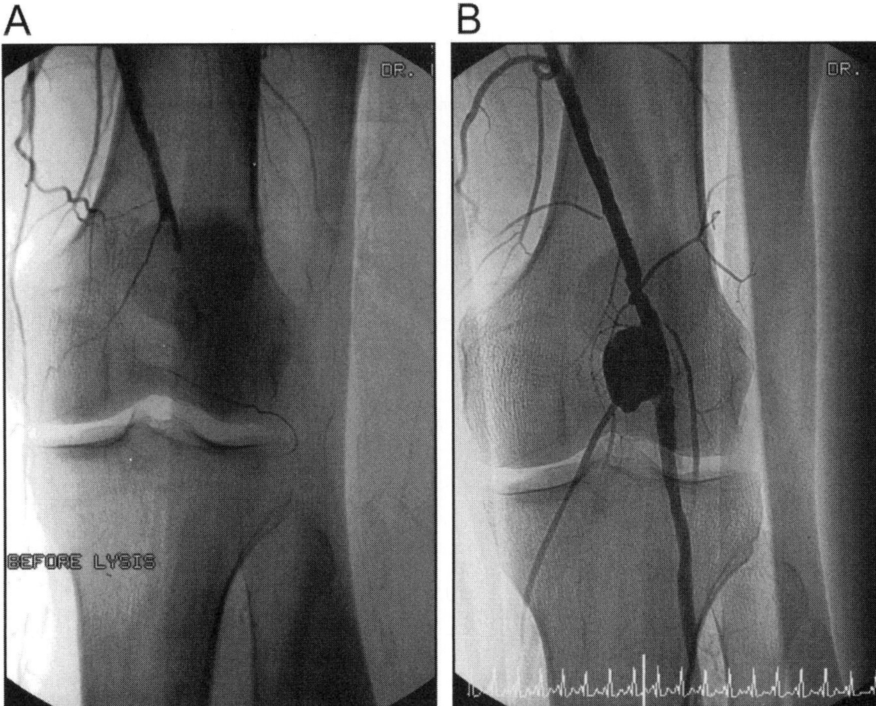

Fig. 29.1 Angiography of thrombosed popliteal aneurysm. *A*, Before lytic therapy. *B*, After lytic therapy.

30-month cumulative patency rate for vein grafts was 69.3% compared with 28.6% for prosthetic grafts.

Risks of Thrombolytic Therapy

The predominant risk associated with thrombolytic therapy is bleeding. The spectrum of complications ranges from minor bleeding from puncture or catheter entry sites to life-threatening bleeding and intracranial hemorrhage. In a retrospective analysis of major bleeding complications for different lytic agents, the incidence of major bleeding complications for streptokinase, reteplase, and UK was 28%, 12%, and 6%, respectively. The incidence of intracranial bleeding was less than 1%.

In another retrospective study of the incidence of in-hospital complications after catheter-directed thrombolysis, patients with lower extremity arterial occlusion (n=527) or venous occlusion (n=126) were treated with UK (4,000 IU/min up to 48 hours), rtPA (0.05-0.1 mg·kg^{-1}·h^{-1} up to 24 hours), or both. Heparin was administered concomitantly to maintain a partial thromboplastin time of 1.5 to 2.0 times control value. Compared with rtPA, UK was associated with lower blood transfusion requirements (12.4% vs 22.2%; P=.04), fewer groin hematomas (21.9% vs 43.8%; P<.001), a lower rate of intracranial hemorrhage (0.62% vs 2.78%; P=.03), and a lower incidence of decompensation requiring transfer to an intensive care setting (1.5% vs 4.9%; P=.02). However, the doses of thrombolytic used in this study were substantially higher than those used by most interventionalists today.

In a pilot study to assess the safety and efficacy of reteplase for treating peripheral arterial and venous occlusion, complete dissolution of thrombus was achieved in 23 (89%) of 26 patients with arterial occlusion (16 native vessels and 10 bypass grafts). The mean infusion time was 19.3 hours. Adjuvant endovascular or surgical procedures were required in 8 patients (31%); limb salvage was achieved in all patients. No patients died during the index hospitalization. Major hemorrhagic complications were seen in 5 patients (19%). For patients with deep vein thrombosis (n=11), mean infusion duration was 31.1 hours, with clinically successful thrombolysis in 10 cases (91%). Periprocedural bleeding complications were observed in 3 of 11 patients.

The National Audit of Thrombolysis for Acute Leg Ischemia represents a series of more than 1,000 consecutive patients who underwent intra-arterial thrombolysis to treat acute limb ischemia in one of 11 centers in the United Kingdom. Outcomes and complications were reviewed for 1,133 thrombolytic events. A total of 852 patients (75.2%) survived the ischemic episode without requiring amputation. Mortality was higher in women, older patients, those with native vessel occlusion or emboli, and in patients with a history of ischemic heart disease. Major hemorrhage requiring transfusion or operation was observed in 87 cases (7.68%), with 5 fatal events. Stroke occurred in 26 patients (2.3%) and was fatal in 20 (77%) of these. Of the strokes that occurred, half were reported as hemorrhagic and half were thromboembolic; most strokes occurred during anticoagulation after thrombolysis.

Practical Applications of Thrombolytic Therapy in Clinical Practice

Specific thrombolytic infusion methods vary and include intravenous, intra-arterial bolus followed by continuous infusion, and pulse-spray techniques. In a study of 40 patients, intravenous delivery of rtPA was less efficacious than intra-arterial administration and carried a significantly higher risk of hemorrhagic complications. Intra-arterial infusion of rtPA produced more consistent and complete thrombolysis. Although continuous end-hole infusions have been used successfully, the development of multiple side-hole catheters that can be positioned across the entire length of thrombus has allowed higher local drug concentration and faster thrombolysis.

Recombinant tPA is now commonly substituted for UK for catheter-directed treatment of peripheral arterial and venous occlusive disease. In cases of moderate ischemia, rtPA is diluted with normal saline to yield a concentration of 0.1 mg/mL for continuous infusion through a multiple side-hole catheter. Starting doses are 2 to 3 mg/h for 2 to 3 hours, then are decreased to 1 to 2 mg/h. The trend has been to use lower infusion rates; adequate thrombolysis has been achieved with infusion rates as low as 0.5 to 1.0 mg/h.

In situations of profound ischemia, many operators advocate a lacing dose of rtPA (5-10 mg) throughout the entire length of the thrombosed segment, followed by a continuous infusion starting at 2 to 4 mg/h followed by a rate of 1 to 2 mg/h after 2 to 4 hours. Less data are available regarding the use of reteplase. Typical concentrations for its use in peripheral arterial occlusive disease include a bolus of 5 units followed by an infusion rate of 0.5 to 1.0 U/h.

The use of heparin along with a thrombolytic agent has varied considerably. Heparin is typically used to prevent thrombus formation around the infusion catheter, as well as to prevent the reaccumulation of thrombus in the treated segment. Several studies have shown that heparin does not increase the efficacy of lysis and in some situations, particularly with higher doses, leads to increased bleeding complications. Many operators either withdraw the heparin or decrease its dose considerably during lytic therapy. Typical heparin dosing is 400 to 600 U/h with a target activated partial thromboplastin time of less than 45 seconds after thrombolysis has been started.

Comparison of Thrombolytic Therapy and Surgery

Several clinical trials suggest that local thrombolysis using UK or tPAs relieves limb ischemia and decreases the need for surgical intervention without an increase in limb loss or mortality. In a study from Rochester, New York, thrombolytic therapy was compared with operative revascularization in the initial treatment of acute peripheral arterial ischemia. Although the trial involved only 114 patients, mortality was significantly lower in the thrombolytic therapy group than in the surgical group—16% versus 42%—at 12 months. No difference was observed in the rate of major amputation, which was approximately 18% at 12 months in each group. The authors concluded that thrombolytic therapy was associated with a decrease in cardiopulmonary complications and mortality.

After the Rochester study, two larger, prospective, randomized trials were performed. The STILE (Surgery versus Thrombolysis for Ischemia of the Lower Extremity) trial compared surgery with thrombolysis using UK or reteplase for acute and chronic lower extremity ischemia. UK and reteplase were equivalent with respect to the outcome measure evaluated. The trial was stopped prematurely because a primary end point was reached; a significantly greater proportion of patients treated with thrombolysis had ongoing or recurrent ischemia compared with patients who underwent surgery. However, subsequent post hoc analysis of a subset of patients with bypass graft occlusions concluded that thrombolytic therapy was associated with significant benefit over primary operation. The thrombolytic therapy group had fewer surgical procedures and a lower amputation rate at 1 year. The benefit was pronounced in patients with acute limb ischemia of less than 14 days' duration (Fig. 29.2).

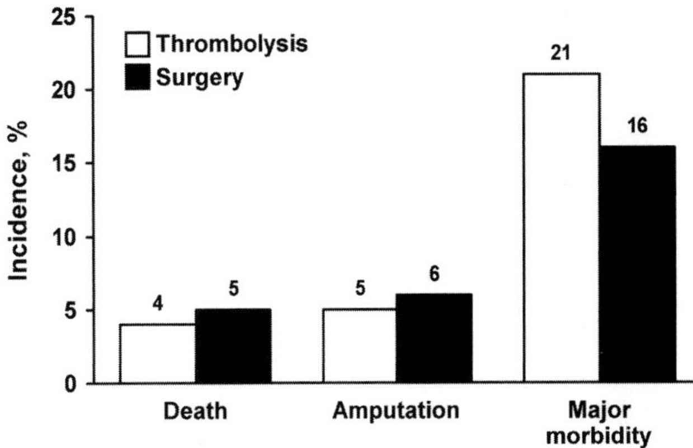

Fig. 29.2 Outcome measures from the STILE trial at 30-day follow-up. Major morbidity was more common in the thrombolysis group, whereas the death and amputation rates were similar between groups. (Data from The STILE Investigators. Results of a prospective randomized trial evaluating surgery versus thrombolysis for ischemia of the lower extremity: the STILE Trial. Ann Surg. 1994;220:251-68.)

The Thrombolysis or Peripheral Arterial Surgery (TOPAS) study compared recombinant UK (rUK) with primary operation in patients with acute lower extremity arterial ischemia. This multicenter trial examined 272 patients in both the rUK and surgical groups. No difference between the groups was found in the rates of major amputation or death within 1 year of follow-up. The TOPAS trial established equivalency of the two treatments (Table 29.2).

Although the STILE trial failed to demonstrate an overall benefit of thrombolytic therapy over surgery, there

Table 29.2 TOPAS Trial Results

	Native artery occlusion (*N*=242)			Bypass graft occlusion (*N*=302)		
Parameter	**Urokinase (*n*=122)**	**Surgery (*n*=120)**	***P* value**	**Urokinase (*n*=150)**	**Surgery (*n*=152)**	***P* Intervention**
Patients with complete dissolution of clot*	67/112 (60)	NA	NA	100/134 (75)	NA	NA
Mean±SE increase in ankle-brachial index	0.44±0.04	0.52±0.04	.15†	0.48±0.03	0.50±0.03	.76†
Mortality, %						
6 mo	20.8	15.9	.33‡	12.1	9.4	.45‡
1 y	24.6	19.6	.36‡	16.2	15.0	.77‡
Amputation-free survival, %						
6 mo	67.6	76.1	.15‡	75.2	73.9	.79‡
1 y	61.2	71.4	.10‡	68.2	68.8	.91‡

NA, not applicable; TOPAS, Thrombolysis or Peripheral Arterial Surgery.
*On final angiogram. Values are *n*/total *n* (%).
†Kaplan-Meier analysis.
‡One-way analysis of variance.
Data from Ouriel K, Shortell CK, DeWeese JA, et al. A comparison of thrombolytic therapy with operative revascularization in the initial treatment of acute peripheral arterial ischemia. J Vasc Surg. 1994;19:1021-30.

were numerous methodologic flaws in the trial. Randomization and analysis were based on "intention to treat." However, many patients who were randomly assigned to thrombolysis were never treated because of technical difficulties that prevented initial catheter placement. Perhaps a larger flaw that affected both the STILE and TOPAS trials was viewing the two treatment modalities conceptually as competitive rather than complementary. Ultimately, the goal of arterial thrombolysis is not to replace surgery but to uncover and more clearly define the etiology of an arterial occlusion. Once accomplished, this can often decrease the magnitude of any subsequent surgical or endovascular intervention.

Mechanical Adjuvants to Thrombolysis

Approximately 20% of patients have a contraindication to thrombolytic therapy. Moreover, thrombolytic therapy may require prolonged infusions and can be associated with significant risk of hemorrhagic complications. The US Food and Drug Administration has approved two mechanical thrombectomy devices for treatment of infra-inguinal acute lower extremity arterial ischemia: a rheolytic thrombectomy catheter and a drug-dispersion catheter. Other devices have been used "off label" to treat peripheral arterial occlusions.

- Approximately 20% of patients have a contraindication to thrombolytic therapy

The rheolytic thrombectomy catheter uses high-velocity saline jets for thrombus maceration and evacuation. The device initially was developed for use in the coronary arteries. A recent retrospective analysis showed the efficacy of this device in 99 patients with limb-threatening ischemia; occlusions were present in 80 native arteries and 19 surgical bypass grafts. Most patients presented within 14 days of symptom onset. A complete result was obtained in 34, a substantial result in 36, and a partial result in 22. Adjunctive catheter-directed thrombolysis was performed in 37 cases. An underlying stenosis that required angioplasty, stenting, or surgery was shown in 81 limbs. Major bleeding occurred in 5 patients. At 30-day follow-up, the amputation rate was 4.0% and the cumulative mortality rate was 7.1%. These results compare favorably with surgical series. A newer design of this catheter features a larger bore and is compatible with a 0.035-in wire system. This larger catheter may decrease the need for adjunctive catheter-directed thrombolysis.

The other system is a 7F drug-dispersion catheter that permits localized infusion of thrombolytic agent by using a proximal and distal occlusion balloon to isolate the treated arterial segment. During infusion, an oscillating wire mechanically fragments the thrombus while dispersing the lytic agent. After the liquefied thrombus is aspirated, angiography can be performed through the infusion catheter. The potential advantages of this system include minimal systemic release of thrombolytic agent, decreased likelihood of distal embolization, and shorter infusion times. In one series of 26 patients with lower extremity ischemia treated with this device, the mean dwell time was 18 minutes. The technical success rate was 92% and the 30-day amputation-free survival rate was 96%. No episodes of major bleeding or intracranial hemorrhage were reported.

Adjunctive mechanical thrombectomy decreases thrombus burden and helps restore antegrade blood flow to the ischemic limb. This technique has allowed for the treatment of profoundly ischemic limbs that in the past would have required emergent surgical revascularization.

A novel development combines thrombolytic agent with rheolytic thrombectomy in a technique described as "power-pulse spray." By occluding the catheter's outflow lumen, lytic solution exits from the distal windows of the device, thereby sending a high-pressure penetrating infusion into the surrounding thrombus without extraction. In a study using this technique with 10 to 20 mg of tenecteplase (group 1) or 1,000,000 units of UK (group 2), procedural success was observed in 92% and 91.6%, respectively, with a mean procedural time of 72 minutes (range, 40-110 minutes). No major hemorrhagic or vascular complications were observed. This technique may allow improved treatment of patients with acute limb ischemia who would not tolerate the longer duration of therapy needed to achieve adequate thrombolysis using more conventional infusion techniques.

Summary

The use of intra-arterial thrombolysis is an important therapeutic modality for the treatment of native vessel and arterial graft occlusions. Currently available plasminogen activators such as rtPA and reteplase show promise in achieving safe and effective thrombolysis. As more experience is gained, more uniform standards can be developed for dosing, technique, and adjuvant therapy to minimize complications and maximize efficacy of thrombolysis.

Thrombolysis for Acute Venous Occlusion

The spectrum of venous occlusive diseases ranges from asymptomatic calf vein deep vein thrombosis (DVT) to extensive iliofemoral DVT resulting in phlegmasia cerulea dolens. The clinical presentation of the patient is largely dependent on the extent of thrombosis. Anticoagulation with heparin or low-molecular-weight heparin, followed by oral warfarin, has been the standard of care.

Despite the difference in thrombus burden between iliofemoral and infrainguinal DVT on clinical presentation, many clinicians treat them as if they were identical problems. Patients with iliofemoral DVT are at much higher risk for post-thrombotic morbidity, including venous hypertension and chronic venous insufficiency.

The use of percutaneous intervention for critical venous occlusive disease remains controversial. Numerous investigators have suggested that thrombus removal in patients with acute DVT is not associated with improved outcome. Proponents of percutaneous intervention maintain that thrombolysis improves the structural and functional integrity of the vein. The combination of venous obstruction and valve incompetence is associated with increased severity of post-thrombotic symptoms. Historically, systemic thrombolytic therapy produced significant or complete lysis in 45% of cases. One study showed that successful lysis of the clot was associated with significant decreases in post-thrombotic morbidity and, to some extent, preservation of venous valve function. Systemically administered thrombolytic therapy has largely been abandoned in favor of the catheter-directed approach. As with intra-arterial therapy, catheter-directed thrombolysis in the venous system allows for accelerated thrombolysis, which increases the likelihood of success and decreases the risk of bleeding complications.

Several reports have shown favorable outcomes after catheter-directed thrombolysis of venous occlusions. The majority (71%) of the 287 patients enrolled in the National Venous Registry presented with iliofemoral DVT. Catheter-directed thrombolysis was performed with UK. Of these 287 patients, 31% had 100% resolution of thrombus, 52% had 50% to 99% resolution, and 17% had less than 50% of the thrombus dissolved; overall, significant thrombolysis was seen for 83% of the patients.

Survival data from the National Venous Registry showed thrombosis-free survival in 65% of the patients at 6 months and 60% of the patients at 12 months. Of the 89 patients with complete clot resolution, 78% had patent veins at 1 year, compared with 37% of those with less than 50% of the clot resolved with thrombolysis. In addition to sustained patency, early success of thrombolytic therapy correlated directly with valve function at 6 months; 62% of patients with less than 50% of the clot burden lysed had venous valvular incompetence, whereas 72% of those with complete lysis had normal valve function.

A recent series used a combination of modalities, including thrombolysis, mechanical thrombectomy, percutaneous venoplasty, and stent placement, to treat 25 patients with critical venous thromboses or occlusions. Resolution of symptoms was achieved in 18 patients (72%) and partial resolution occurred in 4 patients (16%).

On the basis of the limited data available, anticoagulation remains the standard of care for treating most patients who present with acute DVT. Patients with extensive iliofemoral DVT appear to benefit from thrombolytic therapy. Catheter-directed therapy represents an important adjunctive therapy to anticoagulation.

- With the lower rates of effective lysis, systemically administered thrombolytic therapy has largely been abandoned in favor of the catheter-directed approach
- Anticoagulation remains the standard of care for treating most patients with acute DVT with mild or moderate symptoms and extent of thrombosis
- Catheter-directed therapy represents an important adjunctive therapy to anticoagulation

Questions

1. A 63-year-old man presents with right leg pain of 4 hours' duration. The patient has known coronary artery disease and was discharged recently after being treated for an anterior myocardial infarction. On examination, his right leg is cool and mottled below the knee. Strength and sensation are diminished in the right foot. The left foot is warm with a palpable pulse. What is the optimal treatment strategy?
   a. Systemic thrombolysis
   b. Open embolectomy
   c. Intravenous heparin, with a glycoprotein IIb/IIIa inhibitor
   d. Primary below-knee amputation

2. Which of the following predicts successful outcome after catheter-directed thrombolysis of an occluded arterial bypass graft?
   a. Graft occlusion of <14 days
   b. Guidewire cannot traverse the occluded graft
   c. One-vessel runoff
   d. Inflow stenosis >60%

3. Which of the following factors increases the risk of bleeding during catheter-directed thrombolysis?
   a. Use of mechanical thrombectomy device
   b. Low-dose heparin regimen (300 U/h)
   c. Short dwell time
   d. Fibrinogen level <100 mg/dL

4. Which of the following is the least likely sequela of revascularizing a non-viable limb?
   a. Infection
   b. Acute renal failure
   c. Hyperkalemia
   d. Alkalosis

5. A 60-year-old woman presents with acute right lower extremity arterial ischemia. The femoral pulse is palpable. Based on the results of the TOPAS trial, which of the following statements is correct?

a. Survival rates at 1 year are equivalent with surgery or thrombolysis.

b. The major amputation rate at 1 year is higher with surgery than with thrombolysis.

c. Ongoing ischemia is higher with thrombolysis than with surgery.

d. The ankle-brachial index is increased more with thrombolysis than with surgery.

Suggested Readings

Akesson H, Brudin L, Dahlstrom JA, et al. Venous function assessed during a 5-year period after acute ilio-femoral venous thrombosis treated with anticoagulation. Eur J Vasc Surg. 1990;4:43-8.

Allie DE, Hebert CJ, Lirtzman MD, et al. Novel simultaneous combination chemical thrombolysis/rheolytic thrombectomy therapy for acute critical limb ischemia: the power-pulse spray technique. Catheter Cardiovasc Interv. 2004;63:512-22.

Ansel GM, George BS, Botti CF, et al. Rheolytic thrombectomy in the management of limb ischemia: 30-day results from a multicenter registry. J Endovasc Ther. 2002;9:395-402.

Berridge DC, Gregson RH, Hopkinson BR, et al. Randomized trial of intra-arterial recombinant tissue plasminogen activator, intravenous recombinant tissue plasminogen activator and intra-arterial streptokinase in peripheral arterial thrombolysis. Br J Surg. 1991;78:988-95.

Comerota AJ, Aldridge SC. Thrombolytic therapy for acute deep vein thrombosis. Semin Vasc Surg. 1992;5:76-81.

Comerota AJ, Aldridge SC. Thrombolytic therapy for deep venous thrombosis: a clinical review. Can J Surg. 1993;36:359-64.

Dayal R, Bernheim J, Clair DG, et al. Multimodal percutaneous intervention for critical venous occlusive disease. Ann Vasc Surg. 2005;19:235-40.

Earnshaw JJ, Whitman B, Foy C. National Audit of Thrombolysis for Acute Leg Ischemia (NATALI): clinical factors associated with early outcome. J Vasc Surg. 2004;39:1018-25.

Gardiner GA Jr, Harrington DP, Koltun W, et al. Salvage of occluded arterial bypass grafts by means of thrombolysis. J Vasc Surg. 1989;9:426-31.

Hanover TM, Kalbaugh CA, Gray BH, et al. Safety and efficacy of reteplase for the treatment of acute arterial occlusion: complexity of underlying lesion predicts outcome. Ann Vasc Surg. 2005;19:817-22.

Haskal ZJ. Mechanical thrombectomy devices for the treatment of peripheral arterial occlusions. Rev Cardiovasc Med. 2002;3 Suppl 2:S45-52.

Hess H, Mietaschk A, Bruckl R. Peripheral arterial occlusions: a 6-year experience with local low-dose thrombolytic therapy. Radiology. 1987;163:753-8.

Kessel DO, Berridge DC, Robertson I. Infusion techniques for peripheral arterial thrombolysis. Cochrane Database Syst Rev. 2004; No. 1:CD000985.

Laird JR, Dangas G, Jaff M, et al. Intra-arterial reteplase for the treatment of acute limb ischemia. J Invasive Cardiol. 1999;11:757-62.

McNamara TO, Bomberger RA. Factors affecting initial and 6 month patency rates after intraarterial thrombolysis with high dose urokinase. Am J Surg. 1986;152:709-12.

Mewissen MW, Seabrook GR, Meissner MH, et al. Catheter-directed thrombolysis for lower extremity deep venous thrombosis: report of a national multicenter registry. Radiology. 1999;211:39-49. Erratum in: Radiology. 1999;213:930.

Ouriel K, Gray B, Clair DG, et al. Complications associated with the use of urokinase and recombinant tissue plasminogen activator for catheter-directed peripheral arterial and venous thrombolysis. J Vasc Interv Radiol. 2000;11:295-8.

Ouriel K, Katzen B, Mewissen M, et al. Reteplase in the treatment of peripheral arterial and venous occlusions: a pilot study. J Vasc Interv Radiol. 2000;11:849-54.

Ouriel K, Shortell CK, DeWeese JA, et al. A comparison of thrombolytic therapy with operative revascularization in the initial treatment of acute peripheral arterial ischemia. J Vasc Surg. 1994;19:1021-30.

Ouriel K, Veith FJ, Sasahara AA, TOPAS Investigators. Thrombolysis or peripheral arterial surgery: phase I results. J Vasc Surg. 1996;23:64-73.

Sarac TP, Hilleman D, Arko FR, et al. Clinical and economic evaluation of the trellis thrombectomy device for arterial occlusions: preliminary analysis. J Vasc Surg. 2004;39:556-9.

Semba CP, Murphy TP, Bakal CW, et al, The Advisory Panel. Thrombolytic therapy with use of alteplase (rt-PA) in peripheral arterial occlusive disease: review of the clinical literature. J Vasc Interv Radiol. 2000;11:149-61.

The STILE Investigators. Results of a prospective randomized trial evaluating surgery versus thrombolysis for ischemia of the lower extremity: the STILE trial. Ann Surg. 1994;220:251-66.

Sullivan KL, Gardiner GA Jr, Kandarpa K, et al. Efficacy of thrombolysis in infrainguinal bypass grafts. Circulation. 1991;83 Suppl:I99-105.

Weaver FA, Comerota AJ, Youngblood M, et al, The STILE Investigators (Surgery versus Thrombolysis for Ischemia of the Lower Extremity). Surgical revascularization versus thrombolysis for nonembolic lower extremity native artery occlusions: results of a prospective randomized trial. J Vasc Surg. 1996;24:513-21.

Working Party on Thrombolysis in the Management of Limb Ischemia. Thrombolysis in the management of lower limb peripheral arterial occlusion: a consensus document. Am J Cardiol. 1998;81:207-18.

30 Endovascular Treatment of Venous Disease

Robert M. Schainfeld, DO

Venous Thromboembolism

Venous thromboembolism (VTE), which includes deep vein thrombosis (DVT) and pulmonary embolism (PE), is a potentially fatal condition with an estimated annual incidence of 0.1% in white populations. About 400,000 new cases occur annually in the United States, and one-third of patients have recurrent episodes within 10 years. PE accounts for approximately 100,000 to 200,000 deaths per year in the United States. The primary goals of initial treatment of VTE are to limit the extent of thrombus and the long-term sequelae of post-thrombotic syndrome (PTS) related to residual obstruction and valvular incompetence, which frequently results in disability. Clinicians must not only accurately diagnose the disorder but also provide patients with the most appropriate and cost-effective treatment options. Anticoagulation remains the cornerstone of treatment for VTE.

- VTE includes DVT and PE
- The annual incidence of VTE is 0.1% in white populations
- Anticoagulation is the mainstay of therapy

The treatment goals for DVT include decreasing the severity and duration of symptoms, preventing PE, minimizing the risk of recurrence, and preventing PTS and chronic thromboembolic pulmonary hypertension. The complications associated with proximal (iliofemoral) DVT include PE, which develops in 50% of untreated patients within the first few days, and recurrent thrombosis, which commonly occurs early but also has some long-term risk. The incidence of DVT recurrence is up to 10% in the first year in patients with unprovoked ("idiopathic") VTE.

Goals of Therapy for DVT:

- Decrease symptoms
- Prevent PE
- Minimize recurrence
- Prevent PTS and chronic thromboembolic pulmonary hypertension

Prospective natural history studies have shown that patients with DVT can have development of progressive valvular incompetence over time (months to years), with PTS occurring in two-thirds of patients. Manifestations of PTS include pain, edema, hyperpigmentation, or ulceration. Trophic skin changes can be seen in 6 to 7 million people in the United States; 400,000 to 500,000 patients have ulceration, primarily due to chronic venous insufficiency. The underlying pathophysiology of PTS is ambulatory venous hypertension caused by residual venous obstruction and valvular incompetence. The combination of venous obstruction and valvular insufficiency has been shown to be particularly virulent. Valvular damage results in venous reflux and hypertension, which leads to stasis and secondary skin changes, including ulceration. Patients with more extensive DVT involving the proximal segments, including the iliac veins and inferior vena cava (IVC), are more likely to have PTS.

- PTS occurs in two-thirds of patients with antecedent DVT
- Trophic skin changes are observed in 6-7 million people in the United States
- 400,000-500,000 Americans have venous ulcerations

Catheter-Directed Pharmacologic Thrombolysis

Despite standard anticoagulation therapy, symptomatic PTS develops in a substantial number of patients with DVT. It has been proposed that the more rapid and complete thrombus dissolution achieved with pharmacologic thrombolytic therapy could potentially decrease the incidence of this long-term complication. A recent systematic review of thrombolytic therapy showed increased rates of early vein patency, but major hemorrhagic rates were increased compared with unfractionated heparin treatment. Because of methodologic flaws in the reported trials, it is not possible to draw definitive conclusions about the effectiveness of thrombolytic therapy on the incidence of PTS.

An alternative approach to systemic thrombolytic therapy is to administer lytic agents through a catheter introduced into the femoral or popliteal vein—"catheter-directed thrombolysis" (CDT). In hopes of assessing the feasibility of CDT for iliofemoral DVT, a National Venous Thrombolysis Registry was assembled in a prospective, multicenter study that enrolled 473 patients from 63 sites. Complete lysis was seen in 31% and partial lysis in 52%. The degree of lysis was a significant predictor of early and continued patency. Of the patients who had complete clot dissolution, 78% had patent veins at 1 year, compared with 37% of those with less than 50% clot resolution after lytic therapy. In addition, early success of thrombolytic therapy directly correlated with 6-month valvular function. Major bleeding was observed in 11%—39% of these occurred at the access site, and 13% were retroperitoneal bleeds. Minor bleeding was reported in 16%. Major neurologic complications occurred in 0.4% of patients. PE occurred during treatment in 1% of patients, and 2 deaths were reported, for a mortality rate of 0.4% in the entire series.

At present, CDT most likely should be reserved for exceptional circumstances, such as in patients with limb-threatening ischemia caused by phlegmasia cerulea dolens and in young patients with extensive iliofemoral DVT (i.e., those with a favorable risk-benefit ratio). Other candidates who may benefit from CDT are those with multisegment DVT, those with expected long-term survival, and those who remain symptomatic despite therapeutic anticoagulation. Additional randomized trials are warranted to address these specific issues.

- CDT for DVT achieves more rapid lysis, may decrease PTS, preserves valvular competence, and restores vessel patency compared with standard anticoagulation or systemic thrombolytic therapy
- Access via common femoral or popliteal vein
- CDT is associated with an increased risk of hemorrhagic complications
- Indications for CDT include:
  - Phlegmasia cerulea dolens
  - Young patients with iliofemoral DVT
  - Multisegment DVT
  - Expected long-term survival
  - Patient symptomatic despite therapeutic anticoagulation

Contraindications to thrombolytic therapy are stratified into two categories, absolute and relative. Absolute contraindications include stroke within 2 months, bleeding diathesis, active or recent (within 10 days) gastrointestinal tract bleeding, neurosurgery (intracranial or spinal; within 12 months), intracranial trauma within 3 months, or neoplasm. Relative contraindications include cardiopulmonary resuscitation within 10 days, major non-vascular surgery or trauma within 10 days, uncontrolled hypertension (systolic >180 mm Hg or diastolic >110 mm Hg), puncture of non-compressible vessel, intracranial tumor, recent eye surgery, pregnancy, or bacterial endocarditis.

Contraindications

- Absolute:
  - Stroke (<2 months)
  - Bleeding diathesis
  - Active or recent gastrointestinal tract bleeding (<10 days)
  - Neurosurgery (intracranial, spinal; <12 months)
  - Intracranial trauma (<3 months) or neoplasm
- Relative:
  - Cardiopulmonary resuscitation (<10 days)
  - Major non-vascular surgery or trauma (<10 days)
  - Uncontrolled hypertension (systolic >180 mm Hg or diastolic >110 mm Hg)
  - Puncture of non-compressible vessel
  - Intracranial tumor
  - Recent eye surgery
  - Pregnancy
  - Bacterial endocarditis

Several thrombolytic agents are currently available in the United States, although none are Food and Drug Administration (FDA)-approved for the treatment of DVT. Available agents include streptokinase, urokinase, alteplase, reteplase, and tenecteplase. Each agent has different characteristics with respect to fibrin affinity, specificity, and selectivity, half-life, and average time to clot lysis. Despite the widespread availability and increasing use of these agents, no dosage regimens have been universally validated to guide therapy; the most frequently reported regimens are shown in Table 30.1.

After thrombolytic therapy of iliofemoral DVT, an underlying residual stenosis may be identified in the iliac vein, which must be corrected to avoid rethrombosis of the venous segment. This condition, May-Thurner syndrome, results from compression of the left iliac vein by the overlying right iliac artery. The response to percutaneous transluminal angioplasty (PTA) alone is usually

Table 30.1 Thrombolytic Agents and Regimens

Agent	Infusion
Alteplase	0.5-1.0 mg/h
Reteplase	0.5-1.0 U/h
Tenecteplase	0.25-0.5 mg/h
Urokinase	60,000-240,000 U/h

suboptimal; therefore, self-expanding nitinol stents are preferred to avoid potential stent compression, but placement should be restricted to the suprainguinal portion of the iliac vein. On the basis of current evidence, stenting below the lesser trochanter or the inguinal ligament should be avoided.

- Adjunctive PTA and stenting are indicated for residual venous stenosis after lysis
  - Nitinol self-expanding stents are preferable
- Confine deployment to the above-inguinal segment of iliac vein, and avoid stenting below the lesser trochanter
- Duration of antiplatelet and anticoagulant therapy depends on the underlying substrate
- Postprocedural clinical and non-invasive imaging are mandated

Warfarin anticoagulation, in addition to antiplatelet therapy, should be continued for at least 3 to 6 months, depending on the underlying cause, recurrence, or presence of a hypercoagulable state (which may justify indefinite anticoagulation). Clinical and non-invasive imaging (duplex ultrasonography) should be performed post procedure as a baseline, at 6- and 12-month intervals, and annually thereafter. The reported 1-year patency rate is 79% in selected series.

Summary of CDT for DVT

- CDT is a promising therapy that has demonstrated excellent angiographic lysis rates in highly selected patients
- Long-term follow-up data are not available
- There is a need for validation of concepts in controlled, prospective, randomized studies

Percutaneous Mechanical Thrombectomy

Indications

Percutaneous mechanical thrombectomy (PMT) refers to a heterogeneous group of devices and techniques used to fragment, ablate, or extract intravascular thrombus in an effort to produce more rapid lysis and limit repeat angiography. Because outcomes are optimized for maximal clot removal and because thrombolytic agents are less effective or ineffective on subacute or chronic thrombus, mechanical thrombolysis has emerged as a useful adjunct to pharmacologic therapy. In addition, some patients with absolute contraindications to pharmacologic thrombolysis may still be candidates for mechanical thrombectomy. PMT is also a possible alternative or adjunct to CDT for the treatment of DVT. Other potential advantages of PMT are that it has a shorter treatment time to patency, is more cost-effective, and is safer. Numerous devices are already FDA approved for other applications; however, none are currently approved for DVT management.

Technique

The extent of thrombosis is determined by imaging with duplex ultrasonography and computed tomography in selected cases. Cross-sectional imaging can indicate other pertinent anatomic factors such as May-Thurner syndrome, osteophytes, tumors, masses, or the presence of concomitant PE. Access is obtained peripheral to the thrombosed segment, and an antegrade approach is used with ultrasonographic guidance. The tibial or popliteal veins can be punctured with a single-wall technique, and venography is performed to delineate the extent of thrombus. After traversal of the thrombosed vein, options include pharmacologic lysis to remove acute thrombus and preemptive use of a mechanical thrombectomy device, which may provide more rapid partial decompression in the setting of phlegmasia cerulea dolens. If the thrombus is unresponsive to pharmacologic lysis, combined PMT and lysis may be more effective than either therapy alone. The role of retrievable IVC filters is yet to be defined; further investigation is needed to assess their role in patients undergoing PMT for DVT.

- Access for PMT is obtained via tibial or popliteal veins under ultrasonographic guidance
- Combined therapeutic modalities are the norm (e.g., lysis combined with PMT)
- The role of retrievable IVC filters in PMT is yet to be defined

The seventh American College of Chest Physicians Consensus Committee concluded that "the use of thrombolytic agents in the treatment of PE continues to be highly individualized, and clinicians should have latitude in using these agents. In general, patients with hemodynamically unstable PE" or massive iliofemoral thrombosis are the best candidates. Although the authors of this consensus statement recognized the potential benefits of thrombolytic therapy, in the absence of Level I evidence they made no firm recommendations regarding thrombolytic therapy.

Endovascular Therapy for DVT

- Lack of randomized, prospective, controlled data to support it
- Some safety concerns vs standard anticoagulation
- Introduction of device technology despite lack of prior trials
- Lack of accepted reporting system and clinical benefit end points
- No FDA-approved lytic agent or device available

IVC Filters

In the late 1960s, methods were developed that allowed caval interruption devices to be placed into the vena cava percutaneously through the femoral or jugular veins. In the ensuing years, intracaval devices have undergone substantial modification with respect to efficacy, patency, and ease of insertion, and are widely used as both treatment and prophylaxis for thromboembolic disease.

IVC filters now have an important role in the management of venous thromboembolic disease. Indications for IVC filter placement include: contraindications to or complications from anticoagulation; as prophylaxis for patients without VTE or for patients with VTE and anticoagulation; to prevent PE after failure of a previous device; or in concert with thrombectomy, embolectomy, or thrombolytic therapy. Possible indications include chronic thromboembolic disease or large free-floating iliocaval thrombus. Types of IVC filters are shown in Table 30.2.

Complications from IVC filters are related to their insertion, long-term consequences, and subsequent retrieval for cases in which a temporary, removable filter is used. The complications most frequently cited are venous access site thrombosis (2%-3%), filter thrombosis (0%-28%), and recurrent PE (3%-4%). Other rare, albeit potential, complications include filter penetration of the IVC, device fracture or migration, and arteriovenous fistula or guidewire entrapment during subsequent central venous catheter insertion. The contraindications to IVC filter placement are absence of access, IVC thrombosis, bleeding diathesis, and septic emboli or positive blood cultures. All indications, complications, and contraindications must be considered for each patient before device insertion. Patients with IVC filters should be followed up annually to evaluate the mechanical stability of the filter and determine preserved patency of the vena cava.

Table 30.2 Types of Inferior Vena Cava Filters

Product	Indicated use	FDA approval
ALN	Permanent/temporary	No
Simon nitinol	Permanent	Yes
Recovery	Optional	Yes
Vena Tech	Permanent	Yes
Greenfield (stainless steel/titanium)	Permanent	Yes
Bird's nest	Permanent	Yes
Günther tulip	Optional	Yes
Trapease	Permanent	Yes
Optease	Optional	Yes

FDA, Food and Drug Administration.

- IVC filters are important in the management of venous thromboembolic disease
- Indications, complications, and contraindications must be contemplated before filter placement
- Patients with IVC filters should undergo annual follow-up to evaluate mechanical stability of the filter and determine preserved patency of the IVC

Placement of Suprarenal IVC Filters

Certain circumstances preclude the placement of a filter in the infrarenal IVC. These include thrombus extending into the infrarenal IVC, renal vein thrombosis, or pregnancy. The safety of suprarenal filters has been well documented, with no reported instances of renal dysfunction, and when compared with infrarenal filters there are no differences in the rates of filter migration, recurrent PE, or caval thrombosis.

Placement of Superior Vena Cava Filters

The incidence of upper extremity DVT is increasing due to the increased use of short- and long-term upper extremity central venous catheters; because of this, 12% to 16% of all PEs now originate in the upper extremities. In patients who have such a complication or a contraindication to anticoagulation, a filter can be safely placed immediately below the confluence of the innominate veins. The orientation of the filter must be reversed to allow stabilization and thrombus trapping, and special attention must be given to the size of the superior vena cava (SVC) relative to the filter.

Technique

The most common access site for IVC filter placement is the right common femoral vein because it allows relatively direct entry into the vena cava and thus less tilting of the filter during placement compared with using the left common femoral vein. Other access sites, in decreasing frequency of use, include the left common femoral vein, the right and left internal jugular veins, the right and left antecubital veins, and the right and left subclavian veins, in rare instances. Most of the available IVC filters are indicated for use in IVCs with diameters of 28 mm or less.

The filter is typically deployed below the level of the renal veins. The left renal vein is traditionally lower than the right, but this should be confirmed with contrast venography before filter placement.

Chronic Venous Insufficiency

Chronic venous insufficiency is an extremely common condition, with an estimated 27% of the US adult population affected by some form of lower extremity venous disease. Approximately 25 million Americans have varicose veins of varying degrees of severity, with advanced, severe disease in 2 to 6 million adults; 500,000 have had venous ulcers. The true prevalence of varicose veins in a general population is difficult to accurately discern, owing to the lack of uniformity in reporting standards and to other confounding variables in data collection that compromise the integrity of current epidemiologic studies. Chronic venous insufficiency therefore represents a substantial health problem in terms of both expenditures for care and patients' quality of life. Annual health care costs for venous ulcerations in the United States are an estimated $1 billion.

Endovascular Treatment of Chronic Iliac Vein Obstruction

Occlusive lesions of iliac veins can result from thrombosis or extrinsic compression of the vessel and are more common on the left side. Surgical bypass to relieve iliofemoral obstruction traditionally has been used to treat this condition. Several studies have recently reported the results of endovascular management to recanalize obstructed iliac vein segments. In one of the largest series to date, technical success was achieved in 97%. The rate of stent thrombosis was only 8%, and 2-year primary, assisted, and secondary patency rates were 52%, 88%, and 90%, respectively, in patients treated for PTS.

May-Thurner syndrome (iliocaval compression syndrome) is diagnosed in 2% to 5% of patients undergoing evaluation for venous disorders of the lower extremities and, if chronic, may result in intraluminal venous webs. Because of the mechanical nature of the obstruction (left common iliac vein compression by the overlying artery), patients respond poorly to conservative therapy, and in the past, surgical reconstruction was the only available treatment option. Recently, endovascular treatment (PTA and/or stent placement) of this condition has shown promising results. After endovascular therapy, patients with May-Thurner syndrome had 60% primary patency with 100% primary-assisted and secondary patency rates at 2-year follow-up. Between 6% and 60% of patients with PTS (without documented May-Thurner syndrome) were pain free after stent placement, and absence of limb swelling was noted in 3% to 42%. In contrast, 26% to 59% of patients with May-Thurner syndrome were pain free, with comparable rates of edema resolution in the PTS cohort.

- Endovascular treatment of May-Thurner syndrome was associated with excellent technical success, few complications, and excellent primary-assisted and secondary patency rates

Endovascular Treatment of Varicose Veins

Treatment of superficial venous disease has changed substantially in the past 5 years. Previously, elimination of saphenous vein reflux was accomplished surgically (ligation and stripping) or chemically (sclerotherapy). Surgical ligation and stripping has been associated with complications, including hematoma, paresthesias, and recurrence. Sclerotherapy is performed commonly throughout the world with minimal risk but with high failure rates. The currently available treatment options continue to evolve rapidly with the adoption of the latest novel endovenous techniques for ablation of incompetent superficial veins (greater and lesser saphenous); they include radiofrequency ablation (RFA) and endovascular laser ablation (EVLA). The available options for surgical treatment of varicose veins include ligation and stripping, ambulatory phlebectomy, subfascial endoscopic perforator surgery, valvuloplasty, valve transplantation, and percutaneous valve bioprosthesis.

The latest innovations in minimally invasive therapies deliver thermal energy intraluminally to the vein wall to destroy the intima and denature collagen in the media. The result is fibrous occlusion of the vein. Thermal ablation for reflux of the saphenous veins can be achieved by RFA or EVLA and is most commonly applied to the greater and lesser saphenous veins. Patients not suitable for endovascular therapy, including those with multiple comorbid conditions, allergy to lidocaine, thrombophilia, prior DVT with incomplete recanalization, and active superficial thrombophlebitis, are best treated conservatively with compression. Large superficial varicose veins (tributaries of the greater and lesser saphenous) often are best removed surgically; tortuous veins can be challenging because of difficult guidewire navigation. Experience and clinical judgment are essential.

- Endovascular treatment options for varicose veins include RFA and EVLA
- RFA and EVLA result in fibrous occlusion of the vein after destruction of the intima and collagen within the media
- Poor candidates for endovascular or surgical treatment should be managed conservatively

- Superficial and tortuous veins make endovascular therapy undesirable

RFA and EVLA

Percutaneous endovenous ablation procedures are performed using tumescent anesthesia, which avoids skin burns and paresthesias (less than 2% incidence). RFA consists of a bipolar heat generator and a catheter with the capacity to close veins of 2 to 12 mm in diameter. The catheter is introduced percutaneously into the saphenous vein under ultrasonographic guidance and navigated to the saphenofemoral junction. Upon completion of RFA, absence of flow is assessed with ultrasonography, and patent segments are retreated. The clinical results for RFA in a registry study of 1,222 limbs were excellent, with a technical success rate of 98.5% and absence of reflux in 88.2% at 1-year follow-up. Maintenance of occlusion was seen in 87.2% of veins at 5 years, along with an absence of reflux in 83.8% of limbs. The EVOLVeS (Endovenous Radiofrequency Obliteration [Closure] Versus Ligation and Vein Stripping) study was a multicenter, prospective, randomized trial comparing quality-of-life factors between RFA and vein stripping. RFA and vein stripping had identical treatment results: 91.2% versus 91.7% of limbs free of reflux at 2 years. However, in all outcome variables, patients treated with RFA had faster recovery, less postoperative pain, fewer adverse events, and superior quality-of-life scores than did those treated with surgical stripping.

EVLA allows delivery of laser energy directly into the blood vessel using an 810-nm diode laser, which results in destruction of the vein endothelium by selective photothermolysis. Excellent clinical results, similar to those for RFA, have been reported with EVLA. One study showed technical success in 98% of 499 limbs treated. Greater saphenous vein closure was maintained in 93.4% of limbs at 2 years, with no recurrence in 40 limbs at 36 months.

Venous stripping has been associated with postoperative hematomas, paresthesias, and wound complications, with high recurrence rates, presumably because of neovascularization in the groin (approximately 60% at 38 years). After RFA in 63 limbs, no neovascularity was identified at 24 months. The early literature reported failure rates with either RFA or EVLA of approximately 10%, which seemed to occur during the first year. The result appears to be caused by leaving other larger tributaries or perforating veins untreated.

Technique

The greater saphenous vein is accessed percutaneously at the most distal segment of axial vein reflux. The lesser saphenous vein is accessed at the mid calf posteriorly, where the gastrocnemius muscle becomes prominent. Access is obtained with duplex ultrasonographic guidance using a 21-gauge needle for both RFA and EVLA procedures. The laser fiber tips or radiofrequency electrodes are positioned 1 cm distal to the common femoral vein. Complications of RFA and EVLA include paresthesias (12% at 1 week and 2.6% at 5 years), phlebitis (2.9%), edema (2%), skin burn (1.2%), DVT (0.9%), and access site infection (0.2%).

- RFA and EVLA are promising endovascular techniques for treating varicose veins in appropriately selected patients
- RFA has advantages over vein stripping, with less recovery time and postoperative pain, greater safety, and superior quality-of-life scores
- RFA and EVLA have excellent rates of technical success and maintenance of greater saphenous vein closure
- Neovascularization, common after vein stripping, has not been observed with RFA in short-term follow-up
- Endovenous failure, which occurs in approximately 10% of cases at 1 year, can be decreased by ablating all perforating and refluxing veins

Upper Extremity Venous Thrombosis

Upper extremity venous thrombosis accounts for 2% to 4% of all cases of DVT. The axillary and subclavian veins are most frequently involved, although in some cases thrombus propagates to involve more peripheral deep veins. When thrombus propagates into collateral channels or distal superficial veins, symptoms can be further exacerbated. Patients typically present with arm swelling, venous engorgement, skin discoloration, and pain or discomfort involving the arm, shoulder, and neck regions. Axillary-subclavian vein thrombosis (ASVT) can be classified as primary or secondary based on the presence or absence of associated conditions. Primary ASVT has no obvious cause on initial examination. Paget-Schroetter syndrome, or effort-related ASVT, is a potentially disabling condition that typically affects young, healthy persons. Secondary ASVT is the result of various causative factors, which include central venous access catheters, pacemakers, implantable cardioverter-defibrillator devices, malignancy, thrombophilia, and trauma.

The risk of acute PE due to upper extremity thrombosis varies from 11% to 36% with a reported mean of approximately 12%. Long-term sequelae of upper extremity thrombosis result primarily from venous hypertension secondary to obstruction (as opposed to lower extremity DVT, which is mainly a result of venous hypertension due to reflux with or without obstruction). Loss of future vascular access is a concern. Severe cases have been reported in approximately 13% of patients with PTS, owing to the robust venous collateral development of upper extremity venous systems.

- ASVT accounts for 2%-4% of all venous thromboses
- Clinical presentation includes swelling, pain, and discomfort in the upper extremity and neck, with prominent superficial chest veins or collaterals
- Primary ASVT, or Paget-Schroetter syndrome, is characterized by the absence of associated disease or trauma; secondary ASVT has a recognized cause
- PE occurs in approximately 12% of cases
- PTS is seen in approximately 13% of cases

Prompt and accurate diagnosis of ASVT is paramount for guiding treatment. Although no multicenter, randomized trials to date have studied different treatment regimens for upper extremity venous thrombosis, some recommendations can be made. Whereas secondary ASVT is managed conservatively, primary (effort-related) ASVT should be treated expeditiously with catheter-directed fibrinolytic therapy. After successful lysis of the thrombus and achievement of vein patency, immediate surgical decompression of the vein by removal of the offending osseous structures (first or cervical ribs), hypertrophied anterior scalene muscle, or subclavius tendon should be performed to relieve persistent vein narrowing due to extrinsic compression. The role of PTA and endovascular stenting remains controversial. However, if a residual stenosis persists after thrombolysis and definitive surgical decompression, endovascular stenting may be indicated to avoid rethrombosis. Individualized treatment, using the method with the most favorable risk-benefit ratio, is necessary to optimize quality of life.

- The optimal treatment strategy for ASVT is a matter of debate
- Prompt and accurate diagnosis is paramount
- Early local thrombolysis is universally accepted
- Individualized treatment is necessary to optimize quality of life

Superior Vena Cava Syndrome

SVC obstruction produces upper body venous hypertension, which can be associated with clinical consequences of varying severity. Because medical and surgical methods of treating SVC occlusion have been only partially successful, endovascular techniques were initially applied to the palliative treatment of these patients in the 80s. Modern combined endovascular therapy has been extremely successful in relieving pain for patients with venous obstruction of varying causes and in different locations. SVC obstruction can be caused by malignancies or various benign conditions, and this distinction significantly affects the available treatment options and goals of therapy.

Most often, SVC syndrome is seen in the context of thoracic malignancy (80%-90%), with the obstruction caused predominantly by tumor invasion and extrinsic SVC compression, sometimes with a component of radiation fibrosis or central venous catheter–related stenosis. The most common benign causes of SVC syndrome are central venous catheter–related or pacemaker-related stenosis, fibrosing mediastinitis, granulomatous infection, thoracic aortic aneurysm–related compression, and anastomotic stenosis associated with heart or heart-lung transplantation. Treatment options in SVC obstruction include anticoagulation, head elevation, corticosteroids for laryngeal edema, venous bypass, chemotherapy, external beam radiotherapy, and endovascular therapy.

- Malignancy accounts for 80%-90% of patients with SVC syndrome
- Benign causes:
  - Central venous catheter
  - Pacemaker
  - Fibrosing mediastinitis
  - Granulomatous infection
  - Thoracic aortic aneurysm–related compression
  - Anastomotic stenosis associated with heart or heart-lung transplantation
- Treatment options:
  - Anticoagulation
  - Head elevation
  - Corticosteroids
  - Chemotherapy
  - External beam radiotherapy
  - Endovascular therapy

Surgical results for benign SVC obstruction have indicated primary patency rates of 53% to 81% at 5 years and 81% at 10 years in one study using spiral saphenous vein grafts. The role of endovascular therapy for SVC recanalization in patients with benign disease remains to be determined. Technical success is excellent, with reported patency rates at 1 year of 70% to 91% and secondary patency rates of 85% at 18 months. Longer-term results, however, are not yet known for endovascular therapy. Therefore, surgical therapy is an acceptable option in selected patients with benign SVC syndrome.

Although randomized trials have not been performed, other evidence suggests that endovascular therapy is reasonable as a first-line therapy for malignant SVC syndrome. Those data show that endovascular SVC recanalization for malignant obstruction has impressive technical success rates of 95% to 100%, achieves clinical relief within days, and shows secondary patency rates of 93% to 100% at 3 months. Given the poor prognosis of these patients, who usually have metastatic disease, no long-term follow-up data are available.

After diagnosis of SVC syndrome, preprocedural cross-sectional imaging of the chest is recommended, using contrast-enhanced computed tomography or magnetic resonance imaging. Bilateral upper extremity venography via the basilic veins is initially performed to assess patency of the SVC and innominate and subclavian veins, the nature of the occlusion, the length of the occluded segment, and the presence of acute thrombus. If acute thrombus is present, catheter-directed therapy is usually the initial method of reestablishing flow in the involved veins. Adjunctive PMT can be used to macerate and remove the thrombus.

In general, venous stenosis and residual thrombus are best treated with balloon angioplasty followed by endovascular stent placement to facilitate maximal expansion and to avoid restenosis due to recoil in these fibrotic and elastic venous lesions. Because of their high radial strength, precise positioning, and lack of significant foreshortening, balloon-expandable stents are preferred for focal stenosis. If the SVC is extremely capacious, larger-diameter self-expanding nitinol stents may be used. The limitation of nitinol stents is that they do not resist radial compression to the same extent as balloon-expandable stents. Further study is needed to determine long-term patency of SVC stents in patients with long life expectancy.

- Endovascular venous recanalization techniques are excellent options in treating malignant and benign SVC obstruction
- Despite lack of available trials, evidence suggests that endovascular therapy is reasonable as first-line therapy for malignant SVC syndrome
- Short-term patency rates for endovascular recanalization in benign SVC syndrome compare favorably with those of modern surgical bypass methods
- Further study is needed to determine long-term patency of SVC stents in patients with long life expectancy

Questions

1. A 21-year-old lobster fisherman from Maine presented to the emergency department with a 3-day history of left arm and hand swelling and discomfort, without any obvious antecedent trauma. Duplex ultrasonography confirms acute ASVT extending into the basilic vein. What would be the most appropriate management strategy for an optimal clinical outcome?

a. Commencement of anticoagulation with either low-molecular-weight or unfractionated heparin with concomitant warfarin

b. Systemic thrombolysis via peripheral intravenous line

c. CDT via basilic vein followed by PTA and stenting of residual subclavian vein stenosis

d. CDT followed by surgical decompression (first rib resection) after restoring patency of veins

e. Anticoagulation therapy for 3 months, followed by first rib resection of persistently thrombosed axillary-subclavian veins.

2. Which method would be *least* effective in treating an acute DVT of the iliac vein?

a. Catheter-directed thrombolysis

b. Systemic thrombolytic therapy

c. Percutaneous mechanical thrombectomy

d. Surgical thrombectomy

e. Balloon maceration

3. Which of the following candidates would benefit *most* from CDT?

a. A 60-year-old patient with acute iliofemoral DVT of 2 weeks' duration

b. Patient with subacute IVC thrombosis

c. Patient with chronic iliofemoral DVT

d. Patient with progression of thrombus despite therapeutic anticoagulation

e. Patient with phlegmasia cerulea dolens

4. Which of the following statements is true regarding iliac vein revascularization?

a. Thrombolysis is essential in all cases of recanalization.

b. Balloon-expandable stents are preferred.

c. Stand-alone balloon angioplasty has a primary role.

d. Access is obtained via the ipsilateral common femoral or popliteal vein.

e. IVC filters are mandated before endovascular intervention.

5. Which type of IVC filter is removable?

a. Simon nitinol

b. Greenfield

c. Bird's nest

d. Trapease

e. Optease

6. A 43-year-old woman with a history of extensive left leg DVT, which occurred post partum involving the iliofemoral and popliteal veins, presents with a recurrent venous ulcer at the medial malleolus. Despite meticulous local wound care, compression, and a course of antibiotics, the ulcer was recalcitrant to healing. Noninvasive assessment of the deep and superficial venous system showed persistent thrombosis/occlusion of the iliac vein and partial recanalization of the femoral and popliteal veins with reflux/incompetence throughout the deep system. The greater saphenous vein also was shown to be incompetent throughout its course. What is the most appropriate initial course of management to facilitate healing of the ulcer?

a. CDT of the iliac, femoral, and popliteal veins
b. Endovenous ablation of the greater saphenous vein only
c. PTA and stenting of the left iliac vein
d. Popliteal vein valvuloplasty or valve transplantation
e. Saphenous vein ablation followed by PTA/stenting of the iliac vein if no ulcer healing after successful superficial vein intervention

Suggested Readings

Büller HR, Agnelli G, Hull RD, et al. Antithrombotic therapy for venous thromboembolic disease: the Seventh ACCP Conference on Antithrombotic and Thrombolytic Therapy. Chest. 2004;126 Suppl:401S-28S.

Comerota AJ, Throm RC, Mathias SD, et al. Catheter-directed thrombolysis for iliofemoral deep venous thrombosis improves health-related quality of life. J Vasc Surg. 2000;32:130-7.

Frisoli JK, Sze D. Mechanical thrombectomy for the treatment of lower extremity deep vein thrombosis. Tech Vasc Interv Radiol. 2003;6:49-52.

Girard P, Tardy B, Decousus H. Inferior vena cava interruption: how and when? Annu Rev Med. 2000;51:1-15.

Joffe HV, Goldhaber SZ. Upper-extremity deep vein thrombosis. Circulation. 2002;106:1874-80.

Lurie F, Creton D, Eklof B, et al. Prospective randomized study of endovenous radiofrequency obliteration (closure procedure) versus ligation and stripping in a selected patient population (EVOLVeS Study). J Vasc Surg. 2003;38:207-14.

Mewissen MW, Seabrook GR, Meissner MH, et al. Catheter-directed thrombolysis for lower extremity deep venous thrombosis: report of a national multicenter registry. Radiology. 1999;211:39-49. Erratum in: Radiology. 1999;213:930.

Min RJ, Khilnani N, Zimmet SE. Endovenous laser treatment of saphenous vein reflux: long-term results. J Vasc Interv Radiol. 2003;14:991-6.

Semba CP, Razavi MK, Kee ST, et al. Thrombolysis for lower extremity deep venous thrombosis. Tech Vasc Interv Radiol. 2004;7:68-78.

Sevestre MA, Kalka C, Irwin WT, et al. Paget-Schröetter syndrome: what to do? Catheter Cardiovasc Interv. 2003;59:71-6.

Urschel HC Jr, Razzuk MA. Paget-Schröetter syndrome: what is the best management? Ann Thorac Surg. 2000;69:1663-8.

Vedantharn S. Endovascular strategies for superior vena cava obstruction. Tech Vasc Interv Radiol. 2000;3:29-39.

31 Complications of Endovascular Procedures

Alan B. Lumsden, MD, FACS
Imran Mohiuddin, MD
Michael Reardon, MD, FACS
Eric K. Peden, MD

With the number of endovascular procedures being performed increasing rapidly, complications of procedures are being encountered with increasing frequency. Indeed, new and previously unimagined complications are being described in association with new procedures and devices. Examples include ultrafiltration through the first-developed aortic endograft and occlusion of cerebral protection devices. Nevertheless, some complications are common to all endovascular procedures. Endovascular complications can be categorized generally as access site complications, complications related to passage of catheters and devices, or intervention-specific complications.

Access Site Complications

The frequency of groin complications after an endovascular procedure performed via femoral access depends on the type of procedure performed, the size of device inserted, and whether adjunctive antithrombotic therapy is used. Because of the large number of coronary interventions performed compared with peripheral procedures, reports of groin complications tend to be described predominantly after coronary interventions. After cardiac catheterization, the incidence of groin complications is 0.05% to 0.7%, whereas after percutaneous transluminal angioplasty the incidence is much higher (0.7%-9.0%). Peripheral vascular complications include (in descending order of frequency) hematomas, pseudoaneurysms, arteriovenous fistulae, acute arterial occlusions, cholesterol emboli, and infections; these complications occur with an overall incidence of 1.5% to 9%. As a result of the increasing use of groin closure devices, the unusual complication of arterial infection has been reported increasingly. Acceptable threshold incidences for these complications have been described by the Society for Interventional Radiology.

- Peripheral vascular complications include (in descending order of frequency) hematomas, pseudoaneurysms, arteriovenous fistulae, acute arterial occlusions, cholesterol emboli, and infections

Groin Hematoma

The complication of groin hematoma varies from trivial to potentially life threatening (Fig. 31.1). Sudden onset of massive bleeding can occur. Symptoms vary from mild groin discomfort to severe pain, swelling, and potential necrosis of the overlying skin from the pressure of the hematoma. Initially, minimal ecchymosis occurs, but more extensive discoloration subsequently develops over hours to days. As the patient ambulates, the ecchymosis may extend down the thigh, and patients should be cautioned

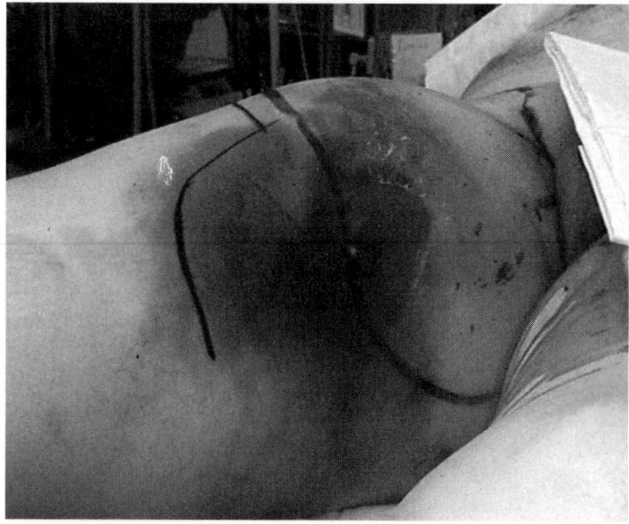

Fig. 31.1 Massive groin hematoma after percutaneous coronary angioplasty. A hematoma of this size is usually associated with immediate hemodynamic instability, compromises skin integrity, and mandates urgent exploration and femoral artery repair.

about these developments. Eventually, the discoloration may extend into the leg below the knee and does not represent new bleeding.

Indications for groin exploration and hematoma evacuation are severe pain, progressive enlargement of the hematoma, skin compromise, or evidence of femoral nerve compression. The incidence of wound infection after hematoma evacuation is high.

Typically, a vertical incision is made over the femoral artery in the groin. Ideally, control of the common femoral or distal external iliac artery is gained by dissecting down the inguinal ligament, perhaps dividing some of its fibers. In some cases the groin hematoma is so large that full exposure of the artery is not feasible; indeed, extensive exposure and control may not be necessary if no attendant pseudoaneurysm is present inside the hematoma. However, the original puncture site may begin bleeding as the artery is dissected. All puncture sites should be oversewn with a single 5-0 prolene suture if groin exploration is warranted, to prevent rebleeding. Drains should be placed, because once the hematoma is evacuated a large potential space remains. Groin infection after hematoma evacuation is common (up to 20%), and the patient should be cautioned about this risk. Antibiotics should be continued for several days.

- Indications for groin exploration and hematoma evacuation are severe pain, progressive enlargement of the hematoma, skin compromise, or evidence of femoral nerve compression
- The incidence of wound infection after hematoma evacuation is high

Arteriovenous Fistula

The most common cause of arteriovenous fistula is inadvertent puncture of the profunda femoris artery and the vein, which crosses in the angle between the profunda femoris and superficial femoral arteries. Fistulae are usually detected clinically by the presence of a palpable thrill in the groin or by auscultating a continuous bruit. Duplex ultrasonography confirms the presence of a fistula, showing the characteristic systolic-diastolic flow pattern with arterialization of the venous signal (Fig. 31.2). Fistulae usually do not close spontaneously and may progressively enlarge with time; therefore, operative repair is indicated when they are detected.

Surgical repair is performed by dissection of the artery until the defect is identified by brisk arterial bleeding. The artery is then controlled either by clamping or digital pressure. Once the defect in the artery is exposed, it is first repaired with interrupted prolene suture, followed by repair of the vein. Usually only one or two horizontal mattress sutures are required in each vessel. Covered stents should not be used in the management of arteriovenous fistulae or pseudoaneurysms. Because the fistula occurs in the groin, stents would be subject to substantial movement during hip flexion and extension; their durability at this location has not been proven. Likewise, coil embolization also is not recommended. These fistulae are typically very short, and coil placement can result in venous or peripheral arterial embolization.

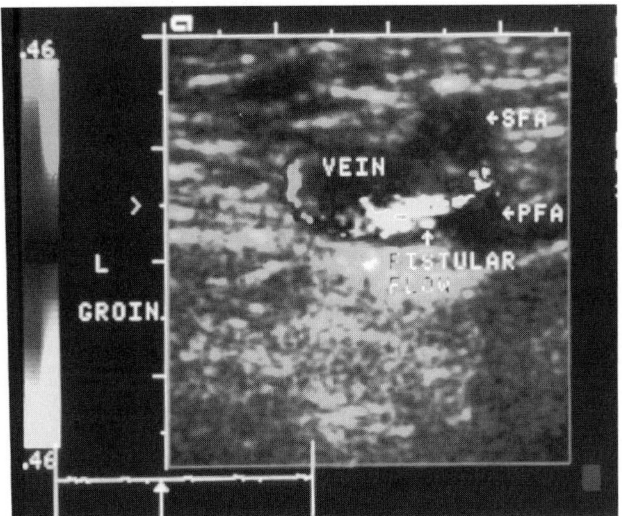

Fig. 31.2 Postprocedural duplex ultrasonography of the groin shows arterialization of the femoral vein with an obvious fistulous communication with the artery. PFA, profunda femoris artery; SFA, superficial femoral artery.

- Fistulae usually do not close spontaneously and may progressively enlarge with time; therefore, operative repair is indicated when they are detected

Pseudoaneurysm

Pseudoaneurysm after arterial puncture results from failure of the arteriotomy site to close, with contained bleeding into the soft tissue around the artery. Pseudoaneurysms can occur in any vessel, although most develop in the femoral artery. They can be difficult to detect if accompanied by a hematoma. However, the presence of expansile pulsation and tenderness should raise suspicion and lead to diagnosis by duplex scanning (Fig. 31.3). The duplex examination should note the size and likely source of the pseudoaneurysm. Some are complex and appear to have multiple lobes; others are a single, simple cavity. The neck of the pseudoaneurysm should be defined, whether it is a single wide neck or a long, tortuous narrow neck (the latter are easier to compress).

Pseudoaneurysm can be treated in several ways. Surgical repair previously was the mainstay of therapy but has been replaced in up to 70% of cases by ultrasonography-

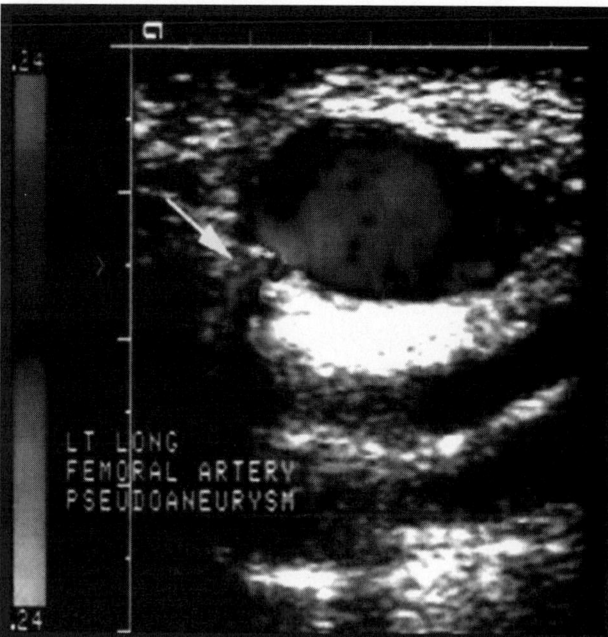

Fig. 31.3 Duplex ultrasonography of a pseudoaneurysm with a long narrow neck. It is unilocular and is ideal for thrombin injection.

guided thrombin injection. When surgery is needed to repair a pseudoaneurysm, the standard operation begins with exposure of the femoral artery through a groin incision by varying techniques. Some surgeons opt to gain full control of the artery before exposing the puncture site. Proximal control can be obtained by sliding down the external oblique muscle and identifying the femoral artery as it enters the thigh. Rolling the inguinal ligament superiorly or dividing the external oblique fibers permits exposure of the external iliac artery. Gaining proximal control is particularly important with a large hematoma or pseudoaneurysm. Because the arterial defect is usually only a 2- to 3-mm puncture site, an alternate approach is to enter the pseudoaneurysm directly, controlling the bleeding digitally and oversewing the puncture site. It is extremely important to ensure that the arterial wall is exposed before repair. A common error is to misidentify a hole in the fascia as the arterial defect and place sutures within the fascia. This can lead to recurrent pseudoaneurysm formation or persistent bleeding. Routine exploration of the posterior wall of the artery is not recommended.

Observation is very reasonable management strategy for small pseudoaneurysms (<2 cm in diameter). Most small pseudoaneurysms thrombose spontaneously within 2 to 4 weeks. However, concurrent anticoagulation decreases the likelihood of spontaneous thrombosis.

Ultrasonography-guided compression is another treatment possibility. The neck of the pseudoaneurysm, identified as a high velocity jet, is localized with duplex ultrasonography, and direct compression applied with the transducer. Pressure is increased until the jet is obliterated, and compression is continued for 20-minute intervals until thrombosis is documented. Mean time to thrombosis is 22 minutes but can be as long as 120 minutes. The increased time, however, may be associated with considerable patient discomfort; therefore, sedation and analgesia may be required. This technique is quite labor intensive because it requires a dedicated technician to apply pressure.

- Surgical repair has been replaced in up to 70% of cases by ultrasonography-guided thrombin injection
- Most small pseudoaneurysms thrombose spontaneously within 2 to 4 weeks

Ultrasonography-guided thrombin injection is an off-label use for thrombin, but it is very successful in inducing thrombosis of pseudoaneurysms, thereby avoiding operative intervention. Sterile gel is applied to the affected groin area and the pseudoaneurysm is identified with the duplex probe. Lidocaine is injected superficial to the pseudoaneurysm. Thrombin is reconstituted and drawn into a syringe with a change of needle to an echogenic biopsy needle to reach appropriate depth of the pseudoaneurysm. While an image of the pseudoaneurysm is obtained on the monitor, the physician inserts the echogenic needle through the skin and into the pseudoaneurysm, directed away from its neck. The syringe is aspirated to confirm appropriate positioning in the sac of the pseudoaneurysm. The aspiration syringe is then changed to a syringe containing thrombin. Small aliquots of thrombin are injected, and constant observation by ultrasonography is maintained during injection. The needle tip is redirected as needed until color flow becomes absent in the pseudoaneurysm and thrombus is seen in the sac of the pseudoaneurysm. The needle is then removed and the groin is rescanned to confirm thrombosis of the pseudoaneurysm and patency of the surrounding arteries and veins. The patient is maintained on bed rest, and follow-up duplex ultrasonography is performed 6 to 12 hours later to confirm continued aneurysm thrombosis.

Retroperitoneal Hematoma

Retroperitoneal hematoma (RPH) after groin puncture is an infrequent (0.15% incidence) but morbid complication. It is perhaps the most feared complication of groin puncture. The term refers to blood contained within the retroperitoneum, but several patterns occur. An iliopsoas hematoma occurs when bleeding enters and is confined within the fascia of the iliopsoas muscle. The psoas muscle contains the lumbar plexus, and this pattern of hematoma may be more likely to be associated with compression neuropathy. In contrast, the space between the peritoneum and retroperitoneal structures is potentially vast and can

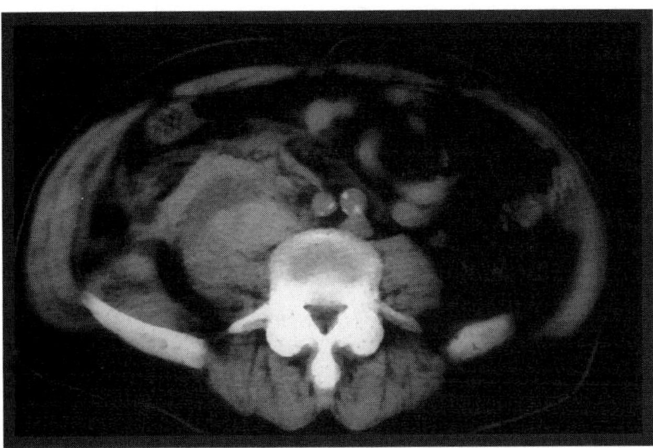

Fig. 31.4 Computed tomography showing a large hematoma extending into and around the psoas muscle. This can result in femoral nerve compression because the lumbar plexus is within the body of the psoas muscle.

contain huge quantities of blood, which may be difficult to detect clinically (Fig. 31.4). These hematomas can lead to pronounced compression of the ipsilateral kidney.

RPH can occur as a result of bleeding from the access site, as a complication of anticoagulation or lysis during an endovascular procedure, or as a consequence of an endovascular procedure (puncture of the renal parenchyma during renal angioplasty). By computed tomography (CT), the source of an RPH complicating groin puncture typically can be traced directly to the punctured artery. However, a high puncture above the inguinal ligament can be associated with a normal groin examination. Fullness in the lower quadrant or tenderness should support early CT. RPH occurring as a result of antithrombotic therapy can occur anywhere in the retroperitoneum, may be bilateral, and usually responds to correction of the underlying coagulopathy. RPH occurring as a consequence of an endovascular procedure (iliac artery rupture during stenting, renal capsule perforation with a guidewire) is best treated with an intervention targeted at the bleeding site, often with an endovascular procedure.

Any patient who has had groin puncture and in whom lower abdominal pain develops should be suspected of having an RPH. Abdominal examination usually shows tenderness only. Occasionally, palpable fullness may be detected. Thigh pain, numbness, or quadriceps weakness should lead to suspicion of RPH and femoral nerve compression and mandates urgent CT and possible decompression. Postcatheterization anticoagulation and high arterial puncture are the principal risk factors. Early recognition is essential and should be prompted by a decreasing hematocrit, lower abdominal pain, or neurologic changes in the lower extremity.

- RPH can occur as a result of bleeding from the access site, as a complication of anticoagulation or lysis during an endovascular procedure, or as a consequence of an endovascular procedure
- Any patient who has had groin puncture and in whom lower abdominal pain develops should be suspected of having an RPH
- Postcatheterization anticoagulation and high arterial puncture are the principal risk factors

The threshold for performing abdomino-pelvic CT (which is diagnostic) in such patients should be low. Management of RPH must be individualized: 1) patients with neurologic deficits in the ipsilateral extremity require urgent decompression of the hematoma; 2) anticoagulation should be stopped or minimized; and 3) hematoma progression by serial CT necessitates surgical evacuation and repair of the arterial puncture site.

Miscellaneous Complications of Femoral Puncture

Acute thrombosis of the femoral artery occurs infrequently and manifests as lower extremity ischemia. Exploration of the femoral artery usually shows disruption of a large posterior plaque by the needle, sheath, or catheter, with thrombosis of the residual lumen. Femoral endarterectomy, patch angioplasty, and balloon-catheter embolectomy of the external iliac and superficial femoral arteries is the most commonly required procedure. Acute occlusion of the artery is occasionally observed after the use of femoral artery closure devices. Numerous such devices now exist; broadly, they can be classified as suture closure devices, which can directly injure the arterial wall. The Angio-Seal vascular closure device involves placement of a biodegradable bar inside the artery, and the Duett system involves injection of thrombin down the access tract. Distal embolization is more commonly caused by passage of catheters and the intervention performed than by groin puncture alone. Rarely, catheter or wire passage can result in arterial perforation and, more rarely, in pseudoaneurysm (Fig. 31.5).

Axillary and Brachial Artery Puncture

All of the complications described above for femoral puncture also have been described for axillary and brachial arterial puncture. However, the incidence of neurapraxia involving the median nerve or other branches of the brachial plexus is higher than the incidence of complications limited to the punctured artery. In a recent prospective study of cardiac catheterization via the femoral artery, damage to the adjacent femoral nerve occurred in 20 of

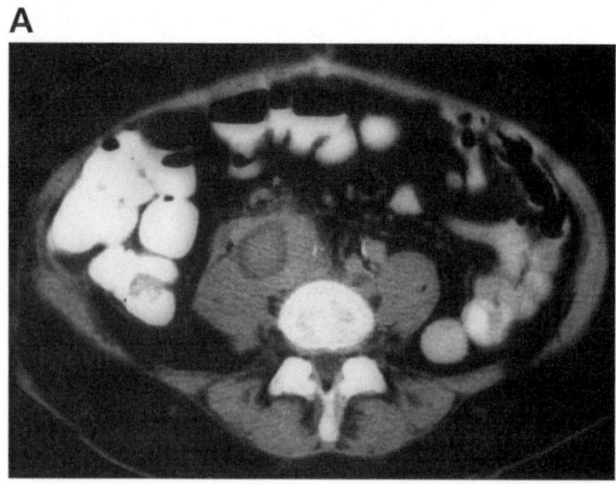

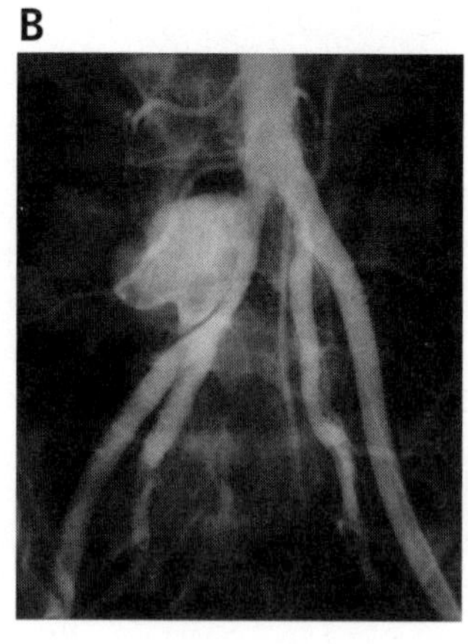

Fig. 31.5 A mycotic iliac pseudoaneurysm, which developed after iliac perforation and retroperitoneal hematoma from passage of a wire and catheter, is shown by computed tomography (*A*) and angiography (*B*). Fortunately, this occurrence is rare.

9,585 cases (0.2%) and, although initially disabling, was reported to be almost completely reversible. Frequency of injury to nerves of the brachial plexus is between 0.4% and 12.7%. The three potential mechanisms of nerve injury are hematoma, direct damage to the nerve, and nerve damage due to ischemia. Hematoma formation is the most common mechanism; the hematoma forms within a fascial compartment containing the neurovascular bundle, which results in nerve compression (Fig. 31.6). Direct nerve damage can be caused by the needle, catheter, or introducer sheath. Nerve damage due to nerve ischemia can be caused by varying degrees of arterial thrombosis.

Fig. 31.6 Magnetic resonance image showing a small but strategically located hematoma (*black arrow*) which compressed the median nerve (*white arrow*) after brachial artery puncture. (From Kennedy AM, Grocott M, Schwartz MS, et al. Median nerve injury: an underrecognised complication of brachial artery cardiac catheterisation? J Neurol Neurosurg Psychiatry. 1997;63:542-6. Used with permission.)

- The three potential mechanisms of nerve injury are hematoma, direct damage to the nerve, and nerve damage due to ischemia
- Pain at the puncture site is the most common symptom
- Muscle weakness accompanied by numbness indicates more severe symptoms and mandates immediate intervention

Symptom onset after nerve damage can occur immediately to 3 days later (mean, 12 hours). Pain at the puncture site is the most common symptom and may radiate down the arm. Muscle weakness accompanied by numbness indicates more severe symptoms and mandates immediate intervention. Swelling from a hematoma is not always obvious; even a small strategically placed hematoma can result in nerve compression. The size of a hematoma or presence of ecchymosis does not correlate with the severity of symptoms or degree of nerve damage.

The treatment principles consist of, first, awareness of the possibility of nerve compression after axillary or brachial artery puncture. Second, the hand should be evaluated post procedure for pain or sensory or motor dysfunction. Third, early surgical decompression should be used for pain in excess of that anticipated from arterial puncture or for presence of a motor or sensory deficit.

The artery should be surgically exposed, any hematoma evacuated, and the puncture site repaired. The fascia of the neurovascular bundle is widely opened and any perineural hematoma evacuated. The deep fascia of the forearm is not closed—only the subcutaneous fat and skin should be approximated.

The functional outcome after a nerve injury that is not identified and treated is poor, and most patients, although having some improvement, report persistent sensory or motor impairment. Disabling pain syndromes can develop in some patients.

Complications Related to Passage of Catheters and Devices

As a wire, catheter, or device is passed through a blood vessel, it can injure the vessel wall directly. Glide wires are notorious for entering the vessel wall and continuing to track in an intramural position. Lack of blood return through a catheter should raise suspicion of dissection. Hand injection of 3 to 5 mL of contrast medium confirms the catheter position by the appearance of a spot of dye that fails to wash out with arterial flow. The catheter should be pulled back until blood return is obtained and a wire used to navigate the true lumen. These types of dissections, when identified, are usually of no clinical consequence. Occasionally, however, large dissections can be created and may be flow limiting. The renal artery is particularly prone to this complication. The interventionalist must make a judgment as to whether the dissection is hemodynamically significant or likely to be self-limiting and consequently whether to repair the affected area. Possible complications in this category include perforation of the main artery, perforation of a side branch, intimal dissection, atheromatous embolization, thrombus embolization from catheter or wire, or air embolization.

Microembolization can occur after passage of any endovascular device (Fig. 31.7). It is particularly likely to happen in patients with severe atheromatous disease. Stroke from catheter manipulation in an atheromatous aortic arch is well recognized. Catheters and wires should be kept out of the arch unless access is necessary for the procedure, and manipulation should be minimized.

- Lack of blood return through a catheter should raise suspicion of dissection
- Microembolization is particularly likely to happen in patients with severe atheromatous disease

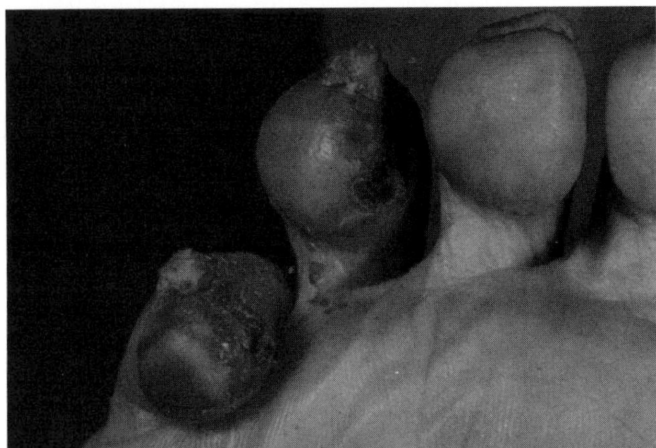

Fig. 31.7 Microembolization (atheroemboli) to the toes is usually associated with palpable pedal pulses because a continuous conduit is usually necessary for such distal embolization to occur.

When wires are passed blindly, they can enter side branches or even the supra-aortic trunks. Even at the femoral access site, wires may deflect inferiorly down the superficial femoral or profunda femoris artery or may deflect superiorly up the circumflex iliac artery. Femoral arterial injury results from attempts at sheath introduction when the wire is misplaced in these positions. Good technique includes imaging of the wire and control of the wire tip. It is possible for inadvertent perforation of organs to occur, such as renal perforation if the wire enters a renal artery and is not visualized. Wires entering the supra-aortic trunks can lead to cerebrovascular accident. Perforation of the renal parenchyma by hydrophilic wires during renal angioplasty and stenting is a well-known complication. It can result in severe RPH, subcapsular hematoma, and compromise of renal function.

When aortic stent grafts were first introduced, the incidence of iliac artery injury was high due to passage of these large stiff devices through the iliac artery. This complication is becoming more frequent again as large endografts are increasingly used to treat thoracic aortic aneurysms. The introducer sheath is up to 24F, and the incidence of avulsion of the external iliac artery has been notable. As interventionalists have become increasingly adept at inserting large-bore devices, the iliac artery injury typically is not manifest until the sheath is removed. This results in an "iliac artery on the stick" phenomenon and can lead to exsanguinating hemorrhage. This complication is best avoided by placing the stent graft through a Dacron graft placed on the iliac artery to avoid having to traverse a small, tortuous, or calcified external iliac artery.

Although catheters and wires are fairly thromboresistant, clot can form on both in patients not treated with anticoagulants. Clot forms particularly on guidewires when outside of the patient and covered in blood. Meticulous technique in catheter flushing and wiping of guidewires is extremely important and should be practiced, regardless of which vascular bed is being manipulated. However, such care is of paramount importance when working in the aortic arch or the supra-aortic trunks. Thrombus on a guidewire is "snowplowed" off the end of the wire when a catheter is inserted and can lead to stroke.

Similarly, meticulous removal of air bubbles from catheters is fundamentally important in minimizing the risk of stroke when working in the carotid circulation. An air bubble in the cerebral circulation may result in stroke.

Intervention-Specific Complications

Intervention-specific complications can be broadly classified as infection, bleeding, rupture, dissection, embolization, occlusion, or restenosis. They can occur with essentially any intervention. However, the frequency and significance of each varies depending on the type of intervention being performed.

Device Infection

Infection of endovascular devices is rare. Given the large number of coronary procedures performed, including stent implantation, reports of infection of these devices are remarkably uncommon. Antibiotic prophylaxis has been sporadic and its necessity questioned. However, the advent of stent grafting clearly has been associated with increasing reports of device infection. Two mechanisms exist: infection at the time of implantation and seeding of an implanted graft via bacteremia. Unlike aortic graft infections, which are indolent, slowly progressive, and present years after implantation, infections of endografts are rapidly progressive and result in rapid conformational changes and rupture of the aneurysm. Patients have the classic signs of sepsis. The device must be removed and aortic reconstruction performed using standard techniques for aortic graft infection.

- The advent of stent grafting clearly has been associated with increasing reports of device infection

Reports of infection in bare stents also have been increasing. This is particularly likely to occur if stents are placed in patients with long catheter dwell times (such as for lysis). Stent infection results in septic arteritis within the wall of the host artery, pseudoaneurysm formation, and rupture.

Another source of stent graft infection is a result of direct erosion of the device into adjacent hollow viscera. Isolated cases of aorto-esophageal and aorto-bronchial fistulae have been reported complicating thoracic aortic stent grafting. In the abdomen, aorto-duodenal fistulae have also been reported from abdominal aortic stent grafting.

Another area of concern for device infection is after the use of groin closure devices. Although this complication is rare, it has essentially introduced a surgical challenge, hitherto only seen in intravenous drug abusers who injected directly into the femoral artery. Mycotic femoral arteritis is a particular challenge for the vascular surgeon, necessitating arterial resection, reconstruction with saphenous vein routed around the infected field, and muscle flap. It is a life- and limb-threatening problem.

Complications of Fibrinolysis

Lytic agents activate plasminogen to form plasmin, which breaks fibrin into fibrin degradation products, resulting in clot lysis. In appropriately selected patient groups, complications of fibrinolysis are minor and most commonly relate to local bleeding at the site of catheter entry, consisting of hematoma, retroperitoneal bleeding, or pseudoaneurysm. In most cases, these may be controlled by local application of pressure. There should be a high index of suspicion of RPH in any patient receiving lytic therapy in whom the hematocrit decreases with no obvious source of blood loss. This can be confirmed easily with abdominal CT. Development of an RPH usually requires discontinuation of fibrinolytic therapy.

- History of a cerebrovascular accident within the preceding 2 months is an absolute contraindication to lytic therapy
- The National Institutes of Health Consensus Panel also recommends against the use of fibrinolytic therapy in patients with sustained systolic blood pressures >200 mm Hg or diastolic pressures >110 mm Hg

Bleeding from an anastomosis is usually a problem only in recently implanted or infected grafts. Distal embolization is, in theory, more likely during graft lysis than lysis of native vessels due to the more extensive thrombus formation. Transgraft bleeding is a concern only in recently placed dacron grafts. Cerebrovascular accident is an uncommon but serious complication of lytic therapy. No specific factors increase this risk, other than a history of cerebrovascular accident. History of a cerebrovascular accident within the preceding 2 months is an absolute contraindication to lytic therapy. The National Institutes of Health Consensus Panel also recommends against the use of fibrinolytic therapy in patients with sustained systolic blood pressures greater than 200 mm Hg or diastolic pressures greater than 110 mm Hg.

Complications of Aortic Stent Grafts

Numerous complications have now been described which are relatively specific for endovascular aortic aneurysm repair. Iliac artery dissection and rupture can occur with device insertion. This is particularly likely in patients with small, calcified iliac arteries, especially those with concurrent occlusive disease. Increasing awareness of this problem has led to the development of alternate approaches, such as insertion of an iliac conduit using a retroperitoneal approach, to avoid such difficult iliac arteries. Misplacement can result in coverage of the renal arteries and lead to development of renal failure. Occlusion of the inferior mesenteric artery or hypogastric arteries can lead to colon ischemia.

Embolization or coverage of the internal iliac arteries results in buttock claudication in 30% of cases. Pelvic ischemia syndromes, including cauda equina ischemia and colon ischemia, can also occur.

Consequences and complications of endoleaks are beyond the scope of this chapter. Graft migration, component separation, and loss of seal at the proximal and distal attachment sites can lead to re-pressurization of the aneurysm sac, resulting in continued aneurysm enlargement and rupture.

Complications of Renal Angioplasty and Stenting

Performance of renal angioplasty can be one of the more technically challenging endovascular procedures. Gaining atraumatic access to the renal artery and establishing a stable platform for intervention are the keys to avoiding complications. Traumatic crossing of a renal stenosis can result in dissection of the renal artery, a condition that must be recognized and is usually successfully treated by renal stenting.

The procedure is set up with the tip of the guidewire always visible in the peripheral image field. Inadvertent advancement of the wire can result in perforation of the renal parenchyma and perinephric hematoma (Fig. 31.8). Most of these hematomas can be managed by anticoagulation reversal and observation, but branch renal vessel embolization may be required.

Microembolization may account for the deterioration in renal function that occurs in some patients after renal stenting. This is usually implied rather than documented, although cholesterol embolization has been documented on renal biopsy.

Renal artery occlusion occurs infrequently, usually as a result of dissection. However, this complication threatens the viability of the kidney and mandates immediate intervention: thrombolysis, stenting, and occasionally surgical bypass grafting.

Restenosis remains the major complication of renal stenting, with rates reported as high as 20%. Restenosis can result in return of hypertension or deterioration in renal function. Repeat angioplasty is required. Surgical bypass can be significantly more complicated if stents extend well beyond the ostia of the renal arteries.

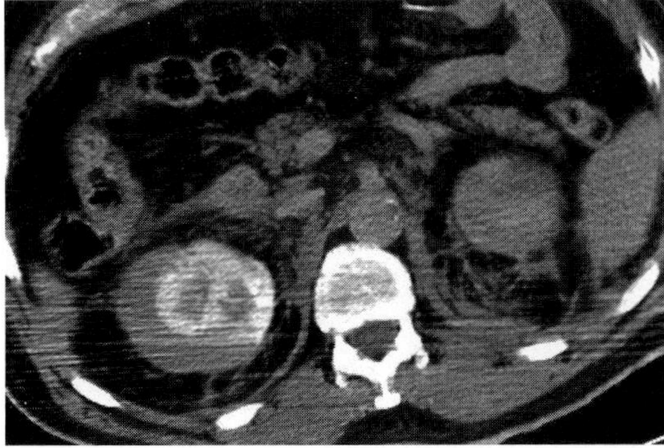

Fig. 31.8 Computed tomography showing a subcapsular hematoma caused by a guidewire perforation during renal angioplasty.

- Microembolization may account for the deterioration in renal function that occurs in some patients after renal stenting
- Restenosis remains the major complication of renal stenting, with rates reported as high as 20%

Complications of Iliac Angioplasty and Stenting

The most common problem encountered with iliac angioplasty is subintimal passage of the guidewire. This is prevented by observing the movement of the wire as it crosses the lesion. Suspicion of subintimal passage is raised by failure to aspirate blood from the catheter and hand injection of 2 to 3 mL of dye that forms a spot in the aortic wall and fails to wash out. The catheter and wire are retrieved and the lesions re-crossed. Failure to recognize that the wire is in a subintimal location can lead to catastrophic problems if devices are then advanced over the wire.

Iliac rupture is remarkably uncommon but is a particular risk in small or calcified iliac arteries, especially the external iliac artery (Fig. 31.9). In these high-risk patients, a stent graft should be immediately available to seal off the rupture. Embolization is uncommon, but the risk is increased when recanalizing total occlusions.

- The most common problem encountered with iliac angioplasty is subintimal passage of the guidewire

Complications of Venous Interventions

Venous angioplasty and stenting is performed for central

A

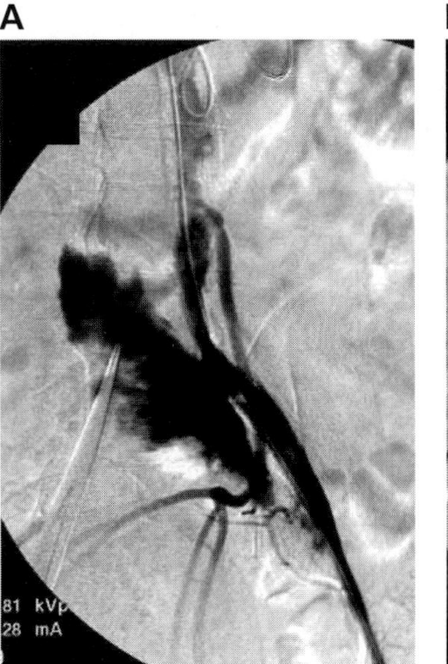

B

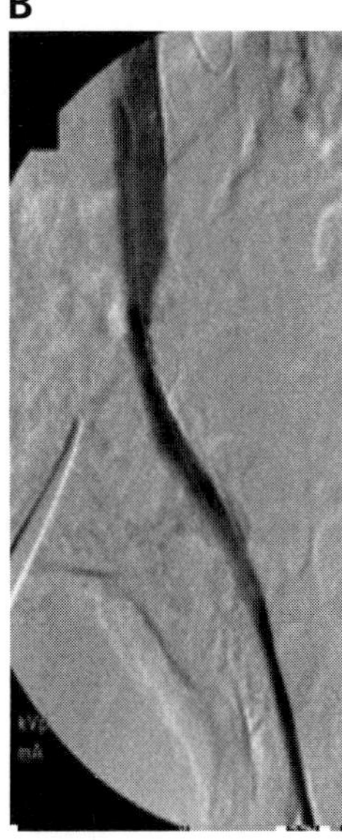

Fig. 31.9 Iliac artery angiography. *A*, Extravasation from the iliac artery after balloon angioplasty and stenting. *B*, The perforation has been sealed by judicious placement of a covered stent.

venous stenoses such as occur with dialysis access or in the left common iliac vein in May-Thurner syndrome. Venous lesions, especially those associated with dialysis access, are notoriously difficult to dilate, often require very high balloon pressures (up to 30 atm), and can result in venous rupture. Most of these venous ruptures are self-limiting and seal either spontaneously or with a few minutes of balloon tamponade.

Stent deployment in central veins is associated with a high incidence of device migration. Because of the highly compliant nature of the veins and their ability to change in diameter substantially, stent migration can occur. Careful measurement, oversizing, and ensuring a secure proximal anchor for the stent are important.

- Stent deployment in central veins is associated with a high incidence of device migration

Inferior vena cava filters are widely used. Specific filter complications include occlusion, caval penetration, filter migration, and improper deployment.

Complications of Carotid Stenting

Carotid artery stenting can be separated into several components, each of which has specific complications: 1) arch angiography and selective catheterization of the common carotid artery; 2) placement and retrieval of an embolic protection device; 3) balloon angioplasty and stenting of the target lesion; and 4) stent thrombosis.

Arch Angiography

The principal risk during arch angiography and selective catheterization of the common carotid artery is of embolization due to dislodgement of plaque during catheter insertion, re-forming reversed-curve catheters within the aortic arch, or engaging the orifice of the target vessel. Patients at particular risk include those with a type III arch, for whom increased catheter manipulation is often required, and patients with extensive atherosclerosis within the arch.

Embolic Protection Devices

Certain unique problems can arise from use of embolic filters. Spasm of the internal carotid artery can occur around the filter, usually due to filter movement stimulating the arterial wall. Occasionally spasm is so severe as to completely collapse the filter. This is treated by intra-arterial administration of 100 μg of nitroglycerin. Angioplasty may be necessary in severe flow-limiting cases that do not respond to nitroglycerin. This is performed after the filter has been removed.

Filter obstruction due to embolization of a large portion of atheroma appears as complete occlusion of the internal carotid artery. A catheter should be used to aspirate debris from the filter before filter retrieval.

Filter separation from the delivery catheter, usually from entanglement of the filter in the stent, can be avoided by maintaining separation of these two devices at all times. Detached filters have been compressed against the vessel wall using a balloon-expandable stent, but surgical conversion may be necessary.

Balloon Angioplasty and Stenting

Angioplasty of the carotid bifurcation can result in bradycardia, asystole, and hypotension. Coughing is usually sufficient to restart the heart, but atropine (0.4 mg intravenously) may be necessary. Pressors should be available should pressure support be necessary. These events can occur with predilation, stent placement, or after dilation of the stent.

- Angioplasty of the carotid bifurcation can result in bradycardia, asystole, and hypotension
- Subacute thrombosis of the stent is more likely if clopidogrel was not administered before the procedure, with inadequate intraprocedural anticoagulation, or with poor dilation of the stent

Stent Thrombosis

Subacute thrombosis of the stent is more likely if clopidogrel was not administered before the procedure, with inadequate intraprocedural anticoagulation, or with poor dilation of the stent. This typically manifests as altered mental status, agitation, or development of focal neurologic deficits.

Questions

1. What is the optimal treatment for a narrow-necked pseudoaneurysm (2 cm in diameter) after femoral puncture?
   a. Surgical repair
   b. Ultrasonography-guided compression
   c. Stent graft of the femoral artery
   d. Ultrasonography-guided thrombin injection

2. What is the most common severe complication of thoracic aortic stent grafting?
   a. Femoral nerve injury
   b. Groin hematoma
   c. Iliac artery injury
   d. Ureteric injury

3. Which of the following complications is(are) associated with renal artery stenting?
   a. Renal artery rupture
   b. Deterioration of renal function
   c. Renal artery dissection
   d. All of the above

4. Which statement is true regarding RPHs?
   a. All should be evacuated
   b. All should be followed up with serial hemoglobin and hematocrit measurements
   c. All require surgical repair of the bleeding source
   d. All are caused by excessive anticoagulation

5. Which of the following is associated with femoral neuropathy caused by an RPH?
   a. Weak knee extension
   b. Inability to dorsiflex the foot
   c. Posterior thigh numbness
   d. Scrotal pain

6. An arteriovenous fistula <2 mm in diameter will usually:
   a. Close spontaneously
   b. Result in a pseudoaneurysm
   c. Progressively enlarge over time
   d. Be easily treated with coil embolization

7. Which of the following symptoms would be an indication(s) for surgical exploration of a large groin hematoma?
   a. Severe pain
   b. Skin compromise
   c. Toe numbness
   d. Hemodynamic instability

Suggested Readings

Baltacioglu F, Cimsit NC, Cil B, et al. Endovascular stent-graft applications in iatrogenic vascular injuries. Cardiovasc Intervent Radiol. 2003;26:434-9.

Basche S, Eger C, Aschenbach R. Transbrachial angiography: an effective and safe approach. Vasa. 2004;33:231-4.

Chitwood RW, Shepard AD, Shetty PC, et al. Surgical complications of transaxillary arteriography: a case-control study. J Vasc Surg. 1996;23:844-9.

Fransson SG, Nylander E. Vascular injury following cardiac catheterization, coronary angiography, and coronary angioplasty. Eur Heart J. 1994;15:232-5.

Lin PH, Dodson TF, Bush RL, et al. Surgical intervention for complications caused by femoral artery catheterization in pediatric patients. J Vasc Surg. 2001;34:1071-8.

Lumsden AB, Miller JM, Kosinski AS, et al. A prospective evaluation of surgically treated groin complications following percutaneous cardiac procedures. Am Surg. 1994;60:132-7.

Parmer SS, Carpenter JP, Fairman RM, et al. Femoral neuropathy following retroperitoneal hemorrhage: case series and review of the literature. Ann Vasc Surg. 2006 Jul;20:536-40. Epub 2006 May 31.

Perings SM, Kelm M, Jax T, et al. A prospective study on incidence and risk factors of arteriovenous fistulae following transfemoral cardiac catheterization. Int J Cardiol. 2003;88:223-8.

Sreeram S, Lumsden AB, Miller JS, et al. Retroperitoneal hematoma following femoral arterial catheterization: a serious and often fatal complication. Am Surg. 1993;59:94-8.

Toursarkissian B, Allen BT, Petrinec D, et al. Spontaneous closure of selected iatrogenic pseudoaneurysms and arteriovenous fistulae. J Vasc Surg. 1997;25:803-8.

Watkinson AF, Hartnell GG. Complications of direct brachial artery puncture for arteriography: a comparison of techniques. Clin Radiol. 1991;44:189-91.

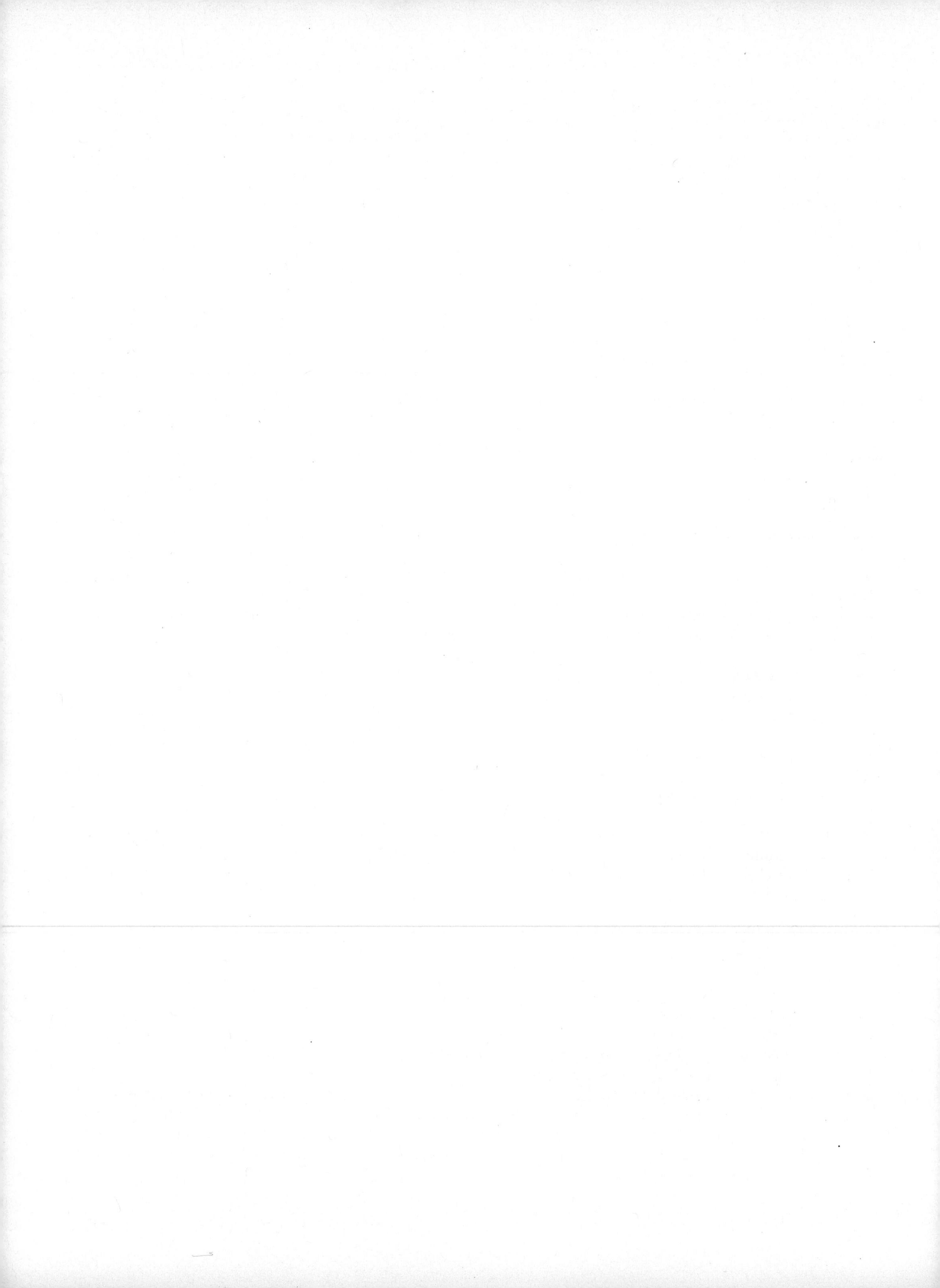

Answers

Chapter 1

1. b. Vascular smooth muscle cells (not endothelial cells) migrate into the intima during atherosclerosis initiation. Endothelin is primarily a vasoconstrictor via the endothelin A receptor on vascular smooth muscle. Endothelin can act on endothelin B receptors on endothelial cells to increase nitric oxide (a potent vasodilator), but the net effect of endothelin on arteries is dominated by the vasoconstrictor effect on endothelin A receptors. The smaller muscular arteries (rather than elastic arteries) regulate resistance. The adventitia contains connective tissue, but the media contains abundant smooth muscle and connective tissue.
2. e. HDL is considered the main transport lipoprotein for reverse cholesterol transport, which removes cholesterol from peripheral tissues.
3. c. Nitric oxide tends to prevent activation of NF-κB. The selectins are most responsible for monocyte rolling, whereas the CAMs are most responsible for monocyte arrest and recruitment into the artery wall. MCP-1 enhances (not blocks) monocyte recruitment.
4. e. All are found in advanced plaques.
5. b and e. Monocytes and leukocytes are more characteristic of atheroma than are neutrophils. Therapies that lower LDL levels usually do not decrease plaque size. Most human studies (intravascular ultrasonographic and angiographic) suggest intensive lipid lowering is associated with small changes in plaque size (generally less than 5%) compared with the large decrease in the risk of clinical events. Calcification is an active (not passive) process that in some cases mimics construction and destruction processes seen in bone.
6. b. Compensatory enlargement refers to the enlargement of the whole artery to accommodate the atherosclerotic plaque to preserve the lumen size. Over time this process is thought to be overwhelmed and the lumen decreases in size. Negative remodeling refers to a decrease in size of the whole artery segment; this tends to contribute to lumen narrowing and the development of stenoses. Metalloproteases are more often found in positively remodeled arterial segments and are thought to contribute to the growth of the artery.

Chapter 2

1. d
2. b
3. c
4. b
5. b

Chapter 3

1. c
2. a
3. d
4. d
5. a
6. d
7. f
8. a

Chapter 4

1. c. The calf pump failure syndrome is caused by either retrograde flow through incompetent perforator veins during calf muscle contraction or ineffective muscle contraction, both of which result in secondary varicose veins.

2. c. May-Thurner syndrome is caused by compression of the left iliac vein by the right iliac artery as the vein crosses over to the left leg. The term "May-Thurner syndrome" is only used when significant venous obstruction is produced by the overlying artery. During pregnancy, an otherwise normal woman may have symptoms of this condition, due to increased intra-abdominal pressure.

3. c. The Trendelenburg test is a simple bedside test that can help distinguish primary from secondary varicose veins and should be performed before consideration of sclerotherapy. She had no symptoms or history of DVT, and duplex ultrasonography would be the preferred diagnostic test to exclude DVT rather than venography. The veins will decompress with elevation, but neither bed rest nor analgesics will resolve her condition in the long term.

4. b. Reducing edema is the most important element of CVI treatment and decreases cutaneous complications. Diuretics only help edema minimally. Small ulcers should be treated first with aggressive medical therapy before consideration of skin grafting. In the SEPS procedure, ligation of perforator veins is performed under endoscopic guidance.

5. c. Filariasis is the most common cause of lymphedema worldwide and is especially prominent in Africa, India, and South America. Lymphedema sometimes secondarily complicates CVI. Milroy disease is a form of familial primary lymphedema.

6. d. This patient has lymphedema praecox, which typically presents during puberty. The patient has swelling that extends into the feet and toes with cutaneous fungal infection, which are characteristics of lymphedema. Stemmer sign is positive if the skin at the base of the toes cannot be pinched. Swelling from lymphedema usually progresses slowly up the leg over time.

Chapter 5

1. e
2. c
3. a
4. d
5. d
6. b

Chapter 6

1. e
2. c
3. c
4. f
5. e
6. d

Chapter 7

1. c. Both PW and CW Doppler instruments can detect forward and reverse flow, but CW Doppler instruments are less costly and simpler to use. The penetration of ultrasound in tissue is primarily dependent on transmitting frequency (with lower frequencies penetrating to deeper depths) and is the same for PW and CW Doppler. Only PW Doppler can distinguish between flow at different sites or depths in tissue.

2. a. Compressibility (or stiffness) should not affect pneumatic cuff pressure measurements in normal tibial and brachial arteries. However, if calcification or atherosclerotic occlusive disease is present in the tibial arteries, they may be less compressible, which leads to erroneously high cuff pressure measurements. The mean arterial pressure decreases as the pulse moves distally, whereas the systolic pressure increases and the diastolic pressure decreases (so the pulse pressure widens). Because the brachial artery site of pressure measurement is closer to the heart, this augmentation or increase in systolic pressure makes the normal ankle pressure greater than the arm pressure and the ABI greater than 1.0. Cuff artifacts should not be significant at the brachial and ankle sites.

3. b. The digital arteries are not affected by medial calcification, even if the tibial arteries are heavily calcified. Toe-brachial indices are in the range of 0.80 to 0.90 in normal persons. It is often difficult to obtain Doppler flow signals from the toes, and PPG is easier to use for this purpose. Although patients with diabetes mellitus are especially prone to medial calcification in the tibial arteries, the digital arteries are not involved, so toe pressure measurements are not different in diabetic and non-diabetic patients.

4. d. The normal segmental plethysmographic waveform is characterized by a rapid steep upstroke, a sharp systolic peak, and a more prolonged downslope that bows toward the baseline. Changes in amplitude alone generally have little diagnostic significance. A prominent dicrotic wave is normally seen on the downslope of the waveform and represents the reverse-flow phase of the arterial flow pulse. Significant arterial occlusive disease proximal to the recording cuff is excluded by the presence of a dicrotic wave.

5. c. The maximum change in ankle pressure after treadmill exercise occurs immediately after walking, so it is important to measure pressures as quickly as possible. A slight increase in ankle pressure after treadmill exercise is often seen in normal persons. Patients with significant arterial occlusive disease typically have symptoms within 5 minutes of walking at 2 mph up a 12% grade, and more prolonged exercise times are rarely necessary. Some mild-to-moderate arterial lesions are not hemodynamically significant at resting flow rates, but they become flow limiting when flow rates are increased by exercise.

Chapter 8

1. b
2. e
3. d
4. a
5. d

Chapter 9

1. c. This patient has intermediate risk factors and is scheduled to undergo a high-risk vascular operation. β-Blockers decrease the risk of adverse preoperative cardiovascular events; this medical management in this situation would result in an outcome similar to coronary revascularization before vascular surgery.
2. a. This patient has an impending rupture of an abdominal aortic aneurysm and requires urgent surgery. Performance of any cardiac tests would delay the operation.
3. d. This patient has a symptomatic carotid stenosis. Carotid endarterectomy, an intermediate-risk procedure, should be performed. She has excellent functional capacity and minimal risk factors. She can proceed directly to surgery with perioperative administration of β-blockers and aspirin because she is at low risk for an adverse cardiovascular event.
4. a. This patient likely has three-vessel coronary artery disease, left ventricular dysfunction, and angina. The popliteal artery aneurysm repair is elective. Regardless of the popliteal artery aneurysm, he should be referred for cardiac catheterization as a prelude to a coronary revascularization procedure.
5. a. According to the ACC/AHA practice guidelines, the presence of symptomatic aortic valvular stenosis, even in the absence of a critical stenosis ($<1.0\ cm^2$), indicates a very high risk that should prompt aortic valve replacement before planned elective vascular surgery.

Chapter 10

1. a
2. c
3. d
4. d
5. c
6. b
7. a

Chapter 11

1. e
2. d
3. d
4. e
5. d
6. e
7. b

Chapter 12

1. c
2. b
3. d
4. a
5. b

Chapter 13

1. e. Although increased levels of LDL are associated with an increased incidence of lower extremity PAD, diabetes mellitus and cigarette smoking are more strongly associated with PAD. Obesity is not as strong a risk factor for PAD as diabetes and cigarette smoking.
2. b. Patients with PAD have a 3.0- to 4.0-fold increased risk of cardiovascular disease mortality compared with patients without PAD.
3. c. Most epidemiologic studies show the sensitivity of the intermittent claudication questionnaire for the diagnosis of PAD to be approximately 10% to 25%.
4. d. Cigarette smoking and diabetes mellitus are the two most important predictors of critical limb ischemia among PAD patients with intermittent claudication.
5. b. Patients with PAD who have rest pain are less likely to require amputation than those who have gangrene or an ulcer.

Chapter 14

1. a
2. c
3. b
4. c

5. c
6. c
7. a

Chapter 15

1. b. Arterial emboli usually lodge at or proximal to arterial bifurcations and predominantly affect the lower extremities. About three-fourths of all cases occur between the aortic and popliteal bifurcation, with the rest affecting the upper limbs and the cerebral and visceral circulation.
2. d. Most patients with clinical atheromatous embolism are men aged 60 years or older. Whites are affected more frequently than blacks.
3. e
4. b. Acute compartment syndrome is especially common in patients with combined arterial and venous injury, due to the added venous hypertension.

Chapter 16

1. b. The most common complication of a fusiform popliteal artery aneurysm is formation of a thrombus, which can embolize to distal vessels. Thrombotic occlusion of the popliteal artery and emboli may cause acute limb ischemia.
2. b. Increased concentration of MMPs has been observed in experimental models of aortic aneurysm and in tissues excised from human aortic aneurysms.
3. d. This aneurysm has expanded 1 cm over the course of 1 year and meets one criterion for repair.
4. d. Of the factors listed, only diabetes mellitus is not associated with aneurysm formation.
5. a. The risk of rupture of TAA increases progressively with expansion, and most studies recommend repair of a descending TAA with a diameter of 6.5 to 7.0 cm. Similar to AAAs, TAAs should be imaged every 6 to 12 months to determine whether the size has increased considerably.

Chapter 17

1. a. Because aortic dissection cannot be excluded, an imaging test must be ordered. The carotid artery and aorta may be imaged well with MRI but not with ultrasonography.
2. d. Pulse deficits are associated with a marked increase in the risk of death for patients with a type B dissection.
3. a. This is a type A IMH in the ascending aorta. The proper management is blood pressure control and rapid repair.
4. c. The factors that most strongly predict need for aneurysm repair are an aortic diameter ≥4.0 cm and a patent false lumen.
5. d. For patients with a type A aortic dissection, pericardiocentesis is associated with higher rates of mortality, and catheterization has not been shown to provide benefit. β-Blockers would be contraindicated in a hypotensive patient.

Chapter 18

1. a. Bilateral RAS is a volume-mediated form of hypertension. Thus, many of these patients have low renin levels and are not angiotensin dependent for filtration. If a diuretic was added, the blood pressure would probably decrease but at the risk of acute renal failure developing.
2. b. Typical medial fibroplasia should be treated with PTA alone. There is no reason for a stent. Branch involvement does not contraindicate PTA. Although the blood pressure may be normalized with medications, the patient is young and may not require any blood pressure medications after PTA.
3. d. The renal-aortic ratio is 5.5 on the right side, and the PSV is greater than 200 cm/s. This indicates a 60%-99% stenosis. The RRIs are normal.
4. c. Answers a, b, and d are not correct because patients with FMD do not require stenting; a creatinine value of 3.5 mg/dL cannot be explained by unilateral RAS; and 40%-60% stenosis is not enough to cause severe hypertension.
5. c. The patient has non-occlusive mesenteric ischemia. This is due to hypoperfusion and not to a fixed obstruction. The diagnosis is made angiographically and the initial treatment is infusion of vasodilators. If peritoneal signs develop, exploration would be the next step, but only after vasodilator infusion.

Chapter 19

1. c. The most common cause of cerebral ischemia is atherosclerotic thrombosis, likely as a result of longstanding hypertension involving the lenticulostriate arteries deep in the brain. CT will show classic abnormalities of a lacunar infarct. The erythrocyte sedimentation rate is an acute-phase reactant used to identify cerebral vasculitis, a rare cause of cerebral ischemia. Transcranial Doppler ultrasonography is useful for de-

termining intracranial collateral pathways in the brain in a patient with extracranial carotid stenosis. Transesophageal echocardiography is used to determine aortic arch atherosclerosis, patent foramen ovale, valvular heart disease, and cardiac chamber thrombi, which are all sources of emboli. Hemoglobin A_{1c} will only identify diabetes mellitus and will not determine the cause of cerebrovascular ischemia.

2. d. The most important clinical clue is clear evidence of a symptom attributable to a moderate or severe carotid artery stenosis. Cervical bruits are markers of atherosclerosis but do not predict the severity of carotid stenosis or indicate the need for revascularization. The absence of a temporal artery pulse suggests clinically significant disease at the carotid artery bifurcation but may represent stenosis of the external carotid artery only. Dermatologic manifestations of familial hypercholesterolemia suggest the need for aggressive lipid-lowering therapy; however, they do not suggest significant carotid stenosis or the need for carotid revascularization. Tobacco use is a risk factor for atherosclerosis, but it does not define the severity of carotid stenosis or the need for revascularization.

3. b. The basic diagnostic algorithm for carotid artery stenosis is a thorough history and physical examination followed by CDUS. If duplex ultrasonography shows severe carotid stenosis in a patient who would benefit from revascularization, digital subtraction arteriography would be the next step. Digital subtraction arteriography should rarely, if ever, be the initial diagnostic test. Diffusion-weighted magnetic resonance imaging is used to evaluate the brain. MRA is an excellent test but requires use of a contrast agent. The two-dimensional time-of-flight images cannot be used alone because the severity of carotid artery stenosis is often overestimated. MRA and multidetector CTA are rarely used together because of the cost.

4. e. A systolic and diastolic cervical bruit caused by extracranial carotid artery stenosis suggests critical bilateral disease. The cardiac valvular pathology that could result in a systolic/diastolic bruit is aortic insufficiency. Impaired left ventricular function and jugular vein thrombosis are unrelated to this physical finding.

5. c. Carotid revascularization is indicated for patients with symptomatic and severe carotid artery stenosis. CAS placement is recommended as an alternative to CEA for patients with high-risk anatomic or medical comorbid conditions. This patient has a severe symptomatic carotid artery stenosis and an anatomic factor (contralateral internal carotid artery occlusion) that places him at high risk with CEA. Combination antiplatelet therapy has not been shown to offer benefit over aspirin alone as the primary medical therapy or after CEA. However, combination antiplatelet therapy is critical for patients who undergo CAS placement to prevent early stent thrombosis.

Chapter 20

1. a
2. b
3. c
4. d
5. b

Chapter 21

1. c. This patient has right subclavian disease involving the ostium. The right subclavian typically projects posteriorly, and the true ostium of the right subclavian artery is frequently eclipsed by the carotid in the LAO and AP views. This anatomy varies depending on the tortuosity and redundancy of the great vessels, particularly in elderly patients, but an RAO view usually provides the best definition of the subclavian ostium.

2. d. CH (Charriere) is synonymous with French size (F). 6F=0.33×6=1.98 mm. 1.98/2.54=0.78 in.

3. c. Shaping the Simmons sidewinder catheter in the aortic arch can put the patient at risk for atheroembolization. Aggressive maneuvers to shape the catheter in the ascending aorta should be avoided. It is generally recommended to first gently advance the catheter over a wire into the left subclavian artery. The wire is then retracted into the secondary curve to provide rigidity at the point of the secondary bend, improving the ease of prolapse as the catheter is advanced forward and assumes its preformed shape. The Simmons sidewinder is the carotid-selective catheter of choice for many operators, but its use has a learning curve and aggressive manipulation in the aortic arch must be avoided.

4. e. The only incorrect answer is increasing the psi threshold and proceeding with an injection. The typical diagnostic catheter has a rated burst of 1,050 to 1,200 psi. By simply increasing the psi threshold of the injector, the catheter could rupture, and the risk is increased of dislodging a thrombus or occlusive material from the catheter into the artery or vein of interest.

5. b. Typically, shaped catheters should be removed over a wire. However, advancing a wire into a diagnostic catheter that has no blood return could result in embolization of the occlusive material through the tip of the catheter as the wire is advanced. If blood cannot be withdrawn from a catheter stationed in a vessel, an attempt should first be made to reposition and make certain the catheter tip is not against the vessel wall or in a small side branch or plaque. After these maneuvers, if the catheter still will not flush and there is no evidence of a kink, attempts to clear the catheter while inside the body using a power injection, forward flush, or guidewire are ill advised.

6. f. Typically, a 65-cm pigtail catheter has a maximal flow rate of 33 mL/s. All of the choices listed would be appropriate on the basis of Poiseuille's law.

7. e. This is the most feared catastrophic complication of simple abdominal angiography. The complication is less common now that image quality has improved and fewer end-hole catheters are being used for non-selective angiography. The complication occurs by inadvertent injection of contrast into a thoracic branch that happens to provide circulation to the anterior spinal artery. The rapid high-pressure injection of contrast is associated with barotrauma to the spinal cord and immediate paralysis. There is some theoretical benefit from venting of the spinal fluid immediately after this complication, but no controlled studies have confirmed change in outcome after venting.

8. d. This is a fairly common normal variant and would not be considered a pathologic finding. If the right subclavian artery originates distal to the left subclavian or contiguous with the left subclavian, this is considered an anomalous origin that can be associated with aneurysmal change or the so-called Kommerell diverticulum (marked by dysphagia and tracheal encroachment).

9. c. This case illustrates the importance of meticulous imaging and of preprocedural physical examination when making decisions within the angiographic suite. Unilateral absence of pedal pulses cannot be explained with the "normal" angiographic findings reported. This patient had an occult popliteal stenosis that was eclipsed by the prosthetic knee. This type of lesion is frequently missed without appropriate image intensifier angulation.

Chapter 22

1. c
2. d
3. b
4. b
5. c

Chapter 23

1. d
2. b
3. b
4. a
5. a

Chapter 24

1. c
2. d
3. c
4. b
5. b
6. a
7. a

Chapter 25

1. c
2. b
3. d
4. a
5. b

Chapter 26

1. c
2. e
3. a
4. c
5. a
6. d

Chapter 27

1. c. On the basis of the MRA, the patient most likely has giant cell arteritis. Because she presented more than 6 hours after symptom onset, immediate intervention with local thrombolytic or angioplasty and stenting would increase the patient's risk of hemorrhagic conversion. Lesions in patients with giant cell arteritis result from inflammation, not atherosclerosis. Thus, atherectomy would not be beneficial. Treatment with corticosteroids should be initiated. Aorta-to-carotid bypass in 5 to 7 days would provide the best revascularization option (Figure).

2. a. In the vast majority of patients, occlusion of the subclavian artery does not lead to serious clinical consequences. If the endograft procedure requires covering the left subclavian artery, preoperative imaging with CTA, MRA, or 4-vessel cerebral angiography is warranted to verify patency of the innominate and right subclavian arteries, assess the size of the vertebral arteries, and determine whether the circle of Willis is intact.

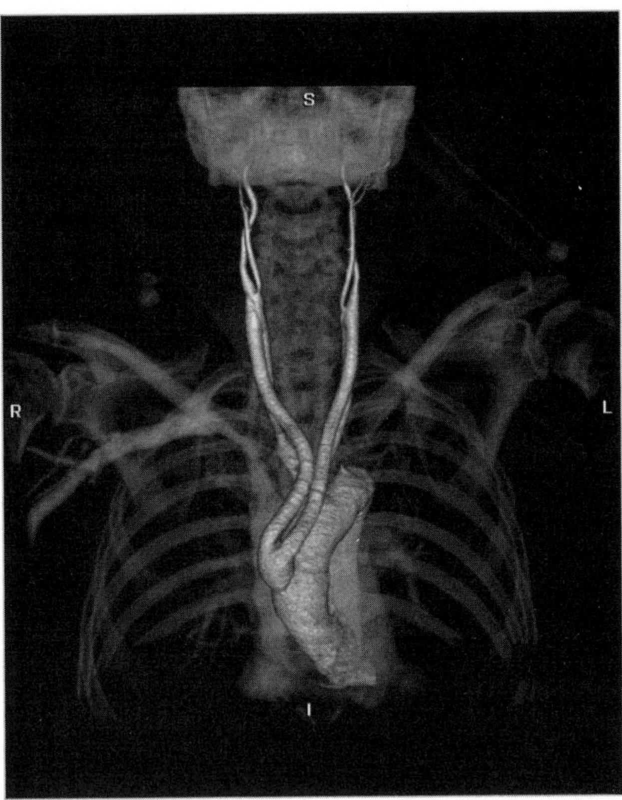

Figure for Answer 1.

3. b. The right aortic arch with aberrant left subclavian artery is the most common form of right aortic arch. It is one of the most common causes of symptom-producing vascular ring.

4. a. Based on results of the WASID study, patients with symptomatic intracranial stenosis should be treated with aspirin. Patients randomly assigned to aspirin (as opposed to warfarin) tolerated the medication better, had a lower incidence of hemorrhage, and had a lower mortality rate.

5. a. CT shows dissection of the left vertebral artery. Most vertebral artery dissections heal spontaneously. Anticoagulation is recommended to decrease the potential for secondary thromboembolic complications. Catheter-based intervention is reserved for patients with ongoing symptoms despite maximal anticoagulation or the presence of an aneurysm causing recurrent thromboembolism or with impending rupture.

Chapter 28

1. c

2. e

3. c

4. a

5. c

Chapter 29

1. b. The most common cause of acute limb ischemia is thromboembolism (75% of cases). The most common source is the left atrial appendage in atrial fibrillation or the left ventricle after an anterior wall myocardial infarction. In some cases, atheromatous material can embolize from the aorta. Typically, patients with an embolic etiology of ischemia have abrupt onset of pain, a recent cardiac event, and no history of claudication. If the etiology is clearly embolic and the site of occlusion can be identified (e.g., the popliteal artery), the patient should undergo surgical embolectomy. Systemic thrombolysis is rarely used. Catheter-directed thrombolysis would be appropriate for patients with thrombosis in situ. Neither intravenous heparin nor a glycoprotein IIb/IIIa inhibitor will dissolve the clot, and amputation is reserved for non-viable limbs.

2. a. Several factors predict successful outcome, including graft occlusion <14 days, ability to traverse the lesion with a guidewire, and two- or three-vessel runoff. Catheter-directed thrombolysis can unmask the etiology underlying the graft failure. Unless the underlying lesion is treated (angioplasty, stenting, or surgical revision), the graft is likely to reocclude.

3. d. Adjunctive use of mechanical thrombectomy devices may avert the need for thrombolysis or permit lower doses of thrombolytic drugs. Low-dose heparin and shorter catheter dwell times decrease bleeding rates. Fibrinogen levels should be checked approximately every 6 hours because levels <100 mg/dL are associated with systemic fibrinolysis.

4. d. In assessing patients with acute limb ischemia, the degree of limb ischemia can be categorized as Category I (viable), IIa (marginally threatened) or IIb (immediately threatened), or III (irreversible). Revascularizing a non-viable limb leads to profound metabolic acidosis, hyperkalemia, myoglobinuria, acute renal failure, and death.

5. a. The TOPAS study compared rUK with primary surgery in patients with acute lower extremity arterial ischemia. The increase in ankle-brachial index was similar in the surgery and thrombolysis arms. There was no difference in the rate of either major amputation or death between the groups within 1 year of follow-up. The TOPAS trial established equivalency of the two treatment arms.

Chapter 30

1. d
2. b
3. e
4. d
5. e
6. e

Chapter 31

1. d
2. c
3. d
4. b
5. a
6. c
7. a, b, and d

Index

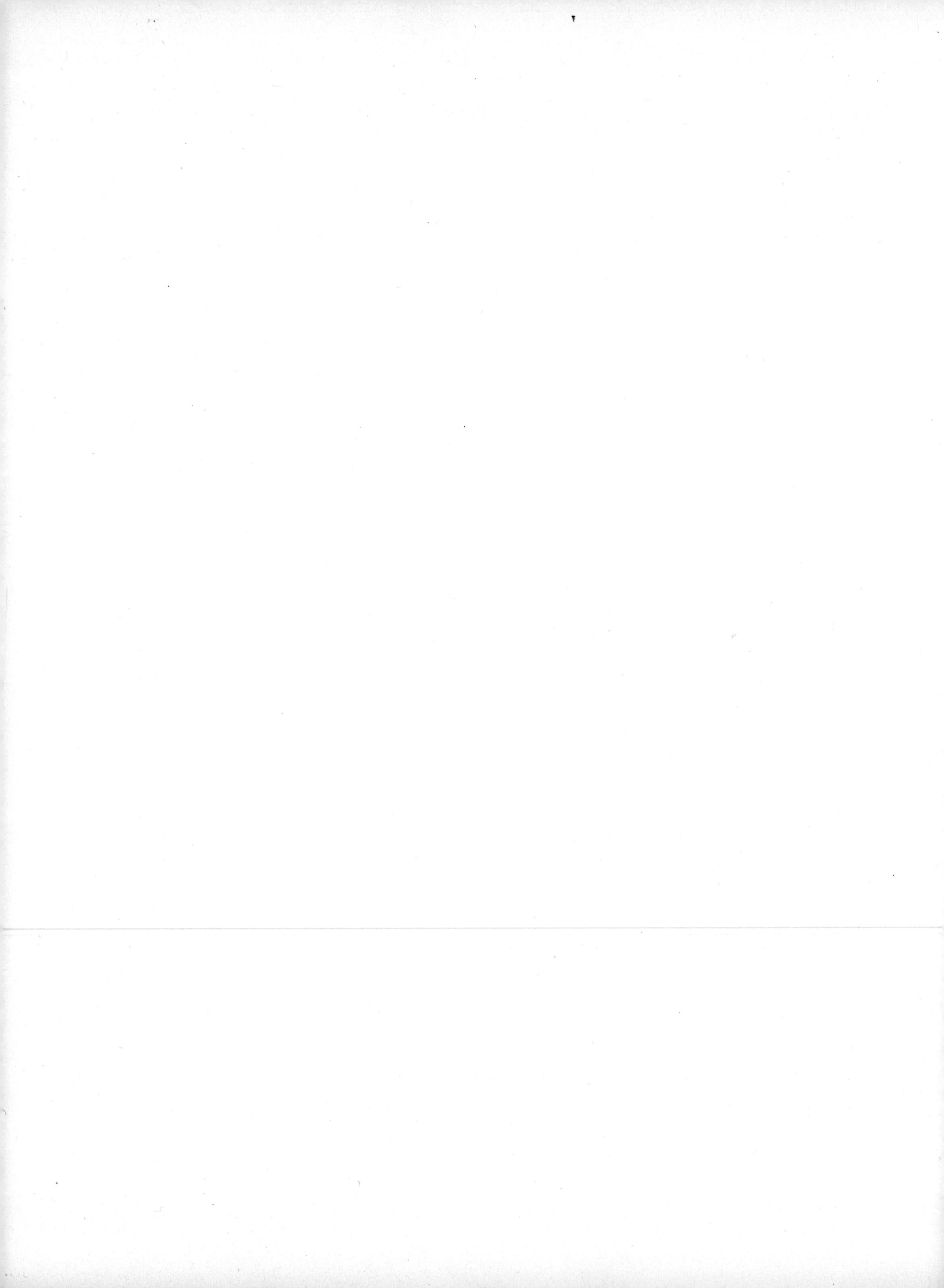